DRUGS, SOCIETY, AND HUMAN BEHAVIOR

DRUGS, SOCIETY, AND HUMAN BEHAVIOR

Eighth Edition

OAKLEY RAY, Ph.D.

Professor, Departments of Psychology and Psychiatry
Associate Professor, Department of Pharmacology
Vanderbilt University and
Vanderbilt University School of Medicine
Nashville, Tennessee

CHARLES KSIR, Ph.D.

Dean of Education
Professor, Departments of Psychology
University of Wyoming
Laramie, Wyoming

Boston Burr Ridge, IL Dubuque, IA Madison, WI New York San Francisco St. Louis
Bangkok Bogotá Caracas Lisbon London Madrid
Mexico City Milan New Delhi Seoul Singapore Sydney Taipei Toronto

WCB/McGraw-Hill

A Division of The **McGraw·Hill** *Companies*

DRUGS, SOCIETY, AND HUMAN BEHAVIOR, EIGHTH EDITION

This book is printed on acid-free paper.

1 2 3 4 5 6 7 8 9 0 VNH/VNH 9 3 2 1 0 9 8

ISBN 0-07-059307-8

Publisher: *Edward E. Bartell*
Developmental editor: *Shirley R. Oberbroeckling*
Senior marketing manager: *Pamela S. Cooper*
Senior project manager: *Peggy J. Selle*
Production supervisor: *Mary E. Haas*
Coordinator of freelance design: *Michelle D. Whitaker*
Photo research coordinator: *Lori Hancock*
Supplement coordinator: *Audrey A. Reiter*
Compositor: *GAC/Shepard Poorman*
Typeface: *10/12 Garth Graphic*
Printer: *Von Hoffmann Press, Inc.*

Freelance cover/interior designer: *Maureen McCutcheon*
Cover image: *Paul Fisch/Stock Illustration Source*

The credits section for this book begins on page 480 and is considered an extension of the copyright page.

Library of Congress Cataloging-in-Publication Data

Ray, Oakley Stern.
    Drugs, society, and human behavior / Oakley Ray, Charles Ksir. — 8th ed.
      p.   cm.
    Includes index.
    ISBN 0-07-059307-8
    1. Drugs of abuse.   2. Drug abuse—Social aspects.
3. Neuropsychopharmacology. I. Ksir, Charles. II. Title.
RM316.R39   1999
362.29—dc21   98-7758
                                 CIP

CONTENTS IN BRIEF

SECTION ONE

Drug Use in Modern Society

1 Drug Use: An Overview, 2
2 Drug Use as a Social Problem, 23
3 Addictions: Theory and Treatment, 37
4 Drug Regulations, 56

SECTION TWO

How Drugs Work

5 The Nervous System, 88
6 The Actions of Drugs, 109

SECTION THREE

Uppers and Downers

7 Stimulants, 134
8 Depressants and Inhalants, 165
9 Psychotherapeutic Drugs, 184

SECTION FOUR

Alcohol

10 **Alcohol in the Body,** 208
11 **Alcohol and Society,** 238

SECTION FIVE

Familiar Drugs

12 Tobacco, 264
13 Caffeine, 290
14 Over-the-Counter Drugs, 311

SECTION SIX

Restricted Drugs

15 Opiates, 334
16 Hallucinogens, 366
17 Marijuana & Hashish, 401
18 Steroids and Other Drugs in Sport, 428

SECTION SEVEN

Reducing the Demand

19 **Breaking the Cycle,** 444

Appendixes, 463
Glossary, 469
Credits, 480
Index, 482

CONTENTS

Preface, xiii

SECTION ONE
DRUG USE IN MODERN SOCIETY, 1

1 Drug Use: an Overview, 2
"The Drug Problem," 2
Talking About Drug Use, 2
FYI: Some Important Definitions—and a Caution! 4
Four Principles of Psychoactive Drugs, 4
How Did We Get Here?, 7
Have Things Really Changed?, 7
Four Pharmacological Revolutions, 7
Recent Cultural Change, 7
Drugs and Drug Use Today, 10
Extent of Drug Use, 10
Your Turn: Methamphetamine Use in Your Community, 10
Correlates of Drug Use, 12
Antecedents of Drug Use, 14
Motives for Drug Use, 18
Up for Debate: Is Drug Use Declining Among Hard-Core Users? 19
Summary, 20
Web Watch, 22

2 Drug Use as a Social Problem, 23
Lassez-Faire, 23
Toxicity, 24
Categories of Toxicity, 24
Drug Abuse Warning Network, 25
Up For Debate: Crack Babies, 26
How Dangerous Is It? 28
AIDS, 29
Drug Addiction, 30
Problems of Definition, 30

Crime and Violence, 31
Does Drug Use Cause Crime? 31
Your Turn: Are Current Laws Fair? 33
Why We Try to Regulate Drugs, 35
Summary, 35
Web Watch, 36

3 Addictions: Theory and Treatment, 37
Drug Addiction, 37
Three Basic Processes, 38
Changing Views of Drug Addiction, 39
The Broad Views of Addictions, 41
Is Addiction Caused by the Substance? 42
Is Addiction Biological? 43
Is There an Addictive Personality? 43
Is Addiction a Family Disorder? 43
Is Addiction a Disease? 44
Assessment of Addictive Disorders, 45
Diagnosis, 45
DSM-IV: Psychiatric Diagnosis of Substance Disorders, 46
Addiction Treatment, 46
Deciding to Quit, 47
Defining Treatment Goals, 48
Treatment Stages, 48
Treatment Approaches, 50
FYI: The Twelve Steps of Alcoholics Anonymous, 52
Is Treatment Effective? 53
Summary, 54
Web Watch, 54

4 Drug Regulations, 56
The Beginnings, 57
Reformism, 57
Problems Leading to Legislation, 57

The 1906 Pure Food and Drugs Act, 59
The Harrison Act of 1914, 60
Two Bureaus, Two Types of Regulation, 61
Regulating Pharmaceuticals, 61
Purity, 61
Safety, 62
Effectiveness, 63
Marketing a New Drug, 63
Narcotics, Dangerous Drugs, and Controlled Substances, 65
After the Harrison Act, 65
Drug Abuse Control Amendments of 1965, 68
Comprehensive Drug Abuse Prevention and Control Act of 1970, 68
State and Local Regulations, 70
FYI: Americans in Prison, 71
Your Turn: What are Your Rights? 72
Paraphernalia, 73
Federal Support for Urine Screening, 74
Military and Federal Employees, 74
Transportation Workers, 74
Private Employers, 74
Testing Methods, 74
Up for Debate: The Special Status of Marijuana, 76
The Impact of Drug Enforcement, 76
Budget, 77
International Programs, 78
Other Federal Agencies, 78
Other Costs, 78
Effectiveness of Control, 80
Summary, 80
Web Watch, 82
Assess Yourself! Drug Use Today, 84–85

SECTION TWO
HOW DRUGS WORK, 87

5 The Nervous System, 88
Chemical messengers, 89
Hormones, 89
Neurotransmitters, 91
Receptors, 91
The Nervous System, 93
Central Nervous System, 93
Somatic Nervous System, 93
Autonomic Nervous System, 94

The Brain, 94
The Whole Brain, 94
Major Structures, 95
Chemical Pathways, 97
FYI: Alzheimer's Disease, 98
Drugs and the Brain, 100
Drugs in the Brain, 100
Life Cycle of a Neurotransmitter, 100
Examples of Drug Actions, 103
Up for Debate: Chemical Causes of Mental Disorders, 105
Chemical Theories of Behavior, 105
Modern Brain Imaging Techniques, 106
Summary, 107
Web Watch, 108

6 The Actions of Drugs, 109
Drugs, 109
Sources of Drugs, 109
Drug Names, 110
Brand Name versus Generic Name, 110
Categorizing Drugs, 110
Your Turn: The Ever-Changing World of Drug Slang, 111
Drug Identification, 113
Drug Effects, 113
Nonspecific (Placebo) Effects, 113
Dose-Response Relationships, 114
Up for Debate: Animal Toxicity Tests, 117
Potency, 118
Time-Dependent Factors in Drug Actions, 118
Getting the Drug to the Brain, 120
A Little "Chemistry," 120
Routes of Administration, 120
Transport in the Blood, 123
Blood-Brain Barrier, 125
Possible Mechanisms of Drug Actions, 125
Drug Deactivation, 126
FYI: Drug-Drug Interactions, 127
Mechanisms of Tolerance and Physical Dependence, 128
Drug Disposition Tolerance, 128
Behavioral Tolerance, 128
Pharmacodynamic Tolerance, 129
Summary, 129
Web Watch, 130
Assess Yourself! How do Drugs Work? 132

SECTION THREE
UPPERS AND DOWNERS, 133

7 Stimulants, 134
  Cocaine, 135
    History, 135
    Coca Wine to Coca-Cola, 136
    Crack, 139
    Basic Pharmacology, 139
    Beneficial Uses, 141
    Causes for Concern, 141
  Up for Debate: the Impact of Maternal Cocaine Use, 144
    Supplies of Illicit Cocaine, 145
    Curent Patterns of Cocaine Use, 145
  Your Turn: Cocaine and Friendship, 146
    Cocaine Treatment, 146
    Cocaine's Future, 147
  Amphetamines, 147
    History, 147
    Basic Pharmacology, 151
    Beneficial Uses, 153
  FYI: Diet Drugs: Out With the New, in With the Newer, 156
  DSM-IV: Diagnostic Criteria for Attention-Deficit Hyperactivity Disorder, 157
    Causes for Concern, 160
    Supplies of Illicit Amphetamine, 162
  Summary, 162
  Web Watch, 163

8 Depressants and Inhalants, 165
  History and Pharmacology, 166
    Before Barbiturates, 166
    Barbiturates, 167
    Meprobamate, 168
    Methaqualone, 169
    Benzodiazepines, 170
  FYI: The Drug-Induced Rape Prevention and Punishment Act, 172
  Mechanism of Action, 172
  Beneficial Uses, 173
    As Sedatives, 173
  Up for Debate: GHB: "Natural" High or Deadly Diversion? 174
    As Sleeping Pills, 175

  Causes for Concern, 176
    Dependence Liability, 176
    Anticonvulsant Effects, 176
  FYI: Sleep Hygiene Techniques for Insomnia, 177
    Toxicity, 178
    Patterns of Abuse, 179
  Inhalants, 179
    Gaseous Anesthetics, 180
    Nitrites, 180
    Volatile Solvents, 181
  Summary, 182
  Web Watch, 182

9 Psychotherapeutic Drugs, 184
  Mental Illness, 184
    The Medical Model, 184
    Classification of Mental Disorders, 185
  DSM-IV: Anxiety Disorders, 186
  DSM-IV: Diagnosis: Schizophrenia, 187
  DSM-IV: Diagnosis: Mood Disorders, 188
  Treatment of Mental Disorders, 188
    Before 1950, 188
    Antipsychotics, 190
  Your Turn: Clozaril: Patient Monitoring versus Cost Containment, 192
    Antidepressants, 193
  FYI: Prozac for Everyone? 196
    Lithium, 197
  The Consequences of Drug Treatments for Mental Illness, 199
  Up for Debate: Catch-22 for the Mentally Ill, 201
  Summary, 202
  Web Watch, 202
  Assess Yourself! Daily Mood Changes, 204

SECTION FOUR
ALCOHOL, 207

10 Alcohol in the Body, 208
  Alcoholic Beverages, 208
    Fermentation and Fermentation Products, 208
    Distilled Products, 209

Alcohol as a Consumer Item, 210
Beer, 210
Wine, 212
Distilled Spirits, 215
Alcohol Pharmacology, 218
Absorption, 218
Metabolism, 218
**FYI: The "Flushing" Reaction and Alcohol
Consumption in Asia, 219**
Central Nervous System Effects, 220
**Up for Debate: Should Beer Labels State
Alcohol Content, 221**
Blackouts, 225
Sexual Behavior, 225
Alcohol Withdrawal—Delirium Tremens, 226
Physiological Effects, 227
Alcohol Toxicity, 228
Hangover, 228
Chronic Disease States, 230
Brain Damage, 230
Liver Disorders, 231
Heart Disease, 232
Cancer, 232
The Immune System, 232
Fetal Alcohol Syndrome, 233
**Your Turn: Protecting the Unborn from
Alcohol, 235**
Summary, 235
Web Watch, 236

11 Alcohol and Society, 238
**Alcohol Use and "The Alcohol
Problem," 238**
The Temperence Movement in America, 239
Prohibition, 240
Regulation after 1993, 243
Up for Debate: Advertising Alcohol, 243
Taxation, 243
Who Drinks? And Why? 244
Cultural Influences on Drinking, 244
Regional Differences in the United
States, 244
Gender Differences, 246
Drinking among College Students, 246
"Time-Out" and Alcohol "Myopia," 247
Social Problems, 247
Driving under the Influence, 247

FYI: Alcohol and Violence, 249
Crime and Violence, 249
Who Is an Alcoholic? 250
Factors Predisposing to Alcoholism, 252
Treating Alcoholism, 254
Alcoholics Anonymous, 254
**FYI: The Twelve Steps of Alcoholics
Anonymous, 255**
Medical Approaches, 256
Behavioral Approaches, 257
Is Controlled Drinking a Realistic Goal? 257
Is Alcoholism Treatment Effective? 259
Summary, 260
Web Watch, 260
**Assess Yourself! How Can You Tell if You
Have a Drinking Problem? 262**

**SECTION FIVE
FAMILIAR DRUGS, 263**

12 Tobacco, 264
Early Medical Uses, 265
Tobacco Use Spreads, 266
Tobacco in Early America, 266
Chewing Tobacco, 266
Cigars and Cigarettes, 267
Current Tobacco Products, 268
Toward a Less Hazardous Cigarette, 270
Trends in Smoking Behavior, 271
Smokeless Tobacco, 273
Cigars Are Back? 274
A Social and Economic Dilemma, 274
Causes for Concern, 276
Adverse Health Effects, 276
Passive Smoking, 278
Smoking and Health in Other Countries, 279
Smoking and Pregnancy, 279
Pharmacology of Nicotine, 281
Absorption and Metabolism, 281
Physiological Effects, 282
FYI: Possible New Painkiller? 282
Behavioral Effects, 283
Addiction to Nicotine, 284
**Up For Debate: Should the Federal
Government Arrange a Settlement
With the Tobacco Companies? 284**
Smoking—How Not To, 285

FYI: Young Children and Cigarette
   Advertising, 286
Summary, 287
Web Watch, 288

13 Caffeine, 290
The World's Most Common
   Psychostimulant, 290
   Coffee, 290
   Tea, 294
   Chocolate, 297
Other Sources of Caffeine, 299
   Soft Drinks, 299
   Over-the-Counter Drugs, 302
Caffeine Pharmacology, 302
   Time Course, 302
   Mechanism of Action, 303
   Physiological Effects, 304
   Behavioral Effects, 304
Up for Debate: Caffeine Dependence
   Syndrome? 305
FYI: Caffeine and Panic Attacks, 306
Causes for Concern, 306
   Cancer, 307
   Benign Breast Disease, 307
   Reproductive Effects, 307
   Heart Disease, 307
   Caffeinism, 308
FYI: How Much Caffeine Do You Use? 308
Summary, 308
Web Watch, 309

14 Over-the-Counter Drugs, 311
FDA Regulation of OTC Products, 311
Simplifying Labels, 313
Over-the-Counter versus Prescription
   Drugs, 313
Up for Debate: Should There Be a Third
   Class of "Pharmacist-Recommended"
   Drugs? 314
Some Psychoactive OTC Products, 314
   Stimulants, 314
   Weight-Control Products, 315
   Sedatives and Sleep Aids, 316
Your Turn: The Medicine Chest, 317

Analgesics, 318
   People and Pain, 318
   Aspirin, 318
   Aspirin Effects: Adverse and Otherwise, 321
   Acetaminophen, 323
   Ibuprofen and Other NSAIDs, 323
Cold and Allergy Products, 324
   The All-Too-Common Common Cold, 324
   Treating Cold Symptoms, 325
FYI: Cold Medications and Kids, 326
Allergy and Sinus Medications, 327
Choosing an OTC Product, 327
FYI: Abuse of OTC
   Dextromethorphan, 328
Summary, 329
Web Watch, 330
Assess Yourself! OTC Products, 331

SECTION SIX
RESTRICTED DRUGS, 333

15 Opiates, 334
History, 335
   Opium, 335
   Morphine, 339
   Heroin, 340
   Opiate Addiction before the Harrison
      Act, 340
   After the Harrison Act, 342
   Eliminating Legal Sources, 342
Up For Debate: Should Heroin be Made
   Available for Medical Purposes? 343
FYI: The Nigerian Connection, 348
Pharmacology of the Opiates, 348
   Chemical Characteristics, 348
   Mechanism of Action, 349
Beneficial Uses, 351
   Pain Relief, 351
   Intestinal Disorders, 351
   Cough Suppressants, 351
Causes for Concern, 352
   Dependence Potential, 352
   Toxicity Potential, 354
   Patterns of Abuse, 355
Treatment of Narcotic Addicts, 358
   History, 358
   Current Medical Approaches, 358

**Your Turn: Tough Moral Stances versus
"Harm Reduction," 362**
Rapid Opiate Detoxification, 363
Summary, 363
Web Watch, 364

16 Hallucinogens, 366
Animism and Religion, 366
Terminology and Types, 367
Phantastica, 367
Indole Hallucinogens, 368
  d-Lysergic Acid Diethylamide (LSD), 369
Your Turn: Attitudes toward LSD, 379
  Morning Glory, 381
  DMT, 381
Catechol Hallucinogens, 382
  Mescaline, 382
  Amphetamine Derivatives, 387
  PCP, 388
**FYI: Ibogaine as an Addiction
Treatment, 391**
Anticholinergic Hallucinogens, 392
  Belladonna, 392
  Mandrake, 393
  Henbane, 393
  Datura, 393
  Synthetic Anticholinergics, 394
Amanita Muscaria, 395
FYI: Toadlicking: An "Urban Legend," 396
Summary, 397
Web Watch, 398

17 Marijuana and Hashish, 401
Cannabis, 401
  The Plant, 401
  Preparations from Cannabis, 402
History, 404
  Early History, 404
  The Nineteenth Century: Romantic
    Literature and the New Science of
    Psychology, 405
  "Marijuana, Assassin of Youth," 406
  The Marijuana Tax Act of 1937, 408
  After the Marijuana Tax Act, 409
Pharmacology, 410
  Cannabinoid Chemicals, 410

  Absorption, Distribution, and
    Elimination, 410
  Mechanism of Action, 411
  Physiological Effects, 411
  Behavioral Effects, 412
Medical Uses of Cannabis, 414
**FYI: Should Medical Patients Have Access
to Marijuana, 416**
  1996 Ballot Inititatives on Medical
    Marijuana, 417
Causes of Concern, 417
  Dependence Potential, 417
  Toxicity Potential, 418
**FYI: Long-Term Effects of Marijuana
Smoke in Monkeys, 421**
Marijuana and American Society, 422
**Your Turn: Use of and Attitudes toward
Marijuana, 422**
Summary, 424
Web Watch, 425

**18 Steroids and Other Drugs in
Sport, 428**
Historial Use of Drugs in Athletics, 429
  Ancient Times, 429
  Early Use of Stimulants, 429
  Amphetamine, 430
  International Drug Testing, 431
  American Football, 431
  Steroids, 431
Your Turn: Winning, 432
  Cocaine Again, 433
**Stimulants as Performance
Enhancers, 433**
Steroids, 435
FYI: Nutritional Ergogenic Aids, 436
Other Hormonal Manipulations, 438
Beta-2 Agonists, 439
**Up for Debate: Did Creatine Kill
Wrestlers? 439**
Summary, 440
Web Watch, 441
Assess Yourself! Street Names, 442

SECTION SEVEN
REDUCING THE DEMAND, 443

19 Breaking the Cycle, 444
    Defining Goals and Evaluating
        Outcomes, 444
    Stages of Prevention, 445
    Prevention Programs in the
        Schools, 446
        The Knowledge-Attitudes-Behavior
            Model, 446
        Affective Education, 447
    FYI: Examples of Values Clarification
        Strategies, 448
        "Just Say No!" 449
        Drug-Free Schools, 449
    Your Turn: Alternatives to Drugs, 450
        Student Assistance Programs, 451
    FYI: Preventing Inhalant Abuse, 452
        Peer Counseling, 452

        Development of the Social Influence
            Model, 452
        DARE, 454
    Peers, Parents, and the
        Community, 456
        Peer Programs, 457
        Parent Programs, 457
        Community Programs, 458
        Prevention in the Workplace, 458
    What Should We Be Doing? 459
    Summary, 459
    Web Watch, 460
    Assess Yourself! Alternatives to
        Drug Use, 462

    Appendix A, 463
    Appendix B, 467
    Glossary, 469
    Credits, 480p
    Index, 482

The first edition of *Drugs, Society, and Human Behavior* was published in 1972, in a time of intense curiosity about psychoactive drugs and little understanding of how they worked and how they related to society. At that time, people were most interested in LSD, marijuana, and amphetamines. This text provided students with factual, unbiased information about those and other drugs in a way that could be understood by those without a background in biology or chemistry. There was a need for such information, and *Drugs, Society, and Human Behavior* met that need for thousands of students. However, perhaps the greater benefit was provided by the historical and social context in which the drug information was presented. Students learned that psychoactive drug use is neither a new nor an isolated phenomenon but rather a feature of every human society. They learned that alcohol, coffee, and cigarettes are drugs also, and they learned to compare the actions, effects, and social roles of these legal drugs with those of the illicit drugs.

RECENT DEVELOPMENTS

Much has changed in the twenty-five-plus years since the publication of the first edition of *Drugs, Society, and Human Behavior*. Whereas the 1970s were a period of widespread experimentation with marijuana and hallucinogens, the 1980s brought increased concern and conservatism, along with decreased use of alcohol, marijuana, and all illicit drugs. Not only did drug-using behavior change, but so did attitudes and knowledge. And of course, over the years,

the particular drugs that have been of immediate social concern have gone through a series of changes: LSD gave way to "angel dust," then to heroin, then cocaine, then "crack." In the 1990s, use of LSD and marijuana has increased, although not yet to the levels of the 1970s. Methamphetamine, associated with the "speed freaks" of the late 1960s, is back—but now more often smoked than injected.

Throughout these changes, our old "standbys," alcohol and tobacco, have remained with us and remained major social issues and major social problems. Regulations have changed, new scientific information is available, new approaches to prevention and treatment are being tried, but throughout these past twenty-five or so years, these substances have continued to be the most widely used drugs in our society.

SUCCESSFUL FEATURES

This text approaches drugs and drug use from a variety of perspectives—behavioral, pharmacological, historical, social, legal, and clinical. This allows the book to appeal to a wide range of students and helps them to apply the content to their own special needs.

This was the first introductory text to expand the coverage of alcohol to two chapters: "Alcohol in the Body" (chapter 10) and "Alcohol and Society" (chapter 11).

NEW IN THE EIGHTH EDITION

- Updated statistics throughout on drug and alcohol use, drug-related emergencies and

fatalities, and dollar sales of alcoholic beverages and drugs, both legal and illegal
- New approaches to the treatment of addiction
- Coverage of date-rape drugs, including rohypnol and GHB
- Coverage of increased use of methamphetamine
- Discussion of the status of medical marijuana
- Updated information on drugs used by athletes, including creatine
- Information on school-based prevention programs that work

PEDAGOGICAL AIDS

- Brief **chapter objectives** are provided as an aid at the beginning of each chapter to alert the student to what he or she will be learning in that chapter.
- **Key terms** are listed at the beginning of each chapter and boldfaced in the text for easy identification.
- **Definition boxes** define key terms and provide pronunciation guides as needed where each term is explained in the text.
- **Web Watch boxes** provide related Internet links for each chapter to help students search for more detailed or late-breaking information
- Each chapter contains **FYI, Up for Debate**, and **Your Turn** boxes, which provide additional content, exercises to involve the student, and information on current concerns and controversies. **DSM-IV** boxes providing the latest psychiatric diagnostic criteria are used when appropriate.
- A **chapter summary** assists students with the review process and reinforces major concepts.
- **Review questions** are provided for each chapter for review and analysis of the material presented.
- **Assess Yourself!** activities and exercises allow the students to apply some of the major concepts learned in that section.

- A comprehensive **glossary** is provided as a reference at the back of the book, listing all key terms.
- **Appendices.** Appendix A provides a list of drug names, allowing for quick reference to determine the type of drug, and a cross-reference to brand and generic names for prescription drugs. Appendix B lists drug information organizations and resources, including addresses and "hot lines" the student can contact for additional information.

SUPPLEMENTARY MATERIALS

Instructor's Manual and Test Bank

Prepared by Michael Havens, Ph.D., of Montana State University, this comprehensive, unique Instructor's Manual is available to qualified adopters of the text. It includes the following practical features:
- A Test Bank of more than 1,000 examination questions, including multiple-choice, true/false, matching, and essay questions
- Chapter overviews
- Chapter outlines with teaching suggestions, key terms, and relevant transparency masters noted in margins
- Student activities, exercises, and assignments, which assist the student in evaluating her or his own values regarding drug use and abuse
- Related issues, including current topics for class discussion
- Current resources lists, including annotated readings, films, and journals
- Transparency masters of the most important and useful illustrations found in the text, as well as some additional illustrations that are not included in the text

Microtest

This software provides a unique combination of user-friendly aids that enable the instructor to select, edit, delete, or add questions, as well as construct and print tests and answer keys. The computerized Test Bank package is available to qualified adopters of the text for IBM DOS and Macintosh computers.

Acetate Transparency Package

Thirty overhead four-color transparencies are provided to assist in classroom presentations of the more difficult concepts in the text. These are available to qualified adopters of the text.

Photo CD for Drugs

The CD includes 39 images on the nervous system, methods of drug administration, alcohol, tobacco, cocaine, opioids, stages of change, and recovery/prevention. Contact your sales representative for details.

HealthQuest

HealthQuest by Fold/Atkinson/Conley/McDermott is an interactive CD-ROM allowing exploration of your health and wellness status. The modules on tobacco, alcohol, and other drugs give you the opportunity to input your criteria and receive feedback on your personal drug level. *HealthQuest* can be packaged with the text. Contact your sales representative for details.

Taking Sides: Clashing Views on Controversial Issues in Drugs and Society

Raymond Goldberg from the State University of New York at Cortland has brought together 36 selections dealing with 18 current controversial drug issues for debate. *Taking Sides* is the perfect tool to encourage critical thinking. *Taking Sides* can be packaged with the text. Call your sales representative for details.

Annual Editions: Drugs, Society, and Behavior

This series of acticles is a collection of facts, issues, and perspectives designed to provide the reader a framework for examining current drug-related issues. *Annual Editions* can be packaged with the text. Your sales representative can help you with the details.

ACKNOWLEDGMENTS

We would like to express our appreciation to the following instructors who reviewed the seventh edition and helped lay the groundwork for the improvements and changes that were needed in the eighth edition:

Brian A. Adrian, Ph.D.
Grand Valley State University

Martin Ayim, Ph.D.
Grambling State University

Karen Ball, Ph.D.
Alma College

Robert W. Bell
Texas Tech University

Angela K. Bray
Illinois State University

Joseph Brown, Ph.D.
Austin Peay State University

Gary L. Chandler, Ed.D.
Gardner-Webb University

Diane L. Clemen
Illinois Wesleyan University

Lou Ebrite, Ph.D.
University of Central Oklahoma

Dale W. Evans, Ph.D.
California State University

Getene Gebrewold, Ph.D.
Western Illinois University

William T. Hey, Ph.D.
Delta State University

Ping Hu, Ph.D.
Florida Atlantic University

Howard Ishisaka, Ed.D.
Indiana State University

John Janowiak, Ph.D.
Appalachian State College

Linda Kryel, RPH
Drake College

Jerry W. Lee, Ph.D.
Loma Linda University

Linda Ludovico, MS
Tyler Junior College

Jennifer McLean
Corning Community College

Edward Meister, Ph.D.
Worcester State College

Patricia A. Miller
Anderson University

Patsy Queen
Gaston College

Kerry Redican, Ph.D.
Virginia Tech

Laurna Robinson, Ph.D.
University of Illinois

Thomas Rowe
University of Wisconsin

Glenn B. Schmidt
Mississippi University for Women

Israel M. Schwartz, Ph.D.
Hofstra University

Sharon Simson
University of Maryland

Barry A. Staples
Lacawanna Junior College

Peggy Trueman, MSN
Gaston College

Martin Turnauer
Radford University

Keeping up with all the changes in this field is a formidable task, one in which we are aided immensely by our continuing to teach courses based on the text and receiving feedback and new information from our students, from students at other institutions, and from other faculty members who use the text. We appreciate (and need!) all that input. Although we also welcome regular mail, in keeping with the information age we invite comments, questions, and criticisms to be sent by electronic mail to cksir@uwyo.edu.

Oakley Ray
Charles Ksir

1

Drug Use in Modern Society

The interaction between drugs and behavior can be approached from two general perspectives. Certain drugs, the ones we call psychoactive, have profound effects on behavior. So part of what a book on this topic should do is describe the effects of these drugs *on behavxior,* and later chapters do that in some detail. Another perspective, however, views drug taking *as behavior.* The psychologist sees drug-taking behaviors as interesting examples of human behavior that are influenced by many psychological, social, and cultural variables. In the first section of this text, we focus on drug taking as behavior that can be studied in the same way that other behaviors, such as aggression, learning, or human sexuality, can be studied.

1 Drug Use: An Overview
Which drugs are being used and why?

2 Drug Use as a Social Problem
Why does our society want to regulate drug use?

3 Addictions: Theory and Treatment
What are the differences among the various approaches to treating alcoholism, opiate addiction, cocaine use, and others? How well do these programs work?

4 Drug Regulations
What are the regulations and what is their effect?

1

Drug Use: An Overview

KEY TERMS	OBJECTIVES

After reading this chapter, you should be able to:

drug
illicit drug
deviant drug use
drug misuse
drug abuse
addiction
psychoactive
marijuana
psychopharmacology
correlate
antecedent
longitudinal study
gateway
reinforcement

- Begin your analysis of "the drug problem" by using a list of six questions.
- Discuss the definition of the term *drug* and distinguish among illicit drug use, deviant drug use, drug misuse, drug abuse, and addiction.
- State four general principles about psychoactive drug effects.
- Describe four pharmacological revolutions that have altered our thinking about drugs, and discuss the impact of recent cultural changes on drug use.
- Describe at least two methods for gathering information

about drug use, and point out some advantages and disadvantages of each method.
- Cite the approximate percentages of high school seniors and adults reporting current use of alcohol, tobacco, marijuana, and cocaine, and describe in general terms the recent trends in overall illicit drug use.
- Name several psychosocial variables that have been found to be related to drug use, and know which are the most highly correlated.

"THE DRUG PROBLEM"

Talking about Drug Use

Phrases such as *the problem is drugs* or *drug and alcohol abuse* are heard almost daily on television or in discussions of social problems. But what do these phrases mean? Before you can meaningfully evaluate the extent of such a problem or propose possible solutions, it helps to define what you're talking about. In other words, it helps to be more specific about just what the problem is. Most of us don't really

view drug use as the problem, if that includes your Aunt Margie taking two aspirins when she has a headache. What we really mean is that some drugs being used by some people or in some situations constitute problems with which our society must deal.

Journalism students are told that an informative news story must answer the questions who, what, when, where, why, and how. Let's see how answering those same questions plus one more question—how much—can help us analyze problem drug use.

- *Who* is taking the drug? We are more concerned about a 15-year-old girl drinking a beer than we are about a 21-year-old woman doing the same thing. We worry more about a 10-year-old boy chewing tobacco than we do about a 40-year-old man chewing it (unless we happen to be riding right behind him when he spits out the window). And although we don't like anyone taking heroin, we undoubtedly get more upset when we hear about the girl next door becoming an addict.

- *What* drug are they taking? This question should be obvious, but often it is overlooked. A simple claim that a high percentage of students are "drug users" doesn't tell us if there has been an epidemic of crack smoking or if the drug referred to is alcohol (more likely). If someone begins to talk about a serious "drug problem" at the local high school, the first question should be "what drug or drugs?"

- *When and where* is the drug being used? The situation in which the drug use occurs often makes all the difference. The clearest example is the drinking of alcohol; if it is confined to appropriate times and places, most people accept drinking as normal behavior. When an individual begins to drink on the job, at school, or in the morning, that behavior is evidence of a drinking problem. Even subcultures that accept the use of illegal drugs might distinguish between acceptable and unacceptable situations; some college-age groups might accept marijuana smoking at a party but not just before going to a calculus class!

- *Why* a person takes a drug or does anything else is a tough kind of question to answer. Nevertheless, we can see that it is important in some cases. If a person takes a narcotic drug because her doctor prescribed it for the knee injury she got while skiing, most of us would not be concerned. If, on the other hand, she takes that same drug on her own just because she likes the way it makes her feel, then we should begin to worry about her developing a dependency. The motives for drug use, as with motives for other behaviors, can be complex. Even the person taking the drug might not be aware of all the motives involved. One of the ways a psychologist can try to answer "why" questions is to look for consistency in the situations in which the

Our concern about the use of a substance often depends on who is using it.

behavior occurs (when and where). If a person drinks only with other people who are drinking, we may suspect social motives; if a person often drinks alone, we may suspect that the person is trying to deal with personal problems by drinking.

- *How* the drug is taken can often be critical. South American Indians who chew coca leaves absorb cocaine slowly over a long period of time. The same total amount of cocaine "snorted" into the nose produces a more rapid, more intense effect of shorter duration and probably leads to much stronger dependence. Smoking cocaine in the form of "crack" produces an even more rapid, intense,

and brief effect, and dependence occurs very quickly.

- *How much* of the drug is being used? This isn't one of the standard journalism questions, but it is important when describing drug use. Often the difference between what one considers normal use and what one considers abuse of, for example, alcohol or a prescription drug comes down to how much a person takes.

Four Principles of Psychoactive Drugs

Now that we've seen how helpful it can be to be specific when talking about drug use, let's look for some organizing principles.

FYI   Some Important Definitions—and a Caution!

Some terms that are commonly used in discussing drugs and drug use are difficult to define with precision, partly because they are so widely used for many different purposes. Therefore any definition we offer should be viewed with caution because each represents a compromise between leaving out something important versus including so much that the defined term is "watered down."

The word **drug** will be defined as "any substance, natural or artificial, other than food, that by its chemical nature alters structure or function in the living organism." One obvious difficulty is that we haven't defined "food," and how we draw that line can sometimes be arbitrary. Alcoholic beverages such as wine or beer may be seen as either drug, food, or both. Are we discussing how much sherry wine to include in beef Stroganoff, or are we discussing how many ounces of wine can be consumed before becoming intoxicated? Since this is not a cookbook but rather

a book on the use of psychoactive chemicals, we will view all alcoholic beverages as drugs.

Illicit drug is a term used to refer to a drug that is unlawful to possess or use. This is complicated by the fact that many of these drugs are available by prescription, but when they are manufactured or sold illegally they are illicit. Traditionally alcohol and tobacco have not been considered illicit substances even when used by minors, probably because of their widespread legal availability to adults. On the other hand, common household chemicals, such as glues and paints, take on some characteristics of illicit substances when people inhale them to get "high."

Deviant drug use is drug use that is not common within a social group *and* that is disapproved by the majority, causing members of the group to take some form of corrective action when it occurs. The corrective action may be informal (making fun of the behavior,

Continued

FYI   Some Important Definitions—and a Caution! Continued

criticizing the behavior) or formal (incarceration, treatment). Some examples of drug use might be deviant in the society at large but accepted or even expected in particular subcultures. We still consider this behavior to be deviant, since it makes more sense to apply the perspective of the larger society.

Drug misuse generally refers to the use of prescribed drugs in greater amounts than, or for purposes other than, those prescribed by a physician or dentist. For nonprescription drugs or chemicals such as paints, glues, or solvents, misuse might mean any use other than the use intended by the manufacturer.

Drug abuse consists of the use of a substance in a manner, amounts, or situations such that the drug use causes problems or greatly increases the chances of problems occurring. The problems may be social (including legal), occupational, psychological, or physical. Once again, this definition gives us a good idea of what we're talking about, but it isn't precise. For example, some would consider any use of an illicit drug to be abuse because of the possibility of legal problems, but many people who have tried marijuana on occasion would argue that they had no problems and therefore didn't abuse it. Another problem is that the use of almost any drug, even under the orders of a physician, has at least some potential for causing problems. The question might come down to how great the risk is and whether the user is recklessly disregarding the risk. How does cigarette smoking fit this definition? In your opinion, should all cigarette smoking be considered drug abuse?

Drug **addiction** is a very controversial term, and in Chapter 3 we review evidence that the scientific view of addiction has changed over the past several years. We find it most convenient to use the term in its original dictionary sense, to "give oneself up to a habit." Drug addiction is thus characterized by frequent use of the drug (usually at least daily) and by the fact that a great deal of the individual's behavior is focused on using the drug, obtaining the drug, talking about the drug, or on paraphernalia associated with the drug's use. We mean this only in a descriptive behavioral way, not necessarily implying anything about physiology or disease. It should be obvious that one could apply this definition to other kinds of behavior, such as watching television or playing some game (e.g., golf or Nintendo), and in common parlance we often do use the term *addiction* in reference to such activities. The controversy discussed in chapter 3 is mainly over whether the addiction to drugs is somehow fundamentally different from these other "addictions."

It might seem that we don't need all of these different definitions since our stereotypical view of addiction usually involves both deviant drug use and drug abuse. However, these definitions allow for the possibility that one might abuse a drug without being an addict (driving while intoxicated is a good example), or that one might be addicted to coffee drinking without engaging in deviant drug use. One of the most active current controversies about cigarettes is that when they are being used in the manner intended by the manufacturer (therefore not misused), they are still potentially dangerous and addictive.

Are there any general statements that can be made about **psychoactive** drugs—those compounds that alter consciousness and affect mood? In fact, there are four basic principles that seem to apply to all of these drugs.

- *Drugs, per se, are not good or bad.* There are no "bad drugs." When drug abuse, drug addiction, and deviant drug use are talked about, it is the behavior, the way the drug is being used, that is being referred to. This statement sounds controversial and has angered some prominent political figures and drug educators. It therefore requires some defense. From the point of view of a pharmacologist, it is difficult to view the drug, the chemical substance itself, as somehow possessing evil intent. It sits there in its bottle and does nothing until we put it into a living system. From the perspective of a psychologist who treats drug addicts, it is difficult to imagine what good there might be in heroin or cocaine. However, heroin is a perfectly good painkiller, at least as effective as morphine, and it is used medically in many countries. Cocaine is a good local anesthetic and is still used for medical procedures, even in the United States. Each of these drugs can also produce bad effects when people abuse them. In the cases of heroin and cocaine, our society has weighed its perception of the risks of bad consequences against the potential benefits and decided that we should severely restrict the availability of these substances. It is wrong, though, to place all of the blame for these bad consequences on the drugs themselves and to conclude that they are simply "bad" drugs. This is very important because many people have a tendency to view some of these substances as possessing an almost magical power to produce evil. When we blame the substance itself, our efforts to correct drug-related problems tend to focus exclusively on eliminating the substance, perhaps ignoring all of the factors that led to the abuse of the drug.

A wide variety of substances can be classified as drugs.

- *Every drug has multiple effects.* Although a user might focus on a single aspect of a drug's effect, we do not yet have compounds that alter only one aspect of consciousness. All psychoactive drugs act on more than one place in the brain, so we might expect them to produce complex psychological effects. Also, virtually every drug that acts in the brain also has effects on the rest of the body, influencing blood pressure, intestinal activity, or other functions.
- *Both the size and the quality of a drug's effect depend on the amount the individual has taken.* The relationship between dose and effect works in two ways. By increasing the dose, there is usually an increase in the same effects noticed at lower drug levels. Also, and frequently this is a more important relationship, at different dose levels there is often a change in the kind of effect, an alteration in the character of the experience.
- *The effect of any psychoactive drug depends on the individual's history and expectations.* Because these drugs act to alter consciousness and thought processes, the effect they have on an individual depends on what was there

initially. An individual's attitude can have a major effect on his or her perception of the drug experience. The fact that some people can experience a real high when smoking oregano and dry oak tree leaves—thinking it's good **marijuana**—should come as no surprise to anyone who has arrived late at a party and felt a "buzz" after one drink rather than the usual two or three. It is not possible, then, to talk about many of the effects of these drugs independent of the user's attitude and the setting.

HOW DID WE GET HERE?

Have Things Really Changed?

Drug use is not new. As we shall see in later chapters, humans have been using alcohol and plant-derived drugs for thousands of years—as far as we know, since *Homo Sapiens* first appeared on the planet. What recorded history we have indicates that some of these drugs were used not just for their presumed therapeutic effects but also for recreational purposes. In some of the highly developed ancient cultures, psychoactive plants played important economic and religious roles. There is also evidence that some people have always overused, misused, or abused these substances.

Drugs play a much different role in modern society than they did even 100 years ago. Major events have occurred in pharmacology and medicine that have produced revolutionary changes in the way in which we view drugs. In addition, recent cultural revolutions have influenced our attitudes and behavior regarding drugs and drug use.

Four Pharmacological Revolutions

One hundred years ago, most Americans had a very different view of medicines than we have today. There were only a few drugs that had powerful effects, and these were used to treat a wide variety of ailments. The idea that a drug could be a specific treatment for a specific disease was only a dream. As a consequence, most people had limited faith in the power of drugs and were cautious about using them. Our modern attitudes about drugs are based to a great extent on several important advances in pharmacology.

The first revolution brought some major communicable diseases well under control. The use of *vaccines,* which began with Pasteur, Jenner, and Koch in the nineteenth century, certainly has had a major impact on our society. The deadly disease smallpox was almost entirely eliminated, and other serious diseases are virtually a thing of the past; diphtheria, polio, and whooping cough are unheard of except when we refer to the vaccines for them. Measles, mumps, and tetanus also are preventable now through the development of specific vaccines. *Vaccines helped convince the public that medicine is capable of producing drugs with very powerful and very selective beneficial effects.*

The second pharmacological revolution resulted from the introduction of *antibiotics:* "sulfa" drugs, penicillin, and then others. First proven effective during World War II, they continue to save lives daily. These drugs not only cure such previously dreaded diseases as syphilis and pneumonia but can also prevent or treat infections resulting from injury or surgery, thus saving both lives and limbs. *Antibiotics helped give us faith in drugs as real cures for serious illnesses.* We now expect that when we get sick we will go to a physician who will prescribe a drug that will make us better.

The first two revolutions might be too pervasive and too close to home for most of us to

---

psychoactive: having effects on thoughts, emotions, or behavior.

marijuana: (mare i *wan* ah) also spelled "marihuana." Dried leaves of the *cannabis* plant.

appreciate their importance. This is not the case with the third pharmacological revolution—the development of **psychopharmacology** that began in the 1950s (see chapter 9). The most important single event was the introduction of the antipsychotic drugs for the treatment of schizophrenia and other major psychotic disorders. These drugs have freed thousands of patients from long-term hospitalization and have helped to restructure our society's approach to mental illness on several levels. One important, but little-studied, effect on our culture came about because these drugs have their primary effect on mental processes. *Because of advances in psychopharmacology, we came to accept the notion that drugs could have powerful and selective effects on our mind, our emotions, and our perceptions.* Perhaps the psychopharmacological revolution of the 1950s helped set the stage for the "psychedelic" experimentation of the 1960s.

The fourth pharmacological revolution, the development of the *oral contraceptive,* contributed to the sexual revolution that was beginning to occur in the 1950s and has not yet stabilized. It is probably true that the opportunity for unmarried couples to engage in sex without fear of pregnancy contributed to a greater sexual freedom in the 1960s and 1970s. That a married woman could be relatively certain for the first time of having several years of her life uninterrupted by pregnancy made it possible for her to commit to more education and to developing her career. Perhaps those social changes were ready to happen without "the pill," but we all began to think in terms of *planning* for pregnancy and childbirth. In fact, this control factor might be one of the most pervasive and subtle influences of the oral contraceptive on our society's view of drugs. *With oral contraceptives, powerful chemicals clearly labeled as drugs were not being used to prevent or treat disease but were being used by healthy people to gain chemical control over their own bodies.* This may have helped pave the way for attempts to control emotions and thoughts by using chemistry in the 1960s.

Recent Cultural Change

America bounded out of World War II with a belief in the future that was untarnished by minor setbacks, such as the Iron Curtain, the Korean War, and an economic recession here and there. Everything seemed to be moving up after the depression of the 1930s and the war of the 1940s. This was the time to make it big, to make up for not having. The bright-eyed boys and girls who applauded the American flag when it appeared in the movies during the world war grew up, got married, and moved to the suburbs. They knew where they were headed. The formula was simple: work hard, and you'll get ahead. Advancement meant a nicer home, a new car, and a college education for the kids. Blue-collar workers also got their share. In the 1950s, miners and assembly-line workers could make their take-home pay cover a house payment and a car payment, with a bit left over to save up for that TV set. This was the good life—and their kids would have it even better!

When those kids of the postwar baby-boom generation began to turn seventeen or eighteen in the early 1960s, American society underwent a rapid change. The kids who grew up in that affluent society without fear of poverty and hunger did not understand the driving ambition of their parents. Partly, television and the information age made it clear that the society their parents had built was far from perfect. In particular, institutionalized racial discrimination in the form of segregated schools and colleges, segregated public transportation, hotels, restrooms, and restaurants, and discriminatory voter registration procedures all existed in 1960. The picture being painted of hard work leading to the better life apparently didn't apply to everyone. The Vietnam War contributed in a major way. Why were we being asked to risk our lives over there? Who were the good guys and who were the bad guys, and why? Automatic acceptance of authority wasn't going to work anymore. It was time to fix American society, to open it up. We needed more understanding and acceptance of those who were different, not more conformity and materialism. Thus was born the hang-loose ethic of the Aquarian age of the 1960s and 1970s. The so-called Protestant ethic, in which a person's worthiness is indicated partly by material success, was replaced by a more existential approach that focused on how people responded to the experiences of life and how well they got along with others. *Peace, love,* and *happiness* were the watchwords. Being, not having, was a basic component of the youth philosophy. Give to others as Aquarius the waterbearer gives; but first know yourself, be yourself, and experience yourself, through drugs if necessary.

Perhaps it's true that when the social pendulum swings that far that fast, it will always swing back again. Maybe it's just that each new generation has to reject their parents' values to forge their own. To reject the Aquarian age you have to tighten your belt and aim for something, and that's what we started to do in the late 1970s. The shift to conservatism began about when the large baby-boom generation entered their thirties and began to constitute the establishment they had earlier criticized. The expansion of individual liberties and civil rights faltered and bogged down.

The mood of the country changed fairly quickly. A study of above-average high school students in late 1981 found a 20 to 30 percent increase in conservatism compared with one or two years earlier.[1] American society in the 1980s became less tolerant of differences, foreigners, pornography, experimental drug use, and young people questioning America's traditional ideals. Congress debated a constitutional amendment to ban the burning of the American flag. Penalties for violating drug laws, which had been loosened in the 1970s, were increased and broadened. The drinking age, which most states had lowered during the 1970s, was increased to 21 again. Authority was back, along with conformity and materialism. College students were being criticized for their focus on the dollar value of their degree rather than on the experience of learning.

If the 1970s were the decade of the "hippie," then the 1980s were the decade of the "yuppie": the young, upwardly mobile professional. The ideal yuppie appeared to be someone with a very nice job, very nice clothes, a very nice car, and a very nice apartment. Married or unmarried, the ideal yuppie had a meaningful relationship with a very nice member of the opposite sex who also had a very nice job, very nice clothes, and so on.

The stereotypical 1980s person was more interested in personal health than previous generations; running shoes, jazzercise, fitness centers, and home exercise equipment became significant indicators of that change. You would expect that these health-conscious individuals would use fewer drugs, and they might have: light beers, low-alcohol beverages, decaffeinated coffee, and soft drinks grew rapidly in popularity. Average consumption of alcohol and cigarettes declined along with drops in per capita intake of sugar and red meat.[2] But the stereotypical yuppies were also status conscious. Imported bottled water quenched their thirst, but sales of designer chocolates and imported cheese also increased. It is ironic that expensive imported beers also sold well, even though they contained more alcohol and calories than their domestic counterparts.[2]

So the yuppie seemed capable of balancing concerns about health with a little self-indulgence, especially if the indulgence was in something chic and expensive. In that context, what was the major new drug of abuse for this generation? Until the 1980s, considered by many to be relatively safe and nonaddicting? Expensive, supposedly glamorous, used by film and TV stars and sport figures? A drug not intended to expand consciousness but to give that

---

psychopharmacology: the study of the behavioral effects of drugs.

extra energy, effort, the competitive edge? "Coke" was it! (And not the kind in the red and white cans.)

It's always easier to look back and characterize a decade than it is to describe one when it is happening. Would the 1990s be a continuation of the conservative 1980s, or would the pendulum swing again? By the late 1990s the jury was in: marijuana use was rising, and two states passed initiatives in favor of medical use of marijuana. The only question now is how far the pendulum will swing, and for how long?

DRUGS AND DRUG USE TODAY

Extent of Drug Use

In trying to get an overall picture of drug use in today's society, we quickly discover that it's not easy to get accurate information. It is not possible to measure with great accuracy the use of, let's say, cocaine in the United States. We don't really know how much is imported and sold, because most of it is illegal. We don't really know how many cocaine users there are in the country, because we have no good way of counting them. For some things, such as prescription drugs, tobacco, or alcohol, we have a wealth of sales information and can make much better estimates of rates of use. Even there, however, our information might not be complete (home-brewed beer would not be counted, for example, and prescription drugs might be bought and then left unused in the medicine cabinet).

Let us look at some of the kinds of information we do have. A large number of survey questionnaire studies have been conducted in junior highs, high schools, and colleges, partly because this is one of the easiest ways to get a lot of information with a minimum of fuss. Researchers have always been most interested in drug use by adolescents and young adults, because this age is when drug use usually begins and reaches its highest levels.

There are a couple of drawbacks to this type of research. The first is that you can use this technique only on the students who are in classrooms. We can't get this information from high school dropouts. Imagine being sent to conduct such a questionnaire survey at a meeting of the local Hell's Angels motorcycle gang!

A second limitation is that we must assume that most of the self-reports are done honestly. In most cases, we have no way of checking to see if Johnny really did smoke marijuana last week, as he claimed on the questionnaire. Nevertheless, if every effort is made to encourage honesty (including assurances of anonymity), we expect that this factor is minimized. To the extent that tendencies to overreport or

Methamphetamine Use in Your Community

Assume that you have just been appointed to a community-based committee that is looking into drug problems. A high school student on the committee has just returned from a residential treatment program and reports that methamphetamine use has become "very common" in local high schools. Some members of the committee want to immediately call in some experts to give schoolwide assemblies describing the dangers of methamphetamine. You have asked for a little time to "check out" the student's story to find out what you can about the actual extent of use in the community and report back to the group in a month. Make a list of potential sources of information and the type of information each might provide. If you could get all the information on your list, how close do you think you could come to making an estimate of how many current methamphetamine users there are in your community? Do you think it would be above or below the national average?

underreport drug use are relatively constant from one year to the next, we can use such results to reflect trends in drug use over time and to compare relative reported use of various drugs.

Let's look first at the drugs most commonly reported by young college students in a recent nationwide sample.[3] Table 1.1 presents data from one of the best and most complete research programs of this type, the Monitoring the Future Project at the University of Michigan. Data are collected each year from more than 15,000 high school seniors in schools across the United States, so that nationwide trends can be assessed. Data are also gathered from eighth- and tenth-graders and from college students. We are presenting three numbers for each drug: the percentage of college students (1 to 4 years beyond high school) who have *ever* used the drug, the smaller percentage who report having used it within the past *30 days,* and the still smaller percentage who report *daily* use for the past 30 days. Note that almost all of these college students have tried alcohol at some time in their lives. Fewer than half have tried marijuana, and most students report never having tried the rest of the drugs listed. Also note that daily use of any of these drugs other than ciga-

rettes can be considered somewhat rare. One especially valuable aspect of this project is that the high school senior survey has been conducted annually since 1975. Figure 1.1 shows trends from 1975 to 1996 in the reported use within the past *30 days* for alcohol and for marijuana, the most commonly used illicit drug.[4] From this we can see that both the number of students reporting current alcohol use and the number reporting current marijuana use reached a peak in approximately 1978 to 1980, and both declined until 1992. From 1992 to 1996, alcohol use remained relatively constant, while marijuana use increased significantly. This decline and subsequent increase in marijuana use has been the subject of many news articles and political debates, but for now it's mainly important for us to realize the dramatic nature of this change over time. From the peak rate of self-reported

TABLE 1.1

Percentage of College Students 1 to 4 Years beyond High School Reporting Use of Seven Types of Drugs (1994)

Drug	Ever used	Used in last 30 days	Used daily for last 30 days
Alcohol	88	68	3.6
Cigarettes	NA	24	13.2
Marijuana/hashish	42	15	1.8
Inhalants	12	1	0
Stimulants	9	2	0.1
Hallucinogens	10	2	0
Cocaine (all)	5	1	0.1
Crack	1	0.1	0

Source: Monitoring the Future Project, University of Michigan[3]

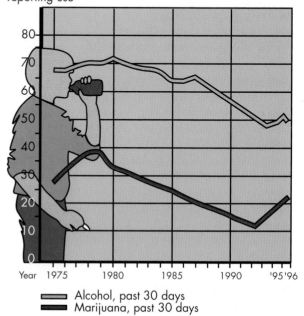

Percentage reporting use

Year

Alcohol, past 30 days
Marijuana, past 30 days

Figure 1.1 Drug use by high school seniors, 1975 to 1996

use in 1978, marijuana use declined by almost 70 percent according to this measure. From its low point in 1992, marijuana use had almost doubled by 1996. It will be interesting for us all to observe whether this statistic will again climb back to the levels of the 1970s or whether it will level off or begin to decline without reaching such high rates.

Since 1986 this same research group has reported data from young adults, sampled from their earlier high school samples. By 1993, data were available for people ranging in age from 19 to 28.[4] In general, these results are similar to the high school senior results, with a decline in marijuana use over the eight-year period, a smaller decline in alcohol use, and an even larger proportional decline in cocaine use. The main difference between these young adults and their high school counterparts is in alcohol use, with reports of use in the past 30 days by 70 percent of young adults aged 19 to 28, compared with 50 percent of high school seniors.

Another way to get broad-based self-report information is with house-to-house surveys. With proper sampling techniques, these studies can estimate the drug use in most of the population, not just among students. This technique is much more time consuming and expensive, it has a greater rate of refusal to participate, and we must suspect that individuals engaged in illegal drug use would be reluctant to reveal that fact to a stranger on their doorstep. Table 1.2 presents recent data from the National Household Survey on Drug Abuse,[5] obtained from over 30,000 randomly selected individuals in carefully sampled households across the country. Data on current use are presented for four age groups: 12 to 17, 18 to 25, 26 to 34, and 35 and older. You may notice that the data for the 18-to-25 group are similar to the comparable data from the high school survey. This kind of cross-checking gives us some additional confidence in the numbers, since different sampling techniques produce similar results. Notice that

TABLE 1.2

Most Commonly Used Drugs among Different Age Groups, 1995 NIDA Household Survey— Percentage Reporting Use in the Past 30 Days

Drug	Age 12–17	Age 18–25	Age 26–34	Age 35+
Alcohol	21	61	63	53
Cigarettes	20	35	35	27
Marijuana	8	12	7	2
Cocaine	0.4	1.3	1.2	0.4

for all age groups, alcohol and cigarettes are the most commonly used of these substances. Although most of the data are not presented in this table, typically the highest rates of illicit drug use are in the 18-to-25 age group. Figure 1.2 shows trends in the *30-day* figures for this age group for alcohol, marijuana, and cocaine since 1974. Again, we see that the peak of reported use of all these substances was in 1980.

Correlates of Drug Use

Once we know that a drug is used by some percentage of a group of people, the next logical step is to ask about the characteristics of those who use the drug as compared with those who don't. Often the same questionnaires that ask each person which drugs they have used also includes several questions about the person completing the questionnaire. The researchers might then send their computers "prospecting" through the data to see if certain personal characteristics might be correlated with drug use. An important point to remember about these studies is that they rarely reveal much about either very unusual or very common types or amounts of drug use. For example, if we sent a computer combing through the data from 1,000 questionnaires looking for characteristics correlated with heroin use, only one or two people in that sample might report heroin use, and you can't correlate much

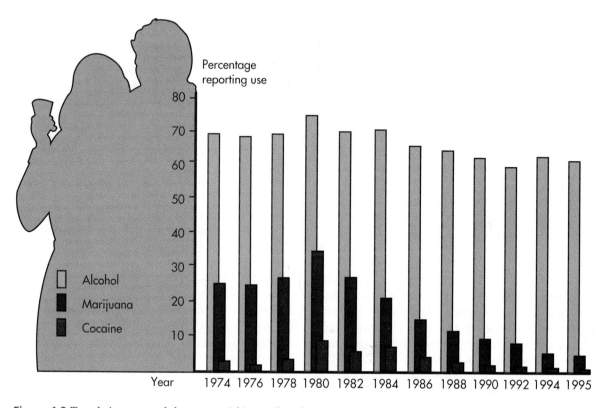

Figure 1.2 Trends in reported drug use within 30 days for young adults ages 18 to 25

based on one or two people. Likewise, it would be difficult to identify distinguishing characteristics of the people who have "ever tried" alcohol, because that group usually represents over 90 percent of the sample.

Much of the research on **correlates** of drug use has used marijuana smoking as an indicator, partly because marijuana use has been a matter of some concern and partly because enough people have tried it so that meaningful correlations can be done. Other researchers focus on early drinking or on the amount of drinking, and others have developed composite "drug use" scores based on use of alcohol and marijuana and experimentation with other substances. We have already seen that age is one factor that re-

lates to drug use; another that shows up consistently is gender. Males of all ages are somewhat more likely to use alcohol or illicit drugs.[5]

You may be surprised at some of the factors that generally do *not* correlate well with alcohol or drug use. One of these is the *socioeconomic status* (SES) of the family. Whether reporting on illicit drug use or level of drinking, most studies find little correlation to the parents' fields of employment (professional, clerical, or blue-collar, for example). These results surprise

---

correlate: (*core* **a let**) a variable that is statistically related to some other variable, such as drug use.

people who think it's the kids with all the money who use drugs and other people who believe that it's the poor kids who use drugs. In fact, most of these studies do not gather enough data on the most economically disadvantaged youth, and when those groups are studied there is a higher rate of drug use.[6] So, very low SES does play a role in drug and alcohol use, but for the vast majority of the population, SES is not a significant factor. Another surprise for most people is the consistent finding that *personality problems* are such poor predictors of drug use. In spite of the fact that many theories of drug use assume that people use alcohol or drugs because of low self-esteem, depression, or anxiety, study after study has found that measures of these characteristics are only weakly correlated with drug use. People often report that they drink or use drugs when they're depressed or anxious, but they are probably referring to a temporary *state* of depression or anxiety, as opposed to a long-term personality *trait*.[6] Self-esteem apparently has complicated relationships to drug use because there is evidence that young people sometimes enhance their self-esteem by becoming involved with a drug- or alcohol-using group.[7] Also, please remember that here we're trying to understand the overall range of drug or alcohol use as found in the population at large, as opposed to looking selectively at that small fraction of people who are addicts or alcoholics.

These studies are also fairly consistent in finding a collection of psychosocial factors that are related to drug use. Those students who are religious, attend school regularly and get good grades, have good relationships with their parents, and do not break the law are the students who report the least drinking and drug use. At the other end of the scale, the picture is that of general *nonconformity* to society, and drug use is one part of that overall picture. This doesn't account for every instance of drug use, but it is the most consistent overall finding. The nonconforming individual often has closer associations with peers than with his or her parents,

and the peers are also likely to be nonconforming. In other words, drug-using youngsters are often part of a *deviant subculture*. Some researchers have begun to think in terms of *risk factors,* that is, indicators that a child or an adolescent has become or is becoming a member of such a deviant subculture. The idea is that no one of these factors is critical, but the more risk factors one has, the more likely one is to be a drug user. An example of this kind of research is given in box 1.1, which describes the significant risk factors derived from a group of about 3,000 California students in seventh, ninth, and eleventh grades, and table 1.3 on p. 16, which shows how drug use was related to the number of risk factors.[8] Those with the most risk factors were much more likely to smoke cigarettes, drink alcohol daily, smoke marijuana daily, and use cocaine and other hard drugs. Notice that even with seven risk factors, less than half the students smoked marijuana daily, and only 7 percent used cocaine. But among those with no risk factors, there was no reported cocaine use and no regular marijuana use.

The other side of this picture is that the same individuals who are at risk for drug abuse are also at risk for other deviant behaviors; fighting, stealing, vandalism, and early sexual activity are correlated with drug use and heavier alcohol use. Therefore the pattern of deviance-prone activity might have both a variety of causes and a variety of behavioral expressions, one of which is drug use.

Antecedents of Drug Use

Finding characteristics that tend to be associated with drug use doesn't help us understand causal relationships very well. For example, do adolescents first become involved with a deviant peer group and then use drugs, or do they first use drugs and then begin to hang around with others who do the same? Does drug use cause them to become poor students and to fight and steal? To answer such questions it is nec-

BOX 1.1

Risk Factors for Substance Abuse in a Group of California Junior High and High School Students

Risk factor and description	Correlation* with composite substance abuse score
Early alcohol intoxication: Intoxication at 12 years of age or younger (23% of respondents)	0.41
Perceived adult drug use: Number of adults you know who have used alcohol at least weekly, pills at least weekly, cannabis or cocaine. Score of 2 or more (30% of respondents)	0.47
Perceived peer approval of drug use: What would your friends think about someone who gets "loaded" on drugs or alcohol? Score of 3 or 4 on 4-point scale (30% of respondents)	0.56
Perceived parent approval of drug use: Two 5-point scales on parent's attitude toward marijuana and alcohol use by the student. Average score of 2 or greater (25%)	0.28
Absence from school: Self-reported absences for reasons other than illness 5 or more times per year (16%)	0.33
Poor academic achievement: Self-reported D or F average (7%)	0.15
Distrust of teacher drug knowledge: (11%)	0.25
Distrust of parent drug knowledge: (11%)	0.25
Low educational aspirations: How much schooling do you plan to complete? Less than a college degree (28%)	0.27
Little religious commitment: How religious are you? Not religious at all (23%)	0.13
Emotional distress: How much were you bothered by each of seven problems during the past month? Each problem rated on a 5-point scale. Average score of 2.1 or more (29%)	0.16
Dissatisfaction with life: Level of satisfaction with eight life areas, each area rated on a 5-point scale. Average of 3 or less (26%)	0.15

*Correlation of 0.0 means no relationship; correlation of 1.0 means perfect predictability.

essary to interview the same individuals at different times and look for **antecedents,** those characteristics that predict later initiation of drug use. For example, one study started with seventh-graders who had not yet tried alcohol

antecedent: (ant eh *see* dent) a variable that occurs before some event such as the initiation of drug use.

TABLE 1.3

Abuse of Five Substances and the Number of Risk Factors

| | Percentage reporting abusing* | | | | | |
| | --- | --- | --- | --- | --- | Abusing at least one substance (%) |
Risk factors	Cigarettes	Alcohol	Cannabis	Cocaine	Hard drugs	
0	1	0	0	0	0	1
1	2	1	0	0	0	3
2	5	1	2	0	1	8
3	11	2	2	1	1	13
4	15	3	11	2	5	25
5	29	7	18	5	7	41
6	34	13	28	6	10	47
7 or more	56	18	40	7	18	71

*Abuse of cigarettes, alcohol, or cannabis was defined as at least daily use, whereas abuse of cocaine and hard drugs was defined as at least weekly use.

and then followed up 3 months and 12 months later.[9] At 3 months, those who had begun heavy alcohol use (more than three drinks per occasion) were most strongly predicted by their earlier association with peers who used marijuana and by their own expectancy that they might also use marijuana. Frequency of heavy drinking at 12 months was best predicted by their drinking behavior at 3 months and by peer approval of cigarette use.

A few scientists have been able to follow the same group of young people at annual intervals for several years in what is known as a **longitudinal study,** and those results have been quite informative. To answer our first question about the deviant peer group, the research results are consistent in reporting that other indicators of deviant behavior generally appear before drug use. For example, children often will be getting poor grades or getting into trouble for fighting or stealing before they first experiment with alcohol, cigarettes, or other substances.[10] This is important because it means that in most cases the conduct problems and grade problems are not caused by drug use. We might not know what the ultimate causes of all these behaviors are, but it is both too simple and obviously

illogical to conclude that all of the problems these kids have are a consequence of their using drugs, because the drug use usually comes later.

Gateway substances

One very important study done in the 1970s[11] pointed out that there was a typical sequence of involvement with drugs. Most of the high school students in that group started their drug involvement with beer or wine. The second stage involved either hard liquor or cigarettes or both, the third stage was marijuana use, and only after going through those stages did they try other illicit substances. Not everyone followed the same pattern, but it is interesting that only 1 percent of the students began their substance use with marijuana or some other illicit drug. It is as though they first had to go through the **gateway** of using alcohol and in many cases cigarettes. Let's keep our logic in order here: Most of the illicit drug users had probably also eaten hamburgers before they smoked marijuana. The point is that students who had not used beer or wine at the beginning of the study were much less likely to be marijuana smokers at the end of the study than the students who had used these substances. Cig-

Gateway substances

arette smokers were about twice as likely as nonsmokers to move on to smoking marijuana. There is evidence that the gateway function of cigarettes continues to be important: in the senior class of 1994, those who were daily smokers of a pack or more of cigarettes were about 15 times as likely as nonsmokers to have used cocaine and about 4 times as likely to have smoked marijuana.[12] From the 1995 Household Survey[13] among youth aged 12 to 17, just over one-third had ever tried cigarettes, but those who had tried cigarettes were more than 10 times as likely to have also tried marijuana. From the self-reported age at which each person first tried cigarettes or marijuana, it was found that 75 percent smoked cigarettes before smoking marijuana.

One possible interpretation of the gateway phenomenon is that young people are exposed to alcohol and tobacco and that these substances themselves somehow make the person more likely to go on to use other drugs. Because most people who use these gateway substances do not go on to become cocaine users, we should be cautious about jumping to that conclusion. What seems more likely is that early alcohol use and cigarette smoking are common indicators of the

general deviance-prone pattern of behavior that also includes an increased likelihood of smoking marijuana or trying cocaine. For example, in the senior class of 1994, a student with a D average was about 14 times as likely as a student with an A average to be a pack-a-day smoker.[12]

Because beer and cigarettes are more widely available to a deviance-prone young person than marijuana or cocaine, it is logical that beer and cigarettes would most often be tried first. The socially conforming students are less likely to try even these relatively available substances until they are older, and they are less likely ever to try the illicit substances. Let's ask the question another way: What if we managed to develop a prevention program that stopped all young people from smoking cigarettes? Would that cut down on marijuana smoking? Most of us think it might because people who don't want to suck tobacco smoke into their lungs probably won't want to inhale marijuana smoke either. Would such a program keep people from getting D averages or getting into trouble of other kinds? Probably not. In other words, we think of the use of gateway substances not as the *cause* of later illicit drug use but instead as an early indicator of the basic pattern of deviant behavior resulting from a variety of psychosocial risk factors.

Parent and peer influences

It is generally true that adolescents are more influenced by their parents when it comes to long-term goals and plans, but their peers have more influence over their immediate lifestyle and day-to-day activities.[14] Also, in early adolescence, parent influences are relatively strong,

---

longitudinal study (lon jeh *too* di nul) a study done over a period of time (months or years).

gateway: one of the first drugs (e.g., alcohol or tobacco) used by a typical drug user.

and as adolescence progresses peer influences become stronger. There is evidence from longitudinal research that both peers and parents influence adolescent drug-use behavior, but in general peer influences are more important. We can imagine situations in which peer and parent influences are in the same direction: a family that encourages school performance and long-term goals or a young person who does well in school and regularly attends religious services and is therefore surrounded by other young people who do well in school and hold similar values. Alternatively, we may have an environment in which one or more parents is an alcoholic, other drugs are used openly, success in school is not valued or encouraged, the family lives in a neighborhood with many such families, and many of the other young people have the same problems. More commonly, we think of a model in which there is a conflict—parents opposing drug or alcohol use and the peer group encouraging such behavior. Two longitudinal studies have tried to examine these influences over time. Although the results are complex, some of the major points can be summarized. As in previous research, the best predictors of drug use were peer variables. In one of the studies, having peers with antisocial attitudes was the strongest predictor of drug use.[10] In the other study, having peers who used marijuana was the best predictor of marijuana use.[14] The use of alcohol by parents did have an impact on alcohol use, but it is not clear whether this is because of direct "modeling" effects. For example, in one study it appeared that adolescents whose parents drank were more likely to have friends who drank, and the drinking pattern of friends was a big influence.[14] In the other study it was argued that heavy drinking by the parent might interfere with parental *monitoring* of the child's activities, and poor monitoring by parents was found to be a major factor in allowing the child to associate with a deviant peer group.[10]

What advice for parents can we draw from all this research? First, encourage and reinforce the value of school and school achievement and of long-term life goals. When day-to-day activities and behavior are incompatible with those long-term goals, point that out. Second, be on the alert for school practices such as remedial "tracks" or after-school detention that might frequently group your child with deviance-prone peers. Third, realize that you do have some influence on the types of peers your child associates with, particularly during childhood and early adolescence. Your child might associate with children who behave the way your family behaves, so it might pay to examine your own behavior. You can encourage or provide support for after-school activities that will bring your child into contact with positive peer groups. Monitoring involves knowing what your child is doing and with whom, as well as showing interest in school activities and accomplishments. This advice comes with no guarantee of success, but it is based on consistent research findings.

Motives for Drug Use

To most of us it doesn't seem necessary to find explanations for normative behavior; we don't often ask why someone takes a pain reliever when they have a headache. Our task is to try to explain the drug-taking behavior that frightens and infuriates—the deviant drug use. There is one fact about human conduct that we should keep in mind throughout this book: In spite of good, logical evidence telling us we "should" avoid certain things, we all do some of them anyway. We know that we shouldn't eat that second piece of pie or have that third drink on an empty stomach. Cool-headed logic tells us so. We would be hard pressed to find good, sensible reasons why we should smoke cigarettes, drive faster than the speed limit, go skydiving, sleep late when we have work to do, flirt with someone and risk an established relationship, or use cocaine. Whether one labels these behaviors sinful or just stupid, they don't seem to be designed to maximize our health or longevity.

UP FOR DEBATE

Is Drug Use Declining Among Hard-Core Users?

Reports of declining numbers of high school students and adults using marijuana and other drugs during the 1980s were accompanied with the warning that use may not have declined among the hard-core addicts who are unlikely to be counted in these surveys.[4] The homeless, high school dropouts, and other groups who might be expected to have a larger number of hard-core users are not well sampled in these studies. The concern is that although casual or experimental use may have decreased in the general population, there may be as many or more addicts as there were ten years ago, especially among the minorities and the poor. However, the scientists who conduct the high school survey have pointed out that self-reported *daily* use of illicit drugs also dropped

dramatically, and daily use cannot be said to be casual or experimental. Declines were seen for all ethnic groups and in all regions of the country. Among the students who are most likely to be dropouts, those who were in school to take the survey but who are frequently truant and have low grades, self-reported use also declined during the 1980s.

We might look at the numbers of people in treatment programs, but those figures are often influenced more by program availability than by the numbers needing treatment. Likewise, the number of arrests for drug use reflect police effort to arrest users more than the number of users who could be arrested. As this chapter explains, it's always harder to estimate the number of addicts than the number of users.

But humans do not live by logic alone; we are social animals who like to impress each other, and we are pleasure-seeking animals as well. These factors help to explain why people do some of the things they shouldn't, including drugs.

The research on correlates and antecedents points to a variety of personal and social variables that influence our drug taking, and many psychological and sociological theorists have proposed models for explaining illegal or excessive drug use. We have seen evidence for one common reason why some people begin to take certain illegal drugs: usually young, and more often male than female, they have chosen to identify with a deviant subculture. These groups frequently engage in a variety of behaviors not condoned by the larger society. Within that group the use of a particular drug might not be deviant at all but might in fact be expected.

Occasionally the use of a particular drug becomes such a fad among a large number of youth groups that it seems to be a nationwide problem. However, within any given community there will still be groups of people of the same age who don't use the drug.

Rebellious behavior, especially among young people, serves important functions not only for the developing individual but also for the evolving society. Adolescents often try very hard to impress other people and may find it especially difficult to impress their parents. An adolescent who is unable to gain respect from people or who is frustrated in efforts to "go his or her own way" might engage in some particularly dangerous or disgusting behavior as a way of demanding that people be impressed or at least pay attention!

One source of excessive drug use may be found within the drugs themselves. Many of

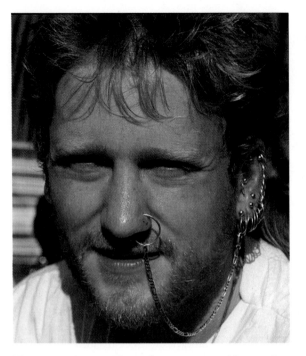

Young people sometimes do outrageous things to impress others. Some of the more dangerous forms of drug use might serve this same purpose.

these drugs are capable of *reinforcing* the behavior that gets the drug into the system. **Reinforcement** means that, everything else being equal, each time you take the drug you increase slightly the probability that you will take it again. Thus with many psychoactive drugs there is a constant tendency to increase the frequency or amount of use. Some drugs (such as intravenous heroin or cocaine) appear to be so reinforcing that this process occurs relatively rapidly in a large percentage of those who use them. For other drugs, such as alcohol, the process seems to be much slower. In many people, social factors, other reinforcers, or other activities prevent the increase from occurring at all. For some, however, the drug-taking behavior does increase and consumes an increasing share of their lives. These are the addicts and alcoholics we sometimes pity and sometimes fear but almost never respect.

Most drug users are seeking an altered state of consciousness, a different perception of the world than is provided by normal day-to-day activities. It is usually impossible to separate this altered state from the reinforcing effect, because the altered state might be the psychological reflection of the reinforcing state. Many of the high school students in the nationwide surveys report that they take drugs "to see what it's like," or "to get high," or "because of boredom."[15] In other words, they are looking for a change, for something new and different in their lives. This aspect of drug use was particularly clear during the 1960s and 1970s when lysergic acid diethylamide (LSD) and other perception-altering drugs were popular. We don't always recognize the altered states produced by other substances, but they do exist. A man drinking alcohol might have just a bit more of a perception that he's a tough guy, that he is influential, that he is well liked. A cocaine user might get the seductive feeling that everything is great and that she is doing a great job (even if she isn't). Many drug-abuse prevention programs have focused on efforts to show young people how to feel good about themselves and how to look for excitement in their lives without using drugs.

Another thing seems clear: although societal, community, and family factors (the outer areas of figure 1.3) play an important role in determining whether an individual will first *try* a drug, with increasing use the individual's own experiences with the drug become increasingly important. For those who become seriously addicted, the drug and its actions on that individual become central, and social influences, availability, cost, and penalties play a less important role in the continuation of drug use.

SUMMARY

▲ Drug use is a form of behavior that has many things in common with other behaviors, and many of the same kinds of controlling variables.

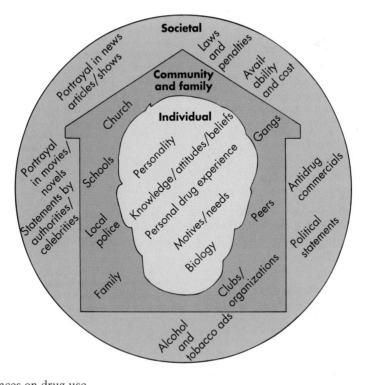

Figure 1.3 Influences on drug use

▲ Any individual drug can have various effects, depending on who has taken it, how much has been taken, and how it is taken.

▲ Drug use and problems caused by drug use are probably as old as humankind.

▲ Changes in American society since the 1950s have influenced fashion in many areas, and recreational drug use is no exception.

▲ Most of the information about current drug use comes from large-scale nationwide surveys done in high schools or house-to-house.

▲ Drug use is greater among those who are more rebellious and who engage in other deviant behaviors, such as heavy drinking.

▲ Psychoactive drugs can be behaviorally reinforcing, produce altered states of consciousness, and help an individual make a social statement about what group he or she belongs to.

REVIEW QUESTIONS

1. Besides asking a person the question directly, what is one way a psychologist can try to determine why a person is taking a drug?
2. What two characteristics of a drug's effect might change when the dose is increased?
3. In what way might the development of oral contraceptives have changed people's views

---

reinforcement: a procedure in which a behavioral event is followed by a consequent event such that the behavior is then more likely to be repeated. The behavior of taking a drug may be reinforced by the effect of the drug.

of drugs to make experimenting with psychoactive drugs more likely?

4. In about what year did the mood in the United States first show a rapid trend away from the Aquarian age toward a more conservative, less tolerant perspective?

5. What are the two types of large drug-use surveys sponsored by the federal government on a regular basis?

6. In about what year did both alcohol use and illicit drug use reach an apparent peak?

7. What is the relationship between SES and illicit drug use or heavy drinking?

8. What is meant by the term *risk factors for drug use,* and what are some of the risk factors?

9. In what sense is cigarette smoking a "gateway" to marijuana or cocaine use?

10. Why would a person purposefully act in ways that frighten and anger others?

Related Internet Sites on Drug Use

National Clearinghouse for Alcohol and Drug Information: Research and Statistics: http://www.health.org:80/survey.htm

Yahoo! drugs page: http://www.yahoo.com/text/Health/Pharmacology/Drugs

And don't miss our own *Drugs, Society, and Human Behavior* web site with updated information and links to other information sources: http://www.uwyo.edu/A&S/psyc/dshb.htm

REFERENCES

1. Conservatism is found in top teen students, *New York Times* p A1, Dec 3, 1981.

2. Sherman SP: America's new abstinence, *Fortune* pp 20–23, Mar 18, 1985.

3. *Preliminary tables from national survey results on drug use, Volume 2, College students and young adults.* Institute for Social Research, 1995, The University of Michigan.

4. Johnston LD, Bachman JG, O'Malley PM: *The rise in drug use among American teens continues in 1996,* press release from the Institute for Social Research, 1996, The University of Michigan.

5. *Preliminary estimates from the 1995 National Household Survey on Drug Abuse.* SAMHSA Advance Report Number 18, Washington DC, August, 1996.

6. Oetting ER, Beauvais F: Common elements in youth drug abuse: peer clusters and other psychosocial factors. In Peele S, editor: *Visions of addiction,* Lexington, Mass, 1988, DC Heath.

7. Stein JA, Newcomb MD, Bentler PM: Personality and drug use: reciprocal effects across four years, *Personality and Individual Differences* 8:419–430, 1987.

8. Newcomb MD and others: Substance abuse and psychosocial risk factors among teenagers: associations with sex, age, ethnicity, and type of school, *American Journal of Drug and Alcohol Abuse* 13:413–433, 1987.

9. Ellickson PL, Hays RD: Antecedents of drinking among young adolescents with different alcohol use histories, *Journal of Studies on Alcohol* 52:398–408, 1991.

10. Dishion TJ, Patterson GR, Reid JR: Parent and peer factors associated with drug sampling in early adolescence: implications for treatment. In Rahdert ER, Grabowski J, editors: *Adolescent drug abuse: analyses of treatment research,* NIDA Research Monograph, No 77, Washington, DC, 1988, US Government Printing Office.

11. Kandel D, Faust R: Sequence and stages in patterns of adolescent drug use, *Archives of General Psychiatry* 32:923–932, 1975.

12. Bachman, JG, Johnston LD, O'Malley, PM: *Monitoring the Future: A Continuing Study of the Lifestyles and Values of youth,* 1994 [Computer file]. Conducted by University of Michigan, Survey Research Center. ICPSR ed. Ann Arbor, MI: Inter-University Consortium for Political and Social Research [producer and distributor], 1996.

13. Greenblatt, J: Analysis shows correlation between smoking cigarettes and marijuana in adolescents. *SAMHSA News,* Substance Abuse and Mental Health Services Administration, Winter, 1997.

14. Kandel DB, Andrews K: Processes of adolescent socialization by parents and peers, *International Journal of the Addictions* 22:319–342, 1987.

15. Johnston LD, O'Malley PM: Why do the nation's students use drugs and alcohol? Self-reported reasons from nine national surveys, *Journal of Drug Issues* 16:29–66, 1986.

2

Drug Use as a Social Problem

KEY TERMS	OBJECTIVES

After reading this chapter, you should be able to:

laissez-faire
toxic
behavioral toxicity
acute
chronic
DAWN
AIDS
HIV

- Explain what is meant by *laissez-faire* and "victimless crimes," and give three general motivations for societal regulation of drug use.
- Define four categories of toxicity and give an example of each.
- Describe the DAWN system and the two basic types of information it collects.
- Explain what is meant by a drug's relative dependence potential.

- State the estimated dependence potential for several psychoactive drugs.
- Give a few brief factual statements about whether heroin addicts become criminals as a result of their addiction.
- Discuss the ways in which alcohol contributes to *violent* crime.

Drugs are widely used, some legally and some illegally. If you hear someone talking about the "drug problem," the reference is probably to those situations in which groups or individuals are using drugs in such a way as to attract the disapproval of the rest of society (in other words, the type of deviant or excessive drug use described at the end of chapter 1). One possible way to look at the "drug problem" is as a social conflict between drug-using or drug-selling individuals and the majority social group.

LAISSEZ-FAIRE

In the 1800s the U.S. government had virtually no laws governing the sale or use of most

drugs. The idea seemed to be that if the seller wanted to sell it and the buyer wanted to buy it, let them do it—**laissez-faire**, in French. This term has been used to characterize the general nature of the U.S. government of that era. Some current thinkers have advocated a return to that attitude.[1] After all, buying and selling marijuana or cocaine can be called, like prostitution, a "victimless" crime. Both parties get what they want from the transaction, and neither party complains. Because that is often true, the only way

> **laissez-faire: (lay say fair)** a hands-off approach to government.

23

society, through its enforcement agencies, can make many arrests for these crimes is to go looking for trouble, by pretending to be either buyer or seller. Instead, why not just look the other way?

In fact, state and federal laws controlling drug sales were passed because it was believed that there were victims in some of these transactions. Three main concerns aroused public interest: (1) *toxicity:* some drug sellers were considered to be endangering the public health and victimizing individuals because they were selling dangerous, toxic chemicals, often without labeling them or putting appropriate warnings on them; (2) *addiction:* some sellers were seen as victimizing individuals and endangering their health by selling them habit-forming drugs, again often without appropriate labels or warnings; and (3) *crime:* the drug user came to be seen as a threat to public safety—the attitude became widespread that drug-crazed individuals would often commit horrible, violent crimes. In chapter 4 we will look at the roots of these concerns and how our current legal structures grew from them. For now, let's look at each issue and develop some ground rules for the discussion of toxicity, addiction, and drug-induced criminality.

TOXICITY

Categories of Toxicity

The word **toxic** means "poisonous, deadly, or dangerous." All the drugs we discuss in this text can be toxic if misused or abused. We will use the term to refer to those effects of drugs that interfere with normal functioning in such a way as to produce dangerous or potentially dangerous consequences. Seen in this way, for example, alcohol could be toxic in high doses because it suppresses respiration—this can be dangerous if breathing stops long enough to induce brain damage or death. But we can also consider alcohol to be toxic if it causes a person

to be so disoriented that for them otherwise normal behaviors, such as driving a car or swimming become dangerous. This latter is an example of something we refer to as **behavioral toxicity.** We make a somewhat arbitrary distinction, then, between behavioral toxicity and "physiological" toxicity—perhaps taking advantage of the widely assumed mind-body distinction, which is more convenient than real. The only reason for making this distinction is that it helps remind us of some important kinds of toxicity that are special to psychoactive drugs, and that are sometimes overlooked.

Another distinction we make for the purpose of discussion is **acute** versus **chronic.** Most of the time when people use the word *acute,* they mean "sharp" or "intense." In medicine an acute condition is one that comes on suddenly, as opposed to a chronic or long-lasting condition. When talking about drug effects, we can think of the acute effects as those that result from a single administration of a drug or are a direct result of the actual presence of the drug in the system at the time. For example, taking an overdose of heroin can lead to acute toxicity. By contrast, the chronic effects of a drug would be those that result from long-term exposure and can be present whether or not the substance is actually in the system at a given point in time. For example, smoking cigarettes can eventually lead to various types of lung disorders. If you have emphysema from years of smoking, that condition is there when you wake up in the morning and when you go to bed at night, and whether your most recent cigarette was five minutes ago or five days ago doesn't make much difference.

Using these definitions, table 2.1 can help give us an overall picture of the possible toxic consequences of a given type of drug. However, knowing what is *possible* is different from knowing what is *likely.* How can we get an idea of which drugs are most likely to produce adverse drug reactions?

TABLE 2.1

Examples of Four Types of Drug-Induced Toxicity

	Acute	Chronic
Behavioral	"Intoxication" from alcohol, marijuana, or other drugs that impair behavior and increase danger to the individual	Personality changes reported to occur in alcoholics and suspected by some to occur in marijuana users (amotivational syndrome)
Physiological	Usually results from taking too much of a drug, as in overdose	Heart disease, lung cancer, and other effects related to smoking; liver damage resulting from chronic alcohol exposure

Drug Abuse Warning Network

In an effort to monitor the toxicity of drugs other than alcohol, the federal government set up the Drug Abuse Warning Network (**DAWN**). This system collects data on drug-related crises from several hundred hospital emergency rooms in metropolitan areas around the country. If an individual comes to the emergency room with any sort of problem that is determined to be related to drug abuse, then each drug involved (up to four) will be recorded as "mentioned" in connection with a medical emergency. For DAWN's purposes, drug abuse includes improper uses of prescription or over-the-counter drugs, and the use of any other substance for psychic effect, dependence, or suicide. Note that the recorded incident could arise because a person swallowed a bottle of aspirin in a suicide attempt or smoked marijuana and then suffered a panic reaction. In the latter case, probably no lasting harm would have occurred, if the person had not gone to the emergency room, but each incident counts as one mention anyway. You can imagine that doing the recordkeeping in any other way would require many subjective judgments on the part of the emergency room physicians: Was it really a serious medical emergency? Was that drug really responsible? This would probably result in systematic differences from one hospital or one city to another. Beginning in 1989, the sampling procedure for

including emergency rooms in the DAWN system was changed to better estimate the total number of episodes in the United States. The numbers for emergency room episodes given on the left-hand side of table 2.2 are these national estimates for 1995.[2]

If a drug is involved in a person's death, the medical examiner (coroner) is expected to report in a consistent way to the DAWN system, and these drug-related deaths form a second set of statistics (with, of course, smaller numbers of mentions). Some of those death statistics are shown on the right-hand side of table 2.2.

Before looking at the specific DAWN results, it is important for us to remember a couple of

---

toxic: poisonous, dangerous.

behavioral toxicity: toxicity resulting from behavioral effects of a drug.

acute: referring to drugs, the short-term effects of a single dose.

chronic: referring to drugs, the long-term effects from repeated use.

DAWN: Drug Abuse Warning Network. System for collecting data on drug-related deaths or emergency-room visits.

Crack Babies

One toxicity issue that has received national attention is the effect of crack use during pregnancy on the unborn child. The image of the "crack baby" is a powerful one: born to a mother who was smoking crack during her pregnancy and up until the time of birth, the infant is addicted at birth, suffers withdrawal agonies, and continues to suffer from developmental abnormalities. In the early 1990s politicians and news media were able to attract our attention by describing the plight of these young victims of drug abuse and by suggesting that large numbers of children would be affected. These tragedies occur at too high a rate no matter how many there are, but just how many are there? How would we find out?

The Partnership for a Drug-Free America is well known for its high-impact television ads, including the famous egg in the frying pan ("This is your brain on drugs"). In 1992 they began running an ad showing crack in a baby bottle, claiming that "a crack baby is born every 5 minutes." This would work out to about 100,000 per year. Are there that many? The 1991 Household Survey data esti-mated that about 280,000 women of all ages may have used crack at some time during the year. Perhaps most of these were of child-bearing age, but most were not using the drug frequently and most were not pregnant, so the 100,000 "crack baby" figure would seem high. A call to the Partnership office revealed that they had gotten the 100,000 figure from the 1989 National Drug Control Strategy published by the White House.[18] The estimated 100,000 "cocaine babies" referred to on p. 44 of that document seems to be an estimate of the number of babies whose mothers used any form of cocaine, even once, at some time during the pregnancy. We have heard people use numbers ranging from 60,000 to over 300,000 per year in referring to crack babies. If we mean only those babies who are born addicted because of recent heavy crack smoking by the mother, then all of these numbers are probably too high. Crack babies are discussed further in chapter 7. Why do you think that politicians and news media tend to "oversell" the latest drug problem to the public?

TABLE 2.2

Drug Mentions in the DAWN System for 1995

	Emergency room episodes				Drug-related deaths		
Rank	Drug name	Number of mentions	Percentage of total episodes	Rank	Drug name	Number of mentions	Percentage of total episodes
1.	Alcohol-in-combination	172,800	32.49	1.	Cocaine	3,465	46.00
2.	Cocaine	142,494	26.79	2.	Alcohol-in-combination	2,944	39.09
3.	Heroin/morphine	76,023	14.29	3.	Heroin/morphine	2,912	38.66
4.	Marijuana/hashish	47,069	8.85	4.	Codeine	880	11.68
5.	Acetaminophen	36,813	6.92	5.	Diazepam (Valium)	640	8.50
6.	Ibuprofen	20,915	3.93	6.	Methadone	431	5.72
7.	Methamphetamine	17,547	3.30	7.	Amitriptyline	414	5.50
8.	Aspirin	17,231	3.24	8.	D-propoxyphene	398	5.28
9.	Alprazolam (Xanax)	17,217	3.23	9.	Marijuana/hashish	359	4.77
10.	Amitriptyline	14,719	2.77	10.	Nortriptyline	335	4.45

important facts. First, alcohol is not counted if it is the only drug mentioned, but it is counted in the category "alcohol-in-combination" if it is mentioned along with other drugs. Second, more than one drug may be mentioned per incident, and each drug will be counted as a separate "mention."

Now let's look at table 2.2, which lists the most frequently mentioned drugs in recent DAWN reports. Probably the most obvious thing is that alcohol-in-combination is near the top in both lists, a place it has held for several years. In fact, if alcohol were counted alone and treated like other drugs in the system, its numbers would so overwhelm both sets of data that all the other drugs would appear to be unimportant beside it. This would seem to indicate that alcohol is a pretty toxic substance. It is, but let us also remember that about half of all adult Americans drink alcohol at least once a month, whereas only a small number of people use cocaine, a drug that is also near the top of both DAWN lists. The DAWN system does not correct for frequency of use but rather gives us an idea of the total impact of a substance on medical emergencies or drug-related deaths. Cocaine has vied with alcohol-in-combination for the top

spot on these lists since the mid 1980s. Methamphetamine has moved into the top ten during the mid 1990s.

You should notice that the three over-the-counter pain relievers acetaminophen, aspirin, and ibuprofen (see chapter 14) would rank between cocaine and heroin in emergency room mentions if they were combined as a group. However, these drugs do not show up among the top ten for drug-related deaths. They are often used in suicide attempts but usually do not result in death. Other suicide-related drugs include alprazolam (Xanax) and diazepam (Valium), which are widely prescribed sedatives (see chapter 8), and amitriptyline, an antidepressant (see chp   33apter 9). For each of these three classes of drugs, suicide was listed as the motive in about 70 percent of the emergency room episodes.

The importance of drug combinations, particularly combinations with alcohol, in contributing to these numbers cannot be overstressed. About half of the emergency room episodes were multiple-drug episodes, whereas three-fourths of the drug-related deaths mentioned multiple drugs. For both heroin and cocaine, alcohol was the most common "other" drug.

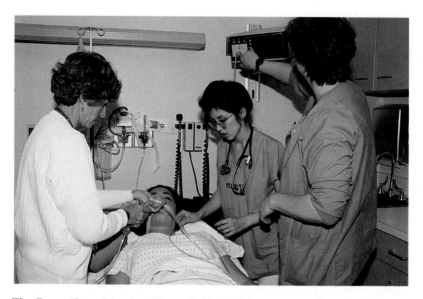

The Drug Abuse Warning Network (DAWN) keeps records of drug-related medical emergencies.

How Dangerous Is It?

Now that we have seen how complex the interpretation of these tables can become, let's see if we can use the information they present to ask some questions about the relative danger to a person of taking one drug versus another. We have seen that the DAWN data do not correct for incidence of use. Let's use the data presented in table 1.2 (see chapter 1, p. 12), obtained from home surveys, as a rough estimate of the relative proportions of use of these drugs in our society. The populations studied are not exactly the same, and there are other reasons why we would not want to use this approach to make fine distinctions among drugs. But we can easily see that marijuana, which was reported to be in current use by about 12 percent of the young adults, did not appear among the top ten drugs for drug-related deaths. About 1 percent of young adults reported using cocaine, but cocaine was more frequently associated with

death than any other substance in the DAWN report. From these statistics we can draw the obvious conclusion, even from imperfect data, that cocaine is many times more deadly than marijuana.

Heroin, which was reported in current use by many fewer people than was cocaine, was mentioned in almost as many drug-related deaths. Can we conclude from this that heroin use is more dangerous than cocaine use? Probably so, given the way each is typically used. Please keep in mind that the amount taken and how a drug is taken can greatly influence toxicity. Heroin was once sold in small doses in tablet form. If it were still available in that form as a prescription drug, many more people would be taking it but almost none of those would die from it, and our estimates of heroin's relative toxicity would drop drastically. Cocaine is most often "snorted" into the nose, less often smoked as crack, and seldom injected, whereas heroin is often injected intravenously. An experiment indicated that rats allowed to intravenously self-inject as much cocaine as they wanted were more likely to die than rats allowed to self-inject as much heroin as they wanted,[3] so it might be that if the two drugs were both taken intravenously by most of their human users, cocaine would cause many more deaths than heroin.

We cannot tell precisely from the DAWN data how many total deaths are related to the use of cocaine or heroin, because not all coroners are included in the system. Data are gathered from metropolitan areas that include about a third of the U.S. population, but they are areas that have higher than average use of illicit drugs. A rough estimate of the total annual number of deaths related to cocaine, for example, might be twice the reported DAWN figure, or about 7,000 per year. The total for all illicit drugs, including cocaine, heroin, marijuana, and phencyclidine hydrochloride (PCP), might be approximately 15,000. In a country in which over two million people die each year, this is a relatively minor cause of death, a fact that is surprising to many people. For comparison, it is estimated that alcohol is responsible for about 100,000 deaths annually (see chapter 11), and more than 400,000 annual deaths are attributed to cigarette smoking (see chapter 12). Of course many more people use those substances, and in terms of *relative* danger of toxicity, heroin and cocaine are probably more dangerous than alcohol or cigarettes. However, in looking at the *total* impact of these drug-related deaths on American society, if you were about to conclude that politicians and the news media have been paying a disproportionate amount of attention to cocaine and heroin-related toxicity, you would be right.

AIDS

There is a great deal of concern about the spread of acquired immunodeficiency syndrome (**AIDS**) among drug abusers. The human immunodeficiency virus (**HIV**) is a blood-borne agent capable of spreading the disease among addicts who share needles. The insidious thing about HIV is that a person can be infected for a year or two with no overt symptoms and during that time spread the disease to others. Both AIDS and hepatitis B, another blood-borne disease, have been responsible for hundreds of deaths among intravenous drug abusers. In large cities around the world, the proportion of intravenous drug users who test positive for HIV might be as high as 40 to 50 percent.[4] Because HIV also can be transmitted sexually, the public at large is at some risk of contracting HIV from intravenous drug users, especially considering that many female drug users earn money through prostitution.

It is important to point out that this type of drug-associated toxicity is not due to the action of the drug itself but is incidental to the sharing of needles, no matter which drug is injected or whether the injection is intravenous or intramuscular. A study of intravenous drug users in Baltimore found that about half the syringes and needles they used were obtained from street dealers and that only about 30 percent came directly from a pharmacy. These needles were commonly used several times.[5] In a sense, the spread through needle sharing is due less to the drug addiction itself than to laws designed to prevent addiction, in particular the laws restricting the sale of hypodermic equipment. Failing to use clean needles is the most significant risk factor leading to new HIV infections in cities with high infection rates.[6] Although the U.S. government does not support needle exchange programs, the number of such programs has grown rapidly during the 1990s. These programs vary from city to city in terms of how

---

AIDS: acquired immunodeficiency syndrome.

HIV: human immunodeficiency virus.

Collecting needles for exchange program in an effort to prevent the spread of HIV among needle using addicts.

they are funded, where the needle exchanges take place, and other operating rules. Typically the programs require a one-for-one exchange of a used needle for a clean one, thus allowing for collection and proper disposal of potentially infected needles. In some communities the programs operate in violation of state laws or local ordinances, whereas in other communities specific legal exemptions have been passed for needle exchange programs. In many European countries and in Australia, needle exchange programs are an important component of government AIDS prevention programs. The primary concern in the United States seems to be that providing clean needles would seem to condone intravenous drug use, or that new users would more readily begin intravenous drug use if the fear of AIDS were lessened. Small-scale studies conducted by needle exchange programs in some cities have not found any evidence for

increased numbers of new users or of a decrease in the average age of users.

DRUG ADDICTION

Problems of Definition

Another of the concerns expressed by those urging passage of drug controls in the early 1900s was for the victims of drug addiction. Those who unknowingly or carelessly took habit-forming drugs risked becoming enslaved by them. The unscrupulous sellers of these drugs were thus assured a steady market, whereas the addicts were forced to continue to endanger their own health and supposedly to undermine their own mental and moral strength. That is one major reason that the habit-forming drugs, such as cocaine and the opiates, were singled out for special taxation and record keeping in 1914 (see chapter 4).

BOX 2.1

Dependence Potential of Psychoactive Drugs

Very High:	Heroin (IV)
	Crack cocaine
High:	Morphine
	Opium (smoked)
Moderate/High:	Cocaine powder
	Tobacco cigarettes
	PCP (smoked)
Moderate:	Diazepam (Valium)
	Alcohol
	Amphetamines (oral)
Moderate/Low:	Caffeine
	MDMA ("Ecstasy")
	Marijuana
Low:	Ketamine (see
	chapter 16)
Very Low:	LSD
	Mescaline
	Psilocybin

LSD, lysergic acid diethylamide; MDMA, methylenedioxy methamphetamine.

The next chapter deals in some detail with the concept of addiction, which has been defined in many ways over the years. As we shall see, addiction to alcohol or another drug involves complex interactions among the individual, the substance, and the social environment. Therefore, questions such as "Is marijuana an addicting drug?" are too simple. Some people have developed what most professionals would agree is an addiction to marijuana, but most marijuana users have not. For most psychoactive drugs, the most accurate answer to the question of whether that drug "is addictive" would be that addiction is possible. It does seem clear that some kinds of drug use are more likely to lead to addiction than other kinds: intravenous use of heroin is more likely to become

addicting than is marijuana smoking or LSD use. Thus we might legitimately ask ourselves which drugs, or which methods of using those drugs, pose the greatest risk for addiction. A recent report[7] reviewed 350 published articles to come up with relative ratings, then had the preliminary tables reviewed by a panel of psychopharmacologists for suggested changes. Based on that report, we can classify psychoactive drugs into seven categories of "dependence potential," from very high to very low (box 2.1). Please remember that such rankings ignore some very important biological, psychological, and social factors that are also major contributors to the development of addiction (see chapter 3).

CRIME AND VIOLENCE

Does Drug Use Cause Crime?

It might seem obvious to a reader of today's newspapers or to a viewer of today's television that drugs and crime are linked. There are frequent reports of killings attributed to warring gangs of crack dealers.[8] Our prisons house a large population of people convicted for drug-related crimes, and there have been several reports that a large fraction of arrestees for non-drug felonies have positive results from urine tests for illicit substances.

The belief that there is a causal relationship between many forms of drug use and criminality probably forms the basis for many of our laws concerning drug use and drug users. The relationship between crime and illegal drug use is complex, and only recently have data-based statements become possible. Facts are necessary because political actions are taken, and laws are enacted, on the basis of what we believe to be true.

The basis for concern was the belief that drug use *causes* crime. The fact that drug addicts engage in robberies or that car thieves are likely to also use illicit drugs does not say anything about causality. Both criminal activity and drug use could well be caused by other factors, producing both types of deviant behavior in the same individuals. There are several senses in which it might be said that drugs cause crime, but the most frightening possibility is that drug use somehow *changes the individual's personality in a lasting way,* making him or her into a "criminal type." For example, during the 1924 debate that led to a complete prohibition against heroin sales in the United States, a testifying physician asserted regarding users that heroin "dethrones their moral responsibility." Another physician testified that some types of individuals will have their mental equipment "permanently injured by the use of heroin, and those are the ones who will go out and commit crimes."[9] Similar beliefs are reflected in the introductory message in the 1937 film *Reefer Madness,* which referred to marijuana as "The Real Public Enemy Number One!" and described its "soul-destroying" effects as follows:

> emotional disturbances, the total inability to direct thought, the loss of all power to resist physical emotions, leading finally to acts of shocking violence . . . ending often in incurable insanity.

Such verbal excesses seem quaint and comical these days, but the underlying belief that drug use changes people into criminals still can be detected in much current political rhetoric. You should remember from chapter 1 that longitudinal research on children and adolescents has led to the conclusion that indicators of criminal or antisocial behavior usually occur before the first use of an illicit drug. Several studies have concluded that criminal activity typically precedes drug use and "suggests that the relationship between drugs and crime is developmental rather than causal."[10]

A second sense in which drug use might *cause* criminal behavior is when the person is *under the influence* of the drug. Do the acute effects of a drug make a person *temporarily* more likely to engage in criminal behavior? There is little good evidence for this with most illicit sub-

stances. In most individuals, marijuana produces a state more akin to lethargy than to crazed violence (see chapter 17), and heroin tends to make its users more passive and perhaps sexually impotent (see chapter 15). Stimulants such as amphetamine and cocaine can make people paranoid and "jumpy," and this can indeed contribute to violent behavior in some cases (see chapter 7). The hallucinogen PCP causes disorientation and also blocks pain, so that users are sometimes hard to restrain (see chapter 16). This has led to a considerable amount of folklore about the dangerousness of PCP users, although actual documented cases of excessive violence are either rare or nonexistent.

If there is some question as to whether the direct influence of illicit drugs produces a person more likely to engage in criminal or violent behavior, there has been less doubt about one commonly used substance: alcohol. A large number of studies indicate that alcohol is clearly linked with violent crime. In many assaults and sexual assaults, alcohol is present in both assailant and victim. You might not know that most homicides are among people who know each other—and alcohol use is associated with over three-fifths of all murders. Of all reported assaults, 40 percent involve alcohol, as do one-third of forcible rape and child-molestation cases.[11] A study of jail inmates found that almost half of those committing violent crimes reported being under the influence of alcohol or a combination of alcohol and other drugs at the time of the offense, whereas fewer than 10 percent reported being under the influence of only drugs other than alcohol.[12] However, the relationship between drinking and violence is complex, and it has recently been argued that alcohol might have been overestimated as a direct cause of violence.[13]

There is a third sense in which drug use may be said to cause crime, and that refers to *crimes carried out for the purpose of obtaining money* to purchase illicit drugs. It has long been noted that heroin addicts constitute a larger proportion of those arrested for robbery than of the general population. A survey of almost 400,000 jail inmates found that almost one-third of all burglaries and robberies were committed to obtain money for drugs, as was almost one-fourth of all fraud. It is interesting that only about one-fifth of all drug-trafficking offenses were reported to be for the purpose of obtaining money to buy drugs.[14]

Although most addicts are criminals first and addicts second, a 1976 survey of heroin addicts found that most reported an increase in the amount of crime they committed, and many started committing new types of crime, after they became addicts. A 1981 report suggests just how much criminal activity increases during periods of addiction. When addicts were not dependent on heroin, their crime rate was 84 percent lower than when they were regularly using the drug.[15] Reducing heroin addiction will certainly result in lower crime rates.

In 1987 the U.S. Justice Department established the Drug Use Forecasting program, which studies urine samples of persons arrested for serious offenses in twenty-four major U.S. cities. The interviewers try to limit the number of arrestees charged with drug sale or possession in the sample, and this undersampling results in fewer than 20 percent of those studied being arrested for drug charges. All interviews and tests are voluntary and anonymous; about 90 percent of the arrestees who are asked agree to an interview, and about 80 percent of those agree to provide urine specimens. In 1994, between 48 and 79 percent of the male arrestees in the various cities tested positive for some illicit drug figure 2.1).[16] Evidence of cocaine use was found in 19 to 68 percent of the men, depending on the city. Marijuana was the next most commonly detected illicit drug in the overall sample. This level of drug use among those arrested for nondrug crimes is quite high; how can we account for it? First, those who adopt a deviant lifestyle might engage in both crime and drug use. Second, because most of these arrests were

for crimes in which profit was the motive, the arrestees might have been burglarizing a house or stealing a car to get money to purchase drugs.

It would be remiss not to point out that the commission of crimes to obtain money for expensive illicit drugs is due, not primarily to a pharmacological effect of the drug, but to the artificially high cost of the drugs, which results from drug controls and enforcement. Both heroin and cocaine are inexpensive substances when obtained legally from a licensed manufacturer, and it has been estimated many times that if heroin were freely available it would cost no more to be a regular heroin user than to be a regular drinker of alcohol. It is the black-market cost of these substances, combined with their addicting nature, that makes the use of cocaine or heroin consume so much money.

There is a fourth and final sense in which drug use causes crime, and that is that *illicit drug*

Are Current Laws Fair?

There are things that people do all the time that are potentially dangerous for themselves and potentially messy and expensive for others. Driving faster than the speed limit, driving without a seat belt, and riding a motorcycle without a helmet are examples, some of which may not be illegal where you live. In what ways are these behaviors similar to a person "snorting" cocaine or injecting heroin into his or her veins? In what ways are they different? Do you feel that the laws as they currently exist in your area are appropriate and fair in dealing with these behaviors? If it were up to you, would you outlaw some things that are now legal, legalize some things that are now controlled, or some of each?

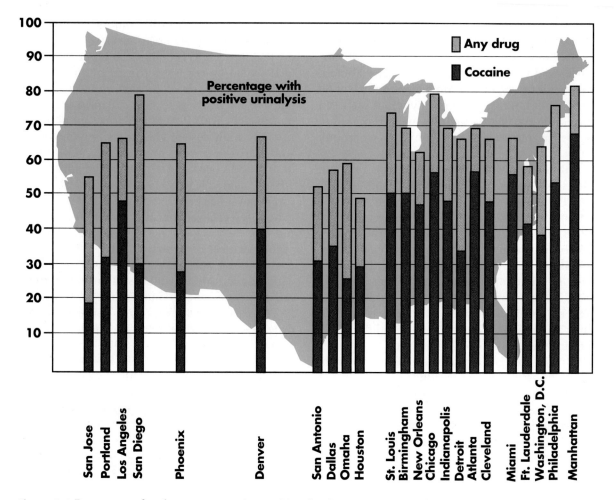

Figure 2.1 Percentage of male arrestees testing positive for drug use, January through December 1995

use is a crime. At first that may seem trivial, but there are two senses in which it is not. First, we are now making over one million arrests for drug-law violations each year, and more than half of all federal prisoners were convicted on drug charges.[17] Thus drug-law violations are one of the major types of crime in the United States. Second, it is likely that the relationship between drug use and other forms of deviant behavior is strengthened by the fact that drug use is a crime. A person willing to commit one type of

crime might be more willing than the average person to commit another type of crime. Some of the people who are actively trying to impress others by living dangerously and committing criminal acts might be drawn to illicit drug use as an obvious way to demonstrate their alienation from society. To better understand this relationship, imagine what might happen if the use of marijuana were legalized. Presumably, a greater number of otherwise law-abiding citizens might try using the drug, thus reducing the correlation between marijuana use and other forms of criminal activity. The concern over possibly increased drug use is, of course, one major argument in favor of maintaining legal controls on the illicit drugs.

WHY WE TRY TO REGULATE DRUGS

We can see that there are reasonable concerns about the potential toxicity and habit-forming nature of some drugs, and even the criminality of some drug users. That does not mean that our current set of laws represents a rationally devised plan to counteract the most realistic of these concerns in the most effective manner. In point of fact, most legislation is passed in an atmosphere of emotionality, in response to some specific set of concerns. Often the problems have been there for a long time, but public attention and concern have been recently aroused and Congress must respond. Sometimes members of Congress or government officials play a major role in calling public attention to the problem for which they offer the solution: a new law, more restrictions, and a bigger budget for some agency. This is what is known in political circles as "starting a prairie fire." As we will see in chapter 4, often the prairie fires include a lot of emotion-arousing rhetoric that borders on the irrational, and sometimes the results of the prairie fire and the ensuing legislation include some unexpected and undesirable outcomes.

SUMMARY

▲ American society has changed from being one that tolerated a wide variety of individual drug use to being one that attempts strict control over some types of drugs. This has occurred in response to social concerns about drug toxicity, addiction potential, and drug-related crime and violence.

▲ Toxicity can refer either to physiological poisoning or to dangerous disruption of behavior. Also, we may distinguish acute toxicity, resulting from the presence of too much of a drug, from chronic toxicity, which results from long-term exposure to a drug.

▲ Addiction means different things to different people in different contexts. Although addiction does not depend solely on the drug itself, the use of some drugs is more likely to result in addiction than the use of other drugs.

▲ The idea that narcotic drugs or marijuana can produce violent criminality in their users is an old and largely discredited idea. Narcotic addicts seem to engage in crimes mainly to obtain money, not because they are made more criminal by the drugs they take. One drug that is widely accepted as contributing to crimes and violence is alcohol.

▲ We can see that the laws that have been developed to control drug use have a legitimate social purpose, which is to protect the society from the dangers caused by some types of drug use. Whether these dangers have always been viewed rationally, and whether the laws have had their intended results, can be better judged after we have learned more about the drugs and the history of their regulation.

REVIEW QUESTIONS

1. The French term *laissez-faire* is used to describe what type of relationship between a government and its people?
2. What three major concerns about drugs led to the initial passage of laws controlling their availability?
3. Long-term, heavy drinking can lead to permanent impairment of memory. What type of toxicity would this be (acute or chronic; physiological or behavioral)?
4. What two kinds of data are recorded by the DAWN system?

5. What drug other than alcohol is mentioned most often in both parts of the DAWN system?
6. Why has AIDS been of particular concern regarding users of illicit drugs?
7. What drugs and methods of using them are considered to have very high dependence potential?
8. What is the apparent dependence potential of hallucinogenic drugs such as LSD and mescaline?
9. What are four ways in which drug use might theoretically cause crime?
10. About how many arrests are made each year in the United States for violations of drug laws?

Web Watch: Related Internet Sites on Toxicity and Crime

DAWN reports: http://www.samhsa.gov/oas/dawn/dwnfiles.htm

Drugs and crime: http://ncjrs.org/drgshome.htm

And don't forget our own *Drugs, Society, and Human Behavior* site with updated information and links to these and other sites of interest: http://www.uwyo.edu/A&S/psyc/dshb.htm

REFERENCES

1. Dennis, RJ: The economics of legalizing drugs, *The Atlantic*, Nov 1990.
2. *Preliminary estimates from the Drug Abuse Warning Network*, SAMHSA Advance Report Number 17, US Department of Health and Human Services, August 1996.
3. Bozarth MA, Wise RA: Toxicity associated with long-term intravenous heroin and cocaine self-administration in the rat, *JAMA* 254:81–83, 1985.
4. Des Jarlais, DC and others: Maintaining a low HIV seroprevalence in populations of injecting drug users. *JAMA* 274:1226–1231, 1995.
5. Gleghorn A and others: Acquisition and use of needles and syringes by injecting drug users in Baltimore, Maryland, *JAIDS*, 10:97–103, 1995.
6. Friedman SR and others: Risk factors for human immunodeficiency virus seroconversion among out-of-treatment drug injectors in high and low seroprevalence cities, *American Journal of Epidemiology* 142:864–874, 1995.
7. Gable RS: Toward a comparative overview of dependence potential and acute toxicity of psychoactive substances used nonmedically, *American Journal of Drug and Alcohol Abuse*, 19:263–281, 1993.
8. Morganthau T and others: The drug gangs, *Newsweek* p 20–27, Mar 28, 1988.
9. Prohibiting the importation of opium for the manufacture of heroin, Hearing before the Committee on Ways and Means, House of Representatives, *Congressional Record*, Apr 3, 1924.
10. Bureau of Justice Statistics: *Drugs, crime, and the justice system*. Washington, DC, 1992, US Department of Justice.
11. *Alcohol and health: Fifth special report to the US Congress*, DHHS Pub No (ADM) 84-1291, Washington, DC, 1984, US Government Printing Office.
12. *Drugs and Crime Data Center: Fact sheet: drug data summary*, Bureau of Justice Statistics, Nov 1991, US Department of Justice.
13. *Alcohol and health: Seventh special report to the US Congress*, DHHS Publication No. (ADM) 90-1656, Washington, DC, 1990, US Government Printing Office.
14. Rouse, BA (editor): *Substance abuse and mental health statistics sourcebook*, DHHS Publication No. (SMA) 95-3064, Washington, DC, Superintendent of Documents, US Government Printing Office, 1995.
15. Ball JC and others: cited in Study stresses link between heroin dependence and incidence of crime, *New York Times* p 22, Mar 22, 1981.
16. National Institute of Justice: *Drug use forecasting 1994 annual report*, Washington DC, 1995, US Department of Justice.
17. The White House Office of National Drug Control Policy: *National drug control strategy*, Washington, DC, 1994.
18. The White House Office of National Drug Control Policy: *National drug control strategy*, Washington, DC, 1989.

3

C H A P T E R

Addictions: Theory and Treatment

KEY TERMS	OBJECTIVES

After reading this chapter, you should be able to:

tolerance
withdrawal syndrome
physical dependence
psychological dependence
catheters
reinforcement
Alcoholics Anonymous
biopsychosicial
DSM-IV
stages of change
abstinence
controlled drinking
detoxification

- Describe three basic processes relating to addiction.
- Explain how the predominant view of addiction has changed during the past thirty years.
- State the contributions and limits of biochemical, personality, family, and disease models of addiction.
- Explain the diagnostic distinction between substance dependence and substance-abuse disorders.
- List the major characteristics of therapeutic community,

medication-assisted, outpatient drug-free, and chemical dependency programs, and explain the differences between these approaches.
- Recognize the twelve steps of Alcoholics Anonymous and explain their relationship to NA and CA.
- Describe some of the cost factors that have been used to determine that addiction treatment is in fact cost-effective.

Thirty years ago, the term *addict* had a pretty narrow meaning for most people: someone who used heroin several times daily and who would suffer terrible withdrawal symptoms if he was late getting his "fix." Now it seems that addiction is everywhere: not only are alcoholics and cigarette smokers referred to as addicts, but we also hear about sex addicts, food addicts, gambling addicts, addictive relationships, and even addictive forms of politics.[1] What do we mean by addiction, and how have models of addiction become important for describing such a wide variety of human conduct?

DRUG ADDICTION

We begin by attempting to define drug addiction, both because this book is primarily about drugs, and also because that's where our current concepts of addiction in general were formed. A leading addiction researcher has offered the following definition of drug addiction: "a behavioral pattern of drug use, characterized by overwhelming involvement with the use of a drug (compulsive use), the securing of its supply, and a high tendency to relapse after withdrawal.[2]

It is important to distinguish the defining component of addictive drug use (overwhelming involvement) from the proposed causes of that behavior. As we proceed, we will find that some people believe addiction to be a function of the drugs themselves and how they affect the user, whereas others believe the key to addiction lies in the individual's physiology and how the drug influences biological processes. Some believe that addiction grows out of early positive experiences with a drug, others believe that addiction is found in the personality of the user, and others find the key to addiction in social structures such as the family, relationships with significant others, or even society itself. Finally, there are those for whom addiction reflects spiritual dysfunction: a mistaken seeking for understanding, peace, or bliss through drugs. We believe that there is value in understanding each of these perspectives. However, the definition of addiction should not depend on its proposed causes, but should be in terms of the behavior that causes us to call it addiction. Once the behavior is defined, we can explore possible causes of that behavior.

Three Basic Processes

There are three basic processes related to addiction that have been important in the history of drug addiction research. Defining these three concepts will help focus our discussion of drug addiction and will also be useful in discussing each drug in more detail in later chapters.

Tolerance

Tolerance refers to a phenomenon seen with many drugs, in which repeated exposure to the same dose of the drug results in a lesser effect. There are many ways this diminished effect can occur, and some examples are given in chapter 6. For now, it is enough for us to think of the body as developing ways to compensate for the chemical imbalance caused by introducing a

drug into the system. As the individual experiences less and less of the desired effect, it is often possible to overcome the tolerance by increasing the dose of the drug. Because individuals often develop a tolerance up to the level at which dangerous effects of these drugs can occur, some regular drug users might eventually build up to taking much more of the drug than it would take to kill a nontolerant individual. Tolerance has been proposed as a key component in some definitions of addiction or dependence.

Physical dependence

Physical dependence is defined by the occurrence of a **withdrawal syndrome**. Suppose a person has begun to take a drug and a tolerance has developed. The person increases the amount of drug taken and continues to take these higher doses so regularly that the body is continuously exposed to the drug for days or weeks. With some drugs, when the person stops taking them abruptly, a set of symptoms begin to appear as the drug level in the system drops. For example, as the level of heroin drops in a heroin addict, that person's nose might run and he or she might begin to experience chills and fever, diarrhea, and other symptoms. When we have a drug that produces a consistent set of these symptoms in different individuals, we refer to the collection of symptoms as a withdrawal syndrome. These withdrawal syndromes vary from one class of drugs to another. Our model for why withdrawal symptoms appear is that the drug initially disrupts the body's normal physiological balances. These imbalances are detected by the nervous system, and over a period of repeated drug use the body's normal regulatory mechanisms compensate for the presence of the drug. When the drug is suddenly removed, these compensating mechanisms now produce an imbalance. You can see that tolerance typically precedes physical dependence. To continue with the heroin example, when it is first used it slows intestinal movement and produces consti-pation. After several days of constant heroin use, other mechanisms in the body counteract this effect and get the intestines moving again (tolerance). If the heroin use is suddenly stopped, the compensating mechanisms produce too much intestinal motility. Diarrhea is one of the most reliable and dramatic heroin with-drawal symptoms.

Because of the presumed involvement of these compensating mechanisms, the presence of a withdrawal syndrome is said to reflect **physical** (or physiological) **dependence** on the drug. In other words, the individual has come to depend on the presence of some amount of that drug to function normally; removing the drug leads to an imbalance, which is slowly corrected over a period of a few days.

Reinforcement

The term *reinforcement* is used in psychology to describe a process: a behavioral act is fol-lowed by some consequence, resulting in an in-creased tendency to repeat that behavioral act. The consequence may be described as plea-surable or as a "reward" in some cases (e.g., pro-viding a tasty piece of food to someone who has not eaten for a while). In other cases the conse-quence may be described in terms of escape from pain or discomfort. The behavior itself is said to be strengthened, or *reinforced,* by its con-sequences. A major contribution of animal experiments performed by behavioral pharma-cologists has been to point out that the adminis-tration of certain drugs can reinforce the be-haviors that led to the drug's administration. Laboratory rats and monkeys have been trained to press levers when the only consequence of lever pressing is a small intravenous injection of heroin, cocaine, or some other drug. Because some drugs and not others are capable of serving this function, it is possible to refer to some drugs as having "reinforcing properties" and to note that there is a general correlation be-

tween those drugs and the ones to which people can become addicted.

Changing Views of Drug Addiction

Until the twentieth century, the most com-mon view of alcoholism or dependence on opi-ates was probably that the addicted individuals were weak-willed, lazy, or immoral. Then med-ical and scientific studies began to be made of alcoholics, and later of narcotic addicts. It seemed as if something more powerful than mere self-indulgence was at work, and the pre-dominant view began to be that addiction is a drug-induced illness.

Early medical models

If heroin addiction is induced by heroin, or alcoholism by alcohol, then why do some people become addicts and others not? An early guess was simply that some people, for whatever reasons, were exposed to large amounts of the substance for a long time. This could happen through medical treatment or self-indulgence. The most obvious changes resulting from long exposure to large doses are the withdrawal symptoms that occur when the drug is stopped. Both alcohol and the narcotics can produce rather dramatic withdrawal syndromes. Thus addiction came to be defined by the presence of

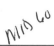

tolerance: reduced effect of a drug after repeated use.

withdrawal syndrome: a consistent set of symptoms that appears after discontinuing use of a drug.

physical dependence: drug dependence defined by the presence of a withdrawal syndrome, im-plying that the body has become adapted to the drug's presence.

physical dependence (a withdrawal syndrome), and enlightened medically oriented researchers went looking for treatments based on reducing or eliminating withdrawal symptoms. According to the most narrow interpretation of this model, the medical addiction itself was cured when the person had successfully completed withdrawal and the symptoms disappeared, although of course there was concern that people often reacquired the addiction.

Pharmacologists and medical authorities continued into the 1970s to define "true" addiction as occurring only when physical dependence was seen. Based on this view, public policy decisions, medical treatment, and individual drug-use decisions could be influenced by the question, "Is this an addicting drug?" If some drugs produce addiction and others do not, then legal restrictions on addicting drugs, care in the medical use of those drugs, and teaching people to avoid the recreational use of addicting drugs would be appropriate. The determination of whether a drug is or is not "addicting" was therefore crucial.

It became a public issue in the 1960s that some drugs, particularly marijuana and amphetamine, were not considered to have well-defined, dramatic, physical withdrawal syndromes. The growing group of interested scientists began to refer to drugs like marijuana, amphetamines, and cocaine as producing **psychological dependence**, whereas heroin produced a "true" addiction, which includes physical dependence. The idea seemed to be that psychological dependence was merely mental, whereas with physical dependence actual bodily processes were involved, subject to physiological and biochemical analysis and possibly to improved medical treatments for addiction. This was the view held by most drug-abuse experts in the 1960s.

Positive reinforcement model

At about this time a remarkable series of experiments began to appear in the scientific literature—experiments in which laboratory monkeys and rats were given intravenous **catheters** connected to motorized syringes and controlling equipment so that pressing a lever would produce a single brief injection of morphine, a narcotic very similar to heroin. In the initial experiments, monkeys were exposed for several days to large doses of morphine, allowed to experience the initial stages of withdrawal, and then connected to the apparatus to see if they would learn to press the lever, thereby avoiding the withdrawal symptoms. As you can see, these experiments were based on the predominant view of addiction as being driven by physical dependence. The monkeys did learn to press the levers. Later experiments sought to determine whether monkeys would make themselves "addicted," and so the initial phase of drug exposure was dropped. Indeed, the monkeys began to press the lever to give themselves morphine, and if doses were large enough and constant access was allowed, the monkeys would eventually display withdrawal symptoms when no longer allowed access to morphine. Thus the monkeys had made "true" drug addicts of themselves.

This research next began to draw on the experience gained from many years of research with animals pressing levers to obtain food. It is not necessary to provide food for every lever press, because once animals have learned to press the lever they will continue if food is given for every other press, then for every third press, then every fifth press, every tenth, and so on. Some scientists began to ask how hard monkeys or rats would "work" to obtain their drug injections, and how that compared with how hard they would work for food. With appropriate scheduling and training, it was possible to show that monkeys would press the lever hundreds of times for each drug injection. When food had been used in such experiments, the amount of food delivered each time was found to be important. A rat or monkey might press only 10 times for a small amount of food, but be willing to press 30 times for a greater amount. Therefore the drug addiction researchers began to vary the amount of morphine given with each delivery, eventually finding that a great deal of lever pressing could be maintained with fairly small injections of drug. As these scientists began to publish their results and as more experiments like this were done, they pointed out some interesting facts. First, monkeys would begin pressing and maintain pressing without first being made physically dependent. Second, monkeys who had given themselves only fairly small doses and who had never experienced withdrawal symptoms could be trained to work very hard for their morphine. In fact, a history of physical dependence and withdrawal didn't seem to have much influence on response rates in the long run. Clearly, the small drug injections themselves were working as "positive reinforcers" of the lever-pressing behavior, just as food can be a positive reinforcer to a hungry rat or monkey. Thus the idea spread that drugs can act as reinforcers of behavior and that this might be the basis of what had been called psychological dependence.[3] Drugs like amphetamines and cocaine could easily be used as reinforcers in these experiments, and they were known to produce strong psychological dependence in humans.

Which is more important, physical dependence or reinforcement?

These results seemed to indicate that the immediate reinforcing effect of a drug might be more important than the development of physical dependence in narcotic addiction, and this led people to examine the lives of heroin addicts from a different perspective. Stories were told of addicts who occasionally stopped taking heroin, voluntarily going through withdrawal so as to reduce their tolerance level and get back to the lower doses of drug they could more easily afford. When we examine the total daily heroin intake of many current addicts, we see that they do not need a large amount and that the agonies

of withdrawal they experience are probably more like a prolonged case of intestinal flu. We have known for a long time that heroin addicts who have already gone through withdrawal in treatment programs or in jail have a high probability of returning to active heroin use. In other words, if all we had to worry about was addicts avoiding withdrawal symptoms, the problem would be much smaller than it actually is.

Reinforcement is increasingly accepted as the real driving force behind drug addiction, and tolerance and physical dependence are now seen as related phenomena that sometimes occur but probably are not critical to the development of addictive patterns of drug-using behavior.

THE BROAD VIEWS OF ADDICTIONS

If we define drug addiction not in terms of withdrawal but in more behavioral or psychological terms, as an overwhelming involvement with getting and using the drug, then might this model also be used to describe other kinds of behavior? What about a man who visits prostitutes several times a day, or someone who eats large amounts of food throughout the day, or someone who places bets on every football and

---

psychological dependence: behavioral dependence; indicated by high rate of drug use, craving for the drug, and a tendency to relapse after stopping use.

catheters: (*cath* a ters) plastic or other tubing implanted into the body.

reinforcement: a procedure in which a behavioral event is followed by a consequent event such that the behavior is then more likely to be repeated. The behavior of taking a drug may be reinforced by the effect of the drug.

basketball game, every horse race or automobile race, and who spends hours each day planning these bets and finding money to bet again? Shouldn't these also be considered addictions? Do the experiences of overeating, gambling, sex, and drugs have something in common, some common change in physiology or brain chemistry, some common personality trait that might lead to any or many of these addictions? Are all of these filling some unmet social or spiritual need? More and more, addiction researchers are looking for these common threads and discussing "the addictions" as a varied set of behavioral manifestations of a common addictive process or disorder.

Is Addiction Caused by the Substance?

Especially with chemical dependence, many people speak as though the substance itself is the cause of the addiction. Certainly some drugs are more likely than others to result in addiction. For example, it is widely believed that heroin and crack cocaine are both extremely addicting, with most users becoming slaves to the habit. In contrast, most users of marijuana report occasional use and little difficulty in deciding when to use it and when not to. Self-administration studies with animals support this view: rats and monkeys readily learn to self-inject either heroin or cocaine, but no one has yet demonstrated reliable self-administration of marijuana in animal models. May we then describe some drugs as "addicting," whereas others are not? We have already seen that this perspective was common in an earlier era, and it played a major role in the establishment of laws intended to limit access to those addicting drugs. Certainly alcohol prohibition in the 1920s was based on the view that alcohol itself was the main culprit in many of society's problems.

The problem is that, although some drugs might be more likely than others to result in addiction, there is no clear distinction between substances that are addicting and those that are

not. What about alcohol, perhaps the most common cause of serious chemical dependence? Most of its users avoid addiction, yet for perhaps one-tenth of drinkers alcohol use becomes an overwhelming habit. Contrary to popular opinion, many users of either heroin or crack cocaine use the drug only a few times a week or less, and not every user becomes overwhelmingly involved. And contrary to the beliefs of some, there are quite a few marijuana users who become addicted, try to stop and cannot, and voluntarily seek treatment for their addiction. Any of these drugs can be "addicting" for some people, and some people can use any of them without becoming addicted. Thus the drug itself cannot be the entire cause of addiction.

When we extend the concept of addiction to other activities such as gambling, sex, or overeating, it seems harder to place the entire blame on the activity, again because many people do not exhibit addictive patterns of such behaviors. Some activities might be more addictive than others—few people become addicted to filling out income-tax forms, whereas a higher proportion of all those who gamble become overwhelmingly involved. Still, it is wrong to conclude that any activity is by its nature always "addicting."

When a chemical is seen as causing the dependence, there is a tendency to give that substance a personality and to ascribe motives to it. When we listen, either to a practicing addict's loving description of his interaction with the drug or to a recovering addict describe her struggle against the drug's attempts to destroy her, the drug seems to take on almost human characteristics. We all realize that is going too far, yet the analogy is so powerful that it pervades our thinking. Alcoholics Anonymous (AA) members often describe alcohol as being "cunning, baffling, and powerful," and admit that they are powerless against such a foe. And those seeking prohibition of alcohol, cocaine, marijuana, heroin, and other drugs have over the years tended to "demonize" those substances, making them into powerful forces of evil. The concept of a "war on drugs" reflects in part such a perspective—that some drugs are evil and war must be waged against the substances themselves.

Is Addiction Biological?

There has been increasing interest in recent years in the possibility that all addictive behaviors might have some common physiological or biochemical action in the brain. For example, many theorists have recently focused on dopamine, one of the brain's important neurotransmitters, which some believe to play a large role in the process of positive reinforcement. The idea is that any drug use or other activity that has pleasurable or rewarding properties releases dopamine in a particular part of the brain. This idea is discussed more fully in chapter 5. Although this theory has been widely tested in animal models and there is much evidence that is consistent with it, there is also considerable evidence that this model is too simple and that other neurotransmitters and other brain regions are also important. A great deal of attention has been given to recent reports from various brain-scanning experiments done on cocaine users, showing that cocaine activates many areas that are widely separated in the brain, including some that are known to be dopamine-rich areas and some that are not.[4] Although these studies show some of the physiological *consequences* produced by cocaine or by even thinking about cocaine, they have not yet been useful in examining the possible biological *causes* of addiction. One important question that remains is whether the brains of people who have used cocaine and not become addicted to it show different responses compared to the brains of cocaine addicts. Ultimately, the strongest demonstration of the power of such techniques would be if it were possible to know, based on looking at a brain scan, whether or not

a person had become an addict or was on the way to becoming an addict. Many previous biological theories of addiction have failed this test: so far no genetic physiological, or biochemical marker has been found that strongly predicts alcoholism or any other addiction.

Is There an Addictive Personality?

Perhaps the explanation for why some people become addicts and others do not lies in their personality—that complex set of attributes and attitudes that develops over time, partly as a result of particular experiences. Is there some common personality factor that is seen in addicts and not in others? This type of research has been conducted for decades, and its value is still controversial.[5] The problem with many studies on practicing or recovering addicts is that it is not possible to know whether the alcohol or other drug use has changed the person's personality. In retrospective studies of personality tests given to college students who later became alcoholics, the prealcoholic students showed what would be considered a "normal" overall personality profile. However, they also tended to be more independent, nonconformist, gregarious, and impulsive. Please note the word *tended.* In all of these studies, although there are statistical differences between the alcoholic and nonalcoholic groups, there is considerable overlap. Once again, personality factors might make some contribution, but they are not the sole cause of alcoholism, or of any other addictive behavior.

Is Addiction a Family Disorder?

Although few scientific studies have been done, examination of the lives of individual addicts, again primarily alcoholics, reveals some typical patterns of family adaptation to the addiction. A common example in a home with an alcoholic father is that the mother enables this behavior, by calling her husband's boss to say

Alcoholism affects the children in the family in various ways.

he is ill, or by making excuses to family and friends for failures to appear at dinners or parties, and generally by caring for her incapacitated husband. The children might also compensate in various ways, and all conspire to keep the family secret. Thus it is said that alcoholism often exists within a dysfunctional family—the functions of individual members adjust to the needs created by the presence of alcoholism. This new arrangement can make it difficult for the alcoholic alone to change his or her behavior, because doing so would disrupt the family system. Some people suspect that certain family structures might actually enhance the likelihood of alcoholism developing. For example, the "codependent" needs of other family members to take care of someone who is dependent on them might facilitate drunkenness.

Much has been written about the effects on children who grow up in an "alcoholic family,"

and there is some indication that even as adults these individuals might tend to exhibit certain personality characteristics. The "adult children of alcoholics" are then perhaps more likely to become involved in dysfunctional relationships that increase the likelihood of alcoholism either in themselves or in another family member. Again, the evidence indicates that such influences are statistical tendencies and are not all-powerful. It is perhaps unfortunate that some people with alcoholic parents have adopted the role of "adult children" and try to explain their entire personalities and all their difficulties in terms of that status.

Is Addiction a Disease?

The most important reason for adopting a disease model for addiction is based on the experiences of the founders of **Alcoholics Anony-**

mous (AA) and is discussed in chapter 11. Briefly, psychiatrists had commonly assumed that alcoholism was secondary to some other disorder, such as neurosis or depression, and often attempted to treat the presumed underlying disorder while encouraging the drinker to try to "cut down." The founders of AA believed that alcoholism itself was the primary problem and needed to be recognized as such and treated directly. This is the reason for the continued insistence that alcoholism is a disease—that it is often the primary disturbance and deserves to stand in its own right as a recognized disorder requiring treatment.

On the other hand, Peele[6] and others have argued that alcoholism does not have many of the characteristics of some classic medical diseases like tuberculosis or syphilis: We can't use an X ray or blood test to reveal the underlying cause, and we don't have a way to treat the underlying cause and cure the symptoms—we don't really know that there is an underlying cause, because all we have are the "symptoms" of excessive involvement. Furthermore, if addiction itself is a disease, then gambling, excessive sexual involvement, and overeating will also be seen as diseases, and the addicts as victims of the disease. This in turn weakens our normal understanding of the concept of disease. Marlatt and Fromme[7] have pointed out that the disease model is perhaps best seen as an analogy—addictions are *like* diseases in many ways, but that is different from insisting that they *are* a disease. If we adopt a **biopsychosocial** perspective, the addiction might be related to dysfunctions of biology, personality, social interactions, or combinations thereof. If by a disease model we imply that there is a single unified cause for all addictions, then such a model would be too simple. If our disease model would include such complex medical disorders as high blood pressure, which we know to be influenced by interactions among genetics, diet, exercise level, and other medical conditions, then it might be a more appropriate analogy.

ASSESSMENT OF ADDICTIVE DISORDERS

Diagnosis

How do we know whether someone's drinking or marijuana smoking or coffee consumption indicates an addiction to that substance? The notion of "overwhelming involvement" is somewhat subjective—do we mean that the person does almost nothing else but get and use the drug and deal with the drug's effects, or that it is the predominant thing the person does, or just that the person does it much more than the "average" user of that substance? How do we distinguish the wine connoisseur, who might read and talk about wines, spend time and lots of money shopping for them, and taste wines frequently, from the alcoholic who becomes intoxicated on a daily basis? Let us begin by examining the closest thing to an "official" method of diagnosis, which comes from the American Psychiatric Association's *Diagnostic and Statistical Manual,* fourth edition *(DSM-IV).*[8] Because of the controversy surrounding the definition of such terms as *alcoholism* or *addiction,* this manual describes "substance dependence," which includes tolerance and physical dependence among its criteria, and "substance abuse," which is based principally on

---

Alcoholics Anonymous: a worldwide organization of self-help groups based on helping each other to stop drinking.

biopsychosocial: a theory or perspective that relies on the interaction of biological, individual psychological, and social variables.

DSM-IV: the *Diagnostic and Statistical Manual* of the American Psychiatric Association, fourth edition. Lists criteria for diagnosing psychiatric disorders, including substance dependence and substance abuse.

DSM IV   Psychiatric Diagnosis of Substance Disorders

Diagnostic Criteria for Substance Dependence

A maladaptive pattern of substance use, leading to clinically significant impairment or distress, as manifested by three (or more) of the following, occurring at any time in the same 12-month period:

1. Tolerance, as defined by either of the following:
   a. A need for markedly increased amounts of the substance to achieve intoxication or desired effect
   b. Markedly diminished effect with continued use of the same amount of the substance
2. Withdrawal, as manifested by either of the following:
   a. The characteristic withdrawal syndrome for the substance
   b. The same (or a closely related) substance is taken to relieve or avoid withdrawal symptoms
3. The substance is often taken in larger amounts or over a longer period than was intended
4. There is a persistent desire or unsuccessful efforts to cut down or control substance use
5. A great deal of time is spent in activities necessary to obtain the substance
6. Important social, occupational, or recreational activities are given up or reduced because of substance use
7. The substance use is continued despite knowledge of having a persistent or recurrent physical or psychological problem that is likely to have been caused or exacerbated by the substance

Diagnostic Criteria for Substance Abuse

A. A maladaptive pattern of substance use leading to clinically significant impairment or distress, as manifested by one (or more) of the following, occurring within a 12-month period:
   1. Recurrent substance use resulting in failure to fulfill major role obligations at work, school, or home
   2. Recurrent substance use in situations in which it is physically hazardous
   3. Recurrent substance-related legal problems
   4. Continued substance use despite having persistent or recurrent social or interpersonal problems caused or exacerbated by the effects of the substance
B. The symptoms have never met the criteria for Substance Dependence for this class of substance

behavioral symptoms (see DSM-IV box). The same basic criteria are used, whether the substance is alcohol, heroin, cocaine, tobacco, a medication, or an inhaled solvent. The manual also describes criteria for substance intoxication and substance withdrawal.

ADDICTION TREATMENT

Every year, hundreds of thousands of Americans undergo treatment for alcoholism or addiction to other substances. The word *treatment* conjures up an image of hospitals, nurses, and physicians, but traditional medical approaches form only a small part of the overall treatment picture. As we shall see, the variety of treatment approaches reflects the variety of substance-abuse problems, as well as the variety of theories about substance abuse.

Deciding to Quit

For many years, the predominant theories on why people seek treatment for addiction were based on the anecdotal experiences of alcoholics. According to the conventional wisdom, most addicts use the defense mechanism of *denial,* and are obstinately unwilling to admit either their drinking or drug use is unusual or that it has serious consequences for themselves or others. In this context, only when the addict "hits bottom"—that is, suffers sufficient consequences that the reality of the problem finally sinks in, will he or she be ready to seek help. If family and friends want to cause this reality to sink in sooner, then they may attempt an *intervention*—a meeting between the addict and several significant friends or family members who describe in specific terms the problems caused by the person's drinking or drug use, and mutually and firmly insist that he or she recognize that the addiction is a problem that needs to be addressed. Certainly this approach has been used many times, and in many cases the result has been that the addict has sought treatment.

Studies on smokers who quit smoking without formal intervention led to descriptions of the cognitive stages they went through in making the decision to change their behavior. These **"stages of change"** have since been described more generally for alcohol and other drug use, as well as for other problem behaviors that might be addressed in psychotherapy.[9] In the *precontemplation* stage the individual does not recognize that a problem exists. In the *contemplation* stage the individual believes that a problem might exist and gives some consider-

ation to the possibility of changing his or her behavior. In the *preparation* stage the person decides to change and makes plans to do so. In the *action* stage, the individual takes active steps toward change, such as entering treatment. Finally, the *maintenance* stage involves activities intended to maintain the change. According to this model, in order to help someone to move from one stage to another you need to know where they are in the decision-making process.

Miller and his colleagues believe that aggressively confrontational approaches (intervention) may actually increase denial and resistance to change. They have developed a method called *Motivational Interviewing,* which employs a thorough assessment of the drinking or drug-using behavior and its consequences, and builds upon the client's own concerns about possible problems. The results of the assessment are shared with the client, who then interprets them in light of her or his own concerns. The motivational interviewer listens and helps the client focus on the concerns and the problem behavior, but does not directly tell the client what to do. Ideally, if the therapist knows which stage of change the client is in, the discussion can be guided appropriately to help move the client to the next stage. This approach is relatively new, and research on its effectiveness is now being carried out.[10]

Defining Treatment Goals

The particular theoretical view one has of alcoholism, narcotic addiction, or substance abuse in general influences not only the treatment ap-

---

stages of change: a model for decision making consisting of precontemplation, contemplation, preparation, action, maintenance.

proaches one is likely to take, but even the goals of treatment. For example, if one accepts the increasingly predominant view of alcoholism as a disease, which someone either "has" or does not have, and which has an inevitable progression to more and more drinking, then the only acceptable treatment goal is total **abstinence.** Other experts view alcoholism as representing one end of a continuum of drinking, with no clear dividing line. For some of these theorists, a possible beneficial outcome of treatment would be **controlled** social **drinking.** Likewise, if one views narcotic addiction as inherently evil, undermining the physical and mental health of its victims (a common view until fairly recently), then abstinence from narcotics would be the only acceptable goal. Americans seem to have come around to accepting addiction to the legal narcotic methadone as preferable to heroin addiction, so the goal has changed from eliminating narcotic use to eliminating heroin use. The case with cigarette smoking is similar; some programs have focused on cutting down on smoking or switching to cigarettes that are lower in tar and nicotine, whereas most programs aim for complete abstinence.

When we look for indicators of a treatment program's success, if we find that some people are still using, but using less, should we claim any benefit? Or should we assume, as some do, that any decreases will be temporary, and that, unless the person quits entirely, there has been no real improvement? The answer depends on your goals. Recently researchers have begun to estimate the cost savings resulting from increased employment and decreased crime after treatment, and comparing these savings with the cost of treatment itself, to develop a cost-benefit analysis of the effectiveness of treatment.

Treatment Stages

To understand how most treatment programs work, it is helpful to think in terms of three stages: *detoxification, active treatment,* and *aftercare.*

Detoxification

If the addict is heavily intoxicated and the last dose has been recent, as might occur in an emergency room admission, then the first concern is the possibility of death from drug overdose. Various measures such as clearing the stomach and giving diuretic drugs to increase urine flow may be used to lower the blood levels quickly. In the case of a narcotic overdose, narcotic antagonists may be used to block the drug's immediate effects (see chapter 15). The most common cause of drug overdose death is the depression of respiration (breathing), so it is important to monitor respiration rate, as well as blood pressure and heart rate. Breathing may need to be supported by some means of artificial respiration. Once the person's respiration has stabilized, it is time to deal with the possibility of withdrawal.

Remember that the early medical model of addiction was based on the development of physical dependence, and that withdrawal symptoms are the indicator of physical dependence. As the addict's body begins to metabolize the alcohol or heroin or other drug and the blood levels drop, withdrawal symptoms might occur. Withdrawal from many kinds of drugs can be exceedingly uncomfortable, but withdrawal from alcohol or depressants is in many cases life threatening. Therefore, it might be necessary to give the addict small doses of a depressant drug to limit the severity of the withdrawal.

The word **detoxification** refers to the process of removing the offending substance (the "toxin") from the body, either by allowing the body to clear the drug by normal metabolism and excretion (see chapter 6), or by more active methods, while preventing medical complications due to overdose or withdrawal. During this initial stage of treatment there might be other medical issues of immediate concern, such as malnutrition, liver dysfunction in an alcoholic, or hepatitis or AIDS in an intravenous drug user. Also, because the addict might be either intoxicated or preoccupied with withdrawal during this first stage, not much in the way of addiction treatment is usually accomplished.

Detoxification is not always necessary, because the client might have been using a type of drug or using small enough quantities that neither overdose nor physical dependence is of much concern. Some clients will have already stopped using the substance days or weeks before entering the treatment program, and thus those immediate concerns will have passed.

Active treatment

Early theories of addiction were based primarily on studying alcoholics and narcotic addicts, so it should come as no surprise that the history of treatment approaches also began with the treatment of alcoholism and narcotic addiction. Some of the specifics of treatment for those problems are described in chapters 11 and 15. In addition to various approaches to treating alcoholism and narcotic addiction, there has been quite a lot of recent research on the treatment of cigarette smokers (see chapter 12) and cocaine addicts (see chapter 7). We describe a variety of general treatment methods later in this chapter. The typical treatment program of the 1990s is not designed for a particular substance, but it treats a variety of types of substance addiction.

Aftercare (relapse prevention)

After the period of active treatment has ended, the long-term issue then becomes avoiding use of the substance on a day-to-day basis. Many treatment programs rely on self-help approaches such as AA and the similarly structured groups Cocaine Anonymous (CA) and Narcotics Anonymous (NA). The treatment program typically ensures that each client is referred to a local group for continued discussion of the recovery process. Some programs host

Methadone maintenance programs require the clients to show up each day to receive the methadone. This makes it easier to keep track of the clients and to counsel them on a regular basis.

such meetings themselves for clients who live in the area, and residential programs often invite their clients to return on a regular basis for weekend sessions.

Medically assisted treatment is, in a sense, aimed at relapse prevention from the start. Methadone maintenance, the most common type of substitution program for heroin addicts, may continue for months or years. Nicotine gum or patches are typically used only during treatment and are not given as long-term maintenance aids. Both narcotic antagonists and disulfiram (Antabuse) for alcoholics are often used for weeks or

---

abstinence: no alcohol or drug use at all.

controlled drinking: the idea that alcohol abusers may be able to drink under control.

detoxification: an initial phase of treatment during which the alcohol or other drug clears out of the system months, but indefinite maintenance for years is unusual with these approaches.

Treatment Approaches

Treatment programs may be divided into two major categories, *residential* and *outpatient*. This distinction is based on whether the client "checks in" to a hospital, group home, or other facility where he or she eats and sleeps during the treatment phase, or whether the client lives elsewhere and comes to the treatment facility only to attend counseling or group meetings or to obtain medication. A further basic distinction is whether the treatment will be *drug-free* or medication-assisted.

Residential treatment

Although it is an oversimplification, we can think of residential programs as having two historical roots. The first was medical hospitalization, which was a common early approach to alcoholism and narcotic addiction. This was partly due to the importance of detoxification, and partly because no other type of treatment facility was available. The second root was the *therapeutic community.*

Synanon. In 1958 Charles Dederick, a recovering alcoholic, felt that an organization similar to AA should be able to help narcotic addicts who wanted to be rehabilitated. From quite meager beginnings, Synanon grew by the 1970s into a large and apparently successful rehabilitation program with a developed philosophy. The Synanon concepts and practices are extensive, but a few points seem crucial. One is the belief that a narcotic addict is never cured (as AA believes an alcoholic is never cured). However, in Synanon that presumption led to the conclusion that the addict should continue forever to live in the Synanon center or, after being clearly stabilized as a former addict, move into nearby living quarters and stay affiliated and involved with the Synanon program. A second premise of this organization is that the addict must really want to be helped to discontinue drug use. To assure this motivation, there is an open-door policy: a member is free to leave at any time. An important practice is the use of former addicts as staff, with professionals being involved only for emergency medical service. Former addicts have several advantages. First, they have "been there," and second, they have beaten addiction. Thus new members have someone to relate to who understands their problems. Former addicts also have the advantage of knowing the tricks of the trade. As a result, they are able to recognize these tricks and demonstrate that they will not be effective at Synanon.

The residents at Synanon are kept busy working. Because of a belief that addicts have difficulty expressing emotions and identifying others' emotions, Dederick established the use of "seminars," or group encounters, several times a week. These encounters are often psychologically quite violent. The positive view of them is that they help addicts learn to stop using destructive guards to protect themselves and teach them to see themselves and others more clearly. A less charitable view is that these sessions serve to threaten or cajole the new members into accepting life at Synanon.

Early reports of Synanon's high rate of success should be examined carefully. The program was not research oriented, and Dederick himself pointed out that thousands had left the program.[11] Most of those returned to addiction, but no precise records were kept of the quitters. Thus the high rates of nonaddiction related only to those who stayed with the program.

As the use of various drugs increased in the 1960s, Synanon grew rapidly and began to include a much greater variety of members. For example, youngsters who were caught smoking marijuana were sometimes sent by their families to be rehabilitated at Synanon. Arrestees, whether for marijuana, LSD, amphetamine, or other drug use, sometimes volunteered to go to Synanon at the urging of their attorneys to avoid a jail sentence. The businesses Synanon started to provide employment for the residents became large and profitable, and Synanon became a major property holder. In the early 1980s, newspaper reports implying that Dederick had himself profited greatly from this "cult" led to threats and to violent encounters between Synanon members and outsiders who began to fear their numbers, wealth, and unanimity. Synanon is still around, but it is much smaller and less notorious than it was several years ago.

Other therapeutic communities. Other residential treatment communities were established in the 1960s, including Daytop Village, Phoenix House, Odyssey House, and Gateway Foundation. Because of the reported successes of such programs (although again such reports were not based on scientific evaluations), their number grew through the 1970s and 1980s. There are now hundreds of residential facilities across the country, serving narcotic addicts, alcoholics, and abusers of other substances. The one major difference between these therapeutic communities and Synanon is the goal of returning their clients to society. Most of their staff usually consists of recovering alcoholics or former addicts or abusers of other drugs, and there is still a focus on group encounter sessions and on keeping the clients busy. Relatively high success rates reported for these therapeutic communities are again based on those who stick with the program for the full course of the treatment, which typically lasts for several months.

The Drug Abuse Reporting Program (DARP), financed by the National Institute on Drug Abuse (NIDA), followed the success of a large number of clients admitted to drug-abuse treatment programs from the years 1969 to 1973. In a 1982 follow-up, over 4,000 of the original sample were contacted and interviewed about their drug use.[12] The data indicate that therapeutic communities do reduce drug use rel-

ative to untreated clients or to those who are detoxified and then released. For example, narcotic addicts who had been treated with either methadone maintenance or a therapeutic community approach had about a 20 percent chance of engaging in daily narcotic use during the last follow-up year, compared with about 30 percent for the untreated or detoxified groups. If clients had been treated for less than 90 days in the therapeutic community, their outcome measures were not more positive than for untreated groups, thus indicating that the length of treatment is an important variable for therapeutic communities. Other variables, such as treatment philosophy or types of services available in the program, did not influence the outcome.

Chemical dependency residential programs

Before the 1980s there was a variety of short-term (3 to 8 weeks) private residential programs, primarily for alcoholics, that combined some features of hospitalization with some features of therapeutic communities. They provided medical support for detoxification and relied for treatment mostly on the twelve-step model of AA (see FYI box). The majority of the staff in these programs consist of "chemical-dependency" counselors who typically are recovering alcoholics with limited formal training. Patients who could afford to go away to "dry out," using either personal finances or medical insurance, kept these facilities in operation. The Betty Ford Clinic, which attracts many wealthy celebrities as clients, is an example of such a facility, although many are less expensive. In the 1980s the increased use of medical insurance to pay for treatment of chemical dependence made this type of program a real growth industry. Besides the traditional residential alcohol programs, which expanded to accept cocaine and other drug users, new private psychiatric hospitals sprang up all over the country, with adolescent drug-abuse clients as their primary

The Twelve Steps of Alcoholics Anonymous

1. We admitted we were powerless over alcohol—that our lives had become unmanageable.
2. Came to believe that a Power greater than ourselves could restore us to sanity.
3. Made a decision to turn our will and our lives over to the care of God *as we understood Him.*
4. Made a searching and fearless moral inventory of ourselves.
5. Admitted to God, to ourselves, and to another human being the exact nature of our wrongs.
6. Were entirely ready to have God remove all these defects of character.
7. Humbly asked Him to remove our shortcomings.
8. Made a list of all persons we had harmed and became willing to make amends to them all.
9. Made direct amends to such people wherever possible, except when to do so would injure them or others.
10. Continued to take moral inventory and when we were wrong promptly admitted it.
11. Sought through prayer and meditation to improve our conscious contact with God *as we understood Him,* praying only for knowledge of His will for us and the power to carry that out.
12. Having had a spiritual awakening as the result of these steps, we tried to carry this message to alcoholics, and to practice these principles in all our affairs.

market.[13] The potential for high profits led to many abuses, including active recruitment of clients who might not have been addicted. Inevitably, insurance companies began to be much more restrictive, and large numbers of these private-pay programs went out of business in the 1990s.

Medication-assisted treatment

Medical approaches have been a small part of the overall treatment picture, but they produce beneficial effects for many addicts, and with the development of new drugs they might play an increasingly important role. Especially with outpatient treatment, drugs might be used to assist the client in maintaining abstinence. There are three basic approaches to using medications for addiction treatment: *antagonism,* or blockade, of the abused substance; *substitution,* or providing a drug that reduces the craving for the abused substance; and giving a drug that is *medically incompatible* with the abused substance. The only example of the last approach is a drug called *Antabuse,* which may be given to alcoholics (see chapter 11). Antabuse blocks the normal metabolism of alcohol, so if a client who is taking Antabuse drinks alcohol, he or she will become very ill. Both narcotic antagonists and the substitute narcotic methadone have been used with heroin addicts (see chapter 15), and nicotine gum or patches have been used to reduce cravings in those quitting the use of tobacco (see chapter 12). There is some evidence that the experimental drug buprenorphine can reduce cravings in both heroin and cocaine addicts, leading to hopes of developing a general-purpose drug for treating a variety of drug addictions.[14] Naltrexone, a narcotic antagonist, was shown to reduce craving in alcoholics and has been approved for such use (chapter 11). And attention has recently focused on a drug once considered a hallucinogen: *ibogaine* has been described by some as useful in reducing addictive cravings from a wide variety of drugs. Although animal research is exploring possible mechanisms of ibogaine action,[15] controlled human trials have not yet been approved.

Outpatient drug-free programs

Outpatient drug-free programs grew from two major sources. In the 1960s, because of a large number of panic reactions to LSD and other illicit drugs, "crisis clinics" were set up in most large communities. These clinics provided alternatives to the emergency room for a person who was frightened and needed someone to talk to until the drug wore off. These facilities ranged from telephone hot lines, to emergency-room associated clinics with medical support available, to "crash pads" where people could sleep off a drug's effects and receive some non-judgmental advice and counseling. Another major source of outpatient services has been the community mental health centers that have been established all over the nation since the early 1960s. Treatment choices of a third kind are affiliated with hospitals, correctional facilities, or large employers and might be available only to specific populations.

Because of the large number of outpatient drug-free programs and their ready availability, they constitute the most popular form of drug-abuse treatment, chosen by more than half of all clients. Services range from drop-in "rap" centers to more formal psychotherapy, group counseling, vocational counseling, or other professional services. In contrast to therapeutic communities, the counselors in these programs are more likely to be professional psychologists, social workers, or trained vocational rehabilitation counselors. Also in contrast to therapeutic communities, clients are less likely to be heroin addicts and more likely to be marijuana or multiple drug abusers. Perhaps because contacting one of these programs does not seem to be as big a step as entering a residential center, outpatient programs might be more likely to contact drug users earlier in their drug-abuse career, which might help their success rates.

Is Treatment Effective?

There is a widespread belief that addiction treatment is often ineffective. We've all heard of well-known athletes who have been in treatment programs and are later found to be using illegal drugs, and we might know an alcoholic who had treatment and began drinking again. What we know is that treatment doesn't work for every client every time, especially if our expectation is that one treatment exposure will eliminate the use of the substance for the rest of the person's life. A more meaningful question is whether treatment programs have any effect at all—and, if they do, are their effects worth their cost? A 1990 report from the Institute of Medicine[16] reviewed the evidence gathered to that point, which was mainly based on studies of heroin addicts. The report concluded: (1) Methadone maintenance pays for itself (in reduced crime and increased employment) during the time it is administered, and posttreatment effects are an economic bonus; (2) although therapeutic communities cost more than methadone maintenance, they result in better employment status after treatment; and (3) outpatient drug-free programs attract more clients without a criminal background and therefore do not reduce criminal activity as much as the other two approaches; they are inexpensive, however, and do produce a net benefit because of increased employment. A 1994 report by the California Department of Alcohol and Drug Programs[17] concluded that, on the average, seven dollars are saved for every dollar invested in treatment of alcohol and other drug abuse. Alcohol and other drug use was reduced by about two-fifths after treatment; treatment for crack, powdered cocaine, and methamphetamine use was just as effective as for alcohol; and criminal activity declined by about two-thirds after treatment. The report concluded that treatment is effective but doesn't eliminate all drug use for every client the first time.

SUMMARY

▲ The view of addiction has changed over the past thirty years and is now based on a behavioral definition and is applied to a wider variety of drugs and other activities.

▲ There is evidence that addiction may be influenced by genetics, biochemistry, personality, experience, and social context, but none of these factors can be called the sole cause of addiction. This idea is referred to as a biopsychosocial perspective on addiction.

▲ The DSM-IV diagnosis of substance dependence relies on tolerance and physical dependence, whereas the diagnosis of substance abuse uses behavioral indicators of excessive involvement.

▲ The addict's decision to seek treatment may involve a series of cognitive "stages of change."

▲ Treatment is often divided into the three stages of detoxification, active treatment, and aftercare.

▲ Therapeutic communities are usually staffed by former substance abusers, and clients generally remain in them for several months.

▲ Outpatient drug-free programs are often associated with community mental health centers and employ trained counselors, psychologists, or social workers.

▲ Chemical dependence residential programs also tend to employ former substance abusers, but treatment is usually limited to 3 to 8 weeks.

▲ A variety of new medical approaches is being developed to treat addicts.

REVIEW QUESTIONS

1. How does physical dependence relate to tolerance?
2. What do we mean when we say that a drug has the ability to serve as a positive reinforcer of behavior?
3. Which is more important to our current understanding of addiction, physical dependence or reinforcement? Why?
4. Why does it make sense to discuss gambling, overeating, and other behaviors in the context of addiction? What problems result from such a broad definition of addiction?
5. Why do we sometimes speak about drugs as being able to cause addiction? What are the pitfalls of carrying the concept too far?
6. What personality variables tend to be stronger in prealcoholic students?
7. Why do some people say that addiction is a disease of the family?
8. Which types of diseases provide poor analogies, and which might provide better analogies, for addiction?
9. How does motivational interviewing relate to "stages of change"?
10. What kind of evidence do we have that treatment for substance abuse works?

Related Internet Sites on Addiction

Web of Addictions: http://www.well.com/ user/woa/

College on Problems of Drug Dependence: http://views.vcu.edu/cpdd/

National Institute on Drug Abuse: http:// www.nida.nih.gov/

Alcoholics Anonymous: http://www.alcoholics-anonymous.org/

And don't forget to check our own *Drugs, Society, and Human Behavior* site for many more links: http://www.uwyo.edu/ A&S/psyc/dshb.htm.

REFERENCES

1. Forbes D: *False fixes,* Albany, NY, 1994, State University of New York Press.
2. Goldstein A: *Molecular and cellular aspects of the drug addictions,* New York, 1989, Springer-Verlag.
3. Kelleher RT, Goldberg SR: Control of drug taking behavior by schedules of reinforcement, *Pharmacol Rev* 27:291, 1976.
4. Maas LC and others: Functional MRI of human brain activation during cue-induced cocaine craving, *American Journal of Psychiatry,* 1997.
5. Kerr JS: Two myths of addiction: The addictive personality and the issues of free choice. *Human Psychopharmacology* 11:suppl, 1996.
6. Peele S, Brodsky A, Arnold M: *The truth about addiction and recovery,* New York, 1992, Fireside Press.
7. Marlatt GA, Fromme K: Metaphors for addiction. In S Peele, editor: *Visions of addiction,* Lexington, Mass, 1988, DC Heath.
8. American Psychiatric Association: *Diagnostic and statistical manual of mental disorders,* ed 4, Washington, DC, 1994, the Association.
9. Belding MA and others: Stages and processes of change among polydrug users in methadone maintenance treatment, *Drug and Alcohol Dependence* 39:45, 1995.
10. Miller W: Motivational interviewing: Research, practice, and puzzles, *Addictive Behaviors* 21:835, 1996.
11. Brecher EM: *Licit and illicit drugs,* Boston, 1972, Little, Brown.
12. Simpson DD, Sells SB: *Evaluation of drug abuse treatment effectiveness: summary of the DARP follow-up research,* DHHS Pub No (ADM)82-1194, Washington, DC, 1982, US Government Printing Office.
13. Cowley G and others: Money madness, *Newsweek,* Nov 4, 1991.
14. Schottenfeld RS and others: Buprenorphine dose-related effects on cocaine and opioid use on cocaine-abusing opioid-dependent humans, *Biological Psychiatry* 34:66, 1993.
15. Sershen H, Hashim A, Lajta A: Ibogaine and cocaine abuse: Pharmacological interactions at dopamine and serotonin receptors. *Brain Research Bulletin* 42:161, 1997.
16. Gerstein DR, Harwood HJ, editors: *Treating drug problems,* Washington, DC, 1990, National Academy Press.
17. Lewis DC: More evidence that treatment works, *The Brown University Digest of Addiction Theory and Application* 13:12, 1994.

C H A P T E R 4

Drug Regulations

KEY TERMS	OBJECTIVES

After reading this chapter, you should be able to:

morphine
cocaine
psychotic
patent medicines
FDA
NDA
IND
DEA
paraphernalia
EMIT
THC

- Discuss the historical factors that led to the passage of the 1906 and 1914 laws that are the basis for our current federal drug regulations.
- Explain how the rules governing pharmaceuticals have evolved since 1906 and what events led to major changes in those rules.
- Describe the process by which a drug company works with the FDA to bring a new drug to market.

- Explain how enforcement of the Harrison Act and subsequent federal laws have helped to shape our current illicit drug problem.
- List the basic provisions of the current federal controlled substance regulations.
- Describe the current federal approach to enforcement of our drug laws and some of its positive consequences and enormous difficulties.

Once upon a time in the United States, there weren't any regulations about drug use—at least there weren't any federal regulations. That lasted for about two years. In 1791, Congress passed an excise tax on whiskey, which resulted in a disagreement that historians call the Whiskey Rebellion. West of the Appalachian Mountains, where most whiskey was made, the farmers refused to pay the tax and tarred and feathered revenue officers who tried to collect it. In 1794, President George Washington called in the militia, which occupied counties in western Pennsylvania and sent prisoners to Philadelphia for trial. The militia and the federal government carried the day. The Whiskey Rebellion was an important test for the new government because it clearly established that the federal government had the power to enforce federal laws within the states.

In chapter 2 we saw that drug regulations are passed mainly for what is perceived to be the public good. As the story of the laws and regulations about drugs unfolds, it will become clear that most of the debate centers on the question, "What is the public good?" Issues of fact, morality, health, personal choice, and social order are intertwined—and sometimes confused. It should surprise no one that our laws about drug use resemble a patchwork quilt reflecting the many social changes that have occurred in this country. If we want to understand our current drug laws, we must see how they have evolved over the years in response to one social crisis after another.

THE BEGINNINGS

Reformism

The current federal approaches to drug regulation can be traced to two pieces of legislation passed in 1906 and 1914. Any student of American history will remember that the nation was moving out of the gilded age of *laissez-faire* capitalism into the reform era in which legislation was passed regulating business and labor practices, meat packing, and food production. We should also remember that this general movement toward improvement of our nation's moral character was to bring us, in 1919, a constitutional amendment prohibiting the sale of alcoholic beverages. Theodore Roosevelt was president from 1901 to 1909 and continued to be influential after that time; his role in involving the federal government in both foreign treaties and domestic regulations was crucial to the development of these early drug laws.

Problems Leading to Legislation

The trend toward reform was given direction and energy by the public discussion of several drug-related problems, and those first laws reflected the problems that fueled their passage. Opium smoking among the Chinese, morphinism, cocaine use, and the peddlers of patent medicines provided the basic fuel used by political figures and newspapers to fire public opinion.

Opium and the Chinese

The roots of Chinese opium smoking and the history of the Opium Wars are discussed in chapter 15. It is important, however, to say that in the mid 1800s many British and some American merchants were engaged in the lucrative sale of opium to the Chinese, and many reformers and world leaders disapproved. In 1833 the United States signed its first treaty agreeing to control international trade in opium, and the regulatory tax on crude opium imported into this country was legislated in 1842.

The United States imported Chinese workers after the Civil War, mainly to help build the rapidly expanding railroads, and some of these people brought with them the habit of smoking opium. As always happens when a new pleasure is introduced into a society, the practice of opium smoking spread rapidly. Also, as always happens, the new practice upset the status quo and caused society to react. A contemporary report in 1882 describes both the spread of opium smoking in San Francisco and the reactions it elicited:

> The practice spread rapidly and quietly among this class of gamblers and prostitutes until the latter part of 1875, at which time the authorities became cognizant of the fact, and finding . . . that many women and young girls, as also young men of respectable family, were being induced to visit the dens, where they were ruined morally and otherwise, a city ordinance was passed forbidding the practice under the penalty of a heavy fine or imprisonment, or both. Many arrests were made, and the punishment was prompt and thorough.[1]

This 1875 San Francisco act was the first U.S. ordinance forbidding opium smoking. In 1882, New York State passed a similar law aimed at opium use in New York City's expanding Chinatown. An 1890 federal act permitted only American citizens to import opium or to manufacture smoking opium in the United States. Although this law is sometimes viewed as a racist policy, it was partly in response to an 1887 agreement with China that also forbade American citizens from engaging in the Chinese opium trade.

As more states and municipalities outlawed opium dens, the cost of black-market opium increased and many of the lower-class opium

A San Francisco opium den

addicts took up morphine or heroin, which were readily available and inexpensive.

Morphinism

The *hypodermic syringe* was introduced to the United States in 1856 and used on a large scale during the Civil War. Injecting **morphine,** the primary active ingredient in opium, gave near-immediate relief from pain. Morphine was used widely, and not always wisely, in the treatment of the two major afflictions in the Civil War—pain and dysentery. So many soldiers became addicted to morphine that morphinism was called the "soldier's disease" or the "army disease" in the years after the war. By the turn of the century most physicians, especially those who were younger and better trained, were aware of the danger of morphine addiction and were much more conservative in their use of this drug.

Cocaine

Pure **cocaine** also became available at about the same time as the hypodermic needle, and physicians experimented with its many uses. It was widely touted as a cure for morphine addiction, and many physicians prescribed cocaine injections for this purpose. Within a few years it was clear that cocaine was itself habit forming and that in high enough doses a dramatic **psychotic** state occurred. By the early 1900s there was considerable medical reaction against the indiscriminate use of cocaine.

Patent medicines

The broadest impact on drug use in this country came from the widespread legal distribution of **patent medicines.** Patent medicines were dispensed by traveling peddlers and were readily available at local stores for self-

Instantaneous cure with cocaine toothache drops.

medication. Sales of patent medicines increased from $3.5 million in 1859 to $74 million in 1904.

Within the boundaries of the United States there was increasing conflict between the steady progress of medical science and the therapeutic claims of the patent medicine hucksters. The alcohol and other habit-forming drug content of the patent medicines was also a matter of concern. One medicine, Hostetter's Bitters, was 44 percent alcohol, and another, Birney's Catarrh Cure, was 4 percent cocaine. In October 1905, *Collier's* magazine culminated a prolonged attack on patent medicines with a well-documented, aggressive series entitled "Great American Fraud."[2]

The 1906 Pure Food and Drugs Act

President Theodore Roosevelt recommended in 1905 "that a law be enacted to regulate interstate commerce in misbranded and adulterated foods, drinks, and drugs."[3] The 1906 publication of Upton Sinclair's *The Jungle,* exposing the horribly unsanitary conditions in the meat packing industry, shocked Congress and America. It provided the necessary heat that five months later led to the passage of the Pure Food and Drugs Act. This 1906 act prohibited interstate commerce in adulterated or misbranded foods and drugs. This brought the federal government full force into the drug marketplace, and subsequent modifications have built on it. A drug was defined as "any substance or mixture of substances intended to be used for the cure, mitigation, or prevention of disease." Of particular importance was the phrasing of the law with respect to misbranding. Misbranding referred *only to the label, not to general advertising,* and covered "any statement, design, or device regarding . . . a drug, or the ingredients or substances contained therein, which shall be false or misleading in any particular."

---

morphine: a narcotic, the primary active chemical in opium. Heroin is made from morphine.

cocaine: a stimulant; the primary active chemical in coca.

psychotic: (sigh *cot* ick) out of touch with reality.

patent medicines: medicines sold directly to the public.

The act specifically referred to alcohol, morphine, opium, cocaine, heroin, *Cannabis indica* (marijuana), and several other agents. Each package was required to state how much (or what proportion) of these drugs was included in the preparation. This meant, for example, that the widely sold "cures" for alcoholism or morphine addiction had to indicate that they contained another addicting drug. However, as long as the ingredients were clearly listed on the label, addicting drugs could be sold and bought with no federal restrictions. The goal was to protect people from unscrupulous merchants, not from themselves. The 1906 Pure Food and Drugs Act provided the rootstock upon which all our modern laws regulating pharmaceuticals have been grafted.

The Harrison Act of 1914

In the early 1900s, Dr. Hamilton Wright, the father of American narcotics laws, decided that the United States could gain favored trading status with China by leading international efforts to aid the Chinese in their efforts to reduce opium importation. At the request of the United States, an international conference met in 1912 to discuss controls on the opium trade. Great Britain, which was giving up a very lucrative business, wanted morphine, heroin, and cocaine included as well, because as opium was being controlled, these German products were replacing it.[4] Eventually an agreement was reached in which several nations agreed to control both international trade and domestic sale and use of these substances. In response, Dr. Wright drafted a bill that was submitted by Senator Harrison of New York, titled "An Act to provide for the registration of, with collectors of internal revenue, and to impose a special tax upon all persons who produce, import, manufacture, compound, deal in, dispense, or give away opium or coca leaves, their salts, derivatives, or preparations, and for other purposes."[5] With a title like that, it's no wonder that this historic law is usually referred to as the Harrison Act!

For the first time, dealers and dispensers of the opiates and cocaine had to register annually, pay a small fee, and use special order forms provided by the Bureau of Internal Revenue. Physicians, dentists, and veterinary surgeons were named as potential lawful distributors if they registered. It is important for modern readers to realize that in 1914 there would have been no support and no constitutional rationale for a federal law prohibiting an individual from possessing or using these drugs. Congress would not have considered such a law, and if it had, the Supreme Court would probably have declared it unconstitutional. The Harrison Act was a tax law, constitutionally similar to the whiskey tax. It was not a punitive act, penalties for violation were not severe, and the measure contained no reference to users of "narcotics."

During congressional debate, some concern was expressed about the tax law's inconvenience to physicians and pharmacists, and it is doubtful that such a law would have been passed in the United States if its purpose had been merely to meet the rather weak treaty obligations of the 1912 Hague Conference. It was not meant to replace existing laws and, in fact, specifically supported the continuing legality of the 1906 Pure Food and Drugs Act and the 1909 Opium Exclusion Act. Dr. Wright had written and lectured extensively, waging an effective, emotional, and in some instances outright racist public campaign for additional controls over these drugs. For example, his claims about the practice of "snuffing" cocaine into the nose, which he said was popular among southern blacks, caused a great deal of concern and fear.[6] Dr. Wright testified before Congress that this practice led to the raping of white women. Combining this depiction with the racially tinged fears about those immoral Chinese opium dens added the necessary heat to make the difference, and the Harrison Act passed and was signed into law in 1914. This law was the seed that has since sprouted into all of our federal controlled substance regulations.

Two Bureaus, Two Types of Regulation

By 1914 the basic federal laws had been passed that would influence our nation's drug regulations up to the current time. It might be significant that the Pure Food and Drugs Act was administered within the Department of Agriculture, whereas the Harrison Act was administered by the Treasury Department—two different federal departments administering two different laws. Many of the drugs regulated by the two laws were the same, but the political issues to which each agency responded were different. The Agriculture Department was administering a law aimed at ensuring that drugs were pure and honestly labeled. On the other hand, the Treasury Department's experience was in taxing alcohol, and they would soon be responsible for enforcing Prohibition. The approach taken by each bureau was further shaped by court decisions, so that the actual effect of each law became something a bit different from what seems to have been intended.

REGULATING PHARMACEUTICALS

The 1906 law called for the government to regulate the purity of both foods and drugs, and evidence had been presented during the congressional debate that thousands of products in both categories were at fault. Where was the task of analyzing and prosecuting to begin? Dr. Harvey Wiley, chief chemist in the Department of Agriculture, had been a major proponent of the 1906 law and had drafted most of it. He was in charge of administering the law, and he influenced the direction its enforcement would take. His first concern was with adulterated food, so most of the initial cases dealt with food products rather than drugs.

Purity

Most large drug manufacturers made efforts to comply with the new law, although they were not given specific recommendations as to how this should be accomplished. The manufacturer of Cuforhedake Brane-Fude modified its label to show that it contained 30 percent alcohol and 16 grains of a widely used headache remedy. The government brought the manufacturer to trial in 1908 on several grounds: The alcohol content was a bit lower than that claimed on the label, and the label seemed to claim that the product was a "cure" and food for the brain, both misleading claims. After much arguing about different methods of describing alcohol content and about the label claims, the manufacturer was convicted by the jury, probably because of the "brane-fude" claim, and paid a fine of $700.[7]

Dr. Wiley went on vigorously testing products and pursuing any that were adulterated or didn't properly list important ingredients, but he also went after many companies on the basis of their therapeutic claims. In 1911, government action against a claimed cancer cure was overturned by arguing that the ingredients were accurately labeled and that the original law had not covered therapeutic claims, only claims about the nature of the ingredients. Congress rapidly passed the 1912 Sherley amendment that outlawed "false and fraudulent" therapeutic claims on the label. Even so, it was still up to the government to prove that a claim was not only false but also fraudulent in that the manufacturer knew it to be false. In a 1922 case, the claim that "B&M External Remedy" could cure tuberculosis was ruled not to be fraudulent because its manufacturer, who had no scientific or medical training, truly believed that its ingredients (raw eggs, turpentine, ammonia, formaldehyde, and mustard and wintergreen oils) would be effective.[7] This seems like an encouragement for the ignorant to become manufacturers of medicines!

From its beginning, the Food and Drug Administration (**FDA**) had adopted the approach of encouraging voluntary cooperation, which it could obtain from most of the manufacturers through educational and corrective actions rather than through punitive, forced compliance. As more and more cases were investigated, it became clear to the FDA officials that many of the violations of the 1906 law were unintentional and caused primarily by poor manufacturing techniques and an absence of quality control measures. The FDA began developing assay techniques for various chemicals and products and collaborated extensively with the pharmaceutical industry to improve standards. The prosperous 1920s, coupled with a friendly Republican administration and increasing scientific know-how, resulted in many voluntary changes by the drug industry that improved manufacturing and selling practices.

In spite of these improvements, many smaller companies continued to bring forth "quack" medicines that were ineffective or even dangerous. The depression of the 1930s increased competition for business, and the Democratic Roosevelt administration took a more critical view of the pharmaceutical industry. FDA surveys in the mid 1930s showed that over 10 percent of the drug products studied did not meet the standards of *The United States Pharmacopeia* or *The National Formulary*. Several attempts were made during the early 1930s to enact major reforms, but opposition by the manufacturers of proprietary medicines prevented these changes from happening.

Safety

The 1930s had seen an expansion in the use of "sulfa" drugs, which are effective antibiotics. In searching for a form that could be given as a liquid, a chemist found that *sulfanilamide* would dissolve in diethylene glycol. The new concoction looked, tasted, and smelled fine, so it was bottled and marketed in 1937. Diethylene glycol causes kidney poisoning, and within a short time 107 people died from taking "Elixir Sulfanilamide." The federal government could not intervene simply because the mixture was toxic—there was no legal requirement that medicine be safe! The FDA seized the elixir on the grounds that a true elixir contains alcohol, and this did not. The chemist committed suicide, the company paid the largest fine ever under the 1906 law, and a public crisis arose that led to passage of the 1938 Food, Drug, and Cosmetic Act.[7]

A critical change in the 1938 law was the requirement that *before* a new drug could be marketed its manufacturer must test it for toxicity. The company was to submit a "new drug application" (**NDA**) to the FDA. This NDA was to include "full reports of investigations which have been made to show whether or not such a drug is safe for use." If the submitted paperwork was satisfactory, the application was allowed to become effective. Between 1938 and 1962 about 13,000 NDAs were submitted and about 70 percent were allowed to be marketed.

The new drug application provision was important in two ways: First, it changed the role of the FDA from testing and challenging some of the drugs already being sold to that of a gatekeeper, which must review every new drug before it is marketed. This increased power and responsibility led to a great expansion in the size of the FDA. Second, the requirement that companies conduct research before marketing a new drug greatly reduced the likelihood of new drugs being introduced by small companies run by untrained people.

The 1938 act also stipulated that drug labels either give adequate directions for use or state that the drug is to be used only on the prescription of a physician. Thus the federal law first recognized a difference between drugs that could be sold over the counter and prescription-only drugs.

Effectiveness

In the late 1950s, Senator Estes Kefauver began a series of hearings investigating high drug costs and marketing collaboration between drug companies. As the hearings progressed, manufacturers, physicians, and the FDA itself were criticized. One major concern was that some of the most widely advertised and sold over-the-counter medications were probably ineffective. For example, Carter's Little Liver Pills consisted of small bits of candy-coated dried liver. It was accurately labeled and made no unsubstantiated therapeutic claims on the label—if you jumped to the conclusion that it was supposed to help your liver, that wasn't the company's fault. And no law required the medicines to actually do anything. Amendments to the Food, Drug, and Cosmetic Act were written but were bottled up in committee. Again it took a disaster that raised public awareness and congressional concern before major reforms were implemented.

Thalidomide, a sedative and sleeping pill, was first marketed in West Germany in 1957. The drug was widely used by pregnant women because it also reduced nausea and vomiting associated with the morning sickness often experienced early in pregnancy. An American company submitted an NDA in 1960 to market thalidomide, but luckily the FDA physician in charge of the application did not approve it quickly. In 1961 and early 1962 it became clear that thalidomide had been responsible for birth defects. In Germany, hundreds of children had been born with deformed limbs. The American company had released some thalidomide for clinical testing, but because its NDA was not approved, a major disaster was avoided in the United States.[7]

The 1962 Kefauver-Harris amendments added several important provisions, including the requirement that companies submit plans for and seek approval of any testing to be done with humans before the clinical trials are conducted. Another provision required advertisements for prescription drugs (mostly in medical journals) to contain a summary of information about adverse reactions to the drug.

The most important change was one requiring that every new drug be demonstrated to be *effective* for the illnesses mentioned on the label. As with the details of safety testing required by the 1938 law, this research on effectiveness was to be submitted to the FDA. The FDA was also to begin a review of the thousands of products marketed between 1938 and 1962 to determine their effectiveness. Any that were found to be ineffective were to be removed from the market. In 1966 the FDA began the process of evaluating the formulations of prescription drugs. By the end of 1974 the FDA had taken action to remove from the market 6,133 drugs manufactured by 2,732 companies.

Marketing a New Drug

To translate the 1962 law on the safety and effectiveness of a new drug, the FDA has established certain regular procedures and standards that must be met by the pharmaceutical company that hopes to market a prescription drug. Developing a compound to the point where it can be marketed is a long and expensive procedure for the drug company, costing an average of $360 million.[8]

The FDA formally enters the picture only when a drug company is ready to study the effects of a compound on humans. At that time the

---

FDA: The United States Food and Drug Administration.

NDA: new drug application. Must be approved before a drug is sold.

company supplies to the FDA a "Notice of Claimed Investigational Exemption for a New Drug" **(IND)**; it is also required to submit all information from preclinical (before human) investigations, including the effects of the drug on animals. The principal purpose of this preclinical work is to establish the safety of the compound.

As minimum evidence of safety, the animal studies must include acute, one-time administration of several dose levels of the drug to different groups of animals of at least two species. There must also be studies where the drug is given regularly to animals for a period related to the proposed use of the drug in humans. For example, a drug to be used chronically requires two year toxicology studies in animals. Again two species are required. The method of drug administration and the form of the drug in these studies must be the same as that proposed for human use.

In addition to these research results, the company must submit a detailed description of the proposed clinical studies of the drug in humans. The company must also certify that the human subjects will be told they are receiving an investigational compound and that the subjects will sign a form stating that they know they are to receive such a compound and that this is acceptable to them. Finally, the company must agree to forward annually a comprehensive report and to inform the FDA immediately if any adverse reactions arise in either animals or humans receiving the investigational drug.

If the FDA authorizes the use of the drug in humans, the company can move into the first of *three phases of clinical investigation.*

- **Phase 1** encompasses studies with very small amounts of the drug on a limited number of healthy people—company employees, medical school personnel, prisoners, and others who volunteer for such trials. At this stage the researchers are primarily interested in learning how their drug is absorbed and excreted in healthy people, and what side effects it may trigger.

- **Phase 2** of the human studies involves patients who have the condition the candidate drug is designed to treat. These studies will probably involve as many as a hundred hospital patients who are chosen because the new agent might help them.

- **Phase 3** is quite extensive and involves administering the drug to larger numbers of individuals than in phase 2 (perhaps thousands) with the disease or symptom for which the drug is intended. If the compound proves effective in phase 3, the FDA balances its possible dangers against the benefits for the patient before releasing it for sale to the public.

There have been relatively few changes to this basic procedure since 1962. In 1983, Congress passed the Orphan Drug Act, offering tax incentives and exclusive sales rights for a guaranteed seven years for any company developing a drug for rare disorders afflicting no more than 200,000 people. Up to that time companies had stayed away from much research on rare disorders because they couldn't earn enough to recover the enormous research costs. By 1990, forty-five drugs developed under this act had received FDA approval.[9] On the "drug war" front, the Prescription Drug Marketing Act of 1987 tightened the procedures whereby drug company salespeople could provide free samples to physicians, after Congress had heard testimony about widespread diversion of samples.[10] Also, because counterfeit and adulterated drugs had found their way into the U.S. market from abroad as shipments of "American goods returned," new regulations were added covering the transfer and reimportation of drugs.

There is one big, continually debated issue surrounding the FDA drug approval system: Why does it take so long? The issue is not just one of concern for the individual who is sick. Pharmaceutical manufacturers have only a seventeen-year patent on a new drug. They usually patent the chemical as soon as there is some evidence that it might be marketable. The manufacturers claim that by the time a drug is cleared for marketing, they have only a few years left on the patent—not long enough to reclaim costs and make a profit. From the mid 1980s to the mid 1990s, the average approval time was reduced from 34 months to 18 months—but the increased speed of the FDA's approval process has been more than offset by an increased amount of time spent by companies in clinical trials—an average of almost seven years![8]

Certain classes of drugs, including drugs for AIDS, are considered for priority review by the FDA. In 1987 the first drug was approved for use in AIDS, and by 1997 there were 42 approved drugs and 122 in clinical trials.[8]

NARCOTICS, DANGEROUS DRUGS, AND CONTROLLED SUBSTANCES

To most Americans the word *narcotics* means drugs that are manufactured and sold illegally. Pharmacologically, the term refers only to drugs having certain effects, with the prototype being the narcotic analgesics derived from opium, such as morphine and heroin. Although the Harrison Act controlled opiates, which are narcotics, and cocaine, which is not, the enforcement effort focused so much on the opiates that eventually the enforcement officers became known as narcotics officers, the office within the Treasury Department officially became the Narcotics Division, and people began to refer to the "Harrison Narcotics Act," though, as we have seen, the word *narcotics* was not in the original title. The meaning of the term changed so much in political use that later federal laws incorrectly classified cocaine and then marijuana as narcotics.

After the Harrison Act

In 1914 it was estimated that about 200,000 Americans—1 in 400—were addicted to opium or its derivatives. One way to administer the new law would have been to allow a continued legal supply of opiates to those individuals through registered physicians and to focus enforcement efforts on the smugglers and remaining opium dens. After all, the Harrison Act stated that an unregistered person could purchase and possess any of the taxed drugs if they had been prescribed or administered by a physician "in the course of his professional practice and for legitimate medical purposes." Early enforcement efforts focused on smugglers and did not result in a large number of arrests. However, one very important arrest was to have later repercussions. It seems that a Dr. Webb was taking telephone orders for narcotics, including some from people he had never seen in person. Evidence was presented that this physician would prescribe whatever amount the caller requested. He was arrested, convicted, and appealed the conviction all the way to the U.S. Supreme Court, which in 1919 upheld his conviction on the grounds that his activity did not constitute a proper "prescription" in the course of the professional practice of medicine. However, many addicts continued to receive narcotics quietly through their private physicians, and in most large cities there were public clinics that dispensed morphine to addicts who could not afford private care.

It is ironic that the single most important piece of legislation that has shaped the federal government's approach to controlled substances wasn't a "drug law" at all, but rather the Eighteenth Amendment prohibiting alcohol. That law was also to be enforced by the Treasury Department, and a separate Prohibition unit was established in 1919. The Narcotics Division was placed within that unit, and Colonel Levi G. Nutt was appointed the first director, with 170 agents at his disposal.[4] Although the Harrison

---

IND: application to investigate a new drug in human clinical trials.

Act itself had not changed, the people enforcing it had. Just as with alcohol, these people believed that the cure for narcotic addiction was to prevent the addict from having access to the drug (in other words, narcotic "prohibition," at least for addicts). The new enforcers interpreted the Webb case to mean that any prescription of a habit-forming drug to an addict was not a "legitimate medical purpose," and they began to charge many physicians under the Harrison Act. They seemed to be right on target when in 1922 the Supreme Court upheld the conviction of another physician, Dr. Behrman, who used the defense that his prescriptions were given not to maintain addiction but as part of a cure program. This defense was not allowed in his case, because evidence was presented that one patient had received the equivalent of 3,000 "ordinary doses."[5]

Because even cure programs were not exempt, the Internal Revenue Service (IRS) moved to close down municipal narcotics clinics in over thirty cities from coast to coast. In the period from 1919 to 1929, the Narcotics Division arrested about 75,000 people, including 25,000 physicians and druggists.[4] The American Medical Association, which was concerned with the reputation of the medical profession, supported the view that reputable physicians would not prescribe narcotics to addicts. Because there was then no legal way for an addict to continue his or her habit, the addict was forced either to stop using narcotics or to look for drugs in the illegal market. Thus this new method of enforcing the Harrison Act resulted in the growth of an illicit drug trade that charged users up to fifty times more than the legal retail drug price. Narcotic addiction came increasingly to be viewed as a police, rather than a medical, problem.

Partly in response to this growing illicit market, in 1922 Congress passed the Jones-Miller Act, which more than doubled the maximum penalties for dealing in illegally imported narcotics to $5,000 and ten years of imprisonment. This act was the first to mislabel cocaine as a narcotic, and it established the Federal Narcotics Control Board to initiate an active program against dealers. Included also was the stipulation that the mere possession of illegally obtained narcotics was sufficient basis for conviction, thus officially making the addict a criminal. Because illegal narcotics were so expensive, many addicts came to prefer the most potent type available, heroin. In 1924 another act entirely prohibited importing opium for the manufacture of heroin. Already by this time several important trends had been set: Addicts were criminals at odds with the regulatory agency, the growth of the illicit market was responded to with greater penalties and more aggressive enforcement, and there was a focus on attempting to eliminate a substance (heroin) as though the drug itself were the problem. In the 1925 Linder case, the Supreme Court declared that it could be legal for a physician to prescribe narcotics for an addict if it was part of a curing program and did not transcend "the limits of that professional conduct with which Congress never intended to interfere."[5] However, the damage had been done, and most physicians would have nothing to do with addicts.

By 1928 individuals sentenced for drug violations made up one-third of the total population in federal prisons. Even though the 1920s were the period of alcohol prohibition, during those years twice as many people were imprisoned for narcotics violations as for liquor violations.[11] In 1929, Congress viewed this enormous expenditure for narcotics offenders as an indicator that something was wrong and decided that addicts should be cured rather than repeatedly jailed. They voted to establish two narcotic farms for the treatment of persons addicted to habit-forming drugs (including marijuana and peyote) who had been convicted of violating a federal law. The farm in Lexington, Kentucky, opened in 1935 and generally held about a thousand patients, two-thirds of whom were prisoners.

Harry Anslinger was commissioner of the Bureau of Narcotics for more than thirty years.

Answering the call for new approaches to addiction, and in response to the end of Prohibition and to charges of corruption in the previous Narcotics Division, in 1930 Congress took several actions that culminated in the formation of a separate Bureau of Narcotics in the Treasury Department. Harry Anslinger became the first commissioner of that Bureau in 1932 and took office with a pledge to stop arresting so many addicts and instead to go after the big dealers. Anslinger became the first "drug czar," although he wasn't called that at the time. To some extent he followed the lead of J. Edgar Hoover, director of the Federal Bureau of Investigation (FBI). Each of these men was regularly reappointed by each new president, and each built up a position of considerable power and influence. Anslinger had almost total control of federal efforts in narcotics education, pre-

vention, treatment, and enforcement for more than thirty years, from 1932 to 1962. No federal or state narcotics law was passed without his influencing it, and he also represented U.S. narcotics interests to international organizations, including the United Nations. He was tough-minded in the area of drug abuse and always opposed any form of "ambulatory" narcotic treatment (treatment outside a secure hospital environment).

The end of Prohibition, combined with depression-era cutbacks, had reduced the number of agents available for enforcement, but not for long. After some newspaper reports linked marijuana smoking with crime, Anslinger adopted this new cause and began writing, speaking, testifying, and making films depicting the evils of marijuana. This effort succeeded in bringing public attention to the fight his bureau was waging against drugs and also resulted in the 1937 passage of the Marijuana Tax Act. Marijuana came under the same type of legal control as cocaine and the opiates, in that one was supposed to register and pay a tax to legally import, buy, or sell marijuana. From 1937 until 1970, marijuana was referred to in federal laws as a narcotic.

World War II caused a decrease in the importation of both legal and illegal drugs. With the end of the war and the resumption of easy international travel, the illegal narcotic trade resumed and increased every year, in spite of the 1951 Boggs amendment to the Harrison Act that established mandatory minimum sentences for narcotic offenses. Testimony before a subcommittee of the Senate Judiciary Committee in 1955 included the statement that inducing drug addiction in U.S. citizens was one of the ways Communist China planned to demoralize the United States. Remember that this was the height of the McCarthy era, during which a mere hint by Senator Joseph McCarthy that someone associated with "known communists" was enough to ruin that person's career. One interesting little naughty bit of history from that time was revealed years later. Anslinger and Hoover were aware that McCarthy, in addition to his widely known alcoholism, was addicted to morphine. Anslinger arranged for McCarthy to obtain a regular supply of his drug from a Washington, D.C., pharmacy without interference from narcotics officers.[4] With both crime and communism to combat, Congress passed the 1956 Narcotic Drug Control Act, with the toughest penalties yet. Under this law, any offense except first-offense possession had to result in a jail term, and no suspension, probation, or parole was allowed. Anyone caught selling heroin to a person younger than eighteen could receive the death penalty. Anslinger commented on that particular provision by saying, "I'd like to throw the switch myself on drug peddlers who sell their poisons to minors."[12]

Drug Abuse Control Amendments of 1965

The early 1960s saw not only an increase in illegal drug use but also a shift in the type of drugs being used illegally. The trend was for the new drug users to be better educated and to emphasize primarily drugs that alter mood and consciousness, such as amphetamines, barbiturates, and hallucinogens. Some hospitals in large cities reported that up to 15 percent of their emergency room calls involved individuals with adverse reactions to these drugs. Although amphetamines and barbiturates were legal prescription drugs, it was felt that they should be under the same types of controls as narcotics. The 1965 Drug Abuse Control amendments referred to these as dangerous drugs and also included hallucinogens such as LSD. The Bureau of Narcotics became the Bureau of Narcotics and Dangerous Drugs. Thus the 1960s saw a number of major changes for this agency. Anslinger had retired, the bureau had new classes of drugs to control, and it was facing widespread disregard of the drug laws by large

numbers of young people who were not all members of the underprivileged and criminal classes.

Comprehensive Drug Abuse Prevention and Control Act of 1970

The Comprehensive Drug Abuse Prevention and Control Act of 1970, usually referred to as the *Controlled Substances Act,* almost lived up to its title. It was comprehensive, because it repealed and replaced or updated all previous laws concerned with both the narcotic and dangerous drugs. This basic law is still in effect, so it is important to understand its structure. The law specifically states that the drugs controlled by the act are under federal jurisdiction regardless of involvement in interstate commerce. The law did not eliminate state regulations; it just made clear that federal enforcement and prosecution is possible in any illegal activity involving controlled drugs.

Prevention and treatment

The law dealt with prevention and treatment of drug abuse by appropriating funds to expand the role of community mental health centers and Public Health Service hospitals in the treatment of those who misuse drugs. It authorized the development of educational material and drug education workshops for professional workers and in public schools.

Control issues resolved

The control aspects of the bill were the most debated portions, and several basic philosophical, ethical, and legal issues were resolved by the law. First, this was a law to control drugs directly rather than through taxes. Enforcement authority was moved from the Treasury Department to the new Drug Enforcement Administration (DEA) in the Department of Justice. A second major issue was the separation of enforcement of the law from the scientific evalu-

X UNDERSTAND BASIC CATEGORIES X

TABLE 4.1

Summary of Controlled Substance Schedules

Schedule	Criteria	Examples
Schedule I	a. High potential for abuse b. No currently acceptable medical use in treatment in the U.S. c. Lack of accepted safety for use under medical supervision	heroin marijuana LSD
Schedule II	a. High potential for abuse b. Currently accepted medical use c. Abuse may lead to severe psychological or physical dependence	morphine cocaine methamphetamine
Schedule III	a. Potential for abuse less than I and II b. Currently accepted medical use c. Abuse may lead to moderate physical dependence or high psychological dependence	amphetamine most barbiturates PCP
Schedule IV	a. Low potential for abuse relative to III b. Currently accepted medical use c. Abuse may lead to limited physical or psychological dependence relative to III	barbital chloral hydrate paraldehyde
Schedule V	a. Low potential for abuse relative to IV b. Currently accepted medical use c. Abuse may lead to limited physical or psychological dependence relative to IV	mixtures having small amounts of codeine or opium

ation of the drugs considered for control. The attorney general is responsible for the administration of the control aspects of the law, but the secretary of the Department of Health and Human Services makes a binding recommendation about which drugs shall be controlled. This separation of enforcement from scientific and medical decisions about what should be controlled was a major victory for those arguing for a rational drug law.

Schedules

After specifically excluding "distilled spirits, wine, malt beverages, or tobacco," the law established five schedules of drugs that must be updated and published regularly. Table 4.1 summarizes the characteristics of drugs in each of the five schedules and gives a few examples. Perhaps the most important distinction is between Schedule I and the others: Schedules II to V consist primarily of prescription drugs that are further controlled by these regulations,

whereas the substances in Schedule I by definition "have no medical use" and are therefore not available by prescription. Notice that cocaine is on Schedule II and marijuana on Schedule I.

Penalties for possession

The penalties for simply possessing a drug became more lenient than before and do not depend on the schedule. Therefore, an individual is theoretically guilty of the same crime whether he or she has a Valium tablet prescribed for another person or a bag of heroin. A first offense of illegal possession of a controlled drug or "distributing a small amount of marijuana for no remuneration" can be punished by

DEA: Drug Enforcement Administration, a branch of the Department of Justice.

up to one year's imprisonment and/or a fine of $1,000 to $5,000. In lieu of this, the court can place the individual on probation for up to a year. If there is no violation of the conditions of probation, the charge is dismissed and the conviction is "erased," except that a nonpublic record of the action is kept to prevent a person from being a "first offender" more than once.

Penalties for selling

The penalties for illegally making or selling controlled substances were not too complicated when the law passed in 1970, and the maximum first-offense penalty for distributing a Schedule I or II "narcotic" drug was fifteen years and $25,000. In 1986 the penalties became much more complex, depending on the individual drug and the amount sold. Mandatory minimum penalties were again introduced as they had been in the 1950s. First-offense sale of a large amount of heroin, cocaine, or several other drugs can, if the sale results in death or serious bodily injury, result in a life sentence and a fine of $4 million. First-offense sale of a small amount of marijuana can result in imprisonment for up to five years and a fine of up to $250,000. No parole is allowed.[13]

Changes in the 1988 law

The 1988 Omnibus Drug Act made some interesting additions and adjustments to the Controlled Substances Act.[14] There were many components to this new law, involving the registration of airplanes, money laundering, firearms sales to felons, and chemicals used to manufacture drugs. One part allowed for the death penalty for anyone who murders someone or orders the killing of someone in conjunction with a drug-related felony. Major sections of the law funded treatment and education programs as well. The most noteworthy change was a toughening of approaches toward drug users, aimed at reducing the *demand* for drugs (as opposed to putting all federal efforts into reducing

the *supply* of drugs). Before this law there were few penalties and little interest in convicting users for possessing small (personal-use) amounts of controlled substances. Under the new law, here are some of the unpleasant possibilities if you are convicted of possession:
- A civil fine of up to $10,000
- Forfeiture of the car, boat, or plane conveying the substance
- Loss of all federal benefits, including student loans and grants, for up to 1 year after a first offense and up to 5 years after a second offense

The 1988 law also removes from public housing the entire family of anyone who engages in criminal activity, including drug-related activity, on or near public-housing premises.

Drug czar

To better coordinate all these federal efforts, the law established the "cabinet-level" position of Director of National Drug Control Policy (commonly referred to as a "drug czar"). This individual is ordered by the legislation to prepare a national drug-control strategy and an annual consolidated drug-control budget for all federal agencies involved, to advise the National Security Council, and to report directly to the president.

STATE AND LOCAL REGULATIONS

It is impossible to describe here all of the varied drug laws in the fifty states.[15] We should remember that most states and many local communities had laws regulating sales of drugs before the federal government got into the act in 1906. Some aspects of those old laws might still be in effect in some areas. Regarding legal sales of prescription and over-the-counter drugs, there is considerable uniformity across the states, but some details do differ. For example, in some states licensed physician's assistants are allowed to prescribe many types of medication,

FYI   **Americans in Prison**

Fueled largely by the increases in drug-law arrests, the number of people held in state and local prisons in the United States has reached record levels. From the 1920s through the mid 1970s, about 1 person was in prison for every 1,000 people in the U.S. population. There were peaks and valleys, with the highest peak in 1939 (the end of the depression) at 1.39 per 1,000 population. From 1974 to 1985 the rate doubled, from 1 to 2 per 1,000. By 1995, over 1 million people were in U.S. prisons, a rate of more than 4 per 1,000 population. Over 3 million were on probation or parole, also record numbers and proportions.[23] The United States now has a greater proportion of its own citizens in prisons than any other country.

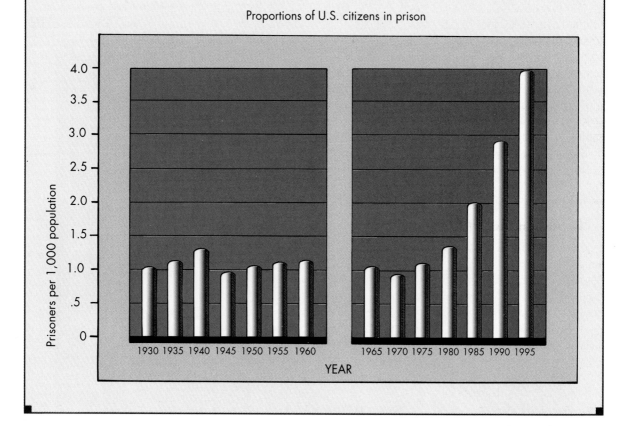

Proportions of U.S. citizens in prison

What Are Your Rights?

Do you know what your own rights and liabilities are under the laws in your area? Suppose you are driving and a police officer stops you for driving erratically. Smelling no alcohol, she suspects some other chemical agent. Can she search your car for drugs? Just the passenger compartment or the trunk as well? Can she search the people in the car? If she finds marijuana in your car, will you be charged? What if the marijuana is found on the person of a passenger in your car? If you don't know the answer to these questions, it might be interesting to find out. You could invite a member of the police force to meet with a group of classmates to talk about this and other issues of drug enforcement. Another idea would be to interview someone from the police force regarding this issue and then write a small article for the campus newspaper.

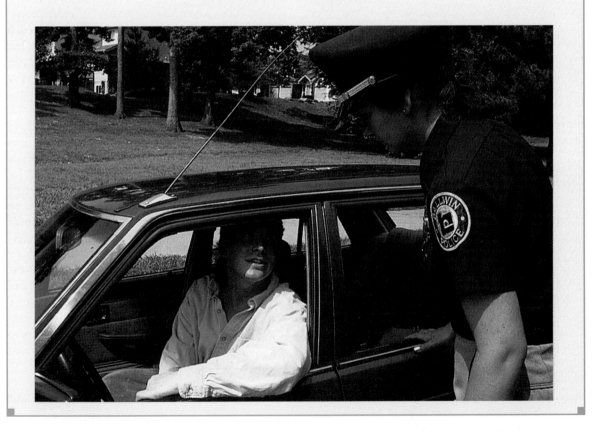

and in a few states pharmacists are now allowed to prescribe a few types of drugs that had previously required prescription by a physician or dentist.

After the passage of the federal 1970 Controlled Substance Act, states began to adopt the *Uniform Controlled Substances Act,* a model state law recommended by the DEA. The same set of schedules is found in these state laws, and they generally follow a similar pattern of penalties, although a given penalty might be greater in one state than in another. This model act was meant to replace all previous drug legislation in each state, but sometimes vestiges of older laws remain. For example, some states define as a special crime the smuggling of intoxicating drugs into a jail or prison. Also, many states have modified the uniform laws since they were originally passed. Some states "decriminalized" possession of marijuana (see chapter 17) by making it a civil offense punishable by a fine, and then later "recriminalized" it. The states have been pressured by the federal government to enact laws setting aside "drug-free school zones"—laws that make delivery penalties higher if the sale occurs near a school. Another federally encouraged action taken by most states is the removal of driver's license privileges for violations of controlled substance laws, even when driving is not involved in the offense.

Paraphernalia

In the mid 1970s a major industry grew up in the United States—the sale of legal items that were in some way related to the use of drugs. Sales of cigarette papers grew, whereas sales of loose cigarette tobacco declined. Water pipes and "bongs" (special pipes for concentrating marijuana smoke) were big items, as were decorative "roach clips," sifters, and scales. These were mainly sold in "head shops," which catered to the drug-using subculture and in many cases were connected to music stores or other youth-oriented businesses. Although the items themselves were not illegal, their obvious relationship to illegal drug use and their visibility to young people raised concerns that drug use was being indirectly condoned and even advertised. Several communities passed ordinances aimed at controlling the sales of drug **paraphernalia,** and in 1977, Indiana passed the first statewide antiparaphernalia law.[16] In 1979 the DEA proposed, at the request of the White House, a model antiparaphernalia act that states could adopt as an amendment to the Uniform Controlled Substances Act. Several have done so.

Interest in drug paraphernalia seemed to peak in about 1979 to 1980, with abundant television and newspaper reports, congressional hearings, and legal action. Concern was fueled by the sale of cocaine freebasing kits and other cocaine-related paraphernalia (straws, spoons, grinders, mirrors, and razors). Virtually every form of antiparaphernalia law has come under legal attack. We can best understand why by looking at the wording of a portion of the DEA's proposed model legislation, which would ban "blenders, bowls, containers, spoons, and mixing devices used, intended for use, or designed for use in compounding controlled substances."[17] Thus a spoon or a bowl might or might not be considered drug paraphernalia, depending on its "intended use." An alligator clip sold as an electronic part would not be paraphernalia, but the same clip sold at a local "head shop" might be, depending on how it is displayed for sale and what the salesperson says about its use. Although some state laws have been thrown out by the courts, most of those based on the Model Act have been upheld. One consequence is that people selling the items have been careful to

---

paraphernalia: (pare a fer *nail* ya) equipment used in conjunction with any activity.

point out their legal intended use. There is now federal law prohibiting the use of the U.S. Postal Service to send drug paraphernalia.

FEDERAL SUPPORT FOR URINE SCREENING

Military and Federal Employees

It wasn't until the 1970s that relatively inexpensive screening tests were invented that could detect a variety of abused substances or their metabolites in urine.[18] The Navy, followed by the other armed forces, was the first to use random urine screening on a large scale. Soon to follow were people in various high-risk or high-profile positions, oil-field workers, air traffic controllers, and professional athletes. In 1986, President Reagan first declared that random urine tests should be performed on all federal employees in "sensitive" jobs. He also urged companies doing business with the federal government to begin testing their employees if they had not already done so.

Transportation Workers

In 1987 a collision between an Amtrak passenger train and a Conrail freight train near Baltimore, Maryland, resulted in the deaths of sixteen people. The wreck was quickly blamed on drug use, because the Conrail engineer and brakeman had shared a marijuana joint shortly before the tragedy. The cause of the wreck can be argued: a warning indicator on the Conrail train was malfunctioning and the backup alarm had been silenced because it was too irritating. The marijuana use could be viewed as a symptom of a general "goofing off" attitude by the Conrail crew, who violated a number of safety procedures. Nevertheless, politicians and the news media saw this tragedy as a clear indication of the need for random urine testing. Transportation workers are now subject to surprise urine testing, and in 1992 this was expanded to interstate truck drivers. In addition,

urine testing has become a common feature for prisoners, both while incarcerated and during probation or parole.

Private Employers

Private corporations, which may require urine testing before hiring a new employee and/or may periodically test employees, have two main reasons for adopting urine tests, but the bottom line in both cases is money. First, companies believe that drug-free workers will be absent less often, make fewer mistakes, have better safety records, and produce more and better work. Second, by spending relatively few dollars on urine tests, they protect the company against negligence suits that might follow if a "stoned" employee hurt someone on the job or turned out a dangerously faulty product. Companies doing business with the federal government have an additional reason, in that they are required to have "drug-free workplace" rules in place.

Testing Methods

What is not widely discussed in the newspaper accounts of such testing programs is which procedures will be used, which drugs will be looked for, and how well the tests work. Most drug screening programs test urine samples using a commercially available kit that is based on a method known as **EMIT** (enzyme multiplied immunoassay test). This method relies on the use of antibodies that react either to the drug in question or to some metabolite (breakdown product) of the drug. A problem with this type of assay is that it is possible that some other drug or chemical might cross-react with the antibody and produce a false positive result.

Although the incidence of such false positives is fairly low, they can occur; therefore it is best to follow up the initial screen with another more selective method, such as gas chromatography/

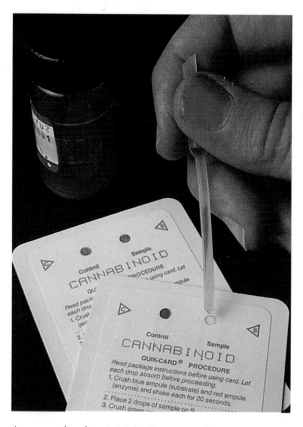

An example of an initial urine screening test

mass spectrometry (GS/MS). This method is more specific and more sensitive but also more expensive: a typical EMIT test can be done for about $20 per sample, but GC/MS tests cost about $100.[19] An early problem with mass screening programs was sloppy handling of the samples, allowing for false reports based on mixups. However, the labs doing this type of work have improved their handling procedures and the companies making the test kits have improved their accuracy, so that it is theoretically possible for a company or government agency to obtain very accurate information. That is not always done in practice, however. For example, several over-the-counter drug products contain ingredients such as ephedrine that are chemi-

cally similar to amphetamine, and someone taking these perfectly legal substances might show up with an EMIT test positive for amphetamine. Until recently, products containing ibuprofen could cause a positive test for marijuana. These false positives can be ruled out if another portion of the same urine sample is subjected to GC/MS, because that test can distinguish between ephedrine and amphetamine or between ibuprofen and marijuana metabolites. But the person paying for the testing has to want to spend the extra money.

EMIT kits can detect marijuana metabolites, the cocaine metabolite benzoylecgonine, PCP, and heroin. However, both the sensitivity and the duration over which the metabolites can be detected vary greatly among these substances. The cocaine metabolite clears within 1 or 2 days after a single use of a moderate amount, and it would probably be impossible to detect cocaine use after more than 3 or 4 days, even in someone chronically using high doses. The outside limit for PCP or heroin would also probably be about 4 days. After a single use of marijuana, metabolites can be reliably detected for 5 days or more, but with chronic use of high doses, tests can be positive for 2 or 3 weeks or as long as 30 days. The point is that it is much easier for these tests to detect marijuana use for long periods of time than to detect other types of drug use. Combined with the much greater frequency of use of marijuana than of these other drugs, the odds are good that if someone "flunks" a drug screen, it is probably because of marijuana metabolites.

The U.S. Justice Department has conducted research on the use of hair samples to detect drug use.[20] This would theoretically allow detection of the use of a drug even weeks in the

---

EMIT: enzyme multiplied immunoassay test, a drug screening urine test.

UP FOR DEBATE

The Special Status of Marijuana

The Controlled Substances Act lists substances under Schedules II through V based on their abuse potential. However, substances with "no medical use" all fall under Schedule I. The active ingredient in marijuana, delta-9-tetrahydrocannabinol **(THC)**, has recently caused some classification headaches for the DEA. For one thing, THC does now have a medical use—treating the nausea caused by cancer chemotherapy agents. Since 1986, under the generic name dronabinol, THC has been legally marketed as a prescription drug. The DEA's response to this has been to reschedule dronabinol *when dissolved in sesame oil and sealed in gelatin capsules,* as a Schedule II controlled substance. Any other preparation of THC is still Schedule I, as is marijuana itself. Marijuana is also being prescribed to some people for the treatment of glaucoma, and the government is even providing "official" marijuana cigarettes for this purpose. Marijuana has also been reported to provide some relief to multiple sclerosis patients. But marijuana cigarettes are not a generally available prescription drug. These prescriptions have been available only to about a dozen people under a "compassionate use" investigation of a new drug application. In 1992 the FDA stopped issuing new compassionate-use approvals for marijuana (see chapter 17).

In 1996 two states, California and Arizona, made the news when they passed citizen referenda allowing marijuana to be used for medical purposes. Because there are no legal sources of marijuana and because the federal government has actively opposed such measures,[22] these referenda have not resulted in widespread availability of legal medical marijuana in those states.

past, if the drug is incorporated into the hair. Although not in widespread use yet, the possibility of such testing raises both practical and ethical concerns.

You should also be aware that all these drug screens can detect the presence of a drug or its metabolite, but they can't tell you anything about the state of impairment of the individual at the time of the test. One person might show up at work Monday morning with a terrible hangover from drinking the night before, be unable to perform well on the job, and pass the drug screen easily. Another person might have smoked some marijuana on Friday night, have experienced no effect for the past day and a half, and yet fail the screen. The general idea of the screens seems to be to discourage illicit drug use more than to detect impairment of performance.

THE IMPACT OF DRUG ENFORCEMENT

We can examine the current efforts at enforcing federal drug laws by asking ourselves three questions: What exactly are we doing to enforce drug laws? How much is it costing us? How effective is it? Although there had been previous "wars" on illicit drugs, the largest efforts to date began in 1982 when President

Customs officers use a trained dog to sniff for drugs in a warehouse.

Reagan announced a renewed and reorganized effort to combat drug trafficking and organized crime. For the first time all federal agencies were to become involved, including the DEA; FBI; IRS; Alcohol, Tobacco and Firearms Bureau; Immigration and Naturalization; U.S. Marshals; U.S. Customs Service; and Coast Guard.[21] In some regions, Defense Department tracking and pursuit services were added. This last item had been legalized earlier in the Reagan administration and signaled an important change in the role of the military. The idea of using our military forces to police our population had long been abhorrent to Americans, who have insisted that most police powers remain at the state and local level. Because of the success of smugglers, we now use Air Force radar and aircraft and Navy patrol boats to detect and track aircraft or boats that might be bringing in drugs. These efforts have continued to expand, and in 1997 the Defense Department was spending almost $1 billion on drug interdiction activities.

Budget

A good overview of the widespread federal efforts can be obtained from the National Drug Control Strategy review and budget prepared

THC: delta-9 tetrahydrocannabinol, the most important psychoactive chemical in marijuana.

each year by the White House.[22] The total requested for the 1998 budget was a record $16 billion. About $10 billion of that was for "supply reduction"—domestic enforcement border control, and international efforts. This is a huge increase from less than $1 billion in 1980.

International Programs

International efforts aimed at reducing the drug supply include State Department programs that provide aid to individual countries to help them with narcotics controls, usually working in conjunction with the DEA. The DEA has agents in more than forty countries, and they assist the local authorities in drug crop eradication, locating and destroying illicit laboratories, and interfering with the transportation of drugs out of those countries. The State Department's International Narcotics Control Program budget for 1998 was $212 million. This included direct aid tied to drug enforcement, and loans and support for South American countries to develop alternative crops and industries. The United States is providing increased military aid in the form of helicopters, "defensive" weapons, uniforms, and other supplies to be used in combating drug trafficking, plus military training to both army and police agencies. This program is restricted to countries that do not engage in a "consistent pattern of gross violations" of human rights. In addition, the State Department must make recommendations to the President, who must then report to Congress each year, regarding each country receiving *any* form of aid from the United States, on whether it can be certified to be cooperating with antinarcotics efforts. All foreign aid is to be suspended to any country that cannot be certified to be cooperating.

Other Federal Agencies

Efforts within the United States have broadened to include activities related to drug trafficking. The Customs Service and IRS were joined in 1990 by a new Financial Crimes Enforcement Network to combat the "laundering" of drug profits through banks and other investments. The Federal Aviation Administration is involved not only in urine testing of pilots and other airline workers but also in keeping track of private aircraft and small airports that might be used for transporting drug shipments. The Department of Agriculture, Bureau of Land Management, and National Park Service are on the lookout for marijuana crops planted on federal land.

Other Costs

Besides the direct budget for drug control strategies, there are other costs, only some of which can be measured in dollars. We are paying to house a large number of prisoners: over 200,000 drug-law violators in state prisons and local jails and over 50,000 in federal prisons.[23] Add to this the cost of thousands on probation or parole, plus various forms of juvenile detention. We should also add the cost of crimes committed to purchase drugs at black-market prices and the incalculable price of placing so many of our state and local police, DEA, FBI, and other federal agents in danger of losing their lives to combat the drug trade, as some have done. A price that has been paid by many law enforcement agencies over the years is the corruption that is ever-present in drug enforcement. Because it is necessary for undercover officers to work closely with and to gain the trust of drug dealers, they must sometimes ignore an offense in hopes of gaining information about more and bigger deals in the future. They may even accept small favors from a drug dealer, and some officers have found it necessary to "use" along with the suspects. Under those circumstances, and given the large amounts of money available to some drug dealers and the small salaries paid to most law officers, the possibility of accepting too large a gift and ignoring too many offenses is always there, and there might be no obvious "line" between doing one's job and becoming slightly corrupted.[24]

There are costs on the international level, also. We are put in an awkward position whenever one of our political allies becomes involved, even unwillingly, in drug trafficking. A great deal of heroin has been flowing through Pakistan, for example, and some might wonder why we haven't cut off aid to them. First, they have been trying to control heroin with our help and their limited resources, but the problem is a large one. From their point of view, perhaps the problem is caused more by our appetite for heroin than by their need for money. Second, we cannot afford to lose them as an ally in that part of the world (they border on Iran and Afghanistan). So we must do the best we can to help them in their drug-control efforts and not

to offend them with too many demands. Our drug-control efforts sometimes find us providing help to repressive governments, and it has been charged that some of our previous narcotics-control aid has been used for political repression, in both Latin America and Southeast Asia. Panama's General Noriega was indicted on drug-trafficking charges by a Florida grand jury before our invasion of that country, and his subsequent trial set a historical precedent: trying another country's deposed leader for violation of our own narcotics laws. To the extent that narcotics control efforts place additional strains on our foreign policy needs in the East, the Caribbean, and Latin America, this also represents a significant cost to our country.

Finally, there is an unquantifiable cost in the loss of individual freedom that is inevitable when we give increased powers to the

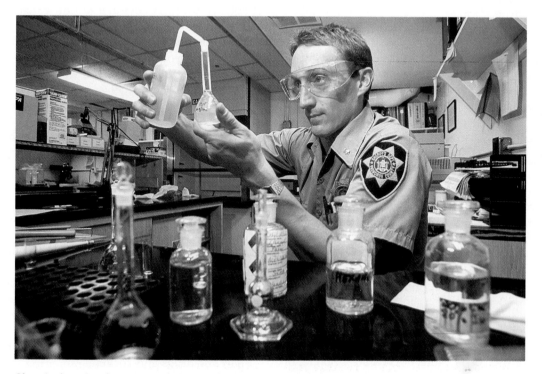

Chemical testing for cocaine being performed at a police Criminalistic Unit.

government. Because of increased drug-control efforts, American citizens are subjected to on-the-job urine tests; searches of homes, land, and vehicles; computer-coded passports that record each international visit; and increased government access to financial records. They are also threatened with seizure of their property and loss of federal benefits.

Given this effort and these costs, are our drug enforcement efforts effective? Do they work? Critics have pointed out that despite escalating expenditures, more agents, and an increasing variety of supply-reduction efforts, the supplies of cocaine, heroin, and marijuana have not dried up; in fact, they may have increased. Although there were record-breaking seizures of cocaine year after year, the price of cocaine did not change much on the streets during the 1980s, and there seemed to be more suppliers than ever. The United States government made a decision in 1924 to make heroin completely unavailable to addicts in this country, and after more than seventy years we can say only that we have been consistent in our failure to accomplish that goal. Our efforts to eradicate illegal coca fields in South America have been described as a failure by the General Accounting Office, which pointed out that many more new acres are being planted in coca each year than are being destroyed by our program.[25] A more recent economic analysis indicated that even if eradication and interdiction efforts could result in massive disruption of a particular source country's production, it would take only about two years for the market to push production back to the previous levels.[26]

Effectiveness of Control

The laws do work at another level. It is estimated that 10 to 15 percent of the illegal drug supply is seized by federal agencies each year. In 1995, for example, U.S. government agencies seized a total of 112 tons of cocaine, 1,300 kg of

heroin, and over 700,000 pounds of cannabis.[22] Efforts to reduce opium supplies and heroin smuggling have made it difficult and expensive to do business as a major importer. Evidence that supply is restricted can be found in the high prices charged on the streets. The price is many times more than the cost of the drug itself if sold legally. It is possible that the high cost is the only thing that regulates the amount taken by some of these addicts, who might otherwise die from overdoses more often than they do. Local efforts make a difference, too. Small pushers forced to work out of sight are less able to contact purchasers, and both the buyer and the seller have a higher risk of being hurt or cheated in the transaction. This not only raises the cost of doing business, it probably deters some people from trying the drugs. For example, suppose you were curious about heroin and wanted to try some. You might take some money to a rough part of one of our larger cities. If you were "lucky" enough to find a dealer, he might not be the sort of person you would trust. The transaction could take place in a nonpublic place, and if you were robbed, beaten, or just sold some worthless junk, you wouldn't be in a position to call the police!

SUMMARY

▲ In the early 1900s, two federal laws were passed on which our modern drug regulations are based.

▲ The 1906 Pure Food and Drugs Act requiring accurate labeling was amended in 1938 to require safety testing and in 1962 to require testing for effectiveness.

▲ A company wishing to market a new drug must first test it on animals, then file an IND. After a three-phase sequence of human testing, the company can file the NDA.

▲ The 1914 Harrison Act regulated the sale of narcotic drugs and cocaine.

▲ The Harrison Act was a tax law, but after 1919 it was enforced as a prohibition against providing narcotics to addicts.

▲ As narcotics became more scarce and their price rose on the illicit market, the illicit market grew. Harsher penalties and increased enforcement efforts, which were the primary strategies of Commissioner of Narcotics Harry Anslinger, failed to reverse the trend.

▲ Marijuana was added to the list of narcotics in 1937, and in 1965 amphetamines, barbiturates, and hallucinogens were also brought under federal control.

▲ The Controlled Substances Act of 1970 first provided for direct federal regulation of drugs, not through the pretense of taxing their sale.

▲ Controlled Substances are placed on one of five "schedules," depending on medical use and dependence potential.

▲ 1988 amendments were aimed at increasing pressure on users, as well as on criminal organizations and money laundering.

▲ Federal support for urine screening began in the military and has since spread to other federal agencies, nonfederal transportation workers, and many private employers.

▲ Current federal enforcement efforts involve thousands of federal employees and include activities in other countries, along our borders, and within the United States.

▲ Most states have adopted some version of the DEA's recommended Uniform Controlled Substances Act. Also, the federal government has mandated a uniform minimum drinking age of 21 years in all states.

▲ Federal, state, and local enforcement limits the supply of drugs and keeps their prices high, but the high prices attract more smugglers and dealers. It will never be possible to completely eliminate illicit drugs.

REVIEW QUESTIONS

1. What four kinds of habit-forming drug use at the turn of the century caused social reactions leading to the passage of federal drug laws?

2. What were the two fundamental pieces of federal drug legislation passed in 1906 and 1914?

3. In about what year did it first become necessary for drug companies to demonstrate to the FDA that a new drug was effective for its intended use?

4. What three phases of clinical drug testing are required before a new drug application can be approved?

5. What historic piece of federal legislation did the most to shape our overall approach to the control of habit-forming drugs in the United States?

6. Who was Harry Anslinger, and what was his role in marijuana regulation?

7. What is the important difference between a Schedule I and a Schedule II controlled substance?

8. What are drug paraphernalia laws, and why have they been subject to court challenges?

9. What are the limitations of the EMIT procedure used in urine screening?

10. Approximately how much is the United States spending per year on federal drug control efforts?

Related Internet Sites in Drug Regulation

Pharmaceutical Research and Manufacturer's Association: http://www.phrma.org

Drug Enforcement Administration: http://www.usdoj.gov/dea/

National Drug Control Strategy: http://www.ncjrs.org/htm/toc.htm

The Drug Reform Coordination Network: http://www.drcnet.org/

And don't forget our own *Drugs, Society, and Human Behavior* web site with updated information and links to these and other information sources: http://www.uwyo.edu/A&S/psyc/dshb.htm

REFERENCES

1. Kane HH: *Opium-smoking in America and China,* New York, 1882, GP Putnam's Sons.
2. Adams SH: The great American fraud, *Collier's,* six segments, Oct 1905 to Feb 1906.
3. *Congressional Record* 40:102 (Part 1), Dec 4, 1905 to Jan 12, 1906.
4. Latimer D, Goldberg J: *Flowers in the blood: the story of opium,* New York, 1981, Franklin Watts.
5. Terry CE, Pellens M: *The opium problem,* New York, 1928, Bureau of Social Hygiene.
6. Courtwright DT: *Dark paradise: opiate addiction in America before 1940,* Cambridge, Mass, 1982, Harvard University Press.
7. Young JH: *The medical messiahs: a social history of health quackery in twentieth-century America,* Princeton, NJ, 1967, Princeton University Press.
8. *Industry Profile 1997,* Washington, DC, 1997, Pharmaceutical Manufacturers Association.
9. Gibbons A: Billion-dollar orphans: prescription for trouble, *Science* 248:678-679, 1990.
10. Greenberg RB: The prescription drug marketing act of 1987, *Am J Hosp Pharm* 45:2118-2126, 1988.
11. Schmeckebier LF: *The bureau of prohibition,* Service Monograph No 57, Institute for Government Research, 1929, Brookings Institute. Cited in King R: Narcotic drug laws and enforcement policies, *Law & Contemporary Problems* 22:122, 1957.
12. *US News and World Report* 41:22, 1956.
13. *Controlled Substances Act as amended, with addenda.* Available from Drug Enforcement Administration, Washington, DC, US Department of Justice.
14. Lawrence C: In its last act, Congress clears anti-drug bill, *Congressional Quarterly* pp 3145-3151, Oct 29, 1988.
15. Bureau of Justice Statistics: *A guide to state controlled substances acts,* Washington, DC, 1991, US Department of Justice.
16. *Community and legal responses to drug paraphernalia,* DHEW Pub No (ADM)80-963, Washington, DC, 1980, US Government Printing Office.
17. National Institute of Justice: *State and local experience with drug paraphernalia laws,* Washington, DC, 1988, US Department of Justice.
18. *Employee drug screening: detection of drug use by urinalysis,* DHHS Pub No (ADM)86-1442, Washington, DC, 1986, US Government Printing Office.
19. Drug testing: the state of the art, *American Scientist* 77:19-23, 1989.
20. *Hair analysis as a drug detector,* Washington, D.C. U.S. Department of Justice, 1995.
21. Organized crime drug enforcement task forces: goals and objectives, *Drug Enforcement,* pp 3-15, Summer 1984.
22. *National drug control strategy,* Washington, DC, 1997, The White House.
23. *Correctional Populations in the United States, 1995,* Washington, DC, US Department of Justice, 1996.
24. Why good cops go bad, *Newsweek,* Dec 19, 1994.
25. Culhane C: US fails in South American drug war, *The US Journal of Drug and Alcohol Dependence* Jan 1989.
26. Riley KJ: *Snow Job?* New Brunswick, NJ, 1996, Transaction.

ASSESS YOURSELF!

Drug Use Today

Drugs and Our Society

Label the bar that corresponds to: (1) the percentage of high school seniors who have ever tried alcohol; (2) the percentage of adults who have smoked a tobacco cigarette within the past month; (3) the percentage of young adults (18 to 25) who have used cocaine within the past month; and (4) the percentage of high school seniors who have used marijuana within the past month.

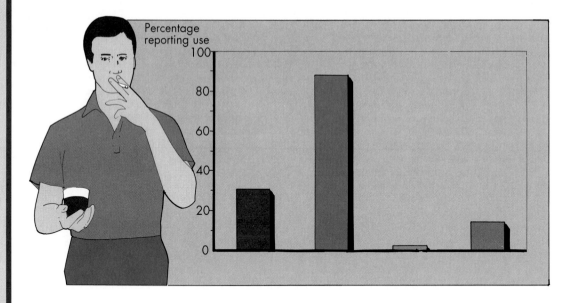

Annual Drug-Related Deaths

On the chart on p. 85, label the areas that correspond to the numbers of annual deaths related to (1) all illicit drugs; (2) alcohol; (3) cigarette smoking.

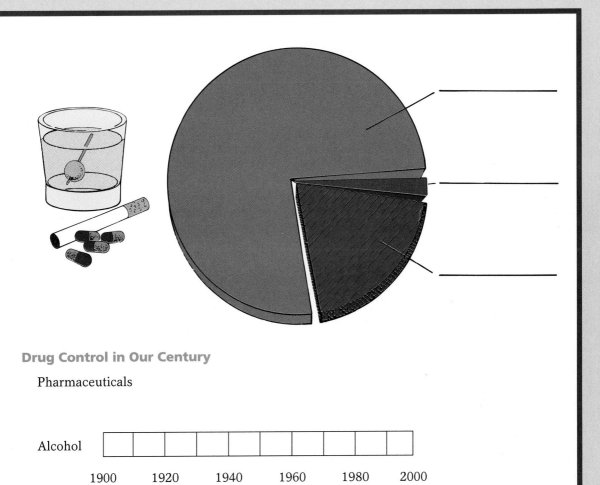

Drug Control in Our Century

Pharmaceuticals

Alcohol

    1900   1920   1940   1960   1980   2000

Illicit drugs

1. Shade in the area on the bar that corresponds to the period of national alcohol prohibition in the United States.
2. Above the time bar, mark the time points corresponding to:
    2a. The Pure Food and Drugs Act
    2b. The law requiring safety testing on all new pharmaceuticals
    2c. The law requiring testing of new drugs for effectiveness
3. Below the time bar, mark the time points corresponding to:
    3a. The Harrison Act taxing narcotics and cocaine
    3b. The Marijuana Tax Act
    3c. The Drug Abuse Control Amendments adding hallucinogens and many prescription drugs to the list of drugs regulated by the Bureau of Narcotics

2

How Drugs Work

A drug is nothing but a chemical substance until it comes into contact with a living organism. In fact, that's what defines the difference between drugs and other chemicals—drugs have specific effects on living tissue.

Because this book is about psychoactive drugs, the tissue we're most interested in is the brain. We want to understand how psychoactive drugs interact with brain tissue to produce effects on behavior, thoughts, and emotions.

Obviously we don't put drugs directly into our brains; usually we swallow them, inhale them, or inject them. In section 2, we will find out how the drugs we take get to the brain, and what effects they might have on the other tissues of the body.

5 The Nervous System
How do drugs interact with the brain and the nervous system?

6 The Actions of Drugs
How do drugs move in the body, and what are the general principles of drug action?

The Nervous System

KEY TERMS	OBJECTIVES

After reading this chapter, you should be able to:

homeostasis
hormones
neurotransmitters
receptors
CNS
autonomic
sympathetic
parasympathetic
basal ganglia
Parkinson's disease
dopamine
nigrostriatal dopamine pathway
mesolimbic dopamine pathway
acetylcholine
norepinephrine
serotonin
GABA
endorphins
precursors
uptake
synthesis
enzyme
reuptake
metabolize

- Explain the need for chemical communication within the body, and explain the similarities and differences between hormonal and neural communication.
- Describe how neurotransmitter chemicals are released from neurons and from what parts, and describe their interaction with receptors.
- Identify the major subdivisions of the nervous system and the functions of the two parts of the autonomic nervous system.

- Name a few of the major structural parts of the brain and some of the chemical pathways along with the general functions served by each path or pathway.
- Describe the "life cycle" of a neurotransmitter molecule and the various ways that psychoactive drugs can interact with it.

Drugs are psychoactive, for the most part, because they alter ongoing functions in the brain. To understand how drugs influence psychological processes, it is necessary to have some knowledge of the normal functioning of the brain and other parts of the nervous system and then to see how drugs can alter those normal functions. A person with little or no background in biology or chemistry can develop a good understanding of these topics at a conceptual level. Learning these concepts and some of the basic terminology will be very helpful in understanding the actions and effects of each of the major types of psychoactive drugs.

CHEMICAL MESSENGERS

Since the first multicellular organisms oozed about in their primordial tidal pools, some form of cell-to-cell communication has been necessary to ensure the organism's survival. Those first organisms probably needed to coordinate only a few functions, such as getting nutrients into the system, distributing them to all of the cells, and then eliminating wastes. At that level of organization, perhaps one cell excreting a chemical that could act on neighboring cells was all that was necessary. As more complex organisms evolved with multicellular systems for sensation, movement, reproduction, and temperature regulation, the sophistication of these communication mechanisms increased markedly. It became necessary for many types of communication to go on simultaneously and over greater distances. Although those early organisms were at the mercy of the sea environment in which they lived, we carry our own sea-water-like cellular environment around with us and must maintain that internal environment within certain limits. This process is known as **homeostasis.** This word can be loosely translated as "staying the same," and it describes the fact that many biological factors are maintained at or near certain levels. For example, most of the biochemical reactions basic to the maintenance of life are temperature dependent, in that these reactions occur optimally at temperatures near 37 °C (98.6 °F). Because we cannot live at temperatures too much above or below this level, our bodies have many mechanisms they can use to either raise or lower temperature: perspiration, shivering, altering blood flow to the skin, and others. Similar homeostatic mechanisms serve to regulate the acidity, water content, and sodium content of the blood; glucose concentrations; and other physical and chemical factors that are important for biological functioning. In humans and other mammals, we find a variety of sophisticated systems for chemical communication within the body; presumably these evolved at different times, forming layers of communication and control that interact with one another at many levels. These chemical messengers can be divided into two broad classes: hormones and neurotransmitters.

Hormones

Hormones are chemicals that are released from specialized groups of secretory cells (often called glands) and that affect other cells, which we think of as "target" cells (figure 5.1). For example, the male sex hormone testosterone is released from the testes into the bloodstream. It then circulates throughout the body, influencing muscular and neural development, sexual and aggressive behavior, and other functions. Another gland, the pituitary (referred to as the master gland), releases several hormones that circulate through the bloodstream, each having specific effects on the appropriate target cells. Many of these target tissues are themselves glands, and the pituitary therefore controls the release of other hormones. Some pituitary hormones have more direct actions. For example, when blood pressure drops, the pituitary releases vasopressin, which signals the kidney to release less fluid into the urine. Drinking alcohol inhibits the release of vasopressin, so the kidney releases more fluid into the urine.

You might be surprised to learn that hormones are still being discovered, many within the past twenty-five years. Each new discovery helps us better appreciate how many mechanisms are at work to coordinate our most basic biological functions.

---

homeostatis: maintenance of an environment of body functions within a certain range (e.g., temperature, blood pressure).

hormones: chemical messengers that send signals over a fairly wide area.

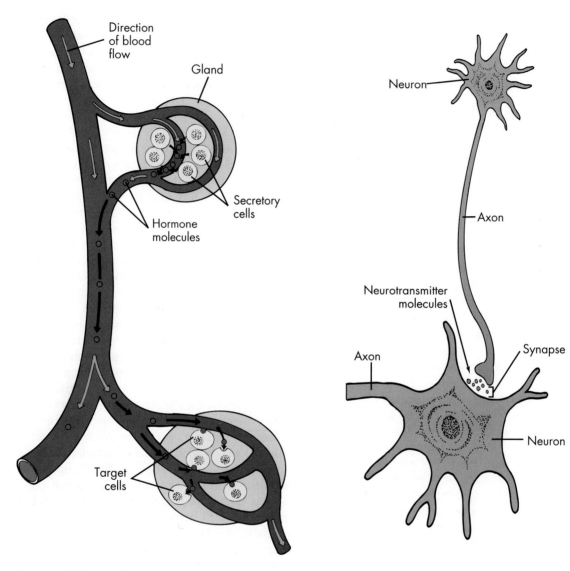

Figure 5.1 Hormonal signaling. Hormone molecules are released by secretory cells in a gland. The molecules are carried by the blood to distant target cells, where they exert their signaling effect.

Figure 5.2 Chemical signaling in the nervous system. When an electrical signal reaches the terminal end of the axon, it causes release of neurotransmitter molecules into the synapse, a small space between the terminal and another neuron. The second neuron is affected by the transmitter molecules, which influences electrical activity in the second neuron.

Neurotransmitters

In the nervous system, more-discrete signals are found (figure 5.2). Neurons act as secretory cells, target cells, and conductors of electrical signals. Each neuron releases one or a few specialized signaling chemicals called **neurotransmitters.** There are about fifty chemicals now believed to act as neurotransmitters, and each neuron is sensitive to one or a few of them.[1, p. 201]

What makes the action of neurotransmitters more discrete than that of hormones is that they are not released into the blood but rather are released into a small space, called a synapse, between two neurons. The chemical released into that synapse affects only one neuron, rather than a whole group of target cells, at once. Because only a small amount of neurotransmitter chemical is released into this small synapse, it can be removed quickly once it has sent its signal. Therefore the signal is discrete in time, as well as in space. This allows the sending of detailed information from one specific place to another in the nervous system. To give some idea of scale, the synaptic space is less than 1/10,000th of an inch across. Several thousand neurotransmitter molecules are released at once, and it takes only microseconds for these molecules to diffuse across the synapse.

Although many neurotransmitters have now been identified, we are concerned mostly with those few that we believe to be associated with the actions of the psychoactive drugs we are studying. Those neurotransmitters include *acetylcholine, norepinephrine, dopamine, serotonin, γ-aminobutyric acid (GABA),* and the endorphins.

Receptors

Chemical signals are useful only if the target cells are able to detect the presence of the signal molecules and then perform some action on the basis of having received that signal. The specialized structures that perform these functions are called **receptors**—subcellular structures that are part of the target-cell membrane.[2] These receptors play an important role in the actions of many of the drugs we discuss in this book, and it is therefore important for you to have a feeling for how they work in the nervous system.

Each of the neurotransmitter chemicals has a unique three-dimensional structure that is characteristic of each of its molecules and different from the molecules of other neurotransmitters. Some parts of the molecule are electrically more positive or negative than other parts, and the locations of these electrical charges also help to make the molecule unique. One analogy that has been used to describe the interaction between the neurotransmitter and its receptor is that of a lock and key: the neurotransmitter fits into a receptor as a key fits into a lock. That model is useful for pointing out the specificity of the interaction based on the three-dimensional structure of the neurotransmitter, but it is difficult to explain the dynamic properties of the interaction using the lock-and-key analogy. In fact, a given molecule might be more or less attracted to a receptor, depending on its degree of fit and the locations of electrical charges on both the molecule and the receptor. This means that molecules will vary widely in their *affinity* for a receptor, whereas we generally think of a key as either fitting or not fitting a lock. Figure 5.3 shows a schematic diagram of a portion of a synapse and depicts neurotransmitter molecules being released from the terminal of one neuron and binding to receptors of another neuron. The schematic diagram indicates that in the process of binding, the receptor structure has to change its shape slightly in order to match up with the neurotransmitter molecule. This change in

---

neurotransmitters: chemical messengers released from neurons and having brief, local efforts.

receptors: recognition mechanisms that respond to specific chemical signals.

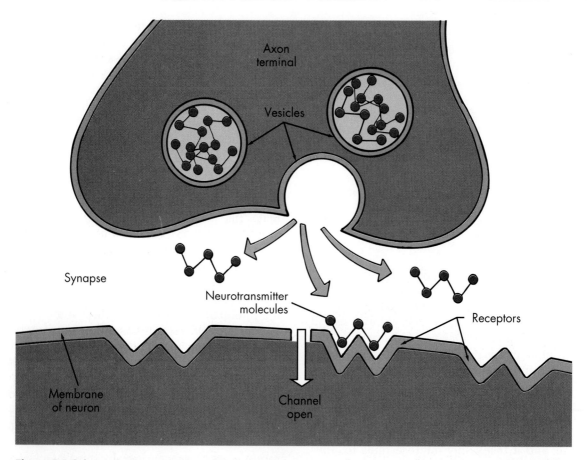

Figure 5.3 Schematic representation of the release of neurotransmitter molecules from synaptic vesicles in the axon terminal of one neuron and of the passage of those molecules across the synapse to receptors in the membrane of another neuron. A neurotransmitter molecule has bound to the center receptor and has distorted it so as to open a channel through the membrane of the second cell. This channel allows the flow of electrically charged ions through the membrane, thus altering the electrical charge on the membrane of the second cell.

shape is the trigger that sets off changes in the electrical activity of the receiving neuron.

In neurons the effect of a neurotransmitter binding to its receptor might be to allow an electrical current to flow across the membrane. Because neurons conduct electrical signals along their membranes, the effect of a particular type of receptor is either to *excite* this electrical activity or to *inhibit* it. Figure 5.4 describes infor-

mation flow in the nervous system. Electrical activity along the nerve membrane conducts information from one place to another, and once that activity arrives at the nerve terminal, it results in the release of a neurotransmitter chemical, which influences the electrical activity of the next neuron. The electrical signal traveling along the membrane is brief—if it is amplified and sent to a loudspeaker, one hears a pop as

| Electrical pulse in axon | → | Electrical pulse in terminals | → | Chemicals released from terminals | → | Chemicals attach to receptor site | → | Chemicals in receptor sites cause changes in electrical activity of dendrite | → | Initiates electrical impulse in axon |

Figure 5.4 Sequence and mode of information movement in the nervous system

the signal travels past the recording electrode. Neurons "fire" these signals several times a second under normal conditions, and excitatory or inhibitory influences may be seen as increasing or decreasing the firing rate of the neuron.

Whether the effect of a neurotransmitter is excitatory or inhibitory depends on the type of receptor. One of the neurotransmitters, GABA, seems to act at only inhibitory receptors. Therefore GABA is often called an inhibitory neurotransmitter. But acetylcholine acts at three or four different types of receptors in the brain, and its action can be either excitatory or inhibitory, depending on the receptor. Most other neurotransmitters also have several different types of receptors, some excitatory, some inhibitory.

THE NERVOUS SYSTEM

Although we often speak of the nervous system, it is perhaps more appropriate to remember that there are several communication and control systems that are based on neurons and neurotransmitters. Some important distinctions among these systems will help us to understand drug actions.

Central Nervous System

The central nervous system (**CNS**) consists of the brain and spinal cord. These two structures form a central mass of nervous tissue, with sensory nerves coming in and motor nerves going out. This is where most of the integration of information, learning and memory, and coordination of activity occur.

Somatic Nervous System

The nerve cells that are on the "front lines," interacting with the external environment, are referred to as the *somatic* system. This consists of a group of peripheral nerves that carry sensory information into the CNS and carry motor (movement) information back out. Cranial nerves that relate to vision, hearing, taste, smell, chewing, and movements of the tongue and face are included, as well as spinal nerves carrying information from the skin and joints and controlling movements of the arms and legs. We think of this system as serving voluntary actions. For example, a decision to move your leg results in activity in large cells in the motor cortex of your brain. These cells have long axons that extend down to the spinal motor neurons. These neurons have long axons that are bundled together to form nerves, which travel out directly to the muscles. The neurotransmitter at neuromuscular junctions in the somatic system is acetylcholine, which acts on receptors that excite the muscle.

CNS: brain and spinal cord.

Autonomic Nervous System

Your body's internal environment is monitored and controlled by the **autonomic** nervous system (ANS), which regulates the visceral, or involuntary, functions of the body, such as heart rate and blood pressure. It is important for us to understand this system, because many psychoactive drugs have simultaneous effects in the brain and on the ANS. The ANS is also of interest because it is where chemical neurotransmission was first studied. If the vagus nerve in a frog is electrically stimulated, its heart slows. If the fluid surrounding that heart is then withdrawn and placed around a second frog's heart, it too will slow. This is an indication that electrical activity in the vagus nerve causes a chemical to be released onto the frog's heart muscle. When Otto von Loewi first demonstrated this phenomenon in 1921, he named the unknown chemical "vagusstoffe." We now know that this is acetylcholine, the same chemical that stimulates muscle contraction in our arms and legs. Because a different type of receptor is found in the heart, acetylcholine inhibits heart muscle contraction.

The ANS is divided into **sympathetic** and **parasympathetic** branches. The inhibition of heart rate by the vagus nerve is an example of the parasympathetic branch; acetylcholine is the neurotransmitter at the end organ. In the sympathetic branch, norepinephrine is the neurotransmitter at the end organ. Table 5.1 gives some examples of parasympathetic and sympathetic influences on various systems. Note that often, but not always, the two systems oppose each other.

Because the sympathetic system is interconnected, it tends to act more as a unit, to open the bronchi, reduce blood supply to the skin, increase the heart rate, and reduce stomach motility. This has been called the "fight or flight" response and is elicited in many emotion-arousing circumstances in humans and other animals. Amphetamines and other diet pills, because they have a chemical structure that resembles norepinephrine, stimulate these functions in addition to their effects on the brain. Those drugs that activate the sympathetic branch are referred to as sympathomimetic drugs.

THE BRAIN

The Whole Brain

Although most of us don't think about it very often, our brain is obviously the most complex organ in our bodies. In fact, it is still the most amazing functional system in the world. We carry around in that small package a machine capable of storing and analyzing more information than the most powerful supercomputers. It might not be as fast at repetitive calculations, but it is able to deal simultaneously with thousands of kinds of input, select the important

TABLE 5.1

Sympathetic and Parasympathetic Effects on Selected Structures

Structure or function	Sympathetic reaction	Parasympathetic reaction
Pupil	Dilation	Constriction
Heart rate	Increase	Decrease
Breathing rate	Fast and shallow	Slow and deep
Stomach and intestinal glands	Inhibition	Activation
Stomach and intestinal wall	No motility	Motility
Sweat glands	Secretion	No effect
Skin blood vessels	Constriction	Dilation
Bronchi	Relaxation	Constriction

from the unimportant, and process images in ways unmatched by the most complex video devices. We might humbly remember that it is this fantastically complex machine that we are tinkering with when we take psychoactive drugs.

The brain has a rich supply of blood from four major arteries, so that drugs circulating in the blood have rapid access to the brain. However, the capillaries in the brain are different from those in the rest of the body—the cells are tightly joined so that some molecules cannot pass freely out of the blood and into the brain. This specialization is part of the blood-brain barrier, which keeps many drugs from reaching the brain. Of course, for a drug to be psychoactive, its molecules must be capable of passing the blood-brain barrier.

The brain contains billions of neurons, and each can influence or be influenced by hundreds of other neurons. If these neurons all looked alike and were connected in random ways, it would be difficult for us to begin to understand anything about the organization of brain activity and function. Therefore it would be impossible to get any understanding of psychoactive drug action by studying the brain. Luckily, study of the brain has revealed both structural and chemical organization that helps us understand many of the functional effects of psychoactive drugs.

Major Structures

Knowing about a few of the major brain structures makes it easier to understanding some of the effects of psychoactive drugs. When looking at the brain of most mammals, and especially of a human, much of what one can see consists of *cerebral cortex*, a layer of tissue that covers the top and sides of the upper parts of the brain (figure 5.5). Some areas of the cortex are known to be involved in processing visual information, and other areas are involved in processing auditory or somatosensory information. Relatively smaller cortical areas are involved in the control of muscles (motor cortex), and large areas are re-

ferred to as association areas. Higher mental processes, such as reasoning and language, take place in the cerebral cortex. In an alert, awake individual, arousal mechanisms keep the cerebral cortex active. When a person is asleep or under the influence of sedating drugs, the cerebral cortex is much less active, whereas other parts of the brain might be equally active whether a person is awake or asleep.

Underneath the cerebral cortex on each side of the brain and hidden from external view are the basal ganglia. The **basal ganglia** are important for the maintenance of proper muscle tone. For example, when you are standing still in a relaxed posture, your leg muscles are not totally relaxed. If they were, you would fall down in a slump. Instead, you remain standing partly because of a certain level of muscular tension, or tone, that is maintained by the output of the basal ganglia. Too much output from these structures results in muscular rigidity in the arms, legs, and facial muscles. This can occur as a side effect of some psychoactive drugs that act on the basal ganglia, or it can occur if the basal ganglia are damaged by **Parkinson's disease.**

The *hypothalamus* is a small structure near the base of the brain just above the pituitary gland. The hypothalamus is an important link between

---

autonomic: part of the nervous system that controls "involuntary" functions such as heart rate.

sympathetic: branch of the autonomic system involved in "flight or fight" reaction.

parasympathetic: branch of the autonomic system that stimulates digestion, slows the heart, and has other effects associated with a "relaxed" physiological state.

basal ganglia: subcortical brain structures controlling muscle tone.

Parkinson's disease: degenerative neurological disease involving damage to dopamine neurons.

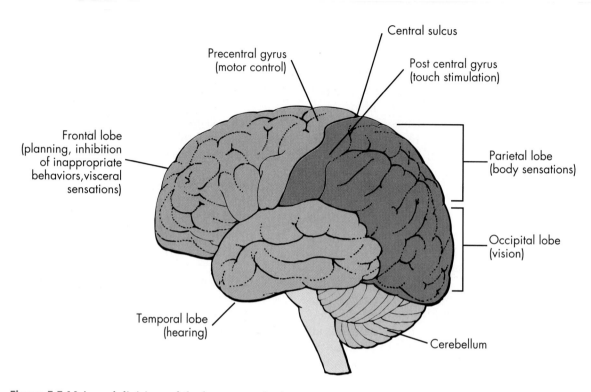

Central sulcus

Precentral gyrus
(motor control)

Post central gyrus
(touch stimulation)

Frontal lobe
(planning, inhibition
of inappropriate
behaviors, visceral
sensations)

Parietal lobe
(body sensations)

Occipital lobe
(vision)

Temporal lobe
(hearing)

Cerebellum

Figure 5.5 Major subdivisions of the human cerebral cortex

the brain and the hormonal output of this master gland (pituitary) and is thus involved in feeding, drinking, temperature regulation, and sexual behavior.

The *limbic system* consists of a number of connected structures that are involved in emotion, memory for location, and level of physical activity. Together with the hypothalamus, the limbic system involves important mechanisms for behavioral control at a more primitive level than that of the cerebral cortex.

The midbrain, pons, and medulla are parts of the brain stem that connect the larger structures of the brain to the spinal cord. Within these brain-stem structures there are many groups of cell bodies (nuclei) that play important roles in sensory and motor reflexes as well as coordinated control of complex movements. Within these brain-stem structures also lie the nuclei that contain most of the cell bodies for neurons

that produce and release the neurotransmitters dopamine, norepinephrine, and serotonin. Virtually all of the brain's supply of these important neurotransmitters is produced by a relatively small number of neurons (a few thousand for each neurotransmitter) located in these brain-stem regions.

In the lower *brain stem* a couple of small areas of major importance are found. One area is the vomiting center. Often when the brain detects foreign substances in the blood, such as alcohol, this center is activated, and vomiting results. It is easy to see the survival value of such a system to those animals, including humans, that have it. Another brain-stem center regulates the rate of breathing. This respiratory center can be suppressed by various drugs, resulting in respiratory depression that can lead to death.

These structures and their functions have been understood in general terms for many

Cerebrum

Frontal lobe
of cerebrum

Medial forebrain
bundle

Hypothalamus

Midbrain

Pituitary gland

Reticular
activating system

Cerebellum

Pons

Medulla oblongata

Figure 5.6 Cross section of the brain: major structures

years. Knowledge about such things comes partly from people who have suffered accidental brain damage and partly from experiments using animals. These basic structures exist in mammals other than humans, with functions and connections that are basically the same, so it is possible to learn a great deal about human brain function from animal experiments.

Chemical Pathways

Dopamine

In some cases, groups of cells in a particular brain region contain a particular neurotransmitter chemical, and axons from these cells are found grouped together and terminating in another brain region. We now think of many psy-

choactive drug actions in terms of a drug's effect on one of these chemical pathways. For example, we know that cells in the basal ganglia receive input from **dopamine** fibers that arise in the substantia nigra in the midbrain, course together past the hypothalamus, and end in the corpus striatum (part of the basal ganglia). This **nigrostriatal dopamine pathway** is what is

> **dopamine:** (*dope ah meen*) a neurotransmitter found in the basal ganglia and other regions.
>
> **nigrostriatal dopamine pathway:** one of two major dopamine pathways; damaged in Parkinson's disease.

Alzheimer's Disease

Alzheimer's disease is a progressive, degenerative disease of the CNS that results in a multifaceted loss of intellectual functioning, personality changes, and eventually death. Its incidence increases dramatically in old age, and it now appears that about half of all cases of senile dementia are a result of Alzheimer's disease. For generations we have accepted forgetfulness and mental confusion as natural consequences of growing old. Now we realize that this mental deterioration is no more natural than other diseases, and considerable efforts are being made to understand the cause of Alzheimer's disease. This may be a genetic disorder, a viral infection, some type of toxin, or some combination of those factors.

Although there are many abnormalities found in the brains of Alzheimer's patients, one has been a selective loss of the nicotinic type of acetylcholine receptors. There is no known relationship between smoking and Alzheimer's disease, and it is not believed that the nicotinic receptor changes are themselves the basic cellular cause of the disorder. However, the loss of those receptors might play a role in the loss of memory and other cognitive functions. Would stimulation of the remaining nicotinic receptors with a drug reverse some of the dementia? Nicotine is a potentially toxic drug, especially in the elderly, so its practical use would probably be quite limited. A recent report of a trial using nicotine patches on a small group of patients found some improvement in a learning task, but no evidence for improved memory or overall cognitive function.[7] Perhaps new drugs designed to act on nicotinic receptors will be more effective.

damaged in Parkinson's disease and also what is affected by the tranquilizers that produce muscular rigidity as a side effect (see chapter 9).

Another important dopamine pathway also begins in the midbrain but projects to areas in the limbic system and frontal cortex. This **mesolimbic dopamine pathway** has been proposed to play a role in some types of psychotic behavior. Also, the most widely studied neurochemical theory of drug dependence is based on the idea that all addictive drugs, from alcohol to heroin to cocaine to nicotine, stimulate dopamine neurons in this mesolimbic system. The mesolimbic system is proposed to be the main component responsible for the "reward" properties of electrical stimulation of the midbrain or limbic system. Thus, according to this theory, drugs lead to psychological dependence because they stimulate this reward system that is responsible for telling the rest of the brain "that's good—do that again."[3]

Acetylcholine

Pathways containing **acetylcholine** arise from cell bodies in the *nucleus basalis* in the lower part of the basal ganglia and project to much of the cerebral cortex. In patients who have died from *Alzheimer's disease,* these cells are damaged and the cortex contains much less acetylcholine than normal. This degenerative disease affects millions of older Americans, causing personality changes, memory loss, and widespread mental deterioration. Because this link with an acetylcholine pathway was only recently discovered, much research activity is currently focused on finding chemical means to diagnose and treat Alzheimer's disease. Acetylcholine has also been one of the main neurotransmitters studied with regard to the initiation of REM (rapid eye movement) sleep, during which most dreaming occurs.

Norepinephrine

Pathways arising from the *locus ceruleus* in the brain stem have numerous branches and project both up and down in the brain, releasing **norepinephrine** and influencing the level of arousal and attentiveness. It is perhaps through these pathways that stimulant drugs induce wakefulness. Norepinephrine pathways play an important role in the initiation of food intake, although other transmitter systems are also involved in the very important and therefore very complex processes of controlling energy balance and body weight.

Serotonin

Serotonin-containing pathways arise from the brain-stem *raphe nuclei* and also have projections both upward into the brain and downward into the spinal cord. Animal research has suggested one or more roles for serotonin in the complex control of food intake and the regulation of body weight. The diet drug fenfluramine, one half of the notorious "fen-phen" combination that became so popular in the 1990s, might cause its (limited) weight-reducing effects in humans by releasing and blocking the reuptake of serotonin.[4] Research on aggressiveness and impulsivity has also focused on serotonin. In studies with monkeys, low levels of serotonin metabolites in the blood have been associated with impulsive aggression as well as with excessive alcohol consumption. And humans who commit suicide or who make serious

---

mesolimbic dopamine pathway: (meh zo *lim* bick) one of two major dopamine pathways; may be involved in psychotic reactions and in drug dependence.

acetylcholine: (eh see till *co* leen) neurotransmitter found in the parasympathetic branch in the cerebral cortex.

norepinephrine: a neurotransmitter that may be important for regulating waking and appetite.

serotonin: (sehr o *tone* in) neurotransmitter found in the raphe nuclei; may be important for impulsivity, depression.

attempts might also show low levels of serotonin metabolites in the blood.[5] The success of selective serotonin reuptake inhibitors such as Prozac in treating major depressive disorder has also led to theories linking serotonin to depression. In all these cases (food intake and weight control, aggression and impulsivity, alcohol use, and depression) it is clear that environmental influences play important roles, and also other drugs that work through different neurotransmitter systems can also influence these behaviors. Therefore it is much too simple to attribute these behavioral problems to low serotonin levels alone. Hallucinogenic drugs such as LSD are believed to work by influencing serotonin pathways.

GABA

GABA is one neurotransmitter that is *not* as neatly organized into discrete pathways or bundles. GABA is found in most areas of the CNS and exerts generalized inhibitory functions. Many sedative drugs act by enhancing GABA inhibition (see chapter 8). Interfering with normal GABA inhibition, such as with the GABA-receptor-blocking drug strychnine, can lead to seizures resembling those seen in epilepsy.

Endorphins

Several chemicals in the brain produce effects similar to those of morphine and other drugs derived from opium. The term **endorphin** was coined in reference to endogenous (coming from within) morphine-like substances. These substances are known to play a role in pain relief, but they are found in several places in the brain as well as circulating in the blood, and their functions are not all known. Although it is tempting to theorize about the role of endorphins in addictions to drug use or other activities, the actual evidence linking addiction to endorphins has not been strong, and other neurotransmitter systems (particularly dopamine and serotonin systems) have also been shown to influence behaviors related to addiction.

DRUGS AND THE BRAIN

Drugs in the Brain

As we have seen, a drug is carried to the brain by the blood supply and, unless it is kept out by the blood-brain barrier, can diffuse out of the blood into the brain tissue. How does each drug know where to go once it gets into the brain? The answer is that the drug doesn't know, it goes everywhere. But because the drug molecules of LSD, for example, have their effect by acting on serotonin systems, LSD affects those brain systems that depend on serotonin. The LSD molecules that reach other types of receptors have no particular effect that we are aware of. Because the brain is so well supplied with blood, an equilibrium develops quickly for most drugs, so that the drug's concentration in the brain is about equal to that in the blood and the number of molecules leaving the blood is equal to the number leaving the brain to enter the blood. As the drug is removed from the blood (by the liver or kidneys) and the concentration in the blood decreases, more molecules leave the brain than enter it, and the brain levels begin to decrease.

We are currently able to explain the mechanisms by which many psychoactive drugs act on the brain. In most of these cases the drug has its effects because the molecular structure of the drug is similar to the molecular structure of one of the neurotransmitter chemicals. Because of this structural similarity, the drug molecules interact with one or more of the stages in the life cycle of that neurotransmitter chemical. We can therefore understand some of the ways drugs can act on the brain by looking at the life cycle of a typical neurotransmitter molecule.

Life Cycle of a Neurotransmitter

The neurotransmitter molecules that are used to communicate are made inside the cell from which they are to be released. This makes sense, because if they were just floating around everywhere in the brain, then the release of a tiny

Tyrosine
*Tyrosine
hydroxylase*

Dopamine
*Dopamine beta
oxidase*

DOPA
Dopa decarboxylase

Norepinephrine

■ carbon   ■ oxygen   ■ hydrogen   ■ nitrogen

Figure 5.7 Neurons use enzymes to synthesize the neurotransmitters dopamine and norepinephrine.

amount from a nerve ending wouldn't have much information value. However, the raw materials, or **precursors,** from which the neurotransmitter will be made are found circulating in the blood supply and generally in the brain. A cell that is going to make a particular neurotransmitter might need to bring in the right precursor in a greater concentration than exists outside the cell, and so machinery is built into that cell's membrane for active **uptake** of the precursor. In this process the cell expends energy to bring the precursor into the cell even though the concentration inside the cell is already higher than that outside the cell. Obviously, this uptake mechanism must be selective and must recognize the precursor molecules as they float by. The precursors themselves are often amino acids that are derived from proteins in the diet, and these amino acids are used in

the body for many things besides making neurotransmitters. In our example diagram of the life cycle of the neurotransmitter norepinephrine (figure 5.7), the amino acid tyrosine is recognized by the norepinephrine neuron, which expends energy to take it in.

GABA: inhibitory neurotransmitter found in most regions of the brain.

endorphins: opiate-like chemicals that occur naturally in the brain of humans and other animals.

precursors: chemicals that will be acted on by enzymes to form neurotransmitters.

uptake: an energy-requiring mechanism by which selected molecules are taken into cells.

After the precursor molecule has been taken up into the neuron, it must be changed, through one or more chemical reactions, into the neurotransmitter molecule. This process is called **synthesis.** At each step in the synthetic chemical reactions, the reactions are helped along by **enzymes.** These enzymes are themselves large molecules that recognize the precursor molecule, attach to it briefly, and hold it in such a way as to make the synthetic chemical reaction occur. Figure 5.8 provides a schematic representation of such a synthetic enzyme in action. In our example diagram of the life cycle of the catecholamine neurotransmitters dopamine and norepinephrine (figure 5.7), the precursor tyrosine is acted on first by one enzyme to make DOPA and then by another enzyme to make dopamine. In dopamine cells the process stops there, but in our norepinephrine neuron, a third enzyme is present to change dopamine into norepinephrine.

After the neurotransmitter molecules have been synthesized, they are stored in small, round packages called *vesicles* near the terminal from which they will be released. This *storage* process also calls for recognizing the transmitter molecules and concentrating them inside the vesicles.

As an electrical signal arrives at the axon terminal, some of the vesicles fuse with the cell membrane and then open, releasing several thousand neurotransmitter molecules at once. This process of neurotransmitter *release* takes place within a few thousandths of a second after the electrical signal reaches the terminal.

Once the neurotransmitter molecules are released into the small synaptic space between neurons, a particular molecule might just float around briefly, or it might be one of the ones that *bind* to the receptor on the membrane of the other neuron (figure 5.3). This receptor is the most important recognition site in the entire process, and it is also one of the most important places for drugs to interact with the natural neurotransmitter. With thousands of neurotrans-

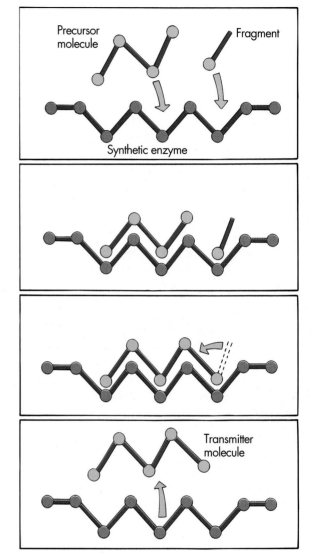

Figure 5.8 Schematic representation of the action of a synthetic enzyme. A precursor molecule and another chemical fragment both bind to the enzyme. The fragment has a tendency to connect with the precursor, but the connection is made much more likely because of the way the enzyme lines the two parts up. After the connection is made, the new transmitter molecule separates from the enzyme.

mitter molecules floating freely in the synapse, some will come near these receptors, bind to them briefly, then float away again. In the process of binding, the neurotransmitter distorts the receptor so that a tiny passage is opened through the membrane, allowing an electrical current in the form of charged ions moving through the membrane (figure 5.3). This opening does not last long, however, and within a few thousandths of a second the neurotransmitter molecule has left the receptor and the ion channel is closed.

The small, localized electrical current found at a single receptor might not have much effect all by itself. However, these electrical currents spread, and if enough receptors are activated at about the same time, then an electrical signal will be sent all the way down the axon to the terminal and a transmitter will be released there. The actual mechanisms by which this electrical current flows and moves along the membrane are too complicated to go into here. For our purposes, we need only remember that electrical signals carry information within a neuron and cause the release of chemical signals that carry information between neurons. These chemical signals in turn cause electrical signals in the next neuron, and so on (figure 5.4).

Because signaling in the nervous system occurs at a high rate, once a signal has been sent in the form of neurotransmitter release, it is important to terminate that signal so that the next signal can be transmitted. Thus the thousands of neurotransmitter molecules released by a single electrical signal must be removed from the synapse. Two methods are used for this. In some cells there is a process of **reuptake,** in which the neurotransmitter is recognized by a part of the membrane on the neuron from which it was released and the releasing neuron then expends energy to recapture its released neurotransmitter molecules. With other neurotransmitters, enzymes present in the synapse **metabolize,** or break down, the molecules (figure 5.9). In either case, as soon as neurotransmitter molecules are

released into the synapse, some of them are being removed or metabolized and never get to bind to the receptors on the other neuron. All neurotransmitter molecules might be removed in less than one hundredth of a second from the time they are released. In the case of our example neurotransmitter, norepinephrine, those molecules are rapidly taken back up into the neuron from which they were released. Once inside the neuron, those molecules are metabolized by an enzyme found in the cell.

Examples of Drug Actions

It is possible to divide the actions of drugs on neurotransmitter systems into two main types. Through actions on synthesis, storage, release, reuptake, or metabolism, drugs can alter the *availability of the neurotransmitter in the synapse.* Either the amount of transmitter in the synapse, when it is released, or how long it remains before being cleared from the synapse will be affected. The second main type of drug effect is *directly on the receptors.* A drug can mimic the action of the neurotransmitter and thus directly activate the receptor (an *agonistic* action), or it can occupy the receptor and prevent the neurotransmitter from activating it (an *antagonistic* action).

reuptake - stored

---

synthesis: the forming of a neurotransmitter by the action of enzymes on precursors.

enzyme: a large molecule that assists in either the synthesis or metabolism of another molecule.

reuptake: the taking back of recently-released neurotransmitter molecules into a neuron.

metabolize: to break down or inactivate a neurotransmitter (or a drug) through enzymatic action.

Figure 5.9 Schematic representation of the action of a metabolic enzyme. The transmitter molecule binds to the enzyme in such a way that the transmitter molecule is distorted and "pulled apart." The fragments then separate from the enzyme.

Drug effects on neurotransmitter availability

The drug L-dopa, which is used in the treatment of the CNS disorder called Parkinson's disease, is actually the normal precursor for dopamine and is converted into dopamine by synthetic enzymes inside the neurons. This makes more dopamine available for release each time the neuron "fires."

Perhaps one of the most interesting mechanisms is interference with the reuptake "pumps" that clear neurotransmitters such as norepinephrine, serotonin, and dopamine from the synapse by bringing them back into the neuron from which they were just released. Both the stimulant drug cocaine and most of the antidepressant drugs block one or more of these reuptake pumps and therefore cause the normally released neurotransmitter to remain in the synapse longer than normal. One of the most exciting research areas in the neurosciences these days is the search for greater understanding of how altering these reuptake processes can produce either cocaine-like or antidepressant effects, depending perhaps on the neurotransmitter systems affected and the time course of the drug's action.

Drug effects on neurotransmitter receptors

One method by which a drug can influence a receptor is to mimic the action of the neurotransmitter molecules. For example, the stimulant drug amphetamine is structurally similar to norepinephrine and dopamine, and one of its effects is to mimic these neurotransmitters at their receptors. Nicotine has effects very similar to the effects of the neurotransmitter acetylcholine (ACh) at some types of cholinergic receptors (they are called *nicotinic* acetylcholine receptors for this reason).

You may remember from figure 5.3 the idea that when the neurotransmitter binds to its receptor, in the process of matching up the structure of the transmitter molecule with the structure of the receptor, the receptor has to "bend" or "stretch" slightly, thus opening a small pore in the membrane. Suppose a drug molecule matched up so well with the receptor that the receptor didn't have to bend or stretch during

UP FOR
DEBATE

Chemical Causes of Mental Disorders

In the past, you may have been only vaguely aware of the number of reports that appear in newspapers and magazines indicating a possible breakthrough in some type of mental illness. Because new brain chemicals are being discovered at a rapid rate, it is inevitable that our hopes are high for new understanding and possible new treatments for schizophrenia, depression, or other major disorders. Chapter 9 presents the current state of our understanding and treatment of these problems.

Now that you have learned some things about the brain and its neurotransmitters and hormones, you will probably pay more attention to such reports in the future. If you want to test and sharpen your understanding of this important approach to understanding human behavior, go to a library and look back over the last year's issues of a magazine, such as *Time, Newsweek,* or *Scientific American.* A list of the brief news reports relating chemicals to mental disorders will probably include quite a few items.

the binding process. That drug molecule would fit the receptor better than the natural neurotransmitter. However, because the receptor doesn't have to change, there would be no effect on the electrical activity of the cell. Such agents are called antagonists, or "blockers," because by occupying the site, they prevent the normal neurotransmitters from having a postsynaptic effect. The antipsychotic (also called neuroleptic or major tranquilizer) drugs such as haloperidol (Haldol) act by blocking receptors for dopamine.

Please remember that when we refer to blocking receptors, only enough drug is given to block some of the receptors some of the time, so the net effect is to modulate or alter the activity in an ongoing system. Generally, if enough drug were given to block most of the receptors most of the time, the result would be highly toxic or even lethal.

Let's see if we can use our understanding of these mechanisms to predict what would happen if we tried to treat a psychotic patient who has Parkinson's disease with both L-dopa and haloperidol. The L-dopa is used to counteract damage to the dopamine systems in Parkinson's disease by making more dopamine available at the synapses. Haloperidol is used to control psychotic behavior, and it acts by blocking dopamine receptors. Thus the drugs seem to have opposing actions. In fact, haloperidol often produces side effects that resemble Parkinson's disease, and L-dopa often produces hallucinations in its users. The two drugs are not used in the same patient because each tends to reduce the effectiveness of the other.

CHEMICAL THEORIES OF BEHAVIOR

Drugs that affect existing biochemical processes in the brain often affect behavior, and this has led to many attempts to explain normal (not drug-induced) variations in behavior in terms of changes in brain chemistry. For example, differences in personality between two people might be explained by a difference in the chemical makeup of their brains, or changes in an individual's reactions from one day to the next might be explained in terms of shifting tides of chemicals. The ancient Greek physician Hippocrates believed that behavior patterns reflected the relative balances of four *humors:* blood (hot and wet, resulting in a sanguine or passionate nature); phlegm (cold and wet, resulting in a phlegmatic or calm nature); yellow bile (hot and dry, resulting in a choleric, bilious, or bad-tempered nature); and black bile (cold and dry, resulting in a melancholic or gloomy nature). The Chinese made do with only two basic dispositions: *yin,* the moon, representing the cool, passive, "feminine" nature; and *yang,* the sun, representing the warm, active, "masculine" nature. Thus any individual personality could be seen as a relative mixture of these two opposing forces. Unfortunately, most of the chemical-balance theories that have been proposed based on relative influences of different transmitters have not really been more sophisticated than these yin-yang or humoral notions of ancient times. Searches for differences in the amounts of norepinephrine, dopamine, serotonin, or other transmitters have not found evidence to relate the levels of these substances to personality differences, psychopathology, or mood swings. It is particularly tempting to speculate that alcoholics or drug addicts differ from "normal" people in the function of some enzyme or neurotransmitter receptor, but, as mentioned in chapter 3, no single biochemical theory of addiction has yet obtained sufficient experimental support to be considered an explanation.

One biochemical theory that still seems to have a lot of merit continues to guide people's thinking about major alterations in moods, such as those seen in clinical depression. Drugs that interfere with the catecholamines (norepinephrine and dopamine) are able to bring on a depressed mood, and drugs like cocaine and amphetamines that stimulate activity in these catecholamine systems produce a temporary mood elevation. Thus the *catecholamine theory of mood* is that too little activity in these systems can cause depression and too much can cause an excited or manic state (seen with high doses of amphetamines or cocaine). Although there is clear evidence that other neurotransmitter systems also play a role in the normal modulation of mood, the catecholamine theory is able to account for many of the basic drug effects on mood.

MODERN BRAIN IMAGING TECHNIQUES

Two techniques were developed during the 1980s for obtaining chemical "maps" of the brains of living humans. These techniques offer exciting possibilities for furthering our understanding of brain chemistry, abnormal behavior, and drug effects.

One of the techniques is positron emission tomography (PET) (figure 5.10). In this technique a radioactively labeled chemical is injected into the bloodstream, and a computerized scanning device then maps out the relative amounts of the chemical in various brain regions. Because all neurons in the brain rely on blood glucose for their energy, a labeled form of glucose can be used to see which parts of the brain are most active, and these will vary depending on what the person is doing. Similarly, blood flow to a particular brain region reflects the activity there, and labeled oxygen or other gases can map regional cerebral blood flow, which also changes depending on what the person is doing. More recently, labeled drugs that bind to dopamine, serotonin, or opiate receptors have been used, and it is therefore possible to "see" where the binding of those chemicals takes place in a living human brain. There is no doubt that our understanding of normal and abnormal brain function and of psychoactive drug effects will be advanced rapidly by these techniques over the next few years. Because these systems are very expensive to operate, they are found in only a few research hospitals.

Magnetic resonance imaging (MRI) is another relatively new brain imaging technique (figure 5.11). Rather than use radioactive labels, the technique relies on applying a strong magnetic field and then measuring the energy released by various molecules as the field is collapsed. The signals are complex, but with the aid of computers it is possible to detect certain chemical "fingerprints" in the signals. This technique gives

Figure 5.10 PET scan

Figure 5.11 MRI scan

a high-resolution image, does not require the administration of expensive radiochemicals, and because it can provide much information not attainable with simple X-ray studies, has been rapidly adopted by the medical community. MRI systems have been installed in most major hospitals. A refinement of this technique (functional MRI) using higher-energy magnetic fields and more complex computational techniques is beginning to be used to study apparent changes in metabolic activity in specific brain regions.[6]

SUMMARY

- Chemical signals in the body are important for maintaining homeostatis. The two types of chemical signals are hormones and neurotransmitters.
- Neurotransmitters act over brief time periods and very small distances because they are released into the synapse between neurons and are then rapidly cleared from the synapse.
- Receptors are specialized structures that recognize neurotransmitter molecules and, when activated, cause a change in the electrical activity of the neuron.
- The nervous system may be roughly divided into the central nervous system, the somatic system, and the autonomic system.
- The autonomic system, with its sympathetic and parasympathetic branches, is important because so many psychoactive drugs also have autonomic influences on heart rate, blood pressure, etc.
- Specialized chemical pathways contain the important neurotransmitters dopamine, acetylcholine, norepinephrine, and serotonin.
- The nigrostriatal dopamine system is damaged in Parkinson's disease, leading to muscular rigidity and tremors.
- The mesolimbic dopamine system is thought by many to be a critical pathway for the dependence produced by many drugs.
- The neurotransmitter GABA is inhibitory and is found in most parts of the brain.

▲ The life cycle of a typical neurotransmitter chemical involves uptake of precursors, synthesis of the transmitter, storage in vesicles, release into the synapse, interaction with the receptor, reuptake into the releasing neuron, and metabolism by enzymes.

▲ Psychoactive drugs have their actions either by altering the availability of a neurotransmitter at the synapse or by directly interacting with a neurotransmitter receptor.

REVIEW QUESTIONS

1. What are some examples of homeostatis in the human body?
2. What are the similarities and differences between hormones and neurotransmitters?
3. Describe the process of neurotransmitter release and receptor interaction.
4. Give some examples of the opposing actions of the sympathetic and parasympathetic branches of the autonomic nervous system. What is the neurotransmitter for each branch?
5. What is the function of the basal ganglia, and which neurotransmitter is involved?
6. What is the proposed role of the mesolimbic dopamine system in drug dependence?
7. Alzheimer's disease produces a loss of which neurotransmitter from which brain structure?
8. What neurotransmitter seems to have only inhibitory receptors?
9. After a neurotransmitter is synthesized, where is it stored while awaiting release?
10. What are the two main ways in which drugs can interact with neurotransmitter systems?
11. PET and MRI are two examples of what relatively new technology?

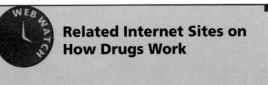

Related Internet Sites on How Drugs Work

   Society for Neuroscience: http://www.sfn.org
   Washington University introduction to PET scanning: http://www.imaging.wustl.edu/NIL/
   Drugs, Society, and Human Behavior: http://www.uwyo.edu/A&S/psyc/dshb.htm

REFERENCES

1. Feldman RS, Meyer JS, Quenzer LF: *Principles of neuropsychopharmacology,* Sunderland, MA, 1997, Sinauer.
2. Cooper JR, Bloom FE, Roth RH: *The biochemical basis of neuropharmacology,* ed 7, New York, 1996, Oxford University Press.
3. Koob GF, LeMoal M: Drug abuse: Hedonic hemostatic dysregulation, *Science* 278:52-58, 1997.
4. Weintraub M: Long-term weight control study: Conclusions, *Clinical Pharmacology and Therapeutics* 51: 586–594, 1992.
5. Azar B: Environment is key to serotonin levels, *Monitor,* American Psychological Association, April, 1997.
6. Maas LC and others: Functional MRI of human brain activation during cue-induced cocaine craving, *American Journal of Psychiatry,* in press, 1997.
7. Wilson AL and others: Nicotine patches in Alzheimer's disease: Pilot study on learning, memory, and safety, *Pharmacology, Biochemistry and Behavior* 51:509-514, 1995.

C H A P T E R

The Actions of Drugs

KEY TERMS	OBJECTIVES

After reading this chapter, you should be able to:

generic
placebo
double-blind procedure
dose-response curve
ataxia
comatose
ED_{50}
LD_{50}
therapeutic index (TI)
safety margin
side effects
potency
time course
cumulative effects
lipid solubility
intravenous (IV)
subcutaneous
intramuscular
blood-brain barrier
metabolite
liver microsomal enzymes
active metabolite
prodrugs
drug disposition tolerance
behavioral tolerance
pharmacodynamic tolerance

- Discuss the plant origins of most drugs.
- Explain the difference between a brand name and a generic name.
- Describe the major categories of psychoactive drugs and give an example of each.
- Distinguish between specific and nonspecific drug effects.
- Describe dose-response relationships and how they are interpreted to reveal effectiveness, safety, and potency.

- Explain how the route of administration, drug distribution, and processes of drug removal are reflected in the time course of a drug's action.
- Name three possible reasons for developing tolerance, and understand how one of them relates to physical dependence.

DRUGS

Sources of Drugs

You're probably already aware that most of the drugs in use fifty years ago originally came from plants. Even now, most of our drugs either come from plants or are chemically derived from plant substances. Have you ever wondered why the plants of this world produce so many drugs? Suppose a genetic mutation occurred in a plant so that one of its normal biochemical processes was changed and a new chemical was produced. If that new chemical had an effect on an animal's biochemistry, when the animal ate the plant the animal might become ill or die. In either case, that plant would be less likely to be eaten and more likely to reproduce others of its own kind. Such a selection process must have taken place many thousands of times in various places all over the earth. Many of those plant-produced chemicals have effects on the intestines or muscles; others alter brain biochemistry. In large doses the effect is virtually always unpleasant or dangerous, but in controlled doses those chemicals might alter the biochemistry just enough to produce interesting or even useful effects. In primitive cultures the people who learned about these plants and how to use them safely were important figures in their communities. Those medicine men (and women) were the forerunners of today's pharmacists and physicians, as well as being important religious figures in their tribes.

Today, the legal pharmaceutical industry is one of the largest and most profitable industries in the United States, with sales well over $50 billion a year.[1] With sales in the billions of dollars, many people expect that there are zillions of drugs. Not so. Over half of all prescriptions are filled with only 200 different drugs.

Drug Names

Commercially available compounds have several kinds of names: *brand, generic,* and *chemical.* The *chemical* name of a compound gives a complete chemical description of the molecule and is derived from the rules of organic chemistry for naming any compound. Chemical names of drugs are rarely used except in a laboratory situation where biochemists or pharmacologists are developing and testing new drugs.

Generic names are the official (i.e., legal) names of drugs and are listed in the *United States Pharmacopeia (USP).* Although a **generic** name refers to a specific chemical, it is usually shorter and simpler than the complete chemical

name. Generic names are in the public domain, meaning they cannot be trademarked.

The *brand* name of a drug specifies a particular formulation and manufacturer, and the trademark belongs to that manufacturer. A brand name is usually quite simple and as meaningful (in terms of the indicated therapeutic use) as the company can make it. For example, the name *Librium* was chosen for an antianxiety drug to indicate that it would liberate the user from worries. However, brand names are controlled by the FDA, and overly suggestive ones are not approved.

Brand Name versus Generic Name

When a new chemical structure, a new way of manufacturing a chemical, or a new use for a chemical is discovered, it can be patented. Patent laws in the United States now protect drugs for twenty years, and after that time the finding is available for use by anyone. Therefore, for twenty years a company that has discovered and patented a drug can manufacture and sell it without direct competition. After that, other companies can apply to the FDA to sell the "same" drug. Brand names, however, are copyrighted and protected by trademark laws. Therefore the other companies will have to use the drug's generic name or their own brand name. The FDA requires these companies to submit samples to demonstrate that their version is chemically equivalent, and also to do studies to demonstrate that the tablets or capsules they are making will dissolve appropriately and result in similar blood levels of the active drug. When a drug "goes generic," the original manufacturer might reduce the price of the brand name product in order to remain competitive.

CATEGORIZING DRUGS

Physicians, pharmacologists, chemists, lawyers, psychologists, and users all have drug classification schemes that best serve their own pur-

The Ever-Changing World of Drug Slang

Some textbooks of this type have attempted in the past to provide a compiled list of "slang terms" or "street names" for drugs. The problem is, as with slang terms for other topics, most of these names are peculiar to certain areas and to certain groups of people. For example, "crack" cocaine was at first also called "rock" in some areas. Some terms are used in popular films or are picked up by the media and become widely known and used, such as "crack" or "ice." But many others are probably not really worth writing down because they would have changed before the text could be printed. The NIDA compiled a list a few years ago, reporting over 150 street names for marijuana and about 75 for cocaine. They also found that the same name might be used in different places to refer to different drugs ("witch" and "white girl" were used for either heroin or cocaine).

Whether or not you drink alcohol, drinking is common in our society. What are some of the terms you and your friends use to refer to such things as a drink ("belt," "snort," "shot"), to becoming intoxicated ("ripped," "fried"), and to vomiting ("tossing your cookies")? You might find it interesting to keep track of the terms you hear for a week. Why do groups come up with terms like that? Do you think it's important for groups to develop expressions that only they can understand? Is that more important if they're talking about some type of illegal activity?

poses. A drug such as amphetamine might be categorized as a weight-control aid by a physician, because it reduces food intake for a period of time. It might be classed as a phenylethylamine by a pharmacologist, because its basic structure is a phenyl ring with an ethyl group and an amine attached. The chemist wastes no time and says flat-out that amphetamine is 2-amino-1-phenylpropane. To the lawyer, amphetamine might be only a controlled substance falling in Schedule III of the federal drug law, whereas the psychologist might say simply that it is a stimulant. The user might call it a diet pill or an upper. The important thing to remember is that any scheme for categorizing drugs has meaning only if it serves the purpose for which the classification is being made.

The scheme presented here organizes the drugs according to their effects on the user, with first consideration given to the psychological ef-

fects. The basic organization and examples of each type are given in Figure 6.1, but it is worthwhile to point out some of the defining characteristics of each major grouping.

At moderate doses, *stimulant drugs* produce wakefulness and a sense of energy and well-being. The more powerful stimulants, such as cocaine and amphetamines, can at high doses produce a manic state of excitement combined with paranoia and hallucinations.

If you know about the behavioral effects of alcohol, then you know about the *depressant drugs.* At low doses they appear to depress inhibitory parts of the brain, leading to disinhibition or

---

generic: (juh *ner* **ic)** a name that specifies a particular chemical but not a particular brand.

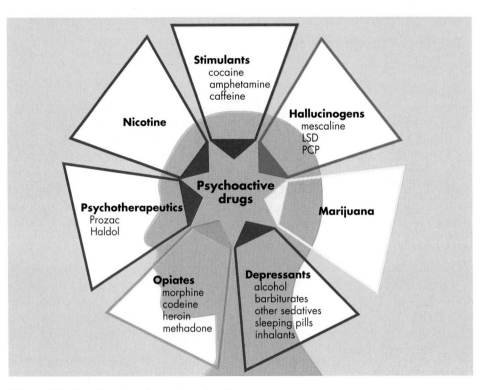

Figure 6.1 Classification of psychoactive drugs

relaxation and talkativeness that can give way to recklessness. As the dose is increased, other neural functions become depressed, leading to slowed reaction times, uncoordinated movements, and "passing out." It should be pointed out that stimulants and depressants do not really counteract one another. Although it may be possible to keep a drunk awake with cocaine, he or she would still be reckless, uncoordinated, and so on. Regular use of depressant drugs can lead to a withdrawal syndrome characterized by restlessness, shakiness, hallucinations, and sometimes convulsions.

Opiates are a group of analgesic (painkilling) drugs that produce a relaxed, dreamlike state; moderately high doses often induce sleep. Pharmacologically, this group is also known as the narcotics, and it is important to distinguish

them from the "downers," or depressants. With opiates there is a clouding of consciousness without the reckless abandon, staggering, and slurred speech produced by alcohol and other depressants. Regular use of any of the narcotics can lead to a withdrawal syndrome different from that of depressants and characterized by diarrhea, cramps, chills, and profuse sweating.

The *hallucinogens* produce altered perceptions, including unusual visual sensations and quite often changes in the perception of one's own body.

The *psychotherapeutic* drugs include a variety of drugs prescribed by psychiatrists and other physicians for the control of mental problems. The *antipsychotics,* such as haloperidol, are also called neuroleptics. They can calm psychotic patients and over time help them to control hallucinations and illogical thoughts. The *antidepressants,* such as fluoxetine (Prozac), help some people to recover more rapidly from seriously depressed mood states. Lithium is used to control manic episodes and to prevent mood swings in manic depressives.

As with any system of classification, there are some things that don't seem to fit into the classes. Nicotine and marijuana are two such drugs. Nicotine is often thought of as being a mild stimulant, but it also seems to have some of the relaxant properties of a low dose of a depressant. Marijuana is often thought of as a relaxant, depressive type of drug, but it doesn't share most of the features of that class. It is sometimes listed among the hallucinogens because it can produce altered perceptions at high doses, but that classification doesn't seem entirely appropriate for the way most people use it.

DRUG IDENTIFICATION

There are many reasons to identify exactly what drug is represented by a tablet, capsule, or plant substance. For example, the *Physician's Desk Reference (PDR)* has for many years published color photographs of many of the legally manufactured pharmaceuticals.[2] In this way a physician can determine from the pills themselves what drugs a new patient has been taking and in what doses. More critically, in emergency rooms it is possible to determine what drugs a person has just taken, if some of the pills are available for viewing. During the late 1960s access to a *PDR* was a big deal for those who were buying and selling amphetamines and barbiturates on the streets, although the later introduction of look-alikes by unscrupulous street dealers made the appearance of the pills a less reliable guide. Police chemistry labs also use the *PDR* to get a preliminary indication of the nature of seized tablets and capsules.

Even illicit drugs can sometimes be identified by visual appearance. Often the makers of illicit tablets containing amphetamines or LSD

mark them, however crudely, in a consistent way so that they can be recognized by their buyers. Such visual identification is far from perfect, of course. Cocaine or heroin powder can also be wrapped and labeled in a consistent way by street dealers. Some plant materials, such as psilocybin mushrooms, peyote cactus, or coca or marijuana leaves, can be fairly easy to identify visually, although again not with perfect accuracy.

If a case involving illicit drugs is to be prosecuted in court, the prosecution will usually be expected to present the testimony of a chemist indicating that the drug had been tested and identified using specific chemical analyses.

DRUG EFFECTS

No matter what the drug or how much of it there is, it can't have an effect until it is taken. For there to be a drug effect, the drug must be brought together with a living organism. After a discussion of the basic concepts of drug movement in the body, you will be better able to understand such important issues as blood alcohol level, the addictiveness of crack cocaine, and urine testing for marijuana use.

Nonspecific (Placebo) Effects

The effects of a drug do not depend solely on chemical interactions with the body's tissues. With psychoactive drugs in particular, the influences of expectancy, experience, and setting are also important determinants of the drug's effect. For example, a good "trip" or a bad trip on LSD seems to be more dependent on the personality and mood of the user before taking the drug than on the amount or quality of drug taken. Even the effect of alcohol depends on what the user expects to experience. *Nonspecific* effects are those that derive from the user's unique background and particular perception of the world. In brief, the nonspecific effects can include anything except the chemical activity of the drug and the direct effects of this activity. Nonspecific effects are also sometimes called **placebo** effects, because they can often be produced by an inactive chemical (placebo) that the user believes to be a drug. Those effects of a drug that depend on the presence of the chemical at certain concentrations in the target tissue are called *specific* effects. One important task for psychopharmacologists is to separate the specific effects of a drug from the nonspecific effects.

Placebo controls

Suppose you design an experiment with two conditions: One group of people receives the drug you're interested in testing, in a dose that you have reason to believe should work. Each person in the control group receives a capsule that looks identical to the drug but contains no active drug molecules (a placebo). It is very important that the people be randomly assigned to the groups and that they be treated and evaluated identically except for the active drug molecules in the capsules of the experimental group. For this reason, tests for the effectiveness of a new drug must be done using a **double-blind procedure.** Neither the experimental subject nor the person evaluating the drug's effect knows whether a particular individual is receiving a placebo or an experimental drug. Only after the experiment is over and the data have all been collected is the code broken so the results can be analyzed.

The double-blind procedure can also be used to compare the effectiveness of two different drugs. One investigator[3] studied the differential effects of two sedatives on anxiety in a group of patients of general practitioners. Neither the patient nor the physician knew which drug was being used, and before the start of medication, both the physician and patient had to indicate whether they were optimistic, indifferent, or pessimistic about the outcome of treatment. After two months, regardless of the drug used, patients for whom the doctors were optimistic

showed a 50 percent reduction in symptoms, whereas those patients for whom the physician had been pessimistic showed only a 20 percent decrease. Optimistic patients showed a 45 percent reduction in their anxiety symptoms, while the patients pessimistic about outcome showed a symptom drop of 35 percent. This experiment demonstrates the strength of nonspecific factors, and how the physician's expectations might be even more influential than the patient's expectations.

Nonspecific effects are not caused by the chemicals we give as drugs, but they are still "real" effects that in some cases might have a chemical basis. In a dental study,[4] some patients receiving a placebo reported a reduction of pain. When they were given a drug whose only effect is to block the opiate receptor in the brain, pain increased (just as it would have if the pain reduction were the result of morphine rather than a placebo). We know (see chapter 15) that the body manufactures chemicals—*endorphins*—very similar to morphine and that these endorphins play an important role in the normal control of pain. The results of the dental study suggest that the placebo (i.e., the belief that the individual was taking a drug that would reduce pain) resulted in an increase in production of endorphins and thus a decrease in pain. However, not all placebo effects on pain are mediated by endorphins. Scientists are now investigating the possible release of other natural chemicals in response to placebos.

Dose-Response Relationships

Perhaps the strongest demonstration of the specific effects of a drug is obtained when the dose of the drug is varied and the size of the effect changes directly with the drug dose. A graph showing the relationship between the dose and the effect is called a **dose-response curve.** Typically, at very low doses no effect is seen. At some low dose there is an observable effect on the response system being monitored.

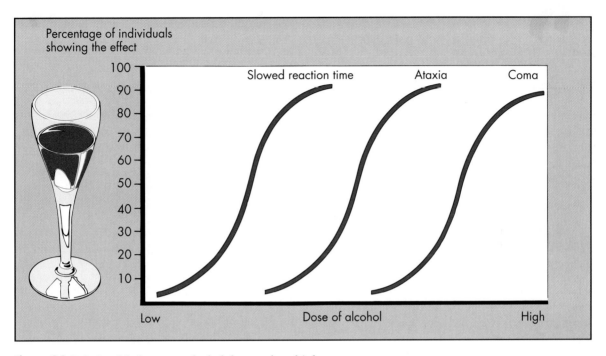

Figure 6.2 Relationship between alcohol dose and multiple responses

This dose is the threshold, and as the dose of the drug is increased, there are more molecular interactions and a greater effect on the response system. At the point where the system shows maximal response, further additions of the drug have no effect.

In some drug-response interactions, the effect of the drug is all-or-none, so that when the system does respond, it responds maximally. There might, however, be variability in the dosage at which individual organisms respond, and as the dose increases, there is an increase in the percentage of individuals who show the response.

Previously, it was mentioned that as the drug dose increases, sometimes new response systems are affected by the drug. This fact suggests that some response systems have higher drug thresholds than others. Figure 6.2 shows a series of dose-response curves for three different

effects of alcohol. As the dose increases from the low end, first a few and then more and more of the individuals show a slowing of their reaction times. If we also have a test for **ataxia** (staggering or inability to walk straight), we see that as the alcohol dose reaches the level at which most individuals are showing slowed

---

placebo: (pluh *see* **bo)** an inactive drug.

double-blind procedure: experiment in which both the doctor and the patient don't know which drug is being used.

dose-response curve: graph comparing the size of response to the amount of drug.

ataxia: (ay *tax* **ee ah)** uncoordinated walking.

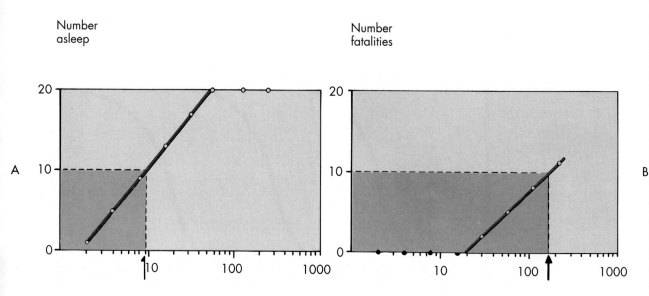

Figure 6.3 Calculation of **A**, effective dose, and **B**, lethal dose.

reaction times, a few are also beginning to show ataxia. As the dose increases further, more people show ataxia and some become **comatose** (they pass out and cannot be aroused). At the highest dose indicated, all of the individuals would be comatose. Note that we could draw curves for other effects of alcohol on such a figure; for example, at the high end we would begin to see some deaths from overdose, and a curve for lethality could be placed to the right of the coma curve.

In the rational use of drugs, there are four questions about drug dosage that must be answered. First, what is the effective dose of the drug for a desired goal? For example, what dose of morphine is necessary to reduce pain? What amount of marijuana is necessary for an individual to feel euphoric? How much aspirin will make the headache go away? The second question is, what dose of the drug will be toxic to the individual? Combining those two, what is the safety margin—how different are the effective dose and the toxic dose? Finally, at the effective dose level, what other effects, particularly ad-

verse reactions, might develop? Leaving aside for now this last question, a discussion of the first three deals with basic concepts in understanding drug actions.

Estimating the safety margin is an important part of the preclinical (animal) testing that is done on any new drug before it is tried in humans. In order to determine an *effective dose* (ED), it is necessary to define an effect in animals that is meaningful in terms of the desired human use. Although in some cases this is difficult, let us use the example of a new sleeping pill (hypnotic), and use several groups of 20 mice each. Each group will receive a different dose of our new hypnotic agent, and an hour later we will check to see how many mice in each group are sleeping. Let us assume that at the lowest dose we tested, only 1 of the 20 mice was asleep, and at the highest doses all were asleep, with other values in between as shown in Figure 6.3. By drawing a line through these points we can estimate the dose required to put any percentage of the mice to sleep. Even if we don't have a dose in our experiment that results

Animal Toxicity Tests

There has been increasing interest in the welfare of laboratory animals, and this has resulted in improved standards for housing, veterinary care, and anesthesia. Some "animal rights" groups have suggested that most types of animal research should be stopped altogether because the experiments are claimed to be either unnecessary or even misleading. The use of the LD_{50} test by drug companies, in which the researchers estimate the dose of a drug required to kill half the animals (usually mice), has been a particular target. The groups have claimed that these tests are outmoded and that toxicity could be predicted from computer models or work on isolated cell cultures.

A pamphlet published by People for the Ethical Treatment of Animals (PETA), one of the most emotional animal rights groups, claims on the one hand that the laboratory animals are sensitive beings with "distinct personalities. Just like you and me . . . ," but on the other hand that toxicity tests on animals are not relevant to humans because of basic biological differences. In reality, most basic biological functions are quite similar among all mammals, whereas the greatest differences between laboratory mice and humans would probably be found in the areas of thoughts, emotions, and "personality."

A specific case cited by PETA was thalidomide testing (see chapter 4), which they claim "passed animal safety tests with flying colors" and later caused thousands of human deformities. Some critical points in that argument were, however, omitted. Thalidomide caused birth defects when taken during pregnancy. Otherwise, its human toxicity was quite low. Thalidomide was not tested on pregnant animals. If it had been, the birth defects would have been detected. And because of thalidomide, the laws were changed thirty years ago to *require* that drugs to be used by humans during pregnancy first undergo testing in pregnant animals.

Admittedly, giving drugs to pregnant animals to see if they produce birth defects or spontaneous abortions may seem cruel. Would you volunteer to be the first living animal to take a new drug whose toxicity had been estimated by a computer model? Which pregnant humans should be the first?

in exactly 10 of the 20 mice sleeping, it is customary to calculate the $\mathbf{ED_{50}}$ (effective dose for 50 percent of the animals, in this case mice, tested).

Toxicity is usually measured in at least one early animal study by determining how many mice die as a result of the drug. Let's say we check each cage the next day to see how many mice in each group died. From such a study we can estimate the $\mathbf{LD_{50}}$ (lethal dose for

---

comatose: (*co mah tose*) unconscious and unable to be aroused.

$\mathbf{ED_{50}}$: effective dose for half of the animals tested.

$\mathbf{LD_{50}}$: lethal dose for half of the animals tested.

50 percent of the mice; see Figure 6.3). The **therapeutic index (TI)** is defined as LD_{50}/ED_{50}. Since the *lethal dose* should be larger than the *effective dose*, the TI should always be greater than 1. The question is, how large should the TI be if the company is going to go forward with expensive clinical trials? The answer is, it depends partly on the TIs of the drugs already available for the same purpose. Also, it should be obvious that the TI will depend on what effect was used to define the effective doses. If the same drug is to be used for surgical anesthesia, a deeper sleep will be required (one from which the mice will not awake when they are poked and prodded). Higher doses would be required for such an effect; thus the ED_{50} would be larger and the TI would be smaller.

This approach of estimating the dose to affect 50 percent of the mice is used in early animal tests because it is statistically more reliable to estimate the 50 percent point using a small number of mice per group than it would be to estimate the 1 percent or 99 percent points. However, with humans we don't do LD_{50} experiments. Also, with some disorders, perhaps the best drugs we have can help only half of the people. What we ultimately want is to estimate the dose that will produce a desired effect in some fraction of the patients (ED_{99}? ED_{60}?), and a dose that we think might be the lowest lethal dose (LD_1), or the lowest dose producing some other unacceptable toxic reaction. The difference between these doses would be called the **safety margin.**

Most of the psychoactive compounds have an LD_1 well above the ED_{95} level, so the practical limitation on whether or not, or at what dose, a drug is used is the occurrence of **side effects.** With increasing doses there is usually an increase in the number and severity of side effects—those effects of the drug that are not relevant to the treatment. If the number of side effects becomes too great and the individual begins to suffer from them, the use of the drug

will be discontinued or the dose lowered, even though the drug may be very effective in controlling the original symptoms. The selection of a drug for therapeutic use should be made on the basis of effectiveness in treating the symptoms with minimal side effects.

Potency

The **potency** of a drug is one of the most misunderstood concepts in the area of drug use. Potency refers only to the *amount of drug* that must be given to obtain a particular response. The smaller the amount needed to get a particular effect, the more potent the drug. Potency does not necessarily relate to how effective a drug is or to how large an effect the drug can produce. Potency refers only to relative effective dose; the ED_{50} of a potent drug is lower than the ED_{50} of a less potent drug. For example, it has been said that LSD is one of the most potent psychoactive drugs known. This is true in that hallucinogenic effects can be obtained with 50 micrograms (μg), compared with several milligrams (mg) required with other hallucinogens (a μg is 1/1000 of a mg, which is 1/1000 of a gram [g]). However, the effects of LSD are relatively limited—it doesn't lead to overdose deaths the way heroin and alcohol do. Alcohol has a greater variety of more powerful effects than LSD, even though in terms of the *dose* required to produce a psychological effect LSD is thousands of times more *potent.*

Time-Dependent Factors in Drug Actions

In the mouse experiment, we picked 1 hour after administering the drug to check for the sleeping effect. Obviously, we would have had to learn a bit about the **time course** of the drug's effect before picking 1 hour. Some very rapidly acting drug might have put the mice to sleep within 10 minutes and be wearing off by 1 hour, and we would pick a 20- or 30-minute time to check the effect of that drug. The time

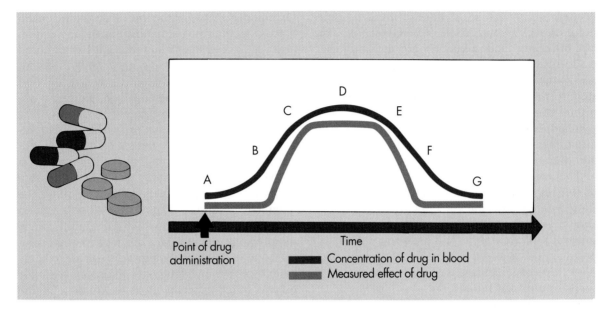

Figure 6.4 Possible relationship between drug concentration in body and measured effect of the drug

course of a drug's action depends on many things, including how the drug is administered, how rapidly it is absorbed, and how it is eliminated from the body.

Figure 6.4 describes one type of relationship between administration of a drug and its effect over time. Between points *A* and *B* there is no observed effect, although the concentration of drug in the blood is increasing. At point *B* the threshold concentration is reached, and from B to *C* the observed drug effect increases as drug concentration increases. At point *C* the maximal effect of the drug is reached, but its concentration continues increasing to point *D*. Although deactivation of the drug probably begins as soon as the drug enters the body, from *A* to *D* the rate of absorption is greater than the rate of deactivation. Beginning at point *D* the deactivation proceeds more rapidly than absorption, and the concentration of the drug decreases. When the amount of drug in the body reaches E, the maximal effect is over. The action dimin-

ishes from *E* to *F,* at which point the level of the drug is below the threshold for effect, although there is still drug in the body up to point G.

It should be clear that if the relationship described in Figure 6.4 is true for a particular

---

therapeutic index (TI): ratio of LD_{50} to ED_{50}.

safety margin: dosage difference between an acceptable level of effectiveness and the lowest toxic dose.

side effects: unintended effects that accompany therapeutic effects.

potency: measured by the amount of drug required to produce an effect.

time course: timing of the onset, duration, and termination of a drug's effect.

drug, then increasing the dose of the drug will not increase the magnitude of its effect. Aspirin and other headache remedies are probably the most misused drugs in this respect—if two are good, four should be better, and six will really stop this headache. No way! When the maximum possible therapeutic effect has been reached, increasing the dose can prolong the effect, but such an increase primarily serves to add to the number of side effects.

The usual way to obtain a prolonged effect is to take an additional dose at some time after the first dose has reached its maximum concentration and started to decline. The appropriate interval will vary from one drug to another. If doses are taken too close together, the maximum blood level will increase with each dose and can result in **cumulative effects.**

One of the important changes in the manufacture of drugs is the development of time-release preparations. These compounds are prepared so that after oral ingestion the active ingredient is released into the body over a six- to ten-hour period. With a preparation of this type, a large amount of the drug is initially made available for absorption, and then smaller amounts are released continuously for a long period. The initial amount of the drug is expected to be adequate to obtain the response desired, and the gradual release thereafter is designed to maintain the same effective dose of the drug even though the drug is being continually deactivated. In terms of Figure 6.4, a time-release preparation would aim at eliminating the unnecessarily high drug level at C–D–E while lengthening the C–E time interval.

GETTING THE DRUG TO THE BRAIN

A Little "Chemistry"

Obviously, if some drugs act quickly and others more slowly, it must be something related to the chemistry of the drug molecules that determines this. One of the most important considerations is the **lipid solubility** of the molecules. You've all seen the demonstration that "oil and water don't mix": shake up some salad oil with some water, let it stand, and the oil will all wind up floating on top. When other chemicals are added, sometimes they "prefer" to be concentrated more in the water or in the oil. For example, if you put sodium chloride (table salt) in with the oil and water and shake it all up, most of the salt will stay with the water. If you crush a garlic clove and add it to the mix, most of the chemicals that give garlic its flavor will remain in the oil. The extent to which a chemical can be dissolved in oils and fats is called its lipid solubility. Most psychoactive drugs dissolve to some extent in either water or lipids, and in our oil-and-water experiment some fraction of the drug would be found in each. The importance of lipid solubility will become clear as we see how molecules get into the brain.

Routes of Administration

We rarely put chemicals directly into our brains. All psychoactive drugs reach the brain tissue by way of the bloodstream. Most psychoactive drugs are taken by one of three basic routes: by mouth, injection, or inhalation.

Oral administration

Most drugs begin their grand adventure in the body by entering through the mouth. Even though oral intake might be the simplest way to take a drug, absorption from the gastrointestinal tract is the most complicated way to enter the bloodstream. A chemical in the digestive tract must withstand the actions of stomach acid and digestive enzymes and not be deactivated by food before it is absorbed. The antibiotic tetracycline provides a good example of the dangers in the gut for a drug. This antibiotic readily combines with calcium ions to form a compound that is poorly absorbed. If tetracycline is

Most drugs are taken orally.

For many heroin users, the preferred route of administration is by intravenous injection.

taken with milk (calcium ions), blood levels will never be as high as if it were taken with a different beverage.

The drug molecules must next get through the cells lining the wall of the gastrointestinal tract and into the blood capillaries. If taken in capsule or tablet form, the drug must first dissolve and then, as a liquid, mix into the contents of the stomach and intestines. However, the more other material there is in the stomach, the greater the dilution of the drug and the slower it will be absorbed. The drug must be water soluble for the molecules to spread throughout the stomach. However, only lipid-soluble and very small water-soluble molecules are readily absorbed into the capillaries surrounding the small intestine, where most absorption into the bloodstream occurs.

Once in the bloodstream, the dangers of entering through the oral route are not over. The veins from the gut go first to the liver (see Figure 6.5, on p. 124). If the drug is the type that is metabolized rapidly by the liver (nicotine is one example), very little may get into the general circulation. Thus nicotine is much more effective when inhaled than when swallowed.

Injection

Chemicals can be delivered with a hypodermic syringe directly into the bloodstream or deposited in a muscle mass or under the upper layers of skin. With the **intravenous (IV)** injection, the drug is put directly into the bloodstream, so the onset of action is much more rapid than with oral administration or with other means of injection. Another advantage is that irritating material can be injected this way, because blood vessel walls are relatively insensitive. Also, it is possible to deliver very high concentrations of drugs intravenously, which can be both an advantage and a danger. A major

cumulative effects: effects of giving multiple doses of the same drug.

lipid solubility: tendency of a chemical to dissolve in oil, as opposed to in water.

Intravenous (IV): (in trah *vee* nuss) injection directly into a vein.

disadvantage to IV injections is that the vein wall loses some of its strength and elasticity in the area around the injection site. If there are many injections into a small segment of a vein, as with an addict who must inject where he or she can see, the wall of that vein eventually collapses, and blood no longer moves through it, necessitating the use of another injection site. The greatest concern about IV drug use is the danger of introducing infections directly into the bloodstream, either from bacteria picked up on the skin as the needle is being inserted or from contaminated needles and syringes containing traces of blood. This risk is especially great if syringes and needles are shared among users, and this has been an important means by which AIDS and other blood-borne diseases have been spread (see chapter 2).

Subcutaneous and **intramuscular** injections have similar characteristics, except that absorption is more rapid from intramuscular injection. Muscles have a better blood supply than the underlying layers of the skin, and thus more area over which absorption can occur. Absorption is most rapid when the injection is into the deltoid muscle of the arm and least rapid when the injection is in the buttock. Intermediate between these two areas in speed of drug absorption is injection into the thigh. There is less chance of irritation if the injection is intramuscular because of the better blood supply and faster absorption. Another advantage is that larger volumes of material can be deposited in a muscle than can be injected subcutaneously. Sometimes it is desirable to have a drug absorbed very slowly (over a period of several days or even weeks). A form of the drug that dissolves only very slowly in water might be injected into a muscle, or the drug might be microencapsulated (tiny bits of drug coated with something to slow its absorption).

One disadvantage to subcutaneous injection is that if the material injected is extremely irritating to the tissue, the skin around the site of injection might die and be shed. This method of injection is not very common in medical practice but has long been the kind of injection used by beginning narcotic users. This is commonly called "skin popping."

Inhalation

Inhalation is the drug delivery system used for smoking nicotine, marijuana, or crack cocaine, for "huffing" gasoline, paints, or other inhalants; it is used medically with various anesthetics. It is a very efficient way to deliver a drug. Onset of drug effects is quite rapid because the capillary walls are very accessible in the lungs, and the drug thus enters the blood quickly. For psychoactive drugs, inhalation can produce more rapid effects than even intravenous administration. This is because of the patterns of blood circulation in the body (Figure 6.5). The blood leaving the lungs moves fairly directly to the brain, taking only 5 to 8 seconds to do so. By contrast, blood from the veins in the arm must return to the heart, then be pumped through the lungs before moving on to the brain, and this takes 10 to 15 seconds. Aerosol dispensers have been used to deliver some drugs via the lungs, but three considerations make inhalation of limited value for medical purposes. First, the material must not be irritating to the mucous membranes and lungs. Second, control of dose is more difficult than with the other drug delivery systems. Last, and perhaps the prime advantage for some drugs and disadvantage for others, there is no depot of drug in the body. This means that the drug must be given as long as the effect is desired, and also that when drug administration is stopped, the effect rapidly decreases.

Other routes

Topical application of a drug to the skin is not widely used because most drugs are not absorbed well through the skin. However, for some drugs this method can provide a slow, steady absorption over many hours. For example, a skin patch has been introduced that results in slow

Inhalation is a very effective means of delivering a drug to the brain.

absorption of nicotine over an entire day. This patch has been found to help prevent relapse in people who have quit smoking. Application to mucous membranes results in more rapid absorption than through the skin because these membranes are moist and have a rich blood supply. Both rectal and vaginal suppositories take advantage of these characteristics, although suppositories are used only rarely. The mucous membranes of the nose are used by most cocaine users, who "snort" or "sniff" cocaine powder into the nose, where it dissolves and is absorbed through the membranes. Also, the mucosa of the oral cavity provide for the absorption of nicotine from chewing tobacco directly into the bloodstream without going through the stomach, intestines, and liver.

Transport in the Blood

When a drug enters the bloodstream, often its molecules will attach to one of the protein molecules in the blood, albumin being the most common protein involved. The degree to which there is binding of drug molecules to plasma proteins is important in determining drug effects. As long as there is a protein-drug complex, the drug is inactive and also cannot leave the blood. In this condition, the drug is protected from inactivation by enzymes.

An equilibrium is established between the free (unbound) drug and the protein-bound forms of the drug in the bloodstream. As the unbound drug moves across capillary walls to sites of action, there is a release of protein-bound drug to maintain the proportion of bound to free molecules. Considerable variation exists among

> **subcutaneous:** (sub cue *tay* nee us) injection under the skin.
>
> **intramuscular:** injection into a muscle.

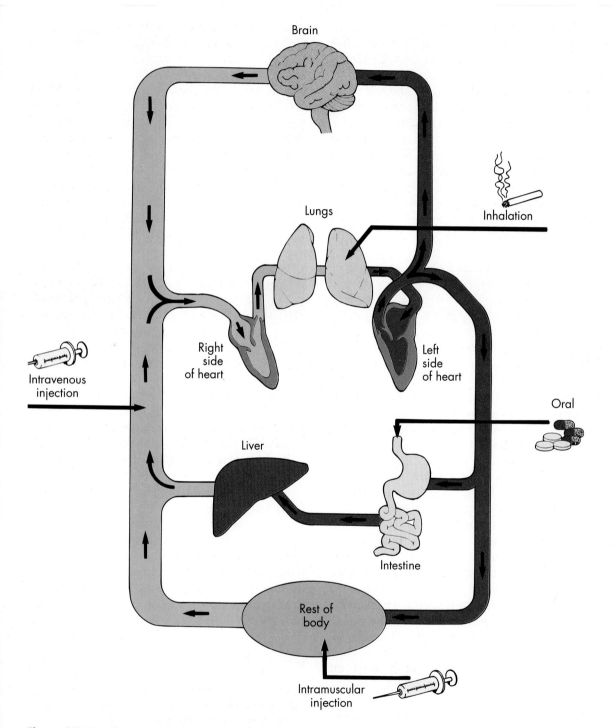

Figure 6.5 Distribution of drugs through the body

drugs in the affinity that the drug molecules have for binding with plasma proteins. Alcohol has a low affinity and thus exists in the blood-stream primarily as the unbound form. In contrast, most the molecules of THC, the active ingredient in marijuana, would be bound to blood proteins, with only a small fraction free to enter the brain or other tissues. If there were two drugs identical in every respect except protein binding, the one with greater affinity for blood proteins would require a higher dose to reach an effective tissue concentration. On the other hand, the duration of that drug's effect would be longer because of the "storage" of molecules in the blood.

Because different drugs have different affinities for the plasma proteins, one might expect that drugs with high affinity would displace drugs with weak protein bonds. And they do. This fact is important because it forms the basis for one kind of drug interaction. When a high-affinity drug is added to blood in which there is a weak-affinity drug already largely bound to the plasma proteins, the weak-affinity drug is displaced and will exist primarily as the unbound form. The increase in the unbound drug concentration helps move the drug out of the bloodstream to the sites of action faster and can be an important influence on the effect the drug has. At the very least, there will be a shortening of the duration of action.

Blood-Brain Barrier

The brain is very different from the other parts of the body in terms of the ability of drugs to leave the blood and move to sites of action. A barrier acts to keep certain classes of compounds in the blood and away from brain cells. Thus some drugs act only on neurons outside the central nervous system, that is, only on those in the peripheral nervous system, whereas others may affect all neurons.

The **blood-brain barrier** is not well developed in infants; it reaches complete devel-

opment only after one or two years of age in humans. Although the nature of this barrier is not well understood, several factors are known to contribute to the blood-brain barrier. One is the makeup of the capillaries in the brain. They are different from other capillaries in the body, because they contain no pores at all. Even small water-soluble molecules cannot leave the capillaries in the brain; only lipid-soluble substances can pass the lipid capillary wall.

If a substance can move through the capillary wall, another barrier unique to the brain is met. About 85 percent of the capillaries are completely covered with glial cells; there is little extracellular space next to the blood vessel walls. With no pores and close contact between capillary walls and glial cells, almost certainly an active transport system is needed to move chemicals in and out of the brain. In fact, known transport systems exist for some naturally occurring agents.

A final note on the mystery of the blood-brain barrier is that cerebral trauma can disrupt the barrier and permit agents to enter that normally would be excluded. Concussions and cerebral infections frequently cause enough trauma to impair the effectiveness of this screen, which normally permits only selected chemicals to enter the brain.

Possible Mechanisms of Drug Actions

Many different types of actions are suggested in later chapters as ways in which drugs can affect physiochemical processes, neuron functioning, and ultimately thoughts, feelings, and other behaviors. It is possible for drugs to affect all neurons, but many exert actions only on very specific presynaptic or postsynaptic processes.

---

blood-brain barrier: structures that prevent many drugs from entering the brain.

Effects on all neurons

Chemicals that have an effect on all neurons must do it by influencing some characteristic common to all neurons. One general characteristic of all neurons is the cell membrane. It is semipermeable, meaning that some agents can readily move in and out of the cell, but other chemicals are held inside or kept out under normal conditions. The semipermeable characteristic of the cell membrane is essential for the maintenance of an electric potential across the membrane. It is on this membrane that some drugs seem to act and, by influencing the permeability, alter the electrical characteristics of the neuron. Some drugs do affect the transport systems involved in maintaining the neuron, but usually the effect is more general.

Most of the general anesthetics have their effects on the central nervous system by a general influence on the cell membrane. Note that the agents that act in this way are depressants and that there are no drugs that increase the cell's activity level by affecting general membrane characteristics. The classical view of alcohol's action on the nervous system is that it has effects similar to the general anesthetics through an influence on the neural membrane. However, recent evidence has pointed to a more specific possible mechanism for alcohol's effects,[5] and in 1991 evidence was presented that even the gaseous anesthetics might be more selective in their action than was previously thought. Thus the entire notion that some drugs act nonspecifically through altering the nerve membrane's electrical properties is now in dispute.[6]

Effects on specific neurotransmitter systems

The different types of psychoactive drugs (e.g., narcotics, stimulants, depressants) produce different types of effects primarily because each type interacts in different ways with the various neurotransmitter systems in the brain. In chapter 5, it was pointed out that the brain's natural neurotransmitters are released from one neuron into a small space called a *synapse,* where they interact with receptors on the surface of another neuron. Psychoactive drugs can alter the *availability* of a neurotransmitter by increasing or decreasing the transmitter chemical's rate of synthesis, metabolism, release from storage vesicles, or reuptake into the releasing neuron. Or the drug might act directly on the *receptor,* either to activate it or to prevent the neurotransmitter chemical from activating it. With over fifty known neurotransmitters, and considering that different drugs can interact with several of these in different combinations, and given the variety of mechanisms by which each drug can interact with the life cycle of a natural neurotransmitter, the potential exists for an endless variety of drugs with an endless variety of actions. However, all of these actions are nothing more mysterious than a modification of the ongoing (and quite complex) functions of the brain.

DRUG DEACTIVATION

Before a drug can cease to have an effect, one of two things must happen to it. It may be excreted unchanged from the body (usually in the urine), or it may be chemically changed so that it no longer has the same effect on the body. Although different drugs vary in how they are deactivated, the most common way is for enzymes in the liver to act on the drug molecules to change their chemical structure. This usually has two effects: one, the **metabolite** no longer has the same action as the drug molecule, and two, the metabolite is more likely to be excreted by the kidneys.

The kidneys operate in a two-stage process. In the first step, water and most of the small and water-soluble molecules are filtered out. Second, most of the water is reabsorbed, along with some of the dissolved chemicals. The more lipid-soluble molecules are more likely to be reabsorbed, so one way in which the liver enzymes can increase the elimination of a drug is by changing its molecules to a more water-soluble and less lipid-soluble form.

FYI   Drug-Drug Interactions

It should be clear that there are many ways in which various drugs can interact with one another: They may have similar actions and thus have additive effects, one may displace another from protein binding and thus one drug may enhance the effect of another even though they have different actions, one drug may stimulate liver enzymes and thus reduce the effect of another, and so on.

Even restricting ourselves to psychoactive drugs, we find that there is such a variety of possible interactions that it would not make sense to try to catalogue them all here. Instead, a few of the most important interactions will be described in hopes that those can be remembered.

Respiratory Depression (Alcohol, Other Depressants, Opiates)

There is no doubt that the single most important type of drug interaction for psychoactive drugs is the effect on respiration rate. All depressant drugs (sedatives such as Valium and Xanax, barbiturates, sleeping pills), alcohol, and all narcotics tend to slow down the rate at which people breathe in and out, because of effects in the brainstem. Combining any of these drugs can produce effects that are additive and in some cases may be more than additive. Respiratory depression is the most common type of drug overdose death: people simply stop breathing.

Stimulants and Antidepressants

Although antidepressant drugs such as amitriptyline (Elavil) and Prozac are not in themselves stimulants, they can potentiate the effects of stimulant drugs such as cocaine and amphetamine, possibly leading to manic overexcitement, irregular heartbeat, high blood pressure, or other effects.

Stimulants and Depressants

It might seem that the "uppers" and "downers" would counteract one another, but that's generally not the case when it comes to behavior. Drugs such as Valium, Xanax, or alcohol may lead to disinhibition and recklessness. When combined with the effects of stimulants, explosive and dangerous behavior are possible!

Cocaine + Alcohol = Cocaethylene

Although this may sound like a special case of combining a depressant and a stimulant (it is), there is another possible interaction in that cocaine can combine chemically with ethyl alcohol to produce a substance called cocaethylene—a potent stimulant that animal studies indicate may be twenty times as toxic as cocaine. The ramifications of this recent discovery are not yet clear (see chapter 7).

The enzymes of the liver that metabolize drugs are quite different from the enzymes in the rest of the body. These **liver microsomal enzymes** do not normally have much to do, since there are no naturally occurring chemicals within the body for them to act on. They seem

metabolite: (muh *tab* oh lite) product of enzyme action on a drug.

liver microsomal enzymes: (my cro *zhome* al) enzymes that metabolize drugs.

to be specialized for inactivating various general kinds of foreign chemicals that the organism might ingest. This is not like the immune system, in which foreign proteins stimulate the production of antibodies for that protein—the enzymes already exist in the liver and are waiting for the introduction of certain types of chemicals. We described earlier how various plants have evolved the ability to produce chemicals that do nothing directly for the plant but serve to kill or make ill any animals that eat the plant. In defense, apparently many animals have evolved mechanisms for eliminating these toxic chemicals once they are eaten.

Although the enzymes are already present, the introduction of a drug may stimulate an increased production of the enzymes and an increase in their activity. Over two hundred drugs have been shown to increase the activity of these drug-metabolizing enzymes: Phenobarbital and DDT have this effect in common. When the enzymes are stimulated, drug metabolism speeds up, and the duration of action of that drug and other drugs in the body is decreased.

Not all of the metabolites of drugs are inactive. Both diazepam (Valium) and marijuana have **active metabolites** that produce effects similar to those of the original (parent) drug, and prolong the effect considerably. In fact, so-called **prodrugs** are being developed that are inactive in the original form and become active only after they are altered by the liver enzymes.

MECHANISMS OF TOLERANCE AND PHYSICAL DEPENDENCE

You should remember that the phenomena of tolerance and physical dependence have historically been associated with drug addiction. *Tolerance* refers to a situation in which repeated administration of the same dose of a drug results in gradually diminishing effects. There are at least three different mechanisms by which a reduced drug response can come about.

Drug Disposition Tolerance

Sometimes the use of a drug increases the drug's rate of metabolism or excretion. This is referred to as **drug disposition tolerance** or pharmacokinetic tolerance. For example, phenobarbital induces increased activity of the liver microsomal enzymes that metabolize the drug. Increased metabolism reduces the effect of subsequent doses, perhaps leading to increased dosage. But additional amounts of the drug increase the activity of the enzymes even further, and the circle continues. Another possible mechanism for increased elimination has to do with the pH (acidity) of the urine. Amphetamine is excreted unchanged in the urine, and the rate of excretion can be increased by making the urine more acidic. Both amphetamine itself and the decreased food intake that often accompanies heavy amphetamine use tend to make the urine more acidic. Amphetamine is excreted twenty times as rapidly in urine with a pH of 5 as compared with a pH of 8.

Behavioral Tolerance

Particularly when the use of a drug interferes with normal behavioral functions, individuals may learn to adapt to the altered state of their nervous system and therefore compensate somewhat for the impairment. In some ways, this is analogous to a person who breaks a wrist and learns to write with the nonpreferred hand—the handwriting probably won't be as good that way, but with practice the disruptive effect on writing will be reduced. A person who regularly drives a car after drinking alcohol will never be as good a driver as he or she would be sober, but with experience the impairment may be reduced. In this type of tolerance, called **behavioral tolerance,** the drug may continue to have the same biochemical effect but with a reduced effect on behavior.

Pharmacodynamic Tolerance

In many cases the amount of drug reaching the brain doesn't change, but the sensitivity of the neurons to the drug's effect does change. This is best viewed as an attempt by the brain to maintain its level of functioning within normal limits (an example of homeostasis). There are many possible mechanisms for this. For example, if the CNS is constantly held in a depressed state through the regular use of alcohol or another depressant drug, the brain might compensate by reducing the amount of the inhibitory neurotransmitter GABA that is released, or by reducing the number of inhibitory GABA receptors (many studies show that the brain does regulate the numbers of specific types of receptors). This adjustment might take several days, and after it occurs the depressant drug doesn't produce as much CNS depression as it did before. If more drug is taken, the homeostatic mechanisms might further decrease the release of GABA or the number of GABA receptors. If the drug is abruptly stopped, the brain now does not have the proper level of GABA inhibition, and the CNS becomes overexcited, leading to wakefulness, nervousness, possibly hallucinations, and the sensation that something is crawling on the skin. In severe cases, brain activity becomes uncontrolled and seizures can occur. These withdrawal symptoms are the defining characteristic of physical dependence. Thus, **pharmacodynamic tolerance** leads not only to a reduced effectiveness of the drug, but also to these withdrawal reactions that indicate physical dependence. After several days the compensating homeostatic mechanisms return to a normal state, the withdrawal symptoms cease, and the individual is no longer as tolerant to the drug's effect.

SUMMARY

▲ Most drugs are derived directly or indirectly from plants.
▲ The legal pharmaceutical industry is one of the largest and most profitable industries in the United States.
▲ Brand names belong to one company; the generic name for a chemical may be used by many companies.
▲ Most psychoactive drugs may be categorized as stimulants, depressants, opiates, hallucinogens, or some type of psychotherapeutic agent.
▲ Drugs can be identified by the appearance of commercial tablets or capsules, in some cases by the packaging or appearance of illicit drugs, or by a variety of chemical assays.

active metabolite: a metabolite that has drug actions of its own.

prodrugs: drugs that are inactive until acted on by enzymes in the body.

drug disposition tolerance: tolerance caused by more rapid elimination of the drug

behavioral tolerance: tolerance caused by learned adaptation to the drug.

pharmacodynamic tolerance: tolerance caused by altered nervous system sensitivity.

- ▲ Specific drug effects are related to the concentration of the chemical; nonspecific effects can also be called placebo effects.
- ▲ Because each drug is capable of producing many effects, many dose-effect relationships can be studied for any given drug.
- ▲ The ratio of LD_{50} to ED_{50} is called the therapeutic index and is one indication of the relative safety of a drug for a particular use or effect.
- ▲ The potency of a drug refers to the amount needed to produce an effect, not to the importance of the effect.
- ▲ The time course of a drug's effect is influenced by many factors, including route of administration, protein binding in the blood, and rate of elimination.
- ▲ The blood-brain barrier prevents many drugs from reaching effective concentrations in the brain.
- ▲ It is now believed that virtually all psychoactive drugs have relatively specific effects on one neurotransmitter system or more, either through altering availability of the transmitter or by interacting with its receptor.
- ▲ The liver microsomal enzyme system is important for drug deactivation and for some types of drug-drug interactions.
- ▲ Drug tolerance can result from changes in distribution and elimination, from behavioral adaptations, or from changes in the responsiveness of the nervous system caused by compensatory (homeostatic) mechanisms. Physical dependence (withdrawal) can be a consequence of this last type of tolerance.

REVIEW QUESTIONS

1. Morton's makes table salt, also known as sodium chloride. Which is the chemical name, which is the generic name, and which is the brand name?

2. Into which major category does each of these drugs fall: heroin, cocaine, alcohol, LSD, Prozac?
3. Why might nonspecific factors influence psychoactive drug effects more than the effect of an antibiotic?
4. Why should LD_{50} always be greater than ED_{50}?
5. Why do people say that LSD is one of the most potent psychoactive drugs?
6. Which route of administration gets a drug to the brain most quickly?
7. If an elderly person has less protein in the blood than a younger person, how would you adjust the dose of a drug that has high protein binding?
8. How might two drugs interact with each other through actions on the liver microsomal enzyme system?
9. Which type of tolerance is related to physical dependence, and why?

Related Internet Sites on Pharmacology

International Union of Pharmacology: http://www.medfac.unimelb.edu.au/iuphar/

Crump Institute Pharmacology: Launching Pad: http://laxmi.nuc.ucla.edu:8000/crump/html_docs/ignarro/Html/Pharmacology.htm

And don't forget to check our own *Drugs, Society, and Human Behavior* site for more links to these and other sites of interest: http://www.uwyo.eud/a&s/psyc/dshb.htm

REFERENCES

1. *Industry profile 1997,* Pharmaceutical Research and Manufacturing Association, Washington, DC.
2. *Physician's desk reference,* Oradell, NJ, annual, Medical Economics Company.
3. Wheatley D: Effects of doctors' and patients' attitudes and other factors on response to drugs. In Rickels K, editor: *Nonspecific factors in drug therapy,* Springfield, Ill, 1968, Charles C Thomas.
4. Fields HL, Levine JD: Biology of placebo analgesia, *Am J Med* 70:745, 1981.
5. Kolata G: New drug counters alcohol intoxication, *Science* 234:1198, 1986.
6. Franks NP, Lieb WR: Stereospecific effects of inhalational general anesthetic optical isomers on nerve ion channels, *Science* 254:427, 1991.

ASSESS YOURSELF

How Do Drugs Work?

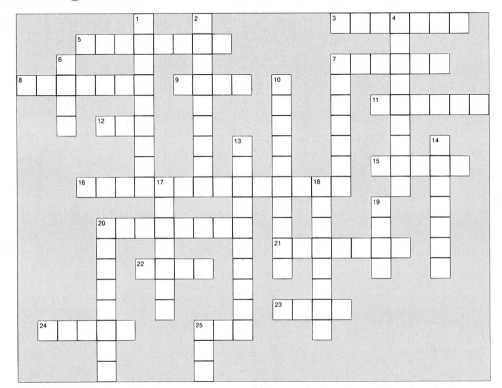

ACROSS

3. Space between two neurons
5. Cause for tobacco dependence
7. Brain part for integration of information, planning
8. Chemical signal carried through the blood
9. Amount of drug given
11. Fastest way to get a drug to the brain
12. Agency responsible for regulating pharmaceuticals
15. Where most drugs are broken down
16. Transmitter in the sympathetic branch
20. Transmitter in the mesolimbic system
21. Most widely used depressant
22. Axons, dendrites are part of the nerve _____ .
23. Most rapid method of injection is into a _____.
24. Potent CNS drugs must be _____ soluble
25. Type of modern brain scan using radioactive chemicals

DOWN

1. Reduced effect of a drug after repeated use
2. Opiate-like substance found in the brain
4. Nervous system controlling heart, pupils of the eye, etc.
6. Chemical that affects a living organism
7. Powerful stimulant derived from a South American plant
10. An _____ signal travels along the axon
13. Drug that makes you drowsy, drunk, uncoordinated
14. Drug name used by several companies
17. Inactive or "fake" drug
18. Opium, morphine, heroin, etc.
19. Neuron part that carries electrical signals to the terminals
20. Neuron part that picks up signals from other neurons
25. Hallucinogen sometimes smoked on marijuana

Uppers and Downers

We start our review of drugs by studying two types that have straightforward actions on behavior. Stimulants generally excite the central nervous system, whereas depressants generally inhibit it. In section 3, we find that most drugs used in treating mental disorders are *not* simply uppers or downers—their action is more complicated. However, this can best be appreciated by comparing them with the stimulants and depressants. Antidepressant drugs, used in treating psychological depression, are *not* stimulants. When taken for several weeks, they can help raise a depressed mood into the normal range, but they don't produce excited, sleepless effects as stimulants do. Likewise, the tranquilizers used in treating psychotic behavior are not depressants and do not always produce the drowsiness that sedatives and sleeping pills do.

7 Stimulants
How do the stimulant drugs, cocaine and amphetamines, act on the body?

8 Depressants and Inhalants
How do the depressants work as sedatives and hypnotics?

9 Psychotherapeutic Drugs
Which drugs are used in the treatment of depression, schizophrenia, and other mental disorders?

7

Stimulants

KEY TERMS	OBJECTIVES

After reading this chapter, you should be able to:

coca
cocaine
crack
rock
coca paste
cocaine hydrochloride
freebase
cocaethylene
ephedrine
sympathomimetic
amphetamine
narcolepsy
speed
crank
ice
ADHD
methylphenidate (Ritalin)

- Discuss the history of the origin and early uses of both cocaine and amphetamine.
- Describe the beginning of legal restrictions on each of these drugs and how illicit use of the two drugs has interacted with legal restrictions over the years.
- Discuss how these drugs work in the brain and how their chemical structures relate to their mechanism of action.

- Describe the previous and current medical uses of cocaine and amphetamine.
- Discuss the use of stimulant drugs as weight reduction medication.
- Discuss the potential for addiction and the possible toxic reactions to each of these drugs.
- Describe the sources of illicit supply for each drug and the current trends in illicit use.

Stimulants are the drugs that can keep you going, both mentally and physically, when you should be tired. There have been lots of claims about the other things these drugs can do for (and to) people. Do they really make you smarter, faster, or stronger? Can they sober you up? Improve your sex life? Are they addicting?

We can divide the stimulants somewhat arbitrarily: the mild stimulants nicotine and caffeine are discussed in chapters 12 and 13; *cocaine* and *amphetamine* are covered in this chapter. These two powerful stimulants produce effects that were virtually unknown to most humans until just over a hundred years ago. Since the widespread introduction of cocaine into western Europe and the United States in the last century, there has always been a fair-sized minority of individuals committed to the regular recreational use of the stimulants, but neither cocaine nor amphetamine has ever achieved widespread social acceptance as a recreational drug.

COCAINE

History

The coca plant

The origin of the earliest civilization in the Americas, the beginning around 5000 B.C. of what was to become the Inca Empire in Peru, has recently been traced to the use of **coca**. Natives of the Andes mountains in Bolivia and Peru today still use coca as their ancestors did: chewing the leaves and holding a ball of coca leaf almost continually in the mouth. The freedom from fatigue provided by the drug is legendary in allowing these natives to run or to carry large bundles great distances over high mountain trails. The psychoactive effects can be made stronger by adding some calcified lime to raise the alkalinity inside the mouth—we now know that this increases the extraction of **cocaine** and allows greater absorption into the blood supplying the inside of the mouth. It appears that humans in the Andes first settled down and formed communities around places where this calcified lime could be mined.[1] Eventually they took up the planting and harvesting of crops in the nearby fields—and one of those important crops was of course coca.

The terrain of the Andes in Bolivia and Peru is poorly suited for growing almost everything. *Erythroxylon coca*, however, seems to thrive at elevations of 2,000 to 8,000 feet (600 to 2,400 meters) on the Amazon slope of the mountains, where over 100 inches (254 centimeters) of rain fall annually. The shrub is pruned to prevent it from reaching the normal height of 6 to 8 feet (1.8 to 2.4 meters), so that the picking, which is done three or four times a year, is easier to accomplish. The shrubs are grown in small, two to three acre patches called cocals, some of which are known to have been under cultivation for over 800 years.

Before the sixteenth-century invasion by Pizarro, the Incas had built a well-developed civilization in Peru. The coca leaf was an important part of the culture, and although earlier

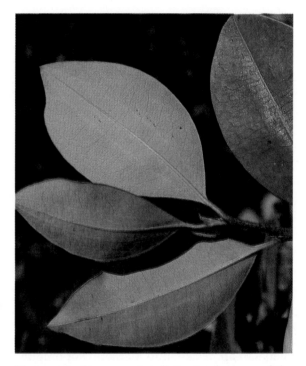

The coca leaf is somewhat distinctive because of the bilateral veins running parallel to the leaf's center.

use was primarily in religious ceremonies, coca was treated as money by the time the conquistadors arrived. The Spanish adopted this custom and paid coca leaves to the native laborers for mining and transporting gold and silver. Even then the leaf was recognized as increasing strength and endurance while decreasing the need for food.

Early European chroniclers of the Inca civilization reported on the unique qualities of this

---

coca: a bush that grows in the Andes and produces cocaine.

cocaine: the active chemical in the coca plant.

plant, but it never interested Europeans until the last half of the nineteenth century. At that time the coca leaf contributed to the economic well-being and fame of three individuals. They, in turn, brought the Peruvian shrub to the notice of the world.

Coca Wine to Coca-Cola

The first of these men was Angelo Mariani, a French chemist. His contribution was to introduce the coca leaf indirectly to the general public. Mariani imported tons of coca leaves and used an extract from them in many products. The quid of leaves was missing, but you could suck on a coca lozenge, drink coca tea, or obtain the coca leaf extract in any of a large number of other products. It was Mariani's coca wine, though, that made him rich and famous. Assuredly, it had to be the coca leaf extract in the wine that prompted the pope to present a medal of appreciation to Mariani. Not only the pope but royalty and the man in the street benefited from the Andean plant. For them, as it had for the Incas for a thousand years and was to do for Americans who drank early versions of Coca-Cola (see chapter 13), the extract of the coca leaf lifted their spirits, freed them from fatigue, and gave them a general good feeling.

Local anesthesia

Coca leaves contain, besides the oils that give them flavor, the active chemical cocaine (up to almost 2 percent). Cocaine was isolated before 1860, but there is still debate over who did it first and exactly when. Simple and inexpensive processing of 500 kilograms of coca leaves yields 1 kilogram of cocaine. An available supply of pure cocaine and the newly developed hypodermic syringe improved the drug-delivery system, and in the 1880s physicians began to experiment with it. In the United States, the second of cocaine's proponents, Dr. W. S. Halsted, who was later referred to as "the father of modern surgery," experimented with the

The tonic in this 1893 advertisement was made from 2 ounces of cola leaves soaked in 18 ounces of red wine. Although the cocaine content of the leaves varied, a typical glass probably contained less than 100 mg (1/10 g) of cocaine.

ability of cocaine to produce local anesthesia and to block sensation from a large area if the drug was injected near a nerve trunk.

Early psychiatric uses

The third famous man to encourage cocaine use was a young Viennese physician named Sigmund Freud, who studied the drug's psycho-

Where is most cocaine grown? ★ PERU ★

logical effects. In 1884 Freud wrote to his fiancée that he had been experimenting with "a magical drug." He had had dazzling success in treating a case of gastric catarrh, and he wrote, "If it goes well I will write an essay on it and I expect it will win its place in therapeutics by the side of morphium, and superior to it. . . . I take very small doses of it regularly against depression and against indigestion, and with the most brilliant success." He urged his fiancée, his sisters, his colleagues, and his friends to try it, extolling the drug as a safe exhilarant, which he himself used and recommended as a treatment for morphine addiction. For emphasis he wrote in italics, *"inebriate asylums can be entirely dispensed with."*[2]

In an 1885 lecture before a group of psychiatrists, Freud commented on the use of cocaine as a stimulant, saying, "On the whole it must be said that the value of cocaine in psychiatric practice remains to be demonstrated, and it will probably be worthwhile to make a thorough trial as soon as the currently exorbitant price of the drug becomes more reasonable." The first of the consumer advocates!

Freud was more convinced about another use of the drug, however, and in the same lecture[3] said:

> We can speak more definitely about another use of cocaine by the psychiatrist. It was first discovered in America that cocaine is capable of alleviating the serious withdrawal symptoms observed in subjects who are abstaining from morphine and of suppressing their craving for morphine. . . . On the basis of my experiences with the effects of cocaine, I have no hesitation in recommending the administration of cocaine for such withdrawal cures in subcutaneous injections of 0.03–0.05 g per dose, without any fear of increasing the dose. On several occasions, I have even seen cocaine quickly eliminate the manifestations of intolerance that appeared after a rather large dose of morphine, as if it had a specific ability to counteract morphine.

Even great men make mistakes. The realities of life were harshly brought home to Freud when he used cocaine to treat a close friend, Fleischl, to remove his addiction to morphine. Increasingly larger doses were needed, and eventually Freud spent a frightful night nursing Fleischl through an episode of cocaine psychosis. After that experience he generally opposed the use of drugs in the treatment of psychological problems.

Besides those three real people, one well-known fictional character reveals that the psychological effects of cocaine, both the initial stimulation and the later depression, were well appreciated by 1890:[4]

> Sherlock Holmes took his bottle from the corner of the mantelpiece, and his hypodermic syringe from its neat morocco case. With his long, white nervous fingers, he adjusted the delicate needle and rolled back his left shirtcuff. For some little time his eyes rested thoughtfully upon the sinewy forearm and wrist, all dotted and scarred with innumerable puncture-marks. Finally, he thrust the sharp point home, pressed down the tiny piston, and sank back into the velvet-lined armchair with a long sigh of satisfaction.
>
> Three times a day for many months I had witnessed this performance, but custom had not reconciled my mind to it. . . .
>
> "Which is it today," I asked, "Morphine or cocaine?"
>
> He raised his eyes languidly from the old black-letter volume which he had opened.
>
> "It is cocaine," he said, "a seven-per-cent solution. Would you care to try it?"
>
> "No, indeed," I answered brusquely. "My constitution has not got over the Afghan campaign yet. I cannot afford to throw any extra strain upon it."
>
> He smiled at my vehemence. "Perhaps you are right, Watson," he said. "I suppose that its influence is physically a bad one. I find it, however, so transcendently stimulating and clarifying to the mind that its secondary action is a matter of small moment."
>
> "But consider!" I said earnestly. "Count the cost! Your brain may, as you say, be roused and excited, but it is a pathological and morbid process which involves increased tissue-change and may at least leave a permanent weakness. You know, too, what

a black reaction comes upon you. Surely the game is hardly worth the candle. Why should you, for a mere passing pleasure, risk the loss of those great powers with which you have been endowed? Remember that I speak not only as one comrade to another but as a medical man to one for whose constitution he is to some extent answerable."

He did not seem offended. On the contrary, he put his finger-tips together, and leaned his elbows on the arms of his chair, like one who has a relish for conversation.

"My mind," he said, "rebels at stagnation. Give me problems, give me work, give me the most abstruse cryptogram, or the most intricate analysis, and I am in my own proper atmosphere. I can dispense then with artificial stimulants. But I abhor the dull routine of existence. I crave for mental exaltation."

Although physicians were well aware of the dangers of using cocaine regularly, nonmedical and quasimedical use of cocaine was widespread in the United States around the turn of the century. It was one of the secret ingredients in many patent medicines and elixirs but was also openly advertised as having beneficial effects. The Parke-Davis Pharmaceutical Company noted in 1885 that cocaine "can supply the place of food, make the coward brave, and silent eloquent" and called it a "wonder drug."[5]

Legal controls on cocaine

With so much going for cocaine, and its availability in a large number of products for drinking, snorting, or injection, it may seem strange that between 1887 and 1914, forty-six states passed laws to regulate the use and distribution of cocaine. One historian provided extensive documentation and concluded:[6]

All the elements needed to insure cocaine's outlaw status were present by the first years of the twentieth century: it had become widely used as a pleasure drug, and doctors warned of the dangers attendant on indiscriminate sale and use; it had become identified with despised or poorly regarded groups—blacks, lower-class whites, and criminals; it had not been long enough established

in the culture to insure its survival; and it had not, though used by them, become identified with the elite, thus losing what little chance it had of weathering the storm of criticism.

Cocaine was included in all sorts of nerve tonics, patent medicines, and home remedies, often without being mentioned on the label, until the 1906 Pure Food and Drugs Act was passed. As we saw in chapter 4, coca and cocaine were included along with opium and its derivatives in the Harrison Act of 1914, which taxed its importation and sale. During the Prohibition era of the 1920s, when the Harrison Act was used by federal Treasury agents as a tool to suppress drug addiction, cocaine became less available and more expensive. Not that it went away: cocaine was sometimes mixed with heroin and injected intravenously (the combination was called a "speedball"), and some of the carefree and wealthy young people of the era dabbled in its use. "Cocaine Lil," a song written in the 1920s, included the line "Lil went to a 'snow' party one cold night, and the way she sniffed was sure a fright." Cole Porter's "I Get a Kick Out of You" in 1934 originally contained the verse:

> I get no kick from cocaine
> I'm sure that if
> I took even one sniff
> It would bore me terrifically too
> But I get a kick out of you.

With the introduction in the 1930s of inexpensive and easily available amphetamine, the use of cocaine declined among both occasional recreational users and serious drug addicts. Little concern was given to cocaine until, at the end of the 1960s when amphetamines became harder to obtain, cocaine use again began to increase. In 1970 it was reported that federal agents were becoming concerned; the amount of cocaine seized by U.S. Customs agents had increased from about 50 pounds in 1967 to almost 200 pounds in 1969.[7] America's second era of flirtation with cocaine grew during the next twenty years, with U.S. seizures reaching a peak of 26,000 pounds in 1989.[8]

Crack

Sometime in the 1970s it was discovered that mixing cocaine with some simple household chemicals, including baking soda, and then drying it resulted in a lump of cocaine in a smokable form. When smoked, a relatively small amount of cocaine can produce a rapid and short-lived high, and during the 1980s the street sales of **crack** or **rock** made this experience available to anyone with $10, a butane torch or lighter, a glass pipe, and access to a dealer. The practice spread rapidly during 1985 and 1986, at first in the ghetto areas of large cities. Cocaine, which had come to symbolize the rich and famous, was now available to the poor.[9]

Basic Pharmacology

Forms of cocaine

As a part of the process of making illicit cocaine, the coca leaves are mixed with an organic solvent such as kerosene or gasoline. After thorough soaking, mixing, and mashing, the excess liquid is filtered out to form a substance known as **coca paste**. In South America this paste is often mixed with tobacco and smoked, but that practice has not caught on in the United States, perhaps because the lingering solvent gives the smoke a unique flavor. The paste can be made into **cocaine hydrochloride,** a salt that mixes easily in water and is so stable that it cannot be heated to form vapors for inhalation. Some U.S. users who want to "smoke" the cocaine convert it into **freebase** by extracting it into a volatile organic solvent, such as ether. The freebase can be heated and the vapors inhaled, but putting fire and ether fumes together can be an enlightening experience, because ether is so explosive. The popularity of this form of freebasing began to decline with the dis-

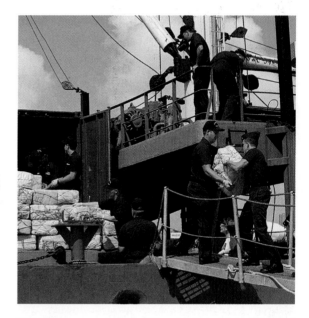

U.S. Customs agents in Miami intercept a shipment of cocaine.

covery that a different type of freebase cocaine could be made by mixing cocaine with baking soda and water as described previously. When a piece of this cocaine crack or rock is heated, cocaine vapors are produced and can be inhaled.

---

crack: a simple and stable preparation of cocaine base for smoking.

rock: another name for crack.

coca paste: a crude extract containing cocaine in a smokable form.

cocaine hydrochloride: the most common form of pure cocaine, it is stable and water soluble.

freebase: a method of preparing cocaine as a chemical base so that it may be smoked.

Crack cocaine and cocaine in powdered form

The chemical structure of cocaine is shown in figure 7.1. This is a fairly complicated molecule that doesn't resemble any of the known transmitters in an obvious way. In fact the structure of cocaine doesn't give us much help at all in understanding how the drug works on the brain.

Mechanism of action

The more we learn about cocaine's effects on brain biochemistry, the more complex its actions seem. Cocaine blocks the reuptake of dopamine, prolonging the effect of each packet of the neurotransmitter that is released. During the 1980s most scientists studying both the stimulant effects and the dependence potential of cocaine focused their research on dopamine neurons. For several years it had been known that cocaine also blocks reuptake of serotonin, and recent experiments indicate the importance of that action as well. New synthetic drugs that block only dopamine reuptake do not produce the same behavioral effects as cocaine. The latest bet is that cocaine's behavioral effects depend on blocking reuptake of both dopamine and serotonin.[10]

Absorption and elimination

People can, and do, use cocaine in many ways. Chewing and sucking the leaves allows the cocaine to be absorbed slowly through the mucous membranes. This results in a slower onset and much lower blood levels than are usually obtained by the most common recre-

■ carbon ■ oxygen ■ nitrogen (hydrogen omitted)

Figure 7.1 Cocaine

ational method of "snorting" or sniffing. In snorting, the intent is to get the very fine cocaine hydrochloride powder high into the nasal passages—right on the nasal mucosa. From there it is absorbed quite rapidly and, through circulatory mechanisms that are not completely understood, reaches the brain rather quickly.

The intravenous use of cocaine delivers a very high concentration to the brain, producing a rapid, powerful, and brief effect. For that reason, intravenous cocaine has been a favorite among compulsive users, many of whom switched from intranasal to IV use. However, for most compulsive users the preferred route produces effects even faster—the smoking of crack. Because the lungs provide a large surface area for absorption, and blood circulation from the lungs to the brain is quite rapid, smoking crack produces more rapid dependence than even IV use (see chapter 6).

The cocaine molecules are metabolized by enzymes in the blood and liver, and the activity of these enzymes is variable from one person to another. In any case, cocaine itself is rapidly removed, with a half-life of about 1 hour. The major metabolites, which are the basis of urine screening tests, have a longer half-life of about 8 hours.

Beneficial Uses

Local anesthesia

The local anesthetic properties of cocaine, that is, its ability to numb the area to which it is applied, were discovered in 1860 soon after its isolation from coca leaves. It was not until 1884 that this characteristic was used medically; the early applications were in eye surgery and dentistry. The use of cocaine spread rapidly because it apparently was a safe and effective drug. The potential for misuse soon became clear, though, and a search began for synthetic agents with similar anesthetic characteristics but little or no potential for misuse. This work was rewarded in 1905 with the discovery of procaine (Novocain), which is still in wide use.

Local anesthetics probably block pain by preventing the generation and conduction of nerve impulses. They seem to act quite specifically on the nerve membrane. By disrupting the membrane processes necessary for the initiation and generation of electrical impulses, impulse conduction and information processing are stopped. Many drugs have been synthesized since 1905 that have local anesthetic properties similar to those of cocaine but have little or no ability to produce CNS stimulation. Those drugs have largely replaced cocaine for medical use. However, because cocaine is absorbed so well into mucous membranes, it remains in use for surgery in the nasal, laryngeal, and esophageal regions.

Other claimed benefits

Because cocaine produces a feeling of increased energy and well-being, it enjoyed an important status among achievers of the 1980s who self-prescribed it to overcome fatigue. It seemed that many athletes and entertainers felt that they could not consistently perform at their peak without the assistance of cocaine, and this resulted in widespread cocaine use among these groups. It should be remembered that cocaine has not been used medically for its CNS effects for many years because its effects are brief, there is a subsequent period of depressed mood, attempts to maintain the euphoria lead rapidly to tolerance and acceleration of the dose, and high doses result in unpleasant restlessness, paranoia, and other side effects. Thus, whereas the drug can provide a brief sense of increased energy, the long-term consequences are frequently disruptive. It seems that enough people experienced these disruptive effects during the 1980s that the drug's popularity has declined considerably since then.

Causes for Concern

Acute toxicity

There is no evidence that occasional use of small amounts of cocaine is a threat to the individual's health. However, many people have increased the amount they used to the point of toxicity. Acute cocaine poisoning leads to profound CNS stimulation, progressing to convulsions that can lead to respiratory or cardiac arrest. This is in some ways similar to amphetamine overdose, with the exception that there is much greater individual variation in the uptake and metabolism of cocaine, so that a lethal dose is much more difficult to estimate. In addition, there are very rare, severe, and unpredictable toxic reactions to cocaine and other local anesthetics in which individuals die rapidly, apparently from cardiac failure. Cocaine can trigger the chaotic heart rhythm called ventricular fibrillation by somehow preventing the vagus nerve from controlling the heartbeat.[11] Intravenous cocaine users might also experience an allergic reaction either to the drug or to some additive in street cocaine. The lungs fill rapidly with fluid, and death can occur.

It was reported in 1992[12] that the combination of cocaine and ethanol (alcohol) in the body can result in the formation of a chemical called **cocaethylene** which might be more toxic than cocaine itself.

Chronic toxicity

Regularly snorting cocaine, and particularly cocaine that has been "cut" with other things, can irritate the nasal septum, leading to a chronically inflamed, runny nose. Because cocaine does have a tendency to decrease food intake, many chronic cocaine users may be malnourished. Use of cocaine in a binge, during which the drug is taken repeatedly and at increasingly high doses, leads to a state of increasing irritability, restlessness, and paranoia. In severe cases, this can result in a full-blown paranoid psychosis in which the individual loses touch with reality and experiences auditory hallucinations.[13] This experience is disruptive and quite frightening. However, most individuals seem to recover from the psychosis as the drug leaves the system.

There has been concern for several years about the effects of chronic cocaine use on the heart muscle. It appears that in some users, frequent, brief disruption of the heart's function can damage the heart muscle itself.[14] It is not clear how often such damage occurs.

Dependence potential

There is no doubt that cocaine can produce powerful psychological dependence in some users, particularly among those who inject it or inhale the vapors of crack, coca paste, or cocaine base. This phenomenon is substantiated by a large number of animal experiments demonstrating that rats or monkeys will rapidly learn to press levers that lead to cocaine injections and that these animals will continue to respond even when large numbers of presses are required for each injection.[15] Thus it appears that cocaine can be a powerfully reinforcing drug: take it and it will make you want to take it again.

Throughout the 1970s the importance of this dependence potential went unrecognized, partly because cocaine was expensive and in short supply and largely because the only common method of using cocaine during this time was snorting it. The 1980s saw an increase in freebasing and then of the more convenient form of smokable cocaine known as "crack" or "rock." As large numbers of people began to smoke cocaine in the mid 1980s, the powerful dependence potential of this form of use became clear to the American public and to the users themselves.

Because at one time addiction was linked to the presence of physical dependence, there have been a number of experiments that asked whether withdrawal symptoms appear after repeated cocaine use. After prolonged daily cocaine administrations in animals there were no obvious withdrawal signs (for example, no diarrhea or convulsions), and many scientists concluded that cocaine produced no physical dependence and was therefore not an addicting

TABLE 7.1

Dependence Liability of Stimulants

Drug and route	Tolerance	Physical dependence	Probability of behavioral dependence
Cocaine, snorted	Yes	At high doses	High
Cocaine, intravenous	Yes	At high doses	Very high
Cocaine, freebase inhaled	Yes	At high doses	Very high
Amphetamines, oral	Yes, short- and long-term	At high doses	Moderate
Amphetamines, intravenous	Yes, long- and short-term	At high doses	Very high

drug. The experiences of large numbers of people in the 1980s has led to a different way of looking at this issue. The cocaine abstinence syndrome has been described as a three-stage process: as cocaine wears off, there is a dysphoric reaction (the cocaine blues). If cocaine use has been prolonged and large doses have been used, this initial period produces a powerful sense of psychological depression, a craving for cocaine, prolonged periods of sleep, and bouts of ravenous food intake. This phase may last for several days, after which mood normalizes. The second stage, which emerges after the initial "crash" and lasts for several weeks, is characterized by anxiety, boredom, lack of motivation, and a reduced ability to experience pleasure. The third phase, which lasts indefinitely, consists of episodes of craving that can be triggered by cues associated with cocaine use (certain places or people, the sight of a large amount of cash). The relative consistency of this withdrawal syndrome demonstrates clearly that physical dependence is possible with cocaine (table 7.1.).

Reproductive effects

Cocaine has been shown in animal studies to restrict blood flow to the placenta, and several human studies have reported that babies are of below-average size when born to women who reported using cocaine during pregnancy or whose urine tested positive for cocaine at the time of birth.[16] The earliest studies reporting

this effect on birth weight and head circumference were not well controlled, in that most of the mothers had also used alcohol and tobacco, and both poor nutrition and lack of prenatal care also characterized the populations studied. These and other reports of babies being born under the influence of cocaine resulted in lurid media accounts of the "crack baby" phenomenon, which unfortunately overstated both the number of such children (see the Up for Debate box on p. 26 in chapter 2) and the expected long-term effects (see the Up for Debate box on p. 144). A follow-up study[17] reported that by 3 months of age the deficiencies in body weight and length were made up for in the cocaine-exposed infants. By 24 months there were no longer any significant differences between cocaine-exposed and control groups. Bayley Scales of Infant Development scores, which measure both mental and psychomotor development, also revealed no differences at 24 months.

In addition to concerns about the long-term effects on the developing fetus, there are more immediate problems associated with cocaine use during pregnancy—there is increased risk for both spontaneous abortions (miscarriages) and a torn placenta.

> **cocaethylene:** (co cah *eth* eh leen) a chemical formed by mixing ethanol and cocaine.

The Impact of Maternal Cocaine Use

Beginning in 1986, highly emotional television and magazine reports appeared relating the horrors of the "crack baby"—infants exposed to cocaine before birth. Not only were the numbers of such children exaggerated (see chapter 2), but the small amount of available data on such infants provided the basis for wild speculation about the eventual health and educational costs associated with this problem: these children would be permanently damaged, intellectually and emotionally retarded, and unable to understand affection or to perform in school. What we actually know is that if the fetus is exposed in utero to cocaine, the baby is likely to be born sooner, to be smaller, and to have a smaller head circumference than babies exposed to no known drugs during pregnancy. The first studies revealed an effect of the same type and approximately the same magnitude as that seen when women smoke cigarettes throughout pregnancy (see chapter 12). Yet the phenomenon was seized on by well-meaning health care providers and educators, some of whom have gone so far as to describe the type of classrooms this "wave" of crack kids would require when they entered school. Substance-abusing mothers have been jailed to protect their unborn children. All of this has been done in the absence of solid information on the long-term effects of cocaine exposure and without comparison with the many other potential risks to the health of the fetus, most of which are more common than prenatal cocaine exposure. One recent study that compared the prenatal effects of alcohol, cigarette smoking, and cocaine found significant effects on birth weight only for alcohol and smoking and concluded that reported effects of cocaine on birth size is "primarily an indirect consequence of shorter gestation and poorer maternal nutrition."[34]

It's natural to react with fear to new threats, even when some old familiar things may actually threaten us more. Because there seem to be new drug threats every few years, keep that in mind when the next one appears. How will you respond to such new (and very real) problems without blowing them out of proportion?

Supplies of Illicit Cocaine

During the 1980s there were only relatively small changes in the price and purity of cocaine on the streets of the United States. Until about 1988 the purity increased slightly and the price decreased slowly, both indicating greater supplies. This trend appeared to reverse in 1989 and 1990, but in 1991 and 1992 the price declined again.[18] Thus, increased efforts to control the supply of cocaine appear to have been countered by increased production and smuggling.

Illicit cocaine comes to the United States primarily from three South American countries: Peru, Bolivia, and Colombia. In 1992 over 200,000 tons of coca leaf were produced in Peru alone, enough to produce about 500 tons of cocaine hydrochloride. Bolivia typically produces about half as much coca as Peru, and Colombia about half as much as Bolivia. In all of these countries, attempts to control production are complex: U.S. DEA agents assist local antinarcotics police, who may be in conflict with army units fighting against local guerrillas. Often the price and availability of coca in these countries are determined more by local politics than by the DEA's eradication and interdiction efforts. Although we might pay some farmers to grow alternative crops, the high profits from growing illicit cocaine draw others to plant new fields. A recent economic analysis of the impact of eradication efforts indicates that even the most successful projects result in at best only temporary shortages.[19]

Large shipments of cocaine were traditionally routed by boat or plane to any of hundreds of islands in the Caribbean, and from there to Miami or other ports in the eastern United States, again by small boat or airplane. Although sea routes continue to be important, the pressure brought by Navy, Air Force, and Coast Guard interdiction efforts has shifted trafficking somewhat more to land routes through Central America and Mexico.

A cocaine user in action with a line of cocaine and a rolled dollar bill.

Current Patterns of Cocaine Use

Cocaine was the drug of abuse for the 1980s. Throughout the early 1980s the national household survey conducted by NIDA (see chapter 1) found that 7 to 9 percent of young adults reported use of cocaine within the past month. By 1993 the comparable figure was just over 1 percent, and all indications were that use of cocaine had dropped significantly in the general population. The annual high school senior survey (see chapter 1) has reported more than an 80 percent decrease in current use of cocaine from 1985 to 1994. However, the DAWN data on emergency-room mentions and cocaine-related deaths did not follow the same pattern, with cocaine-related emergencies and deaths continuing to rise in the early 1990s. The concern is that the type of drug use shifted in this period to a more dangerous form (crack), along with a shift to younger and poorer users who are more often unemployed and black.

A study of crack use among newly arrested individuals found that, contrary to the popular view of crack users being slaves to their pipes all day every day, most of the users reported

Cocaine and Friendship

Imagine you have a good friend who has been using cocaine off and on for a year. However, in the past couple of months it seems the use has become more and more frequent. You have had to stop lending your friend money because it never gets paid back. When you hinted that the cocaine use might be getting out of hand, there was no response. When you tried direct confrontation, you got angry denial that there was any problem. You are still good friends. You certainly don't want to turn your friend in to the police, but you are getting pretty worried. What do you think you should do?

Obviously there is no correct answer to this problem, but it might be interesting to discuss this hypothetical situation with a group of people who are your friends. Find out how they would want to be treated under the circumstances. How would you yourself want to be treated?

smoking fewer than three "rocks" per day on the average. The effect of each rock only lasts for a few minutes, so most of these users were not "high" continuously. In fact, many crack users are occasional users. Crack might be more addicting than other forms of cocaine, but that still doesn't mean that all users become addicted.[20]

Cocaine Treatment

The 1980s saw an enormous increase in the number of people seeking treatment for cocaine dependence. Although cocaine use declined in the general population in the 1990s, the shift to crack cocaine use ensured a steady demand for treatment in many areas of the country.

Cocaine overdose is potentially lethal, and medical treatments have been developed to deal with the acute emergencies resulting from excessive cocaine use. Beta-adrenergic blocking drugs such as propranolol can be used to treat rapid, irregular heart rate and high blood pressure. Psychotic symptoms can be controlled with haloperidol (Haldol). If seizures occur, they can be controlled with intravenous diazepam (Valium).

During the withdrawal phase, patients usually become depressed and feel lethargic and irritable. Antidepressant drugs have been tried and do help some to reduce the depression. Buprenorphine, an experimental drug with some opiate-like effects, has been shown to reduce cocaine self-administration in animals and is being tested in human cocaine users.[21]

After the initial detoxification period, treatment is designed to prevent any attempts to try cocaine use again. Mandatory urine screening at three-day intervals has been suggested as a useful monitoring device. Group therapy, support groups (groups calling themselves Cocaine Anonymous are available in many areas), and individual psychotherapy, job, and family counseling are all important components of current cocaine treatment programs. Promotion of exercise and general health consciousness fit in with current American trends and are felt to help reduce the "hunger" for cocaine.

For cocaine users who are middle- or upper-class individuals with both money and status, a behavioral management technique known as "contingency contracting" has been successfully employed. In this approach, an individual who is highly motivated to stop cocaine but who fears impulsive use signs a contract agreeing that using cocaine (as determined by a urine test) will result in the loss of something of great significance (an automobile, a professional license, a large cash deposit) or automatic notification of an employer. Although such contracts must be established with care, if one freely enters into it and if the contingency is sufficiently important, it can be an important aid to behavioral management.

A promising approach to cocaine addicts that has not yet come into widespread use in treatment focuses on the conditioned stimuli in the addict's environment that become associated with the use of cocaine. For example, seeing a white powder of any kind or seeing a large amount of cash can be so strongly conditioned to cocaine use that these stimuli elicit conditioned cravings, withdrawal symptoms, or excitement. By monitoring the client's emotional and physiological responses while discussing such stimuli or while actually presenting stimuli, it is possible to determine which stimuli elicit the strongest emotional responses and are therefore most likely to lead to relapse. The therapists then use "systematic desensitization," a form of extinction procedure, to reduce these conditioned responses. The clients are induced to relax, then to talk about these situations or to imagine step-by-step the sight of drugs, getting ready to use the drug, and so on, all the time remaining calm and relaxed. It is hoped that by breaking the emotional reactions to these conditioned stimuli, the stimuli will no longer elicit cravings and lead to relapse.

As with other drugs, treatment is probably more effective than no treatment, but the failure rate is still high. It will be several years before the effectiveness of different approaches to cocaine dependence can be evaluated.

Cocaine's Future

In attempting to predict the future, we can learn from two writers who have made successful predictions about cocaine use in the past. The first, writing in the early 1970s, pointed out that historically as cocaine use declined, amphetamine use increased. Looking at the decline in amphetamine use in the late 1960s, he predicted the increased use of cocaine that we saw in the 1970s and early 1980s.[7] The other writer[5] pointed out that at the height of

cocaine use in 1986 we were reliving an earlier cycle of cocaine use that occurred around the turn of the century. As you know, when cocaine was first introduced in the 1880s, the experts had mostly positive opinions about its effects, and it was regarded as a fairly benign substance. In the second stage (1890s), more and more people used cocaine, and its dangers and side effects became well known. In the third stage, in the early 1900s, society turned against cocaine and passed laws to control it. After many years with little cocaine use, in the early 1970s the drug again had the reputation of being fairly benign and not truly addicting. In the 1980s we were in the second stage, in which widespread use eventually made us all aware of the dangers. This comparison led to the prediction that Americans would again turn away from cocaine and would pass increased legal restrictions on it. This prediction certainly came true during the 1990s. As the rejection of cocaine continues, we would not expect increases in cocaine use for several years in the future. But thirty years have passed since the peak of amphetamine's popularity and widespread concerns about it. We therefore made the prediction in the previous edition of this text that the next wave of illicit stimulant use would see increases in the use of amphetamine. Unfortunately, that prediction is now coming true.

AMPHETAMINES

History

Development and early uses
For centuries the Chinese have made a medicinal tea from herbs they call *ma huang*, which we classify in the genus *Ephedra*. The active ingredient in these herbs is called **ephedrine**, and

ephedrine: (eh *fed* rin) sympathomimetic drug used in treating asthma.

it is used to dilate the bronchial passages in asthma patients. Bronchial dilation can be achieved by stimulating the sympathetic branch of the autonomic nervous system, and that is exactly what ephedrine does (it is referred to as a **sympathomimetic** drug). Of course, this drug also has other effects related to its sympathetic nervous system stimulation, such as elevating blood pressure. In the late 1920s, researchers synthesized and studied the effects of a new chemical that was similar in structure to ephedrine: **amphetamine** was patented in 1932.

All major effects of amphetamine were discovered in the 1930s, although some of the uses developed later. Amphetamine's first use was as a replacement for ephedrine in the treatment of *asthma*. Quite early it was shown that amphetamine was a potent dilator of the nasal and bronchial passages and could be efficiently delivered through inhalation. The Benzedrine (brand name) inhaler was introduced as an over-the-counter (OTC) product in 1932 for treating the stuffy noses caused by colds.

Some of the early work with amphetamine showed that the drug would awaken anesthetized dogs. As one writer put it, amphetamine is the drug that won't let sleeping dogs lie! This led to the testing of amphetamine for the treatment of **narcolepsy** in 1935. Narcolepsy is a condition in which the individual spontaneously falls asleep five, ten, fifty times a day (even outside the classroom). Amphetamine enables these patients to remain awake and function almost normally. In 1938, however, two narcolepsy patients treated with amphetamine developed acute *paranoid psychotic* reactions. The paranoid reaction to amphetamine has reappeared regularly and has been studied (as is discussed later).

In 1937, amphetamine became available as a prescription tablet, and a report appeared in the literature suggesting that amphetamine, a stimulant, was effective in reducing activity in hyperactive children. Two years later, in 1939, notice was taken of a report by amphetamine-treated narcolepsy patients that they were not hungry when taking the drug. This *appetite-depressant* effect became the major clinical use of amphetamine. A group of psychology students at the University of Minnesota began experimenting with various drugs in 1937 and found that amphetamine was ideal for "cramming," because it allowed them to stay awake for long periods of time. Truck drivers also noted this effect, and they used "bennies" to stay awake during long hauls.

Wartime uses

In 1939, amphetamine went to war. There were many reports that Germany was using stimulants to increase the efficiency of its soldiers. A 1944 report in the *Air Surgeon's Bulletin* titled "Benzedrine Alert"[22] stated, "this drug is the most satisfactory of any available in temporarily postponing sleep when desire to sleep endangers the security of a mission." Some studies were reported, including one in which

> . . . one hundred Marines were kept active continuously for sixty hours in range firing, a twenty-five mile forced march, a field problem, calisthenics, close-order drill, games, fatigue detail and bivouac alerts. Fifty men received seven 10-milligram tablets of benzedrine at six hour intervals following the first day's activity. Meanwhile, the other fifty were given placebo (milk sugar) tablets. None knew what he was receiving. Participating officers concluded that the benzedrine definitely "pepped up" the subjects, improved their morale, reduced sleepiness and increased confidence in shooting ability. . . . It was observed that men receiving benzedrine tended to lead the march, tolerate their sore feet and blisters more cheerfully, and remain wide awake during "breaks," whereas members of the control group had to be shaken to keep them from sleeping.

Amphetamines were widely used in Japan during World War II to maintain production on the home front and to keep the fighting men going. To reduce large stockpiles of methamphetamine after the war, the drug was sold without prescription, and the drug companies advertised them for "elimination of drowsiness and repletion of the spirit." Such widespread use was accompanied by considerable overuse and abuse. In 1948 and again in 1955, strict controls on amphetamine were put into force, along with treatment and education programs. Although the Japanese government claimed to have "eliminated" the amphetamine-abuse problem before 1960, there were smaller Japanese "epidemics" of methamphetamine use in the 1970s and 1980s.

In 1944 in Sweden, because such a large number of people were using oral amphetamines, prescriptions became tightly controlled. This resulted in a significant decline in amphetamine sales and a decrease in the total number of individuals using the amphetamines. But those who were heavy abusers would not be denied, so there arose a black market in amphetamines and an amphetamine subculture similar to our American heroin subculture. To get the most value out of their expensive black-market amphetamine, some Swedes began injecting it intravenously. In 1968, Sweden banned virtually all prescriptions for amphetamines and related stimulants. The black market, of course, continued to flourish.[8]

Postwar concerns in the United States

There was only slight concern over nonmedical use of amphetamine in the United States after World War II. A 1946 article, "On a Bender with Benzedrine,"[23] in a popular national magazine made explicit just how one could get amphetamine without a prescription:

> After I bought an inhaler, Hal worked off the perforated cap and pulled out the medicated paper, folded accordion-wise. . . . "Like this—" Hal took the innocent looking scrap of paper he had torn away and held it between thumb and finger. He alternately dunked and squeezed this paper into his glass of beer.

Each inhaler contained 250 mg of amphetamine, so a considerable dose could be obtained if taken all at once. It was not until 1959 that the FDA banned the use of amphetamine in inhalers.

The "speed scene" of the 1960s

Most of the misuse of amphetamines until the 1960s was through the legally manufactured and legally purchased oral preparation. In 1963 the AMA Council on Drugs stated, "At this time, compulsive abuse of the amphetamines is a small problem."[24] But at exactly this time, trouble was brewing in California. It is difficult to pinpoint exactly when intravenous abuse of the amphetamines began in the United States, but it was probably among IV users of heroin and cocaine. In the 1920s and 1930s, when IV use of those drugs was spreading among the drug subculture, the combination of heroin and cocaine injected together was known as the "speedball," presumably because the cocaine rush or flash occurs rapidly after injection, thus speeding up the high. So, on the streets, one name for cocaine was "speed." When the amphetamines became so widely available after World War II, some of these enterprising individuals discovered that they could get an effect similar to that of cocaine if they injected amphetamine along with the heroin. Thus slowly and out of the awareness of most Americans, the amphetamines came to be known as **speed** by that small drug underground that used heroin intravenously. By the 1960s, amphetamines became so

---

sympathomimetic: (sim path o mih *met* ick) a drug that stimulates the sympathetic branch of the autonomic nervous system.

amphetamine: a synthetic CNS stimulant and sympathomimetic.

narcolepsy: a disease that causes people to fall asleep suddenly.

speed: street name for amphetamine.

widely available at such a low price that more IV drug users were using them, either in combination with heroin or alone. Although they were prescription drugs, it was not difficult to obtain a prescription to treat depression or obesity.

The most desired drug on the streets was methamphetamine, which was available in liquid form in ampules for injection. Hospital emergency rooms sometimes used this drug to stimulate respiration in patients suffering from overdoses of sleeping pills (no longer considered an appropriate treatment), and physicians also used injectable amphetamines intramuscularly to treat obesity. In the San Francisco Bay area, reports appeared in the early 1960s of "fat doctors" who had large numbers of patients coming in regularly for no treatment other than an injection of methamphetamine.

Because some heroin addicts would inject amphetamines alone when they could not obtain heroin, some physicians also felt that methamphetamine could serve as a legal substitute for heroin and thus be a form of treatment. In those days, amphetamines were not considered to be addicting, so these physicians were quite free with their prescriptions.[7] Reports of those abuses led to legislation, including federal regulation of amphetamines within the new concept of dangerous drugs in the 1965 law. Unfortunately, all of the publicity associated with these revelations and the ensuing legislation fell on the ears of young people whose identity as a generation was defined largely by experimentation with drugs their parents and government told them were dangerous. To the Haight-Ashbury district of San Francisco came the flower children, to sit in Golden Gate Park, smoke marijuana, take LSD, and discuss peace, love, and the brotherhood of man. They moved in next door to the old, established drug subculture in which IV drug use was endemic. That mixture resulted in the speed scene and young people who became dependent on IV amphetamines. Although in historical perspective the speed scene of the late

Variety of ephedrine stimulants

1960s was relatively short-lived and only a small number of people were directly involved, it was the focus of a great deal of national concern, and it helped to change the way the medical profession and society at large viewed these drugs that had been so widely accepted.

As use of the amphetamines began to be considered abuse, physicians prescribed less and less of the drugs. Their new legal status as dangerous drugs put restrictions on prescriptions and refills, and in the 1970s there were limits placed on the total amount of these drugs that could be manufactured. Thus within less than a decade, amphetamines went from being widely used and accepted pharmaceuticals to being less widely used, tightly restricted drugs associated in the public mind with drug-abusing "hippies."

As controls tightened on legally manufactured amphetamines, there were at least three reactions that continued to affect the current drug scene. The first reaction was that a market began to develop for "look-alike" pills: legal, milder stimulants (usually caffeine or ephedrine) packaged in tablets and capsules that are virtually identical in color, shape, and markings to prescription amphetamines. Later the makers of look-alikes began to expand the variety of shapes and sizes to attract a wider market. Because these pills contain legally available, OTC ingredients, their sellers could not be prosecuted. By the early 1980s these products were so popular that the odds were good that if someone bought "speed" pills from a street dealer they were actually getting look-alikes. The national high school survey had to apply a correction factor to their data to account for these look-alikes and get a more accurate measure of actual amphetamine use. The FDA began to crack down on manufacturers and distributors of pills containing large amounts of caffeine or mixtures of caffeine and other legal stimulants, and states passed regulations making it illegal to distribute any substance that is misrepresented to be a controlled substance.

The reduced availability of legally manufactured amphetamines had a second important effect. As the price went up and the quality of the available speed became more questionable, the drug subculture began, slowly and without fanfare, to rekindle its interest in a more "natural," reportedly less dangerous stimulant—cocaine. By 1970, federal agents in Miami reported that "the traffic in cocaine is growing by leaps and bounds."[7] And as we now know, they were seeing only the small beginnings of a cocaine trade that would swell to much greater size by the mid 1980s.

The return of methamphetamine

The third reaction to limited amphetamine availability was an increase in the number of illicit laboratories making methamphetamine, which acquired the name *crank*. Both the process for making methamphetamine and the name **crank** have been around on the streets since the 1960s, and illicit laboratories have been raided every year. By the late 1980s the increasing number of confiscations by authorities led some to wonder if this would be the next drug fad.

In 1989 the media began to describe what many claimed would be America's next drug epidemic: the "smoking" of methamphetamine hydrochloride crystals, also known by the street name **ice.** The practice had been reported among youth in Hawaii and was said to be spreading into California. Along with the scare of a potential new menace came unsubstantiated reports that ice produced effects lasting for a day or more, compared with a few minutes for cocaine (such reports make no sense in terms of the half-life of methamphetamine). Concerns about methamphetamine use increased considerably in the 1990s when rates of methamphetamine seizures increased dramatically and the DAWN reports indicated large relative increases in methamphetamine-related emergency room admissions and deaths.[25] Much of the concern has focused on the rural West, where small clandestine laboratories are making methamphetamine, supplemented by increasing importation of both raw materials and finished product from Mexico.[26]

Basic Pharmacology

Chemical structures

Take a couple of minutes to look at figure 7.2. We're not trying to make medicinal chemists out of anyone, but we want you to see some similarities in the structures of amphetamines and related drugs. First, note the similarity between the molecular structures of the catecholamine neurotransmitters (dopamine and norepinephrine) and the basic amphetamine molecule. It does appear that amphetamine produces its effects because it is recognized as one of these catecholamines at many sites in both the central and the peripheral nervous systems. The amphetamine molecule has both "left-handed" and "right-handed" forms (*l* and *d* forms). The original Benzedrine was an equal mixture of both forms. The *d* form is several times more potent in its CNS effects, however, and in 1945 d-amphetamine was first marketed as Dexedrine for use as an appetite suppressant. Next, look at

---

crank: street name for illicitly manufactured methamphetamine.

ice: street name for crystals of methamphetamine hydrochloride.

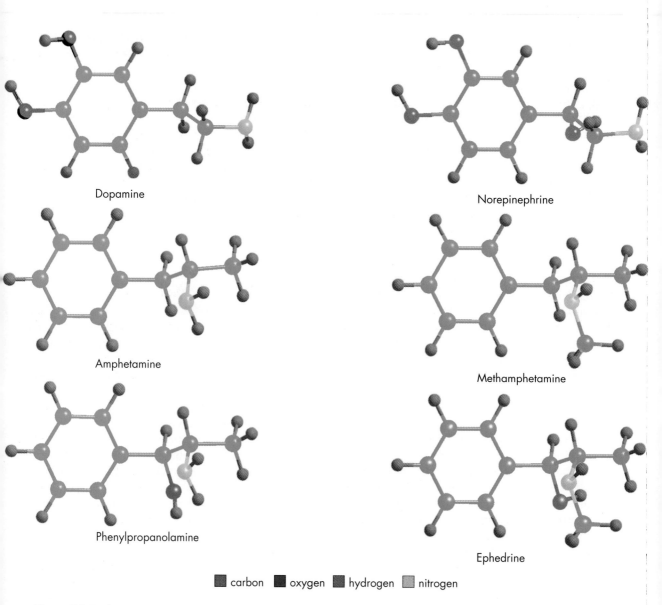

Figure 7.2 Molecular structures of stimulants

the methamphetamine molecule, which simply has a methyl group added to the basic amphetamine structure. This methyl group seems to make the molecule cross the blood-brain barrier more readily and thus further increase the CNS potency. (If more of the molecules get into the brain, then fewer total molecules have to be given.)

We're not through with the molecules yet! Next, look at the structures for ephedrine, the old Chinese remedy that is still used to treat asthma, and for phenylpropanolamine (PPA). PPA is an ingredient in all OTC weight-control preparations (see chapter 14) and in many of the look-alikes mentioned previously. Both of these molecules have a structural addition that makes them not cross the blood-brain barrier as well, and therefore they produce peripheral effects without as much CNS effectiveness.

Mechanism of action

The stimulant types of amphetamine have at least two effects on catecholamine (dopamine and norepinephrine) synapses. The presynaptic storage mechanism recognizes and tries to store amphetamine molecules, which results in the leakage of catecholamines into the synapse, where they can interact with the receptor. Second and probably less important is the ability of amphetamine molecules to occupy the reuptake mechanism so that catecholamines released into the synapse are not taken back up as readily and therefore stay longer in the synapse. Both of these mechanisms produce increased stimulation of the dopamine and norepinephrine receptors.

Exactly which of amphetamine's effects are related to which neurotransmitter is controversial, but current theories can be summarized. Stimulation of the norepinephrine neurons arising from the locus ceruleus would produce the alerting and antifatigue effects, and stimulation of the mesolimbic dopamine pathway would produce euphoria and increased motor activity. Higher doses would activate the nigrostriatal dopamine pathway to produce stereotyped, repetitive movements. Too much activity in the mesolimbic system could be responsible for the paranoid psychotic reaction seen with very high doses.

Absorption and elimination

Amphetamines can be taken by a variety of routes. When taken orally, the peak effects are found 2 to 3 hours after ingestion. The half-life is 10 to 12 hours, so that a fairly stable blood level can be achieved with oral administration at 4- to 6-hour intervals, and virtually complete elimination of the drug would occur within two days after the last dose. With IV injection, peak effects are much more rapid. With higher doses a tachyphylaxis (rapid tolerance) may be seen. Because amphetamine produces its effects largely by displacing the catecholamine transmitters from their storage sites, with large doses the catecholamines might be sufficiently depleted so that another dose within a few hours may not be able to displace as much catecholamine, and a reduced effect will be obtained.

Beneficial Uses

Previous use for depression

During the 1950s and early 1960s, amphetamines were prescribed for depression and feelings of fatigue. If we look at an individual's mood as potentially ranging from very depressed, up through sadness into a normal range, and then into euphoria and finally the excited, manic range (figure 7.3), we can better understand amphetamine's effects on mood. Note that the person who is seriously depressed is not just sad; he or she feels helpless and hopeless with no energy and might think of suicide. Amphetamines are capable of temporarily moving the mood up the scale so that a depressed person might, for a few hours, move into a normal range. The problem is that when the drug wears off, that person doesn't stay "up." The mood drops, often below the predrug level. To keep the mood up, one needs to keep taking amphetamine. Amphetamine does interfere with sleep, so some physicians prescribed sleeping pills for nighttime. These patients often went for a daily "ride" on an emotional roller coaster, waking up depressed and taking a pill to get going in the morning, and either coming off the drug or taking a "downer" at night. As we shall see in chapter 9, other treatments are now used for depression, and amphetamines are not recommended.

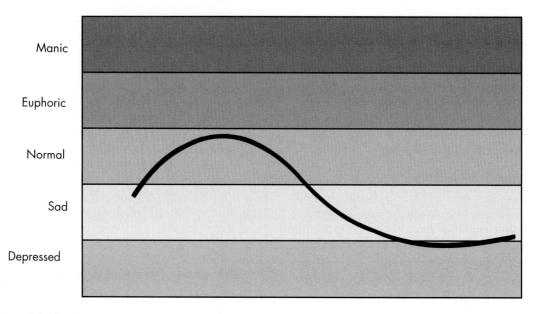

Manic

Euphoric

Normal

Sad

Depressed

Figure 7.3 Mood ranges

Weight control

Probably the most common medical use for the amphetamines through the mid 1960s was for weight control. It is clear that amphetamine can reduce food intake and body weight. This is obvious in people of normal or below-average weight who take the drug for other reasons, and especially obvious in those who take very large doses. Studies on rats show without doubt that amphetamine reduces food intake and body weight compared with rats given a placebo. With one-third of Americans overweight, there is a vast market for a pill that would help us lose weight. For years the common medical response was some form of amphetamine or related sympathomimetic stimulant. Physicians dispensed prescriptions for pills and some gave injections, and some people did lose some weight. But in the 1960s, when people began to view the amphetamines with greater concern, it was also clear that some people who took these stimulants regularly were still overweight.

To understand the role of stimulant drugs in weight control, let's imagine a typical experiment to test the value of amphetamine in treating obesity. Patients who meet some criterion for being overweight are recruited for the study. All are brought to a hospital or clinic where they are weighed, interviewed, given physical examinations, and given a diet to follow. Half are given amphetamine and half a placebo in a double-blind design. Each week the patients return to the hospital, where they are interviewed, weighed, and given their supply of drug for the next week. After two months the drug code is broken and the amount of weight loss in each group is calculated. This type of study virtually always finds that both groups lose weight, mostly in the first 2 or 3 weeks. After that, the weight loss is much slower. This initial weight loss by both groups probably is a result of beginning a new diet and being involved in a medical study in which they know they will be weighed each week. Over the first 2 or 3 weeks the amphetamine group will lose a little more weight than the placebo group. The difference between the two groups after 2 or 3 weeks might be about two or three pounds, which is statistically significant but probably not medically or cosmetically important. The interesting thing is that as the study goes on, the gap doesn't widen, but stays about the same. In other words, in such studies the amphetamine effect is real but small and limited in duration. Even with moderate dose increases, 4 to 6 weeks seems to be the limit before tolerance occurs to this effect. Increasing to high doses might produce some further effect, but these experiments don't allow that, and it would be foolhardy as a treatment approach. The use of amphetamines for weight reduction came under attack from various sources, and the FDA in 1970 restricted the legal use of amphetamines to three types of conditions: narcolepsy, hyperkinetic (hyperactive) behavior, and "short-term" weight reduction programs.

Current use in weight reduction

Over the years from 1970 to the mid 1990s, amphetamine and several related stimulant drugs continued to be used for weight control. Preparations of *d*-amphetamine and methamphetamine were available by prescription for short-term weight loss, as were the other sympathomimetics diethylpropion, phentermine, phenmetrazine, phendimetrazine, and some related but slightly different drugs, fenfluramine and mazindol. The FDA allowed the sale of all these drugs even though experts pointed out that the drugs made a clinically trivial contribution to the overall weight reduction seen in the experiments. The package insert for each of these drugs includes the following FDA mandated statements:

> The natural history of obesity is measured in years, whereas most studies cited are restricted to a few weeks duration; thus, the total impact of drug induced weight loss over that of diet alone must be considered clinically limited. . . . [Drug

name] is indicated in the management of exogenous obesity as a short-term (a few weeks) adjunct in a regimen of weight reduction based on caloric restriction. The limited usefulness of agents of this class must be weighed against possible risk factors inherent in their use.[27]

The prescribing situation changed dramatically beginning in 1992 with reports that a combination of two of these drugs, fenfluramine and phentermine (later called "Fen-Phen") could be more effective than either drug alone.[28] The results of these experiments followed the same general pattern as earlier studies, except that the drug-related increase in weight loss lasted for up to three months and resulted in a greater weight loss in the drug group. Although the benefit of the combination reached its maximum at three months of use and maintenance of the weight loss might require continued use of the drugs indefinitely, many thousands of people asked for and received prescriptions for the fen-phen combination before the associated health risks were publicized and fenfluramine was withdrawn from the market (see FYI box).

Narcolepsy

As described previously, narcolepsy is a sleep disorder in which individuals do not sleep normally at night and in the daytime experience uncontrollable episodes of muscular weakness and falling asleep. Although there has been increased interest in sleep disorders in general and sleep-disorder clinics are now associated with almost every major medical center in the United States, the best available treatment still seems to be to keep the patient awake during the day with amphetamine or methylphenidate, a related stimulant. There is no doubt that some individuals who receive stimulants from a general practitioner under the diagnosis of narcolepsy are actually suffering from some other sleep disorder or from depression, which often includes disruptions of normal sleep patterns. Accurate diagnosis of narcolepsy requires checking in to a sleep-disorder clinic for some sleep

---

FYI   Diet Drugs: Out with the New, in with the Newer

The introduction in 1992 of a new combination of two old drugs, fenfluramine and phentermine, as a more effective aid to weight loss[27] started the well-known "fen-phen" craze and renewed public interest in the use of prescription stimulants as appetite suppressants. This was followed in 1996 by the introduction of a new relative of fenfluramine, dexfenfluramine (Redux). However, in August 1997 the FDA began warning physicians and the public that the fen-phen combination had been associated with damage to heart valves, and that several patients had also developed a serious lung disease. By September 1997 it was clear that the culprit was fenfluramine (Pondimin) and also that its new relative dexfenfluramine (Redux) might have the same effects. As warnings went out from the FDA to stop taking these medications, the manufacturer removed them from the market.

Then in November 1997 another new weight-control drug, sibutramine (Meridia), was introduced.[29] Intended for use only in those who are extremely overweight, this drug is believed to act by blocking reuptake of both norepinephrine and serotonin, which would make its mechanism more similar to some of the antidepressants (chapter 9) than to the more traditional stimulants.

---

recordings on an electroencephalogram (EEG). However, for these recordings to be accurate, the programs usually require that the patient be drug-free for two to three weeks preceding the recordings.

Hyperactive children

Even though it has been more than fifty years since the first report that amphetamine could reduce activity levels in hyperactive children, and even though hundreds of thousands of children are currently being treated with stimulant drugs for this problem, we still have controversy over the nature of the disorder being treated, we still don't understand what the drugs are doing to reduce hyperactivity, and we still don't have a widely accepted solution to the apparent paradox: What's a "stimulant" drug doing producing what appears to be a "calming" effect?

The disorder itself was referred to as childhood hyperactivity for many years, and the children who received that label were the ones who seemed absolutely incapable of sitting still and paying attention in class. Many of these children had normal or even above-average IQ scores yet were failing to learn. During the 1960s it was proposed that lead toxicity or early oxygen deprivation might be the cause of a small amount of brain damage. Pointing out that many of these children exhibit "soft" neurological signs (impairments in coordination or other tests that are not localizable to a particular brain area), the term *minimal brain dysfunction* (MBD) became popular. By 1980 there was a feeling that there had been too much focus on activity levels and that the basic disorder was a deficit in attention, which usually, but not always, was accompanied by hyperactivity. Thus the *Diagnostic and Statistical Manual* of the American Psychiatric Association used the term *attention deficit disorder*. However, the latest revision of that manual, the 1994 *DSM-IV*, recognizes the strong relationship between attention

DSM IV Diagnostic Criteria for Attention-Deficit Hyperactivity Disorder

A. Either (1) or (2):

(1) Six (or more) of the following symptoms of inattention have persisted for at least 6 months to a degree that is maladaptive and inconsistent with developmental level:

Inattention

    a. Often fails to give close attention to details or makes careless mistakes

    b. Often has difficulty sustaining attention in tasks or play

    c. Often does not seem to listen when spoken to directly

    d. Often does not follow through on instructions and fails to finish schoolwork, chores, or duties

    e. Often has difficulty organizing tasks and activities

    h. Is often easily distracted by extraneous stimuli

    i. Is often forgetful in daily activities

(2) Six (or more) of the following symptoms of hyperactivity-impulsivity have persisted for at least 6 months to a degree that is maladaptive and inconsistent with developmental level:

Hyperactivity

    a. Often fidgets with hands or feet or squirms in seat

    b. Often leaves seat in classroom or in other situations in which remaining seated is expected

    c. Often runs about or climbs excessively in situations in which it is inappropriate

    d. Often has difficulty playing or engaging in leisure activities quietly

    e. Is often "on the go" or often acts as if "driven by a motor"

    f. Often talks excessively

Impulsivity

    g. Often blurts out answers before questions have been completed

    h. Often has difficulty awaiting turn

    i. Often interrupts or intrudes on others

B. Some hyperactive-impulsive or inattentive symptoms that caused impairment were present before age 7 years.

C. Some impairment from the symptoms is present in two or more settings.

D. There must be clear evidence of clinically significant impairment in social, academic, or occupational functioning.

E. The symptoms do not occur exclusively during the course of a Pervasive Developmental Disorder or other disorder and are not better accounted for by another mental disorder.

---

deficit and hyperactive behavior by using the term *attention-deficit hyperactivity disorder* (**ADHD**).[30] The criteria used to diagnose this disorder are listed in the DSM-IV box above.

The cause or causes of the disorder are not known. One idea that attracted a lot of attention was that it is the additives in the foods we eat that are the basis for ADHD. Many studies were done, and in 1982 a blue-ribbon panel handed down the verdict on diets without food additives:

ADHD: attention-deficit hyperactivity disorder.

"there is no firm evidence that the diets work. Claims that the diets produce dramatic effects simply did not hold up in well-designed clinical trials."

Some hyperactive children have histories of difficult births or contracting encephalitis when very young. Some reports indicate a higher incidence of abnormal EEGs in these children than in children who do not have ADHD. There are as many children with ADHD, however, who do not show abnormal EEGs or medical histories, so the importance of these factors is not clear. There is also no evidence that a large percentage are mentally retarded, although school achievement is usually quite poor. Some believe that children with ADHD suffer only from a maturational lag: they are exhibiting behavior that is typical of children several years younger.

It is interesting that the disorder is at least three times more common in boys than in girls, though that fact hasn't helped us to understand its cause. Also, in many cases the problems seem to be reduced once the child reaches puberty. It was once thought that this was an absolute developmental change, but now we recognize that as many as one-third of the children continue to have hyperactivity problems even into adulthood, and there are arguments as to whether the disorder fades in the other children or just changes its character to something else, such as antisocial personality disorder.

Regardless of the cause, there is clear evidence of the beneficial effect of both amphetamine and **methylphenidate (Ritalin)**. Methylphenidate is now considered the drug of choice for treating ADHD. It is a milder stimulant than amphetamine, with a potency between that of the amphetamines and that of caffeine. Why either type of stimulant drug should work is still not known. One theory that has been around for years is worth considering, even if it is has been difficult to test experimentally: Assume that the child with ADHD is receiving inadequate sensory input to the CNS, and that his noisiness, rocking movements, run-

ning, and crashing into things are an effort to obtain sensory stimulation. The stimulant drugs might arouse the CNS partly by allowing sensory information more direct access to the thalamus and cerebral cortex. Thus, children treated with stimulants could better attend to environmental stimuli and would have less need for hyperactivity and noisiness. Although this theory is plausible, please understand that there are other theories and none has yet been widely accepted.

One of the more disturbing side effects of stimulant therapy is a suppression of height and weight increases during drug treatment. Amphetamine produces a slightly greater effect in most studies than methylphenidate. If drug treatment is stopped over the summer vacation, there is a rebound and a growth spurt that makes up for most of the suppressed height and weight gain.

The seemingly indiscriminate but medically prescribed use of stimulant drugs to influence the behavior of school-age children has evoked much social protest and commentary. After widespread publicity about the use of amphetamines for this purpose in the late 1960s, coinciding with public reaction against amphetamine use, there was a decline in stimulant prescriptions for children and a switch to methylphenidate. More recently there has been a considerable increase in the number of school-children receiving stimulant medication for hyperactivity, and it is now estimated that over a million children are receiving such treatment in the United States.[31] What is not clear is whether this increase represents more awareness of the disorder and its proper treatment or whether more children are being given the medication inappropriately. Whenever drug therapy is used, it should be only one component of an effective treatment program.

"Smart pills"

In the 1960s there were a number of studies that seemed to show that rats learned faster and

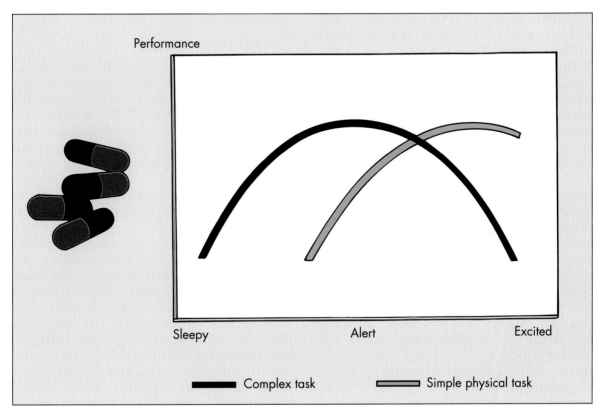

Figure 7.4 Effects of stimulants on performance

performed better if they were given amphetamine or some other stimulant. Abbott Laboratories obtained a patent for the stimulant they named Cylert, which they were testing as a "smart pill." A great deal of animal and human research has since been done on the role of stimulants in improving mental performance, and it is now possible to summarize the ideas that have come from that work. One way to represent the effects of stimulants can be seen in figure 7.4, which schematically relates degree of mental performance to the arousal level of the CNS. At low levels of arousal, such as when the individual is sleepy, performance suffers. Increasing the arousal level into the normal range with a stimulant could then improve perfor-

mance. At the very high end of the arousal scale the person is so maniacal or so involved in repetitive, stereotyped behavior that performance suffers, even on the simplest of tasks. In the region of the graph labeled "excited," it can be seen that some simple tasks can be improved above normal levels, but complex or difficult tasks are disrupted because of difficulty in concentrating, controlling attention, and making careful decisions. Cylert never made it to the

---

methylphenidate (Ritalin): (meth il *fen* ih date) a stimulant used in treating ADHD.

market as a smart pill, but the company later introduced it as an alternative to Ritalin in the treatment of ADHD.

From the schematic in figure 7.4 we can see that anyone trying to improve her mental performance level with amphetamines or other stimulants is taking a chance. Depending on the type of task, predrug performance level, and dose, one might obtain improvement or disruption. A small dose could be beneficial to a tired person driving alone at night on a deserted interstate highway, but would probably only add to the confusion of a school bus driver trying to negotiate a Los Angeles freeway interchange at 7:30 A.M. with a load of noisy students. As for the students themselves, a small dose of a stimulant might help keep a student awake to study when he should be sleeping, but a larger dose? There's an ancient (at least thirty years old) piece of college folklore recounting something that probably never happened but has the ring of possible truth to it. It involves a student who stayed awake for days studying with the help of amphetamines, went into a final exam "wired up," wrote feverishly and eloquently for two hours, and only later when he received his exam back with an F saw that he had written the entire answer on one line, using the line over and over so that it was solid black and the rest of the paper was blank.

Athletics

Under some conditions the use of amphetamine or other stimulants at an appropriate dose can produce slight improvements in athletic performance. The effects are so small as to be meaningless for most athletes, but at the highest levels of competition even a 1 percent improvement can mean the difference between winning a medal or coming in sixth. The temptation has been strong for athletes to use amphetamines and other stimulants to enhance their performances, and this topic is discussed in more detail in chapter 18.

this topic is discussed in more detail in chapter 18.

Causes for Concern

Acute toxicity

During the period of amphetamine intoxication with above-normal doses, what dangers are caused by the altered behavior patterns (acute behavioral toxicity)? As we have seen, even at moderate doses complex decision making can be impaired. At higher doses there is a tendency to be easily panicked and to become suspicious to the point of paranoia. Combine this with increased feelings of power and capability, and there is concern that incidents of violence may increase.

There were multiple reports of the association of amphetamine use and violence and aggression in the late 1960s and early 1970s. Those reports have returned along with increased amphetamine use in the 1990s. Users of large amounts of amphetamine are good people to stay away from. The triad of paranoid ideas, impulsive behavior, and hypersensitivity is directly related to the pharmacological actions of the amphetamines and will occur no matter what the personality of the user. Although the amount of demonstrated violence due to amphetamine use cannot compare with that resulting from alcohol use, it is still a matter of concern, especially when the two are combined. Stimulants and alcohol do not counteract one another in most behavioral effects, and in the case of violence they combine to form an especially explosive mixture.

At one time there was concern that high doses of amphetamines would push the blood pressure so high that small strokes would occur and cause some slight brain damage, which would of course be cumulative for repeated high-dose users. However, no direct human evidence has been obtained indicating this to be a problem. More recently, it was demonstrated in rats that high doses of methamphetamine result in the production in the brain of a chemical that selectively destroys catecholamine neurons.[32]

The possible long-term behavioral consequences for humans could be great from such damage, but as of yet we have no evidence that this occurs in human amphetamine users.

Chronic toxicity

The development of a paranoid psychosis has been long known to be one of the effects of sustained cocaine use. The first amphetamine psychosis was described in 1938, but little attention was given this syndrome until the late 1950s. There have been many suggestions as to the reason for the psychosis: that heavy methamphetamine users have schizoid personalities or that the psychosis is really caused by sleep deprivation, particularly dream-sleep deprivation. The question of the basis for the amphetamine psychosis was resolved by the demonstration that it could be elicited in the laboratory in individuals who clearly were not prepsychotic and who did not experience great sleep deprivation. It seems, then, that the paranoid psychosis after high-dose IV use of amphetamine is primarily the result of the drug and not the personality predisposition of the user. There is evidence that the paranoid psychosis results from dopaminergic stimulation, probably in the mesolimbic system. In some cases in which paranoid psychoses have been produced by amphetamines, the paranoid thinking and loss of touch with reality have been slow to return to normal, persisting for days or even weeks after the drug has left the system. There is no good evidence for permanent behavioral or personality disruption.

There is another behavior induced by high doses of amphetamine: compulsive and repetitive actions. The behavior might be acceptable (the individual might compulsively clean a room over and over) or it might be bizarre (one student spent a night counting corn flakes). There is a precedent for this stereotyped behavior in animal studies using high doses of amphetamine; it probably results from an effect of amphetamine on dopaminergic systems in the basal ganglia.

Dependence potential

Theories about the addictive nature of amphetamines parallel the history of such theories regarding cocaine. For years experts argued about whether the amphetamines were truly "addicting." Because amphetamine withdrawal didn't produce the kinds of obvious physical symptoms seen with heroin or barbiturate withdrawal, most people decided that amphetamine did not produce physical dependence. Yet there is evidence that repeated use of high doses of amphetamine produces a consistent set of withdrawal symptoms: Several hours after the last dose the user "crashes." Mood and energy level drop dramatically, and the user might then sleep for twenty-four hours or more. On awakening, the user is in a depressed mood that can last for days. During this time the individual feels helpless, worthless, and as though she or he could "just sit there and die." Talk of death is common during this period. Of course, taking amphetamine again seems the most rapid way to overcome this mood and get high again. Because this set of symptoms occurs reliably after high-dose amphetamine use, and because it can, within limits, be reversed by taking amphetamine, it does fit our definition of a withdrawal syndrome. Therefore use of high doses of amphetamine can lead to physical dependence (see table 7.1).

It has been known for years that amphetamines could be habit forming, that is, produce psychological dependence. Until a few years ago that was not considered very important. Amphetamine was even considered by some to be a so-called soft drug. It was available by prescription, and it produced only psychological dependence, which most users did not develop. The idea seemed to be that although it could be habit forming in some individuals, its potential for abuse was limited. Now we realize that important factors such as dose and route of administration were not being taken into account. Small doses (5 or 10 mg) taken orally by people acting under their physician's orders for some purpose other than achieving a high rarely resulted in dependence. A larger dose injected intravenously for the purpose of getting high results in very rapid development of strong psychological dependence. Taken in this way, amphetamine is as addicting as any drug we know. Animal studies reveal that rats or monkeys will quickly learn to press a lever that produces IV injections of amphetamine. If required to do so, an animal will press hundreds of times for a single injection.[33]

Supplies of Illicit Amphetamine

Illicit amphetamine for U.S. consumption is primarily produced in small "stovetop laboratories" that might exist for only a few days at a time in some remote area before moving on. Most of these labs produce methamphetamine, although some produce amphetamine itself. For the past several years, law enforcement officers have seized an average of more than 500 of these small methamphetamine labs per year.[8] One reaction to this pressure has been an increase in the importation of "Mexican meth," made in larger laboratories in Mexico and shipped across the border using the methods established for smuggling marijuana and cocaine.

Current patterns of amphetamine abuse

These days there are many fewer people using prescription amphetamines, and the main concern of law enforcement and treatment officials is methamphetamine (crank) made in illicit laboratories. The drug of the 1960s urban hippie has become associated with biker gangs and with laboratories in rural areas of the West.[26] Methamphetamine can be smoked, snorted, or injected, but it is used by only a small fraction of the population. Current use of amphetamine was reported by less than 1 percent of the population in the 1995 Household Survey and the 1996 High School Senior Survey. However, as we said earlier, this number may be expected to increase somewhat within the next few years, and the impact of increased methamphetamine abuse is already being felt in treatment programs and criminal prosecutions.

SUMMARY

- The most effective CNS stimulants are cocaine and amphetamine.
- The stimulants can reverse the effects of fatigue, maintain wakefulness, and temporarily elevate the mood of the user.
- Cocaine is derived from the coca plant. Coca leaves have been chewed for centuries.
- Cocaine's earliest uses in the United States were as a local anesthetic and in psychiatry.
- Coca paste and crack are smokable forms of illicit cocaine.
- Cocaine appears to act by blocking reuptake of both dopamine and serotonin.
- Excessive cocaine use can result in a paranoid psychotic reaction.
- Cocaine and amphetamine produce both psychological and physical dependence.
- Use of cocaine has declined in the general population since 1985.
- Amphetamine is a synthetic sympathomimetic similar to ephedrine.
- The amphetamine-like drugs are similar in structure to dopamine and norepinephrine.
- Amphetamine is used in short-term weight reduction, narcolepsy, and ADHD (methylphenidate is preferred for ADHD, however).
- Illicit use of amphetamine has been associated with violent behavior.
- Illicit methamphetamine is primarily made in small laboratories or imported from Mexico.
- Amphetamine use is currently at a low level in the general population.

REVIEW QUESTIONS

1. At about what periods in history did cocaine reach its first and second peaks of popularity, and when was amphetamine's popularity at its highest?
2. How did Mariani, Freud, Halsted, and Conan Doyle popularize the use of cocaine?
3. How are coca paste, freebase, crack, and ice similar?
4. What similarities and what differences are there in the toxic effects of cocaine and amphetamine?
5. What effect would there be on medical practice if both cocaine and amphetamine were placed on Schedule I?
6. Contrast the typical "speed freak" of the 1960s with the typical cocaine user of the early 1980s and with our stereotype of a 1990s crack smoker.
7. How does the chemical difference between methamphetamine and amphetamine relate to the behavioral effects of the two drugs?
8. Compare the dependence potential of cocaine with that of amphetamine.

Related Internet Sites on Cocaine and Methamphetamine

NIDA: http://www.nida.nih.gov/Drug.Abuse.html

Web of Addictions: http://www.well.com/user/woa/aodsites.htm

And don't neglect our own *Drugs, Society, and Human Behavior* site: http://www.uwyo.edu/a&s/psyc/dshb.htm

REFERENCES

1. Dillehay TD and others: The Nanchoc tradition: The beginnings of Andean civilization, *American Scientist* 85:46-55, 1997.
2. Taylor N: *Flight from reality*, New York, 1949, Duell, Sloan & Pearce.
3. Freud S: *On the general effect of cocaine*, lecture before the Psychiatric Union on March 5, 1885. (Reprinted in *Drug Dependence* 5:17, 1970).
4. Doyle AC: The sign of the four. In *The complete Sherlock Holmes*, New York, 1938, Garden City Publishing.
5. Musto DF: Opium, cocaine and marijuana in American history, *Scientific American*, p 40, July 1991.
6. Ashley R: *Cocaine: its history, uses and effects*, New York, 1976, Warner Books.
7. Brecher EM: *Licit and illicit drugs*, Boston, 1972, Little, Brown.
8. US Drug Enforcement Administration, National Narcotics Intelligence Consumers Committee: *The supply of illicit drugs to the United States*, Washington, DC, June 1991, US Government Printing Office.
9. Witkin G: The men who created crack, *US News & World Report*, p 44, Aug 19, 1991.
10. Feldman RS, Meyer JS, Quenzer LF: *Principles of neuropsycholpharmacology*, Sunderland, MA, 1997, Sinauer.
11. Williams S: Cocaine's harmful effects, *Science* 248:166, 1990.
12. Randall T: Cocaine, alcohol mix in body to form even longer lasting, more lethal drug, *JAMA* 267:1043, 1992.
13. Brady, KT and others: Cocaine-induced psychosis, *J Clin Psychiatry* 52:509, 1991.
14. Bunn WH, Giannini AJ: Cardiovascular complications of cocaine abuse, *Am Fam Physician* 46:769, 1992.
15. Johanson CE: Assessment of the dependence potential of cocaine in animals. In Grabowski J, editor: *Cocaine: pharmacology, effects, and treatment of abuse*, NIDA Research Monograph No 50, Washington, DC, 1984, US Government Printing Office.
16. Zuckerman B and others: Effects of maternal marijuana and cocaine use on fetal growth, *N Engl J Med* 320:762, 1989.
17. Zuckerman B: "Crack kids": not broken, *Pediatrics* 89:337, 1992.
18. *National drug control strategy*, February 1994, Washington, DC, The White House.
19. Riley KJ: *Snow job?* New Brunswick, NJ, 1996, Transaction.
20. Martz L: A dirty secret: hyping instant addiction doesn't help, *Newsweek*, p 74, Feb 19, 1990.
21. Strain EC and others: Buprenorphine versus methadone in the treatment of opioid-dependent cocaine users, *Psychopharmacology* 116:401, 1994.

22. Benzedrine alert, *Air Surgeon's Bulletin* 1(2):19-21, 1944.

23. On a bender with Benzedrine, *Everybody's Digest* 5(2):50, 1946.

24. JAMA 183:363, 1963.

25. Proceedings released from symposium on methamphetamine use, *SAMHSA News*, Summer, 1997, U.S. Department of Health and Human Services.

26. Bai M: White storm warning, *Newsweek*, March 30, 1997.

27. Physician's Desk Reference Medical Economics, Ordell, NJ. Annual.

28. Weintraub M: Long-term weight control, *Clinical Pharmacology & Therapeutics* 51:581-594, 1992.

29. *Weight loss drug receives FDA clearance*, Press release, November 24, 1997.

30. *Diagnostic and statistical manual of mental disorders*, ed. 4, Washington, DC, 1994, American Psychiatric Association.

31. O'Toole K and others: Effects of methylphenidate on attention and nonverbal learning in children with attention-deficit hyperactivity disorder, *Journal of the American Academy of Child and Adolescent Psychiatry* 36:531-537, 1996.

32. Marek GJ and others: Dopamine uptake inhibitors block long-term neurotoxic effects of methamphetamine upon dopaminergic neurons, *Brain Res* 513:274, 1990.

33. Griffiths RR and others: Predicting the abuse liability of drugs with animal self-administration procedures: psychomotor stimulants and hallucinogens, in Thompson T, Dews P, editors: *Advances in behavioral pharmacology*, vol 2, New York, 1979, Academic Press.

34. Jacobson JL and others: Effects of alcohol use, smoking, and illicit drug use on fetal growth in black infants, *J Pediatr* 124:757, 1994.

8

Depressants and Inhalants

After reading this chapter, you should be able to:

sedatives
hypnotics
depressants
benzodiazepines
barbiturates
inhalants
rohypnol
GABA
GHB
epilepsy

- Distinguish among barbiturates, benzodiazepines, alcohol, inhalants, and other classes of depressant drugs and state something of the history of each major group.
- Explain the mechanism of action of the barbiturates and the benzodiazepines in relation to the neurotransmitter GABA.
- Describe the usefulness and some of the practical limitations of sedative-hypnotic drugs in treating

anxiety, insomnia, and epilepsy.
- Discuss the ability of these drugs to produce both psychological and physical dependence and describe the withdrawal syndrome.
- Discuss the ability of these drugs to produce both behavioral and physiological toxicity.
- Describe typical patterns of sedative abuse and contrast them with inhalant abuse.

Downers, depressants, sedatives, hypnotics, gin-in-a-pill: known by many names, these prescription drugs all have a widespread effect in the brain that can be summed up as decreased neural activity. What are the behavioral effects? As suggested by one of the proposed names, if you know what alcohol does, you know what these drugs do. They come from several different chemical classes but are grouped together because of their common psychological effects. At low doses these drugs might be prescribed for daytime use to reduce anxiety (as **sedatives**). At higher doses many of the same drugs are prescribed as sleeping pills (**hypnotics**).

This group of prescription drugs is often referred to as *sedative-hypnotics,* part of a larger group of substances considered to be CNS **depressants.** The most widely *used* depressant is alcohol, which is discussed in detail in chapters

sedatives: drugs used to relax, calm, or tranquilize.

hypnotics: drugs used to induce sleep.

depressants: drugs that slow activity in the CNS.

165

10 and 11. The most widely *prescribed* types of sedative-hypnotics fall into the chemical grouping called the **benzodiazepines,** which in the past thirty years have largely replaced the **barbiturates.** A similar depressant effect is produced by most of the **inhalants**—the glues, paints, solvents, or gasoline fumes that some young people (and a few older people) breathe to get "high."

HISTORY AND PHARMACOLOGY

Before Barbiturates

- **Chloral hydrate.** The "knockout drops" (or "Mickey Finn") they used to slip in the sailor's drink in those old movies were a solution of chloral hydrate. First synthesized in 1832, chloral hydrate was not used clinically until about 1870. It is rapidly metabolized to trichloroethanol, which is the active hypnotic agent. When taken orally, chloral hydrate has a short onset period (30 minutes), and 1 to 2 g will induce sleep in less than an hour. This agent does not cause as much depression of the respiratory and cardiovascular systems as a comparable dose of the barbiturates and has fewer aftereffects.

  In 1869, Dr. Benjamine Richardson introduced chloral hydrate to Great Britain. Ten years later he called it "in one sense a benef-

icent, and in another sense a maleficent substance, I almost feel a regret that I took any part whatever in the introduction of the agent into the practice of healing."[1] He had learned that what humankind can misuse, some will abuse. As early as 1871 he referred to its non-therapeutic use as "toxical luxury" and lamented that chloral hydrate addicts had to be added to "alcohol intemperants and opium-eaters." Chloral hydrate addiction is a tough way to go; it is a gastric irritant, and repeated use causes considerable stomach upset.

- **Paraldehyde.** Paraldehyde was synthesized in 1829 and introduced clinically in 1882. Paraldehyde would probably be in great use today because of its effectiveness as a CNS depressant with little respiratory depression and a wide safety margin, except for one characteristic: It has an extremely noxious taste and an odor that permeates the breath of the user. Its safety margin and its ability to sedate patients led to widespread use of paraldehyde in mental hospitals before the 1950s. Anyone who ever worked in, was a patient in, or even visited one of the large state mental hospitals during that era probably still remembers the odor of paraldehyde, which was often detectable on entering the building.

- **Bromides.** Bromide salts were used so widely in patent medicines to induce sleep in the nineteenth century that the word *bromide* entered our language as a reference to any person or story that was tiresome and boring. The bromides are little used today, now that they have been removed from OTC sleep preparations. Bromides accumulate in the body, and the depression they cause builds up over several days of regular use. There are serious toxic effects with repeated hypnotic doses of these agents. Dermatitis and constipation are minor accompaniments; with increased intake, motor disturbances, delirium, and psychosis can develop. Very low (ineffective) doses of bromides remained in some OTC medicines until the 1960s.

Chloral hydrate

Barbiturates

Over 2,500 barbiturates have been synthesized. Barbital (Veronal) was the first to be used clinically, in 1903. Its name gave rise to the practice of giving barbiturates names ending in *-al.* The second barbiturate in clinical use, phenobarbital (Luminal), was introduced in 1912. Amobarbital (Amytal) in 1923, as well as pentobarbital (Nembutal) and secobarbital (Seconal), both introduced in 1930, are well-established examples of the barbiturates.

As table 8.1 indicates, barbiturates are typically grouped on the basis of the duration of their activity. In general the drugs that are the most lipid-soluble are the ones that have both the shortest time of onset (i.e., they are absorbed and enter the brain rapidly) and the shortest duration of action (i.e., they leave the brain quickly and tend to be more rapidly metabolized). These different time courses are important for our understanding of the different uses of these drugs and their different tendencies to produce dependence.

Various barbiturates

Suppose you want a drug to keep a person calm and relaxed during the daytime (a sedative). You don't want the person to become drowsy, and you want to produce as stable and smooth a drug effect as possible. Therefore you would choose a *low* dose of a *long-acting* barbiturate, say 30 to 50 mg of phenobarbital. On the other hand, for a sleeping-pill (hypnotic) effect, you want the person to become drowsy, you want the drug to act fairly quickly after it is taken, and you don't want the person to still be groggy the next morning. Therefore you would choose a *higher* dose of a *shorter-acting* drug, say 100 to 200 mg of amobarbital or secobarbital. Both of these types of prescription were fairly common thirty years ago, before the introduction of the benzodiazepines.

TABLE 8.1

Groupings of Available Barbiturates

Type	Time of onset	Duration of action (hours)
Short-acting Pentobarbital (Nembutal) Secobarbital (Seconal)	15 minutes	2 to 3
Intermediate-acting Aprobarbital (Alurate) Amobarbital (Amytal) Butabarbital (Butisol)	30 minutes	5 to 6
Long-acting Mephobarbital (Merbaral) Phenobarbital (Luminal)	1 hour	6 to 10

benzodiazepines: (ben zo die *ay* zah peens) a chemical grouping of sedative-hypnotics.

barbiturates: (bar *bitch* er ates) a chemical group of sedative-hypnotics.

inhalants: volatile solvents inhaled for intoxicating purposes.

Although a large fraction of phenobarbital is excreted unchanged in the urine, the majority of this drug and nearly all of the shorter-acting drugs is metabolized in the liver. The barbiturates are one of the classes of drugs that stimulate the activity of the microsomal enzymes of the liver. Some of the tolerance that develops to the barbiturates is the result of an increased rate of deactivation caused by this stimulation. The induction of these enzymes by the barbiturates might also cause the more rapid metabolism of other drugs, perhaps requiring an adjustment of the dose.

Tolerance can develop to the barbiturates, as well as both psychological and physical dependence. In addition, they depress respiration and, in large doses or in combination with alcohol, can completely stop one's breathing. For many years barbiturate sleeping pills were chosen above all others by people wishing to commit suicide. Also, accidental overdoses occurred when sleeping pills were taken after an evening of heavy drinking.

Although the majority of individuals who took barbiturates were not harmed by them, there was a great deal of concern about both the addiction liability and the danger of overdose. These concerns led to the ready acceptance of new sedative or hypnotic agents that appeared to be safer.

Meprobamate

The first modern antianxiety agents (*anxiolytics*) developed from a muscle relaxant called mephenesin, which was patented in 1946 and was a commercial success but had a short duration of action. One compound patented in 1952 not only was longer lasting but was believed to be a unique type of CNS depressant. Clinical trials in 1953 supported this belief, and the compound was approved by the FDA and released for prescription use in 1955. Meprobamate, the generic name, became widely

Meprobamate

known by the brand name Miltown, and it represented the drug revolution of the 1950s to many people.

The boom in meprobamate use was tremendous. In the year it was introduced, sales of Miltown went from $7,500 in May to over $500,000 in December. The happy pills had arrived! A publicity agency and excessive prescribing by physicians combined to make Miltown a public nuisance and the unnamed object of comment concerning overuse by the American Psychiatric Association and the World Health Organization in 1957. *Miltown* became such an overused word that physicians began prescribing meprobamate under its other brand name, Equanil.

It gradually became clear that meprobamate, like the barbiturates, can also produce both psychological and physical dependence. Physical dependence can result from taking a bit more than twice a normal daily dose. In 1970, meprobamate became a Schedule IV controlled substance, and although it is still available for prescription under several brand names, the benzodiazepines have largely replaced it.

Although reports of overdose deaths from meprobamate alone are rare, in retrospect it seems ironic that the medical community so readily accepted meprobamate as being safer than barbiturates. Meprobamate was sold only in anxiolytic doses for daytime sedation. Barbiturates produce physical dependence at doses above 400 mg, or twice a maximum *hypnotic* dose. If barbiturates had been sold only as 30 mg phenobarbital for daytime sedation, many fewer cases of physical dependence or overdose would have been reported. Let this be an object lesson: by deciding that the "barbiturates" were addicting and deadly, the focus was on the chemical class, rather than on the dose and the manner in which the drug was used. Thus a new, "safer" chemical was accepted without considering that its safety was not being judged under the same conditions. This mistake has occurred frequently with psychoactive drugs. In fact, it occurred again with methaqualone.

Methaqualone

With continued reports of overdoses and physical dependence associated with secobarbital and amobarbital sleeping pills, in the 1960s the market was wide open for a hypnotic that would be less addicting and less dangerous. Maybe it was too wide open.

The methaqualone story is one where everyone was wrong—the pharmaceutical industry, the FDA, the DEA, the press, and the physicians. No one can claim to be without sin. Methaqualone was originally synthesized in India, tested, and found to be ineffective as an antimalarial drug. But it was a good sedative, so in 1959 it was introduced as a prescription drug in Great Britain. It never sold well, but after the thalidomide disaster, there was increased interest in a "safe" nonbarbiturate sleeping pill.

Mandrax (250 mg of methaqualone and 25 mg of an antihistamine) was introduced in 1965 in a massive advertising campaign to physicians. The campaign worked, and two million prescriptions were issued for Mandrax in 1971 in Great Britain. The drug had already found its way into the street, where it was widely abused: by heroin users, by high school students, by anyone who wanted a cheap but potent "down." Misuse was so great that Great Britain tightened controls on it in 1970 and then again in 1973.

Germany introduced methaqualone in 1960 as a nonprescription drug, had its first methaqualone suicide in 1962, and discovered that 10 to 22 percent of the drug overdoses treated in this period were a result of this drug. In 1963, Germany reduced the problem by making methaqualone a prescription drug. In 1960 to 1964, Japan experienced a major epidemic of methaqualone abuse, causing over 40 percent of all overdoses admitted to hospitals. Japan tightened controls almost to the maximum possible on methaqualone and stemmed the tide.

Apparently no one in the United States was paying much attention to these problems in other countries, because in 1965, after three years of testing, Quaalude and Sopor, brand names for methaqualone, were introduced in the United States as prescription drugs with a package insert that read, "Addiction potential not established." In June 1966 the FDA Committee on the Abuse Potential of Drugs decided that there was no need to monitor methaqualone, since there was no evidence of abuse potential! Thus from 1967 to 1973 the package insert read, "Physical dependence has not clearly been demonstrated."

In the early 1970s in this country, *ludes* and *sopors* were familiar terms in the drug culture and in drug-treatment centers. Physicians were overprescribing a hypnotic drug that they believed to be nonaddicting and safer than the barbiturates. Most of the methaqualone sold on the street was legally manufactured and then either stolen or obtained through prescriptions. At any rate, sales zoomed, and front-page reporting of its effects when misused helped to build its reputation as a drug of abuse. In 1973, 8 years after it was introduced into this country, 4 years after American scientists began saying it was addicting, 11 years after the first suicide, methaqualone was put on Schedule II. By 1985, methaqualone was no longer available as a prescription drug, and it is now listed on Schedule I.

Was methaqualone really very different from the barbiturates? For a while physicians thought it was safer. Street users referred to it as the "love drug" (one of many drugs to have been called this) or "heroin for lovers," implying an *aphrodisiac* effect. In reality the effect is probably not different from the disinhibition produced by alcohol or other depressants. Methaqualone causes the same kind of motor incoordination as alcohol and the barbiturates. Both psychological and physical dependence can develop to methaqualone as easily and rapidly as with the barbiturates, and for a few years methaqualone was also near the "top of the charts" for drug-related deaths (DAWN coroners' reports). If it was different, it wasn't much different.

Benzodiazepines

The first of the benzodiazepines was chlordiazepoxide, which was marketed under the trade name Librium (possibly because it "liberates" one from anxieties). Chlordiazepoxide was synthesized in 1947, but it was ten years before its value in reducing anxiety was suggested, and it was not sold commercially until 1960. The discovery of this class of drugs was a triumph for behavioral research; a drug-company pharmacologist found that mice given the right dose of chlordiazepoxide would loosen their grip on an inclined wire screen and fall to the floor of the test cage. When this experiment had been done with barbiturates, the mice promptly fell asleep. With Librium, the relaxed mouse con-

Benzodiazepines, from top to bottom: diazepam, chlordiazepoxide, flurazepam, clonazepam, clorazepate, lorazepam, and oxazepam

tinued to walk around sniffing the cage in a normal manner.[2] This drug was marketed as a more selective "antianxiety" agent that produced less drowsiness than the barbiturates and had a much larger safety margin before overdose death occurred in animals. Clinical practice bore this out: physical dependence was almost unheard of, and overdose seemed not to occur except in combination with alcohol or other depressant drugs. Even strong psychological dependence seemed rare with this drug. The conclusion was reached that the benzodiazepines were as effective as the barbiturates and much safer. Librium became not only the leading psychoactive drug in sales but also the leading prescription drug of all. It was supplanted in the early 1970s by diazepam (Valium), a more potent (lower-dose) agent made by the same company. From 1972 until 1978 Valium was the leading seller among all prescription drugs. Since then no single benzodiazepine has so dominated the market, but Xanax (a brand name for alprazolam) is currently the most widely prescribed brand name among this class of drugs.

As these drugs became widely used, reports again appeared of psychological dependence, occasional physical dependence, and overdose deaths. Diazepam was one of the most frequently mentioned drugs in the DAWN system coroner's reports, although almost always in combination with alcohol or other depressants. What happened to the big difference between the barbiturates and the benzodiazepines? One possibility is that it might not be the chemical class of drugs that makes the big difference, but the dose and time course of the individual drugs. It's obvious that *overdose* deaths are more likely when a drug is sold in higher doses, such as those prescribed for hypnotic effects. *Psychological dependence* develops most rapidly when the drug "hits the brain" quickly, which is why intravenous use of heroin produces more dependence than oral use, and why smoking crack produces more dependence than chewing coca leaves. So a drug that has a rapid onset of action will be more likely to produce psychological dependence than a slow-acting drug. *Physical dependence* occurs when the drug leaves the system more rapidly than the body can adapt—one way to reduce the severity of withdrawal symptoms is to reduce the dose of a drug slowly over time. Drugs with a shorter duration of action leave the system quickly and are much more likely to produce withdrawal symptoms than longer-acting drugs.

Figure 8.1 gives a schematic picture of the time course of the depressant actions of some of these drugs. Secobarbital, a short-acting barbiturate, has a relatively rapid onset that should make it more likely than other barbiturates to produce psychological dependence. Also, because its depressant action is terminated fairly quickly, withdrawal symptoms would be quite dramatic if the person had been taking large doses. Because this drug was primarily used as a sleeping pill, relatively large doses were prescribed. Thus in the days when barbiturates were widely prescribed, secobarbital was associated with overdoses and both physical and

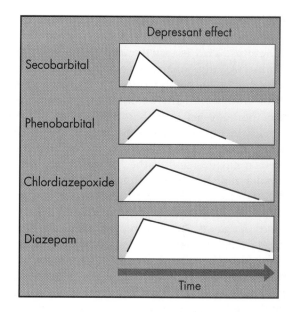

Figure 8.1 Schematic diagram of the relative time courses of two barbiturates and two benzodiazepines after oral administration

psychological dependence. Phenobarbital, a long-acting barbiturate, has a slower onset of action that should be less likely to produce psychological dependence. Because the depressant action is terminated more slowly, drug clearance occurs slowly and withdrawal symptoms are minimized. Because phenobarbital was prescribed mostly in low sedative doses, it was rarely associated with overdose.

The first benzodiazepine was chlordiazepoxide, which was sold in low doses for daytime use and has a slow onset of action and an even longer duration of action than phenobarbital. Chlordiazepoxide produced few problems with either compulsive use or withdrawal symptoms, and overdoses were almost unheard of. Diazepam has a more rapid onset than chlordiazepoxide, but because of slow metabolism and the presence of active metabolites, it also has a long duration of action. We might expect a drug with these characteristics to produce more psychological dependence than chlordiaz-epoxide, but only rarely to produce withdrawal symptoms. This is exactly what happened. To summarize this pharmacology object lesson, there might be greater differences among the barbiturates and among the benzodiazepines than there are between these two classes.

As if to underscore the basic similarity that exists among all the depressant drugs, in the 1990s a new version of the "Mickey Finn" was popularized. **Rohypnol** (flunitrazepam), a benzodiazepine sold as a hypnotic in many countries around the world but not in the United States, hit the news when reports surfaced of its being put into the drinks of unsuspecting women by their dates. The combination of rohypnol and alcohol was reputed to produce a profound intoxication during which the woman would be highly suggestible and also unable to

remember what happened to her. Thus, rohypnol became widely known as the "date-rape" drug (see FYI box). In 1997, the drug's manufacturer changed the formulation of the pill so that when it dissolves in a drink it produces a characteristic color.[3]

MECHANISM OF ACTION

An important key to understanding the effects of these sedative-hypnotic agents was found in 1977 when it was reported that radioactive diazepam molecules had a high affinity for specific receptor sites in brain tissue. Other benzodiazepine types of sedatives also bound to these receptors, and the binding affinities of these various drugs correlated with their behavioral potencies in humans and other animals. These benzodiazepine receptors did not bind any of the

---

FYI   The Drug-Induced Rape Prevention and Punishment Act

In 1996 the U.S. Congress debated what to do in response to widespread concerns about the use of rohypnol as a "date-rape" drug (see text). One proposal was to make the drug a Schedule I controlled substance—after all, it was not a prescription drug in the United States and therefore could be considered to have "no medical use," one of the defining criteria for inclusion in Schedule I. However, the drug was legally available in more than sixty other countries, and Schedule I status would compel the United States to pressure those countries to outlaw it also. Instead, Congress passed the Drug-Induced Rape Prevention and Punishment Act. This act makes it a federal crime to give someone a controlled substance without the recipient's knowledge, with the intent of committing a violent crime. During the debate it was af-

firmed that rape is considered to be a crime of violence. Under this law, the maximum penalty is twenty years in prison and a $250,000 fine. A urine test is available for rohypnol, so any woman who suspects that she may have been given the drug can request that the test be conducted. It would then be possible, under this act, to charge the person suspected of giving her the drug. Even if no rape took place, it might be difficult for the drug-giver to argue that such was not his intention, given the reputation this drug has.

You might start a discussion among a group of your friends about date rape. What is their perception of this problem? What drugs have they heard about in conjunction with date rape? Are they aware of this federal law and its implications?

known neurotransmitters, nor did they bind any of the barbiturates. However, it was soon noticed that the benzodiazepine receptors were always near receptors for the amino acid neurotransmitter *g*-aminobutyric acid (**GABA**). It now appears that when benzodiazepines bind to their receptor site, they enhance the normally inhibitory effects of GABA on its receptors. The barbiturates act at a separate binding site nearby and also increase the actions of GABA on its receptors. The picture emerges of a GABA receptor *complex*, which includes the barbiturate binding site and the benzodiazepine receptor.[4] Drug companies quickly began developing new drugs based on their ability to bind to these sites, and several new sedative-hypnotics have reached the market in recent years.

Although there have been intensive efforts to isolate an endogenous Valium-like substance from brain tissue, so far none has succeeded. A diazepam-binding inhibitor (DBI) peptide has been isolated from brain tissue, but when this substance is administered it has effects opposite to those of diazepam, apparently producing excitement and increased anxiety in some animal tests. Perhaps the brain does not contain a substance that enhances GABA's inhibitory effect and only contains modulators that diminish GABA inhibition. The benzodiazepines and barbiturates would then have an effect opposite to that of the endogenous modulators. Another possibility is that there are endogenous sedative-hypnotic substances that have yet to be discovered.

BENEFICIAL USES

As Sedatives

> Raze out the written troubles of the brain,
> and with some sweet oblivious antidote
> Cleanse the stuff'd bosom of that perilous stuff
> Which weighs upon the heart . . .

As these lines from Shakespeare's *Macbeth* reveal, humans have often sought a "sweet oblivious antidote" to the cares and woes of

TABLE 8.2	
Some Popular Benzodiazepines	
Type	Half-life (hours)
Anxiolytics	
Alprazolam (Xanax)	6–20
Chlordiazepoxide (Librium)	5–30
Clorazepate (Tranxene)	30–200
Diazepam (Valium)	20–100
Lorazepam (Ativan)	10–20
Oxazepam (Serax)	5–15
Hypnotics	
Flurazepam (Dalmane)	40–250
Temazepam (Restoril)	5–25
Triazolam (Halcion)	1.7–3

living. Alcohol has most frequently been used for that purpose, but the sedative drugs also play a major role in modern society. In the United States in recent decades the barbiturates, then meprobamate, and then the benzodiazepines have been among the most widely prescribed medications. Xanax is the most popular of these, ranking in the top ten in sales among all prescription drugs.[5] Also, both diazepam and lorazepam are among the most popular generic drug prescriptions (table 8.2)

The combined sales of the benzodiazepines make them one of the most widely prescribed drug classes. Why? Most psychiatrists refer to the benzodiazepines as antianxiety agents, or anxiolytics. And most psychiatrists seem to accept the widely held view that various types of dysfunctional behavior (e.g., phobias, panic attacks, obsessive-compulsive disorders, psychosomatic problems) might result from various forms of psychological stress that can be lumped under the general classification of "anxieties." So

---

rohypnol: a benzodiazepine; the "date-rape drug."

GABA: an inhibitory neurotransmitter.

if anxieties produce dysfunctional behavior and these drugs can reduce anxieties, then the drugs will be useful in reducing the dysfunctional behavior. In fact these disorders are now officially referred to as "anxiety disorders" (see chapter 9). Although this approach seems logical, in reality not all of these conditions respond well to antianxiety drugs. For specific phobias (e.g., fear of spiders), behavior therapy is a more effective treatment. And for obsessive-compulsive disorder, certain antidepressant drugs seem to be most effective. Most of the prescriptions for antianxiety medications are not written by psychiatrists nor are they written for patients with clearly defined anxiety disorders. In addition, many patients take the drugs on a daily basis for long periods of time. What disorder is being treated with such prescriptions? Galen, the second-century Greek physician, estimated that about 60 percent of the patients he saw had emotional and psychological, as opposed to physical, illness. It is currently estimated that for a typical general practitioner, about half of the patients have no treatable physical ailment. Many of these patients who complain of nervousness, distress, or vague aches and pains will be given a prescription for a sedative such as Xanax. One way to look at this is that the patients may be suffering from a low-level generalized anxiety disorder, and the sedative is reducing the anxiety. A more cynical way of looking at it is that some patients are asking to be protected from the cares and woes of daily living. The physician prescribes something that is relatively

UP FOR DEBATE
GHB: "Natural" High or Deadly Diversion?

Here is a surefire formula for creating a new drug scare: Take a substance that most people have not heard of before, add a group of young people partying and acting wild, mix with the usually present alcohol, along with the typically associated fighting and sexual activity, and someone is going to get hurt. Many drugs can be serious problems in combination with alcohol, but with **GHB** (gamma-hydroxybutyrate) several fatal or near-fatal overdoses and other serious reactions have occurred among young partiers. What proportion of these problems should be attributed to alcohol rather than GHB is not yet clear, but because alcohol is familiar and GHB is not, most of the blame seems to be placed on GHB. What is this stuff? It is a chemical that is found naturally in our brains, and in the 1980s it was being sold in health food stores as a "natural" sleep aid and for other purposes as well. The FDA cracked down on such claims in 1990, after which it became less freely available. Its use as a party drug for young people dates to around this same time, when it was prominently associated with the "rave" scene. Warnings about its potential deadliness have competed with a widespread belief among many young people that this is just an inexpensive, "natural" high.[22] GHB is fairly easy to make and is not a controlled substance under federal law, although a few states have passed laws banning its possession. Most of what we know for certain about this drug can be accounted for by considering it to be another general CNS depressant, which at low doses can result in disinhibition just as is seen with alcohol.

safe and can make the patient feel better in a general way. The patient doesn't complain as much and comes back for more pills, so everyone is happy.

Although most physicians would agree that the benzodiazepines are probably overprescribed, in any individual case it may be impossible to know whether the patient just enjoys getting a "feel-good pill" or feels better because of a specific anitanxiety effect. Whatever the reason for each individual, based on past history there will continue to be a very large and profitable market for prescription sedatives.

As Sleeping Pills

Although one or two beers might relax a person and reduce inhibitions a bit, the effect of larger amounts is more dramatic. If you consume several beers at an active, noisy party, you might become wild and reckless. But if you consume the same number of beers, go to bed, and turn off the lights, you will probably fall asleep fairly quickly. This is essentially the principle on which hypnotic drug therapy is based: the drug is not given in an anesthetic dose but in a large enough amount to help you get to sleep more quickly.

Insomnia is a fairly common symptom, and one nationwide household survey found that about one out of three adults reported some trouble falling asleep, staying asleep, or both.[6] About half of these people felt that their insomnia was serious, but fewer than 10 percent had used a prescription hypnotic drug within the past year. People who complain of insomnia often overestimate how long it takes them to get to sleep and underestimate how much time they actually sleep. Partly because physicians know this and partly because of concern about tolerance, rebound insomnia, dependence, and "hangover" effects, fewer hypnotics are prescribed now than thirty years ago, and they are usually taken for only a few nights at a time rather than continually.

Since 1976, when flurazepam (Dalmane) became the leading hypnotic agent, the benzodiazepines have increasingly displaced the barbiturates in the sleeping-pill market. The shorter-acting drug triazolam (Halcion) is now the most commonly prescribed brand of hypnotic. There is an interesting story in this: When barbiturates are used, they produce a fairly rapid tolerance, so that after a few nights of regular use they are no longer effective. To regain the hypnotic effect it becomes necessary to increase the dose, leading to concerns about addiction. One reason that Dalmane became the hypnotic drug of choice was that research indicated that it still produced hypnotic effects after four weeks of daily use. Dalmane, however, has an active metabolite with a long half-life (well over a day; See table 8.2). With nightly use there is a buildup of this metabolite in the body. Perhaps the reason Dalmane still works after four weeks is that the total dose of metabolite plus Dalmane is quite large by that time. There is concern that this buildup of Dalmane plus its metabolite might impair the individual's performance during the daytime. Halcion has replaced Dalmane because it has a short half-life, no active metabolite, and should not build up in the body. Most patients are instructed to avoid daily use, but in some cases of severe insomnia chronic use is indicated. Can the short-acting benzodiazepines work under chronic treatment conditions without tolerance or withdrawal symptoms (e.g., rebound insomnia)? There are conflicting reports, but one large study indicated that short-acting benzodiazepines could still be effective after three months of chronic use with no evidence of rebound insomnia on withdrawal.[7]

Although the number of prescriptions for hypnotics has declined considerably over the

---

GHB: gamma-hydroxybutyrate; potentially deadly when mixed with alcohol.

past twenty-five years, when a new drug is introduced it displaces some of the older ones and then new concerns are raised about the newer drug and its side effects. By the early 1990s Halcion sales had reached $100 million per year in the United States and $250 million worldwide. However, concerns were raised about the safety of the drug, and Upjohn, the drug's manufacturer, was sued by a woman who claimed the drug made her so agitated and paranoid that she had killed her own mother. That case was settled out of court, but it brought attention to the drug and to other claims that it produced an unusual number of adverse psychiatric reactions in patients. Halcion has been banned in five countries because of these side effects, but it has survived two FDA reviews in the United States and remains on the market.[8] Although sales have no doubt been harmed by the adverse publicity, Halcion remains the most popular sleeping pill in the United States.

The newest benzodiazapine-like hypnotic on the U.S. market is zolpidem (Ambien). Although it binds only to one subtype of benzodiazepine receptor and has therefore been suggested to be a more specific hypnotic agent,[9] clinically it appears to be similar to Halcion, with rapid onset and short duration of action.

If you or someone you know has trouble sleeping, before resorting to the use of medication it would be wise to follow the suggestions given in the FYI box on p. 177. These tactics will probably help most people deal with their concerns about sleeplessness.

Anticonvulsant Effects

A thorough description of seizure disorders (the **epilepsies**) is beyond the scope of this book. However, you should know that both the barbiturates and the benzodiazepines are widely used for the control of epileptic seizures. They are effective in reasonably low doses and are often combined with other anticonvulsant drugs for even better effectiveness. There are some practical problems associated with this use, and by now you could guess what some of them are.

Anticonvulsant medications are given chronically, so there is a tendency for tolerance to develop. The dose should be kept high enough to control the seizures without producing undesirable drowsiness. Abrupt withdrawal of these drugs is likely to lead to seizures, so medication changes should be done carefully. In spite of these problems, the sedative drugs are currently a necessary and useful treatment for epilepsy.

CAUSES FOR CONCERN

Dependence Liability

Psychological dependence

Most people who have used either barbiturates or benzodiazepines have not developed habitual use patterns. However, it was clear with the barbiturates that some individuals do become daily users of intoxicating amounts. Again, the short-acting barbiturates seemed to be the culprits. When Librium, the first benzodiazepine, was in its heyday, relatively little habitual use was reported. As Librium was displaced by the newer, more potent Valium, we saw increasing reports of habitual Valium use, perhaps because its onset, although slower than that of the short-acting barbiturates, is more rapid than that of Librium. Then Xanax, another rapid-acting benzodiazepine, became the most widely prescribed sedative, and reports of Xanax dependence appeared.[10]

Animals given the opportunity to press a lever that delivers intravenous barbiturates will do so, and the short-acting barbiturates work best for this. Animals will also self-inject several of the benzodiazepines, but at lower rates than with the short-acting barbiturates.[11] When

> **epilepsy:** a disorder characterized by uncontrolled movements (seizures).

FYI Sleep Hygiene Techniques for Insomnia

Careful adherence to the following rules can lead to substantial improvement in sleep and can help prevent the development of chronic intractable insomnia.

- Establish and maintain a regular bedtime and a regular arising time. Try to wake up and get out of bed at the appointed time, even if you had trouble sleeping the night before. Avoid excessive sleep during holidays and weekends.
- When you get into bed, turn off the lights and relax. Avoid reviewing in your mind the day's stresses and tomorrow's challenges.
- Exercise regularly. Follow an exercise routine, but avoid heavy exercise late in the evening.
- Prepare a comfortable sleep environment. Too warm a room disturbs sleep; too cold a room does not solidify sleep. Occasional loud noises can disturb sleep without fully awakening you. Steady background noise, such as a fan may be useful for masking a noisy environment.
- Watch what you eat and drink before bedtime. Hunger may disturb sleep, as may caffeine and alcohol. A light snack may promote sleep, but avoid heavy or spicy foods at bedtime.
- Avoid the use of tobacco.
- Do not lie awake in bed for long periods of time. If you cannot fall asleep within 30 minutes, get out of bed and do something relaxing before trying to fall asleep again. Repeat this as many times as necessary. The goal is to avoid developing a paired association between being in bed and restlessness.
- Do not nap during the day. A prolonged nap after a night of insomnia may disturb the next night's sleep.
- Avoid the chronic use of sleeping pills. Although sedative-hypnotics can be effective when used as part of a coordinated treatment plan for certain types of insomnia, chronic use is ineffective at best and can be detrimental to sound sleep.

THE WIZARD OF ID   Brant parker and Johnny hart

By permission of Johnny Hart and Creators Syndicate, Inc.

human drug abusers were allowed an opportunity to work for oral doses of barbiturates or benzodiazepines on a hospital ward, they developed regular patterns of working for the drugs. When given a choice between pentobarbital and diazepam, the subjects generally chose pentobarbital.[12] These experiments indicate that these sedative drugs can serve as reinforcers of behavior, but that the short-acting barbiturates are probably more likely to lead to dependence than are any of the benzodiazepines currently on the market.

Physical dependence

A characteristic withdrawal syndrome can occur after chronic use of large enough doses of any of the sedative-hypnotic drugs. This syndrome is different from the narcotic withdrawal syndrome and quite similar to the alcohol withdrawal syndrome. An early description of the withdrawal from barbiturates is an excellent example:

> Upon abrupt withdrawal of barbiturates from individuals who have been ingesting 0.8 gm. or more daily of one of the shorter-acting barbiturates (secobarbital, pentobarbital, amobarbital), signs of barbiturate intoxication disappear in the first 8-12 hours of abstinence, and, clinically, the patient seems to improve. Thereafter, increasing anxiety, insomnia, tremulousness, weakness, difficulty in making cardiovascular adjustments on standing, anorexia, nausea and vomiting appear. One or more convulsions of *grand mal* type usually occur during the second or third day of abstinence. Following the seizures a psychosis characterized by confusion, disorientation in time and place, agitation, tremulousness, insomnia, delusions and visual and auditory hallucinations may supervene. The psychosis clinically resembles alcoholic delirium tremens, usually begins and is worse at night, and terminates abruptly with a critical sleep.[13]

This syndrome is different in character from the narcotic withdrawal syndrome, longer lasting, and probably more unpleasant. In addition, withdrawal from the sedative-hypnotics or alcohol is potentially life-threatening, with death occurring in as many as 5 percent of those who withdraw abruptly after taking large doses.

There has been considerable controversy over the frequency, nature, and severity of withdrawal symptoms after chronic use of the benzodiazepines. Animal experiments using large intravenous doses show clearly that a barbiturate-like withdrawal syndrome can be produced with benzodiazepines, with an onset that varies with the half-life of the drug. With Librium and Valium, especially when used in low doses, clinical reports of withdrawal were rare. Several reports have not generated sufficient data for us to be sure that benzodiazepine withdrawal symptoms can occur in patients especially in those who have been taking the drug for a year or more. Although the use of short-half-life benzodiazepines began much later than the use of the long-half-life forms, there are a few studies indicating more rapid and more severe withdrawal after the shorter-half-life compounds as would be expected.[14] The symptoms are rarely as severe as those seen with barbiturates and often consist of increased anxiety, irritability, or insomnia, which can be confused with a return to the predrug conditions of anxiety or insomnia for which the drug was initially prescribed.

Because there is a cross-dependence among the barbiturates, the benzodiazepines, and alcohol, it is theoretically possible to use any of these drugs to halt the withdrawal symptoms from any other depressant. Drug treatment is often used, and a general rule is to use a long-acting drug, given in divided doses until the withdrawal symptoms are controlled. Typically one of the benzodiazepines is used during detoxification from any of the CNS depressants.[15]

Toxicity

The major areas of concern with these depressant drugs are the behavioral and physiological problems encountered when high doses of the drug are present in the body (acute toxicity). Behaviorally, all these drugs are capable of producing alcohol-like intoxication with impaired judgment and incoordination. Obviously, such an impaired state vastly multiplies the dangers involved in driving or other activities, and the effects of these drugs combined with alcohol are additive, so that the danger is further increased. On the physiological side the major concern is the tendency of these drugs to depress the rate of respiration. With large enough doses, as in accidental or intentional overdose, breathing ceases entirely. Again, the combination of these depressants and alcohol is quite dangerous. Although diazepam is usually quite high on the list of drugs associated with deaths in the DAWN coroners' reports, in almost every case the culprit is diazepam in combination with alcohol or some other drug rather than diazepam alone.[16]

Patterns of Abuse

Almost all of the abuse of these sedative-hypnotic agents has historically involved the oral use of legally manufactured products. Two characteristic types of abusers were associated with barbiturate use, and these two major types probably still characterize a large fraction of sedative abusers. The first type of abuser is an older adult who obtains the drug on a prescription, either for daytime sedative use or as a sleeping pill. Through repeated use, tolerance develops and the dose is increased. Even though some of these individuals visit several different physicians to obtain prescriptions for enough pills to maintain this level of use, many would vehemently deny that they were "drug abusers." This type of chronic use can lead to physical dependence. The other major group tends to be younger and consists of people who obtain the drugs simply for the purpose of "getting high." Sleeping pills might be taken from the home medicine cabinet, or the drugs might be purchased on the street. These younger abusers

tend to take relatively large doses or to mix several drugs or to drink alcohol with the drug, all for the purpose of becoming intoxicated. With this type of use, the possibility for acute toxicity is particularly high.

INHALANTS

It sometimes seems that some people will do almost anything to escape reality. Gasoline, glue, paint, lighter fluid, spray cans of almost anything, nail polish, and liquid paper all contain volatile solvents that, when inhaled, can have effects that are similar in an overall way to the depressants. High-dose exposure to these fumes makes users intoxicated, often slurring their speech and causing them to have trouble walking a straight line, as if they were drunk on alcohol.

Although most people think first of the abuse of volatile solvents such as glues, paints, and gasoline, other types of substances can be abused through sniffing or inhaling in a similar manner (table 8.3). Besides a wide variety of solvents and gases, two other major groups are the gaseous anesthetics and the nitrites.

Many common household products have been used as inhalants, in spite of their toxicity.

TABLE 8.3

Some Chemicals Abused by Inhalation

Substances	Chemical Ingredients
Volatile solvents	
Paint and paint thinners	petroleum distillates, esters, acetone
Paint removers	toluene, methylene chloride, methanol, acetone
Nail polish remover	acetone, ethyl acetate
Correction fluid and thinner	trichloroethylene, trichloroethane
Glues and cements	toluene, ethyl acetate, hexane, methyl chloride, acetone, methyl ethyl ketone, methyl butyl ketone trichloroethylene, tetrachloroethylene
Dry-cleaning agents	tetrachloroethylene, trichloroethane
Spot remover	xylene, petroleum distillates, chlorohydrocarbons
Aerosols, propellants, and gases	
Spray paint	butane, propane, toluene, hydrocarbons
Hair spray	butane, propane
Lighters	butane, isopropane
Fuel gas	butane, propane
Whipped cream, "whippets"	nitrous oxide
Anesthetics	
Current medical use	nitrous oxide, halothane, enflurane
Former medical use	ether, chloroform
Nitrites	
Locker Room, Rush, poppers	isoamyl, isobutyl, isopropyl nitrite, butyl nitrite, cyclohexyl

Gaseous Anesthetics

Gaseous anesthetics have been used in medicine and surgery for many years, and abuse of these anesthetics occurs among physicians and others with access to these gases. One of the oldest, nitrous oxide, was first used in the early 1800s, and quite early acquired the popular name "laughing gas" because of the hilarity exhibited by some of its users. During the 1800s there were traveling demonstration of laughing gas, during which members of the audience would volunteer to become intoxicated for the amusement of others. Nitrous oxide is also one of the safest anesthetics when used properly, but it is not possible to obtain good surgical anesthesia unless the individual breathes almost pure nitrous oxide, which leads to suffocation through a lack of oxygen. Nitrous oxide is still used for light anesthesia especially by dentists. It is also often used in combination with one of the more effective inhaled anesthetics, allowing the use of a lower concentration of the primary anesthetic. Nitrous oxide is also found as a propellant in whipping-cream containers and is sold in small bottles ("whippets") for use in home whipping-cream dispensers. Recreational users have obtained nitrous oxide from both sources.

Nitrites

The chemicals amyl nitrite and butyl nitrite cause a rapid dilation of the arteries and reduce blood pressure to the brain, thus resulting in a brief period of faintness or even unconsciousness. These chemicals have an unpleasant odor and were sold under such suggestive brand names as "Locker Room" and "Aroma of Men." The male-sounding names might also reflect the popularity of these products among some homosexual males who used these "poppers" during sex to enhance the sense of lightheadedness at orgasm. Although many surveys have not separated nitrites from other inhalants, the high school survey began to do so in 1979. It appears that the popularity of the nitrites declined throughout the 1980s, and in the class of 1996 fewer than 2 percent reported ever having used them. Since 1988 the Consumer Product Safety Commission has taken steps to remove these various nitrites from the market.

Volatile Solvents

The modern era of solvent abuse, or at least of widely publicized solvent abuse, can be traced to a 1959 investigative article in the Sunday supplement of a Denver, Colorado, newspaper. This article reported that young people in a nearby city had been caught spreading plastic model glue on their palms, cupping their hands over their mouths, and inhaling the vapors to get high. The article contained warning about the dangers of accidental exposure to solvent fumes, and an accompanying photograph showed a young man demonstrating another way to inhale glue vapors—by putting the glue on a handkerchief and holding it over the mouth and nose. The article described the effects as similar to being drunk.

That article both notified the police, who presumably began looking for such behavior, and advertised and described the practice to young people: within the next six months the city of Denver went from no previously reported cases of "glue-sniffing" to fifty cases. More publicity and warnings followed, and by the end of 1961 the juvenile authorities in Denver were seeing about "30 boys a month." The problem expanded further in Denver over the next several years, while similar patterns of publicity, increased use, and more publicity followed in other cities. In 1962 the magazines *Time* and *Newsweek* both carried articles describing how to sniff model glue and warning about its dangers, and the Hobby Industry Association of America produced a film for civic groups that warned about glue sniffing and recommended that communities make it illegal to sniff any substance with an intoxicating effect. Sales of model glue continued to rise as the publicity went nationwide.[17]

Since that time it seems that recreational use of various solvents by young people has occurred mostly as more localized fads. One group of kids in one area might start using cooking sprays, the practice will grow and then decline over a couple of years, and meanwhile in another area the kids might be inhaling a specific brand and even color of spray paint.[18]

Although some "huffers" are adults (e.g., alcoholics without the funds to buy alcohol), most are young. The ready availability and low price of these solvents make them attractive to children. In the high school senior class of 1994, 18 percent of the students reported having used some type of inhalant at some time, whereas 12 percent of the eighth-graders reported using an inhalant within the past year. In fact, although most types of drug use declined from 1985 to 1994, inhalant use increased somewhat over that period.[19] Inhalant use has traditionally been more common among poor Hispanic youth and on Indian reservations.[20]

Because so many different solvents are involved, it is impossible to characterize the potential harm produced by abuse of glues, paints, correction fluids, etc., except to say that several of the solvents have been linked to kidney damage, brain damage, and peripheral nerve damage,[21] and many of them produce irritation of the respiratory tract and result in severe headaches. However, several users of various inhalants have simply suffocated. Although most of the children who inhale solvents do so only occasionally and give it up as they grow older and have more access to alcohol, some become dependent and a few will die.

Laws to limit sales of these household solvents to minors or to make it illegal to use them to become intoxicated have been passed in some areas, but typically they have little effect. There are simply too many products too readily available. Look around your own home or on the shelves of a supermarket or discount store—how many products have a warning about using them in an enclosed place? That warning is used by some people to indicate an inhalant to try! This is one type of substance abuse that families and communities should attack with awareness, information, and direct social intervention.

SUMMARY

▲ The barbiturates, benzodiazepines, inhalants, and other depressant drugs all have many effects in common with each other and with alcohol.

▲ Depressants may be prescribed in low doses for their sedative effect or in higher doses as sleeping pills (hypnotics).

▲ Over the past twenty years the barbiturates have been mostly displaced by the benzodiazepines.

▲ The benzodiazepines are the most widely prescribed type of psychoactive drug.

▲ The barbiturates and benzodiazepines both act to increase the inhibitory neural effects of the neurotransmitter GABA.

▲ Drugs that have a rapid onset are more likely to produce psychological dependence.

▲ Drugs that have a short duration of action are more likely to produce withdrawal symptoms

▲ Overdoses of these depressant drugs can cause death by inhibiting respiration, particularly if the drug is taken in combination with alcohol.

▲ The abused inhalants include a variety of volatile solvents, gaseous anesthetics, and certain nitrites.

▲ Abuse of inhalants, especially of the volatile solvents, can lead to organ damage, including neurological damage, more readily than with alcohol or other psychoactive substances.

REVIEW QUESTIONS

1. What was the foul-smelling drug that was so widely used in mental hospitals before the 1950s?
2. A prescription of 30 mg of phenobarbital would probably have been for which type of use?
3. What is the relationship between psychological dependence and the time course of a drug's action?
4. What was the first benzodiazepine?
5. What is the current legal and medical status of methaqualone?
6. The barbiturates and benzodiazepines act at which neurotransmitter receptor?
7. Why should hypnotic drugs usually be prescribed only for a few nights at a time?
8. What are the characteristics of the sedative-hypnotic withdrawal syndrome?
9. What happens to a person who takes an overdose of a sedative-hypnotic?
10. How are the effects of the nitrites different from the effects of inhalant solvent fumes?

Related Internet Sites on Drug Dependence and Psychopharmacology

College of Problems of Drug Dependence: http://views.vcu.edu/cpdd/

Psychopharmacolgy Tips: http://uhs.bsd.uchicago.edu/ ~ bhsiung/tips/tips.html

Last but not least, don't forget to visit our own *Drugs, Society, and Human Behavior* site: http://www.uwyo.edu/A&S/psyc/dshb.htm

REFERENCES

1. Richardson BW: Chloral and other narcotics, I, *Popular Science* 15: 492, 1879.
2. Rosenblatt S, Dobson R: *Beyond Valium*, New York, 1981, GP Putnam's Sons.
3. Drug linked to assaults is reformulated, *The New York Times*, Oct 19, 1997.
4. Feldman RS, Meyer JS, Quenzer LF: *Principles of neuropsychopharmacology*, Sunderland, MA, 1997, Sinauer.
5. Top 200, *American Druggist*, Feb 1994, p 27.
6. Mellinger GD, Balter MB, Uhlenhuth EH: Insomnia and its treatment: prevalence and correlates, *Arch Gen Psychiatry* 42:225–232, 1985.
7. Allen RP and others: Efficacy without tolerance or rebound insomnia for midazolam and temazapam after use for one to three months, *J Clin Pharmacol* 27:768–775, 1988.
8. More Halcion headaches, *Newsweek*, March 7, 1994.
9. Woods JH, Katz JL, Winger G: Abuse and therapeutic use of benzodiazepines and benzodiazepine-like drugs. In FE Bloom and DJ Kupfer, editors: *Psychopharmacology: The fourth generation of progress*, New York, 1995, Raven Press.
10. Eicher D: Xanax tranquilizer proves addictive, *The Denver Post*, February 27, 1989.
11. Griffiths RR and others: Self-injection of barbiturates and benzodiazepines in baboons, *Psychopharmacology* 75:101–109,1981.
12. Griffiths RR, Bigelow G, Liebson I: Human drug self-administration: double-blind comparision of pentobarbital, diazepam, chlorpromazine and placebo, *J Pharmacol Exp Ther* 210:301–310, 1979.
13. Fraser HF and others: Death due to withdrawal of barbiturates, *Ann Intern Med* 38:1319–1325, 1953.
14. Roy-Byrne PP, Hommer D: Benzodiazepine withdrawal: overview and implications for the treatment of anxiety, *Am J Med* 84:1041–1052, 1988.
15. Gitlin M. *The psychotherapist's guide psychopharmacology,* New York, 1996, The Free Press.
16. *Preliminary estimates from the Drug Abuse Warning Network,* SAMHSA Advance Report Number 17, U.S. Department of Health and Human Services, August, 1996.
17. Brecher EM: *Licit and illicit drugs*, Boston, 1972, Little, Brown.
18. Beauvais F: Volatile solvent abuse: trends and patterns, In Sharp CW and others, editors: *Inhalant abuse: a volatile research agenda*, NIDA Research Monograph 129, NIH Publ No 93-3480, Washington, DC, 1992.
19. *Drug use continues to climb*, News release from the University of Michigan's Monitoring the Future Project, December 8, 1994.
20. Crider RA, Rouse BA: *Epidemiology of inhalant abuse: an update*, NIDA Research Monograph 85, DHHS Publ No (ADM) 88-1577, US Public Health Service, 1988.
21. Rosenberg N, Sharp CW: Solvent toxicity: A neurological focus. In Sharp CW and others, editors: *Inhalant abuse: A volatile research agenda*, NIDA Research Monograph 129, NIH Publ No 93-3480, Washington, DC, 1992.
22. Rosenberg D: Death of the party, *Newsweek*, Oct 27, 1997.

9

Psychotherapeutic Drugs

KEY TERMS	OBJECTIVES

After reading this chapter, you should be able to:

anxiety disorders
psychosis
schizophrenia
bipolar disorder
depression
phenothiazines
neuroleptic
antipsychotic
monoamine oxidase (MAO)
  inhibitor
tricyclic
SSRI
lithium

- Explain the medical model of mental disorders and how that model relates to drug therapy.
- Describe the major symptoms associated with anxiety disorders, psychosis, and the mood disorders.
- Discuss some of the approaches to drug treatment that were used before 1950.

- List the names of some of the antipsychotic and antidepressant drugs, and know how they work and how effective they are.
- Explain why lithium was introduced late to the U.S. market and for what conditions it is now used.

For most of today's mentally ill the primary mode of therapy has become drug therapy. Powerful psychoactive medications help to control psychotic behavior, depression, and mania in thousands of patients, reducing human suffering and health care costs. Yet these drugs are far from cures, and they often have undesirable side effects. Should mental disorders be approached with chemical treatments? Do these treatments work? How do they work? What can these drugs tell us about the causes of mental illness? Although we don't yet have complete answers for any of these questions, we do have partial answers for all of them.

MENTAL ILLNESS

The Medical Model

The use of a term such as *mental illness* seems to some to imply a particular model for behavioral disorders or dysfunctions. The medical model has been attacked by both psychiatrists (who are medical doctors) and psychologists (who generally hold nonmedical doctorates such as a Ph.D. or Psy. D).

According to this model the *patient* appears with a set of *symptoms*, and on the basis of these symptoms a *diagnosis* is made as to which *disease* the patient is suffering from. Once the disease is known, its *cause* can be determined and the patient provided with a *cure*. In general terms the arguments for and against a medical model of mental illness are similar to those for and against a medical model of addiction presented in chapter 3. For an infectious disease such as tuberculosis or syphilis, a set of symptoms suggests a particular disorder, but a specific diagnostic test for the presence of certain bacteria or antibodies is used to confirm the diagnosis, identify the cause, and clarify the treatment approach. We know in such cases that once the infection is cleared up, the disorder is cured.

For mental disorders a set of behavioral symptoms is about all we have to define and diagnose the disorder. A person might be inactive, not sleep or eat well, and not say much, and what little they do say might be quite negative. This behavior might lead us to call the person depressed. Does that mean that the person has a "disease" called depression, with a physical cause and a potential cure? Or is to call someone depressed really only to give a description of how they're acting, in the same way as we might call someone "crabby" or "friendly" or "nerdy"? The behaviors that we refer to as indicating depression are varied and probably have many different causes, most of them not known. And we are far from being able to prescribe a cure for depression that will be generally successful in eliminating these symptoms.

In spite of these attacks on the medical model, it still seems to guide much of the current thinking about behavioral disorders. The fact that psychoactive drugs can be effective in controlling symptoms, if not in curing diseases, has lent a great deal of strength to supporters of the medical model. If chemicals can help normalize an individual's behavior, a natural assumption might be that the original problem resulted from some chemical imbalance in the brain—and that measurements of chemicals in urine, blood, or cerebrospinal fluid could pro-

vide more specific and accurate diagnoses and give direction to our efforts at drug therapy.[1] This kind of thinking gives scientists great hope, and many experiments have attempted to find the searched-for chemical imbalances, so far with very little success.

Classification of Mental Disorders

Because human behavior is so variable and because we do not know the causes of most mental disorders, classification of the mentally ill into diagnostic categories is difficult. Nevertheless, there are some basic divisions that are widely used and important for understanding the uses of psychotherapeutic drugs. In 1994 the American Psychiatric Association published the fourth edition of its *Diagnostic and Statistical Manual of Mental Disorders* (referred to as the *DSM-IV*).[2] This manual provides criteria for classifying mental disorders into hundreds of specific diagnostic categories. Partly because this classification system has been adopted by major health insurance companies, its terms and definitions have become standard for all mental health professionals.

Anxiety is a normal and common human experience: anticipation of potential threats and dangers often helps us avoid them. However, when these worries become unrealistic, resulting in chronic uneasiness, fear of impending doom, or bouts of terror or panic, they can interfere with the individual's daily life. Physical symptoms may also be present, often associated with activation of the autonomic nervous system (e.g., flushed skin, dilated pupils, gastrointestinal problems, increased heart rate, or shortness of breath).

The term *neurosis* was traditionally used as a general term to refer to such problems as psychosomatic complaints, phobias, and obsessive-compulsive disorder. The *DSM-IV* doesn't use the term *neurosis* but refers to these and other

DSM IV   Anxiety Disorders

Panic Disorder (with or without agoraphobia)

Panic disorder is defined by recurrent unexpected panic attacks, and by subsequent concern about future attacks or about the meaning of the attacks. Panic attacks may include shortness of breath, dizziness or faintness, palpitations or accelerated heart rate, trembling, sweating, choking, numbness, fear of dying, or fear of going crazy or doing something uncontrolled.

The agoraphobia *(fear of the marketplace)* that often accompanies panic disorders is a fear of being in places or situations from which escape might be difficult or where help might not be available in the event of either a panic attack or some other incapacitating or embarassing situation (e.g., fainting or losing bladder control). The person with agoraphobia might avoid going outside the home alone or be afraid of being in a public place or standing in a line.

Specific Phobia

Excessive or unreasonable fear of a specific object or situation (e.g., elevators, flying, heights, or some type of animal).

Social Phobia

A marked and persistent fear of social or performance situations (e.g., public speaking, entering a room full of strangers, or using a public restroom).

Obsessive-Compulsive Disorder

Obsessions are recurrent and persistent thoughts, impulses, or images that are intrusive and inappropriate, and that cause marked anxiety or distress. Compulsions are urgent repetitive behaviors, such as handwashing, counting, or repeatedly "checking" to make sure that some dreaded event will not occur (e.g., checking that all doors and windows are locked, then checking again and again).

Posttraumatic Stress Disorder

The person has been exposed to an event that involved actual or threatened death or serious injury, and the person reacted with intense fear, helplessness, or horror. The traumatic event is persistently reexperienced through recollections, dreams, or a sudden feeling as if the event were occurring.

Generalized Anxiety Disorder

Excessive anxiety and worry about a number of events or activities, such as school or work performance or finances, lasting for a period of six months or longer.

---

problems as **anxiety disorders** (see the DSM-IV box).

Perhaps because these disorders all seem to have some form of anxiety associated with them, and perhaps because psychiatrists often refer to the sedatives as *antianxiety drugs* (see chapter 8), we all have a tendency to think of anxiety not as a behavioral symptom but rather as an internal state that *causes* the disorders. That view fits well with the medical model, but we should guard against easy acceptance of the view that these disorders are caused by anxiety and that therefore we can treat them using antianxiety drugs. For one thing, most "antianxiety" drugs have not been demonstrated to be very useful in the treatment of specific phobias, panic disorder, or obsessive-compulsive disorder.

Psychosis refers to a major disturbance of normal intellectual and social functioning in which there is loss of contact with reality. Not knowing the current date, hearing voices that aren't there, or believing that you are Napoleon or Christ are only some examples of this withdrawal from reality. Many people refer to psychosis as reflecting a primary disorder of *thinking,* as opposed to mood or emotion.

Psychotic behavior may be viewed as a group of symptoms that can have many possible causes. One important distinction is between the *organic* psychoses and the *functional* psychoses. An organic disorder is one that has a known physical cause, and psychosis can result from many such things, including brain tumors or infections, metabolic or endocrine disorders, degenerative neurological diseases, chronic alcohol use, and high doses of stimulant drugs such as amphetamine or cocaine. Functional disorders are simply those for which there is no known or obvious physical cause. A person suffering from a chronic (long-lasting) psychotic condition for which there is no known cause will probably receive the diagnosis of **schizophrenia**. There is a popular misconception that schizophrenia means "split personality" or refers to individuals exhibiting multiple personalities. Instead, schizophrenia should probably be translated as *shattered mind*. See the DSM-IV box for the diagnostic criteria for schizophrenia.

Mood disorder refers to the appearance of depressed or manic symptoms. Look back at figure 7.3 on p. 154 for one schematic representation of mood in which depression is shown as an abnormally low mood and mania as an abnormally high mood. The important distinction in DSM-IV, and in the drug treatment of mood disorders, is between **bipolar disorder**, in which both

---

DSM IV	**Diagnosis: Schizophrenia**

A. Characteristic symptoms: Two or more of the following:
1. Delusions (irrational beliefs)
2. Hallucinations (e.g., hearing voices)
3. Disorganized speech (incoherent, frequent changes of topic)
4. Grossly disorganized behavior (inappropriate, unpredictable) or catatonic (withdrawn, immobile)
5. Negative symptoms (lack of emotional response, little or no speech, doesn't initiate activities)

B. Interference with social or occupational function

C. Duration of at least six months

---

manic and depressive episodes have been observed at some time, and major **depression,** in which only depressive episodes are reported. See the DSM-IV box "Diagnosis: Mood Disorders" for diagnostic criteria for manic episode and major depressive episode.

---

anxiety disorders: mental disorders characterized by excessive worry, fears, or avoidance.

psychosis: (sy *co* sis) a serious mental disorder involving loss of contact with reality.

schizophrenia (skitz o *fren* ee yah) a type of chronic psychosis.

bipolar disorder: a type of mood disorder also know as manic-depressive disorder.

depression: a major type of mood disorder.

DSM IV	Diagnosis: Mood Disorders

I. **Manic Episode**
   A. Abnormally and persistently elevated, expansive, or irritable mood
   B. At least three of the following:
      1. Inflated self-esteem or grandiosity
      2. Decreased need for sleep
      3. More talkative than usual or pressure to keep talking
      4. Flight of ideas or feeling that thoughts are racing
      5. Distractibility
      6. Increase in activity
      7. Excessive involvement in pleasurable activities that have a high potential for painful consequences (shopping, sex, foolish investments)
   C. Mood disturbance is sufficiently severe to cause marked impairment in functioning

II. **Major Depressive Episode**
   A. Five or more of the following, including either No. 1 or No. 2:
      1. Depressed mood most of the day, nearly every day
      2. Diminished interest or pleasure in most activities
      3. Significant changes in body weight or appetite (increased or decreased)
      4. Insomnia or hypersomnia nearly every day
      5. Psychomotor agitation (increased activity) or retardation (decreased activity)
      6. Fatigue or loss of energy
      7. Feelings of worthlessness or excessive guilt
      8. Diminished ability to think or concentrate
      9. Recurrent thoughts of death or suicide, or a suicide attempt or plan for committing suicide
   B. The symptoms cause clinically significant distress or impairment
   C. Not due to a drug or medical condition, and not a normal reaction to the loss of a loved one

Keep in mind that individual human beings often don't fit neatly into one of these diagnostic categories, and in many cases assigning a diagnosis and selecting a treatment are as much a matter of experience and art as they are of applying scientific descriptions. For example, suppose a person displays both abnormal mood states and bizarre thinking. If it is assumed that the disturbance of thinking is the primary problem and that the person is elated or depressed because of a bizarre belief, then the individual may be diagnosed as schizophrenic. Another professional might see the mood disorder as primary, with the crazy talk supporting a negative view of the world, and give the individual a primary diagnosis of depression.

TREATMENT OF MENTAL DISORDERS

Before 1950

Over the centuries mental patients have been subjected to various kinds of treatment, depending on the views held at the time regarding the causes of mental illness. Because we are concerned with drug therapy, a good place to begin our history is in 1917, when a physical treatment was first demonstrated to be effective in serious mental disease. In those days a great proportion of the psychotic patients were suffering from *general paresis*, a syphilitic infection of the nervous system. It was noticed that the fever associated with malaria often produced marked improvement, and so in 1917 "malaria therapy" was introduced in the treatment of general paresis. Of course, the later discovery of antibiotics that could cure syphilis has virtually eliminated this particular type of organic psychosis.

In the 1920s, some of the wealthier patients could afford to go in for a course of "narcosis therapy," in which barbiturates and other depressants were used to induce sleep for as long as a week or more. Another use for sedative drugs was in conjunction with psychotherapy: an intravenous dose of thiopental sodium, a rapid-acting barbiturate, would relax a person and produce more talking during psychotherapy. The theory was that such a reduction in inhibitions would enable the patient to express repressed thoughts; thus the term *truth serum* came to be used for thiopental sodium or for scopolamine, an anticholinergic drug used similarly. Anyone who has ever listened to a person talking after drinking a good bit of alcohol will tell you that although the talk might be less inhibited, it isn't always more truthful. So-called truth serum apparently worked about as well.

In 1933, Manfred Sakel of Vienna induced comas in some schizophrenics by administering insulin. The resulting drop in blood glucose level caused the brain's neurons to first increase their activity and produce convulsions and then decrease their activity and leave the patient in a coma. A course of 30 to 50 of these treatments over a two-to-three month period was believed to be highly effective, and discharge rates of 90 percent were reported in the early years of insulin-shock therapy. Later studies demonstrated that the relapse rate was quite high, and this treatment was abandoned.

Ladislas von Meduna believed, incorrectly, that no epileptic was schizophrenic, and no schizophrenic ever had epilepsy. Reasoning that epileptic convulsions prevented the development of schizophrenia, he felt that inducing convulsions might have therapeutic value for schizophrenic patients. His first convulsant drug was camphor, but it had the disadvantage of a lag time of several hours between injection and the convulsions. In 1934 he started using pentylenetetrazol (Metrazol), which induced convulsions in less than thirty seconds and reported improvement rates in schizophrenics of 50 to 60 percent.

The use of a drug was not ideal for inducing convulsions, because even a thirty second interval between injection and loss of consciousness (with the convulsion) produced much anguish in the patient. Ugo Cerletti, after experimenting on pigs in a slaughterhouse, developed the technique of using electric shock to induce convulsions. This method has the advantage of inducing loss of consciousness and convulsion at the moment the electric shock is applied.

Electroconvulsive therapy (ECT) is hardly ever used now with schizophrenics. Although early work in the 1930s and 1940s suggested high improvement rates, later studies found a reduction of schizophrenic symptoms in only about half of the patients, and the relapse rates were quite high. However, ECT is still used with severely depressed patients who do not respond to medication.[3]

By the 1950s, probably the major drug in use for severely disturbed patients in the large mental hospitals was paraldehyde, a sedative introduced in chapter 8. Although it produces little respiratory depression and therefore is safer than the barbiturates, the drug has a characteristic odor that is still well remembered by those who worked in or visited the hospitals of that era. Sedation of severely disturbed patients by drugs that make them drowsy and slow them down has been referred to as using a "chemical straitjacket."

Antipsychotics

A number of people were involved in the discovery that a group of drugs call the **phenothiazines** had special properties when used with mental patients. Credit is usually given to a French surgeon, Henri Laborit, who first tested these compounds in conjunction with surgical anesthesia. He noted that the most effective of the phenothiazines, chlorpromazine, did not by itself induce drowsiness or a loss of consciousness, but it seemed to make the patients unconcerned about their upcoming surgery. He reasoned that this effect might reduce emotionality in psychiatric patients and encouraged his psychiatric colleagues to test the drug. The first report of these French trials of chlorpromazine in mental patients mentioned that not only were the patients calmed, but the drug seemed to act on the psychotic process itself. This new type of drug action attracted a variety of names: in the United States the drugs were generally called tranquilizers, which some now think is an unfortunate term that focuses on the calming action and seems to imply sedation. Another term used was **neuroleptic**, meaning "taking hold of the nervous system," a term implying an increased amount of control. Although both of these terms are still in wide use, most medical texts now refer to this group of drugs as **antipsychotics**, reflecting their special ability to reduce psychotic symptoms without necessarily producing drowsiness and sedation.

One of the early reports (1955) dealing with the side effects of chlorpromazine on a large number of hospitalized psychotic patients stated:

> It produces marked quieting of the motor manifestations. Patients cease to be loud and profane, the tendency to hyperbolic associations diminished, and the patients can sit still long enough to eat and take care of normal physiological needs . . .
>
> In the more chronic psychotic states, the effect of the drug is much less immediately dramatic, but for those experienced with the relief of psychotic

symptoms from other measures, the use of the drug produces results that are equally gratifying when compared with results in the more acute situations.[4]

The tremendous impact of phenothiazine treatment on the management of hospitalized psychotics is clear from a 1955 statement[5] by the director of the Delaware State Hospital:

> We have now achieved . . . the reorganization of the management of disturbed patients. With rare exceptions, all restraints have been discontinued. The hydrotherapy department, formerly active on all admission services and routinely used on wards with disturbed patients, has ceased to be in operation. Maintenance EST (electroshock treatment) for disturbed patients has been discontinued. . . . There has been a record increase in participation by these patients in social and occupational activities.
>
> These developments have vast sociological implications. I believe it is fair to state that pharmacology promises to accomplish what other measures have failed to bring about—the social emancipation of the mental hospital.

Treatment effects and considerations

Along with an increase in the use of phenothiazines in the treatment of the mentally ill came an increase in the sophistication of experimental programs that evaluate the effectiveness of various drugs. Results from these studies show clearly that phenothiazine-treated patients improve more than patients receiving placebo or no treatments. In an NIMH study, after six weeks 75 percent of acute schizophrenics receiving phenothiazines showed either moderate or marked improvement, whereas of those receiving placebos, only 23 percent improved. Over the years many more studies have demonstrated consistently that, although phenothiazines are far from a complete cure for every patient, they are significantly better than placebo treatments in reducing psychotic behaviors. The issue of what to call this new type of drug arose early on:

The inappropriateness of the term "tranquilizer" is evident when the pattern of response produced by antipsychotic drugs is examined. They certainly do more than simply calm patients or put them in a "chemical straitjacket." The core symptoms of schizophrenia are consistently improved: emotional withdrawal, hallucinations, delusions and other disturbed thinking, paranoid projection, belligerence, hostility and blunted affect. On the other hand, somatic complaints, anxiety and tension, symptoms which might ordinarily be favorably affected by a "tranquilizer," are not much changed.[6]

Another aspect of evaluating the effectiveness of drug treatment is determining the incidence of relapse or symptom recurrence when treatment is discontinued. It is most likely that discontinuation of drug therapy will lead to relapse in 75 to 95 percent of patients within a year and in more than 50 percent of patients in six months. Almost all studies report that when medication is resumed, there is again a reduction in symptoms.[7]

In the years since 1950, many new phenothiazines have been introduced and several completely new types of antipsychotic drugs have been discovered. The ones on the U.S. market are listed in table 9.1.[8] These drugs vary considerably in how much sedation accompanies their antipsychotic effect, and physicians tend to select among the drugs depending partly on how much sedation they feel is called for. For example, two commonly used antipsychotics are thioridazine (Mellaril), one of the most sedating, and haloperiodol (Haldol), one of the least sedating. The drug clozapine (Clozaril) deserves special comment, because it is useful in treating patients who do not respond to other antipsychotics, but it carries a big risk of dangerous side effects (see the Your Turn box on p. 192). In 1994 another new type of antipsychotic drug was introduced. Whereas all previous antipsychotics had acted to reduce the so-called *positive symptoms* of schizophrenia (hallucinations, delusions, "crazy" behavior), the drug risperidone (Risperdal) was reported not only to cause fewer

TABLE 9.1
Antipsychotic Drugs

Generic name	Brand name	Usual dose range (mg/day)
Phenothiazines		
Chlorpromazine	Thorazine	100–2000
Thioridazine	Mellaril	100–600
Mesoridazine	Serentil	100–400
Trifluoperazine	Stelazine	5–60
Fluphenazine	Permitil, Prolixin	5–60
Perphenazine	Trilafon	8–64
Prochlorperazine	Compazine	10–150
Other chemical clases		
Clozapine	Clozaril	100–900
Haloperidol	Haldol	2–100
Loxapine	Loxitane	30–250
Molindone	Moban	10–225
Olanzepine	Zyprex	5–20
Risperidone	Risperdal	4–16
Thiothixene	Navane	5–60

side effects but also to improve the *negative symptoms* such as social isolation and lack of emotional responsiveness.[9] Risperidone was joined in 1996 by another "atypical" antipsychotic, olanzepine (Zyprex).

Mechanism of antipsychotic action

For several years it was difficult to know which of the many biochemical effects of these drugs was responsible for their antipsychotic action. The phenothiazines tend to block the receptors for norepinephrine, dopamine, acetylcholine, serotonin, and histamine. The antipsychotic drugs vary widely in how much drug

phenothiazines: (feen o *thigh* uh zeens) a group of drugs used to treat psychosis.

neuroleptic: (noor o *lep* tick) a general term for antipsychotic drugs.

antipsychotic: a group of drugs used to treat psychosis; same as neuroleptic.

Clozaril: Patient Monitoring versus Cost Containment

Clozapine, marketed as Clozaril by Sandoz in 1989, has been found to be useful in treating patients who do not respond to other antipsychotics. The problem is that clozapine also can cause agranulocytosis in 1 to 2 percent of the patients who use it. Agranulocytosis is a loss of the white blood cells needed to fight infections and can be fatal if not detected early. At first, Sandoz would only sell the drug in conjunction with its Clozaril Patient Monitoring System, in which the patient has a blood sample taken each week in exchange for the next week's medication, at a cost of $172 per week. This cost was criticized by the Veteran's Administration, Medicaid agencies, and insurance companies as too high. The FDA and Sandoz finally agreed in 1991 that the drug could be sold without the specific monitoring system provided by Sandoz, as long as some other form of blood testing system were required. This didn't reduce costs for most private patients, because the test cost about the same no matter which laboratory is carrying them out.

Think about this issue from the point of view of the company selling clozapine (remember their liability if someone is harmed by their drug), then from the point of view of an insurance company trying to keep costs down, and finally from the point of view of a patient whose life has been severely disrupted by psychosis and for whom other antipsychotics are ineffective. Are there ways to reduce the costs for the patients who require such a drug?

it takes to produce a clinical response (clinical potency) and in biochemical affinity for these various receptors, so it was possible to demonstrate a strong correlation between dopamine-receptor binding and clinical potency. It is therefore now accepted that the primary antipsychotic effect is probably a result of blockade of dopamine receptors. However, the recently approved atypical antipsychotics risperidone and olanzepine also block a subtype of serotonin receptor (the $5\text{-}HT_2$ receptor), which might help account for their slightly different profile of effects.[3]

Side effects of antipsychotics

Two positive aspects of the antipsychotics are that they are not addictive and it is extremely difficult to use them to commit suicide. Some allergic reactions might be noted, such as jaundice or skin rashes. Some patients exhibit photosensitivity, a tendency for the skin to darken and burn easily in sunlight. These reactions have a low incidence and usually decrease or disappear with a reduction in dosage. *Agranulocytosis*, low white blood cell count of unknown origin, can develop in the early stages of treatment. Because white blood cells are needed to fight infection, this disorder has a high mortality rate if it is not detected before a serious infection sets in. It is extremely rare with most of the antipsychotics other than clozapine.

The most common side effect of antipsychotic medication involves the nigrostrial dopamine pathway (see chapter 5). The major effects include a wide range of movement disorders from facial tics to symptoms that resemble those of Parkinson's disease (tremors of the hands when they are at rest, muscular rigidity, including a masklike face; and a shuffling walk). You might remember that Parkinson's disease results from damage to the dopamine neurons in the basal ganglia and that it is now treated with a dopamine precursor, L-dopa. The antipsychotic-drug-induced pseudoparkinsonism is a result of the blockade of dopamine receptors in the basal ganglia. L-dopa is not used to treat these symptoms because it has a tendency to worsen psychotic symptoms. However, before the introduction of L-dopa, Parkinson's disease was treated with anticholinergic drugs that block receptors in the output pathways from the basal ganglia. These anticholinergic antiparkinson drugs are used to control the movement disorders produced by the antipsychotic medications.

The antipsychotic medications vary considerably in their tendency to produce movement disorders, but for most of the drugs this is due to the variance in the amount of anticholinergic activity that the drugs themselves possess. For example, thioridazine, which produces very few movement disorders, is about seven times as potent an anticholinergic as chlorpromazine (Thorazine), which is about nine times as anticholinergic as trifluoperazine (Stelazine), which produces many movement disorders. Haloperidol is almost purely a dopamine antagonist with little anticholinergic activity: it too produces a high incidence of movement disorders. Although some physicians prefer to use antipsychotic drugs that produce fewer movement disorders, others prefer to treat the psychotic symptoms with a purer dopamine antagonist and to separately treat the movement disorders as necessary with an anticholinergic such as benztropine (Cogentin).[10] Clozapine and risperidone might diminish movement disorders through a different mechanism, by blocking serotonin receptors.

Tardive dyskinesia is the most serious complication of antipsychotic drug treatment. Although first observed in the late 1950s, it was not viewed as a major problem until the mid 1970s, twenty years after these drugs were introduced. The term *tardive dyskinesia* means "late-appearing abnormal movements" and refers primarily to rhythmic, repetitive sucking and smacking movements of the lips; thrusting the tongue in and out ("fly-catching"); and movements of the arms, toes, or fingers. The fact that this syndrome usually occurs only after years of antipsychotic drug treatment, and that the symptoms persist and sometimes increase when medication is stopped, raised the possibility of irreversible changes. The current belief is that tardive dyskinesia is the result of supersensitivity of the dopaminergic receptors. Although reversal of the symptoms is possible in most cases, the best treatment is prevention, which can be accomplished through early detection and an immediate lowering of the level of medication.

A recent meta-analysis of several large trials of long-term antipsychotic drug treatment using a total of over 1,600 patients found that pseudoparkinsonism was reported as an adverse reaction in about 20 percent of the patients, whereas tardive dyskinesia was reported for only about 2 percent. Echoing a general principle mentioned in chapter 1, patients maintained on high doses did not show more improvement than patients on lower doses, but the high-dose patients had more adverse side effects.[11]

Antidepressants

Monoamine oxidase inhibitors

The story of the antidepressant drugs starts with the fact that tuberculosis was a major chronic illness until about 1955. In 1952, preliminary reports suggested that a new drug, isoniazid, was effective in treating tuberculosis; isoniazid and similar drugs that followed were responsible for the emptying of hospital beds. One of the antituberculosis drugs was iproniazid, which was introduced simultaneously with isoniazid but was withdrawn as too toxic. Clinical reports on its use in tuberculosis hospitals emphasized that there was considerable elevation of mood in the patients receiving iproniazid. These reports were followed up, and the drug was reintroduced as an antidepressant agent in 1955 on the basis of early promising studies with depressed patients.

Iproniazid is a **monoamine oxidase (MAO) inhibitor**, and its discovery opened up a new class of compounds for investigation. Although several MAO inhibitors were introduced over the years, toxicity and side effects have limited their use and reduce their number. Iproniazid itself was removed from sale in 1961 after being implicated in at least 54 fatalities. Currently there are two MAO inhibitors on the U.S. market (table 9.2). A major limitation to the use of the MAO inhibitors is that they alter the normal metabolism of a dietary amino acid, tyramine, such that if an individual consumes foods with a high tyramine content while taking MAO inhibitors, a hypertensive (high blood pressure) crisis can result. Because aged cheeses are one source of tyramine, this is often referred to as the "cheese reaction." A severe headache, palpitations, flushing of the skin, nausea, and vomiting are some symptoms of this reaction, which has in some cases ended in death from a stroke (cerebrovascular accident). Besides other foods and beverages that contain tyramine (chianti wine, smoked or pickled fish, and many others), patients taking MAO inhibitors must also avoid sympathomimetic drugs such as amphetamines, methylphenidate, and phenylpropanolamine (PPA), the ingredient in OTC weight-control products.

MAO is an enzyme involved in the breakdown of serotonin, norepinephrine, and dopamine, and its inhibition results in increased availability of these neurotransmitters at the synapse. This was the first clue to the possible mechanism of antidepressant action.

Tricyclic antidepressants

Sometimes when you are looking for one thing, you find something entirely different. The MAO inhibitors were found among antituberculosis agents, and the phenothiazine antipsychotics were found while looking for a better antihistamine. The **tricyclic** antidepressants were found in a search for better phenothiazine antipsychotics. The basic phenothiazine structure consists of three rings, with various side chains for the different antipsychotic drugs. Imipramine resulted from a slight change in the middle of the three rings and was tested in 1958 on a group of patients. The drug had little effect on psychotic symptoms, but improved the mood of depressed patients. This was the first tricyclic antidepressant, and many more have followed (see table 9.2). Although these drugs are not effective in all patients, most controlled clinical trials do find that depressive episodes are less severe and resolve more quickly if the patients are treated with one of the tricyclic antidepressants than if they are given a placebo.

TABLE 9.2

Antidepressant Drugs

Generic name	Brand name	Usual dose range (mg/day)
MAO inhibitors		
Phenelzine	Nardil	45–75
Tranylcypromine	Parnate	20–30
Tricyclics		
Amitriptyline	Elavil, Endep	100–200
Amoxapine	Asendin	200–300
Desipramine	Norpramin	75–200
Doxepin	Sinequan, Adapin	100–200
Imipramine	Tofranil	100–200
Nortriptyline	Pamelor	75–150
Protriptyline	Vivactil	15–40
SSRIs		
Fluoxetine	Prozac	20–40
Paroxetine	Paxil	20–50
Sertraline	Zoloft	50–200
Venlafaxine	Effexor	75–375
Others		
Bupropion	Wellbutrin	200–300
Mirtazapine	Remeron	15–45
Nefazodone	Serzone	200–600
Trazodone	Desyrel	150–200

The first tricyclics were discovered to interfere with the reuptake into the terminal of the neurotransmitters norepinephrine, dopamine, and serotonin. This results in an increased availability of these neurotransmitters at the synapse. Because MAO inhibition also results in increased availability of the same neurotransmitters, there has been considerable speculation that the antidepressant actions of both classes of drugs result from increased synaptic availability of one or more of these neurotransmitters. One of the effective antidepressants, desipramine, was found to have a much greater effect on the reuptake of norepinephrine than on the reuptake of either dopamine or serotonin, so for a time most theories of antidepressant action focused on norepinephrine.

Selective serotonin reuptake inhibitors

The introduction in 1987 of fluoxetine (Prozac) ushered in the era of the *selective serotonin reuptake inhibitors* (**SSRIs**). Trazodone had already been available and was known to have a greater effect on serotonin than on norepinephrine reuptake, calling the norepinephrine theory into question. Fluoxetine was followed to market by sertraline (Zoloft), paroxetine (Paxil), and venlafaxine (Effexor), and all of these have highly selective effects on serotonin reuptake. These four drugs constitute the new category of SSRIs. The most successful of these was Prozac, which rapidly became the most widely prescribed antidepressant drug ever marketed. Prozac is safer than the tricyclic antidepressants in that it is less likely to lead to overdose deaths, so physicians feel more confident about prescribing it. In spite of reports in the early 1990s of unusual violent or suicidal reactions, which may have reduced sales temporarily, the manufacturer reported record high sales in 1994. One factor in its popularity might be that, whereas the tricyclics often lead to weight gain, Prozac use is more often accompanied by weight loss.

Depression is a serious, debilitating disorder that often responds to antidepressant medication.

Mechanism of antidepressant action

It now seems clear that antidepressants might work by increasing the availability of either norepinephrine or serotonin at their respective synapses. However, the antidepressant effect of MAO inhibitors, tricyclics, or SSRIs exhibits a "lag period": the patients must be treated for about two weeks before improvement is seen even though the biochemical effects on MAO or on reuptake occur in a matter of minutes. Although it has been suggested that some patients might benefit more from one type than from another, experiments have so far failed to reveal

monoamine oxidase (MAO) inhibitor: a type of antidepressant drug.

tricyclic: (try *sike* lick) a type of antidepressant drug.

SSRI: selective serotonin reuptake inhibitor, a type of antidepressant drug.

FYI   Prozac for Everyone?

When Prozac (fluoxetine) was introduced in 1987 as a new, safer antidepressant, no one expected it to become as successful as it did as quickly as it did. People took it, liked it, told their friends about it, and more people took it. It quickly became the nation's most popular antidepressant drug ever. But few have been as outspoken in favor of widespread us of Prozac as psychologist Jim Goodwin of Wenatchee, Washington. According to a 1994 story by Associated Press writer Aviva Brandt, Goodwin has been called the "Pied Piper of Prozac."

Citing the safety and effectiveness of the drug and its limited side effects, Goodwin, who has taken the drug himself since 1989, has recommended it to virtually all the 700 clients he has seen. Because as a psychologist he couldn't prescribe it himself, he admitted that he was "rather aggressive" in suggesting to people that they obtain a prescription from their family physician. Although Prozac and other antidepressant drugs have been approved for the treatment of major depressive disorder, Goodwin believes that most people suffer from mild depression and can benefit from using the drug. He was quoted as saying, "All of us could probably use a little bit of help with our depressions."

Goodwin's fame and his approach to treating mild depression have generated a storm of criticism from psychiatrists and other psychologists. After all, do most people really need some sort of pill to deal with the trials and tribulations of daily life?

any rational basis for choosing among the drugs in any individual case, and overall the effectiveness of the drug does not seem to depend on which of the neurotransmitters is more affected.

Current theories of the antidepressant action of these agents focus less on the direct biochemical effects of the drugs than on the reaction of the neurons to those direct effects. For example, after prolonged exposure to all of the antidepressants, there is a decreased number of receptors for both norepinephrine and serotonin, as well as other changes that have been measured and no doubt some that have not[12]. It might be these long-term adjustments of the brain tissue that result in the antidepressant action.

Well over half of the prescriptions written for antidepressants are written by nonpsychiatrists. This is unfortunate, because these practitioners frequently prescribe too little for too short a time to decrease the depression It is understandable, though, because the tricyclics can cause severe side effects: About one user in twenty will have disorientation, hallucinations, or other anticholinergic effects. Large doses of the tricyclics can be lethal, so quantities prescribed to suicidal patients need to be restricted. Even with such restrictions and with more patients taking the safer SSRIs, the tricyclic amitriptyline was among the top ten drugs mentioned in drug-related deaths in the 1995 DAWN system (see table 2.2, p. 27). The relative safety of fluoxetine (Prozac) is one major reason for its wide acceptance and prescription, again more often than not written by nonpsychiatrists (family physicians, general practitioners, or internists).

There has been some excitement among those working in laboratories and hospitals about a diagnostic laboratory test for primary unipolar depression: the dexamethasone suppression test (DST). The details need not concern us here, but you should know that the test is only about 40 to 60 percent accurate in identifying patients who are primary unipolar depressives. However, it eliminates about 90 percent of those who are not; that is, it produces few false positive results, but it does produce false negative results. With such a large proportion of depressed people showing a negative (normal) response to this test, one question is whether those who do respond abnormally are either more or less likely to improve when treated with medication. Several studies have found only very slight and inconsistent differences in treatment success between normal and abnormal responders to the dexamethasone test.[13] It appears that this test is of little value in the diagnosis or management of individual patients.

Probably the single most effective treatment for the depressed patient is electroconvulsive shock therapy (ECT). One report summarized the available good studies and showed that in 7 of 8 studies ECT was more effective in relieving the symptoms of depression than was placebo. Further, in 4 studies ECT was more effective than the most effective class of anti-depressant drugs, and in 3 other studies the two treatments were equal. One factor that makes ECT sometimes the clear treatment of choice is its more rapid effect than that found with current antidepressant drugs. Reversal of depression might not occur for two or three weeks with drug treatment, but with ECT results sometimes are noticed almost immediately. When there is a possibility of suicide, ECT is thus the obvious choice, and it is possible to use both drug and ECT treatment simultaneously.[3]

Lithium

In the late 1940s two medical uses were proposed for salts of the element **lithium**. In the United States, lithium chloride, which tastes much like sodium chloride (table salt), was introduced as a salt substitute in heart patients. However, above a certain level lithium is quite toxic, and because there was no control over the dose, many users became ill and several died. This scandal was so great in the minds of American physicians that a proposed beneficial use published in 1949 by an Australian, John Cade, produced little interest in this country.

Cade had been experimenting with guinea pigs, examining the effects of lithium on urinary excretion of salts. Lithium appeared to have sedative properties in some of the animals, so he administered the compound to several disturbed patients. The manic patients all improved, whereas there seemed to be no effect on depressed or schizophrenic patients. This was followed up by several Danish studies in the 1950s and early 1960s, and it became increasingly apparent that the large majority of manic individuals showed dramatic remission of their symptoms after a lag period of a few days when treated with lithium carbonate or other salts.

Three factors slowed the acceptance of lithium in the United States. First, of course, was the salt-substitute poisonings, which gave lithium a bad reputation as a potentially lethal drug. Second, mania was not seen as a major problem in the United States. Remember that manic patients feel energetic and have an unrealistically positive view of their own abilities, and such people are unlikely to seek treatment on their own. Also, patients who became quite manic and lost touch with reality would probably have been called schizophrenic in those days, perhaps at least partly because a treatment existed for schizophrenia. In fact, the antipsychotic drugs can control mania in most cases. The third and possibly most important factor is

lithium: (*lith* ee um) a drug used in treating mania and bipolar disorder.

economic and relates to the way new drugs are introduced in the United States: by companies who hope to make a profit on them. Lithium is one of the basic chemical elements (number 3 on the periodic chart) and its simple salts had been available for various purposes for many years, so it would be impossible for a drug company to receive an exclusive patent to sell lithium. A company generally must go to considerable expense to conduct the research necessary to demonstrate safety and effectiveness to the FDA. If one company had done this, as soon as the drug was approved any other company could also have sold lithium, and it would have been impossible for the first company to recoup its research investment. After several years of frustration, the weight of the academically conducted research and the clinical experience in Europe was such that several companies received approval to sell lithium in 1970.

Treatment with lithium requires ten to fifteen days before symptoms begin to change. Lithium is both safe and toxic. It is safe because the blood level can be monitored routinely and the dose adjusted to ensure therapeutic, but not excessive, blood levels. Patients develop tolerances to the minor side effects of gastrointestinal disturbances and tremors. Excessively high blood levels cause confusion and loss of coordination, which can progress to coma, convulsions, and death if lithium is not stopped and appropriate treatment instituted.

The clinical use and effectiveness of lithium has had some interesting effects in several areas. The mechanism of action is still not clear, but one biochemical effect is that lithium increases the synthesis of serotonin in the brain. Of primary importance in the therapeutic use of lithium is the realization that lithium acts as a mood-normalizing agent in individuals with bipolar (manic-depressive) illness. Lithium will prevent both manic and depressed mood swings. It has only moderate effects on unipolar depressions.

TABLE 9.3

Drug Treatment 2-Year Outcome in Unipolar and Bipolar Patients

	Percentage of patients with relapses during treatment.	
	First 4 months	Next 20 months
Unipolar subjects		
Lithium	30	41
Imipramine	32	29
Placebo	73	85
Bipolar subjects		
Lithium	22	18
Imipramine	46	67
Placebo	54	67

These very selective clinical effects of lithium have forced better diagnostic decisions and have given a new basis for belief that unipolar and bipolar mood disorders are not the same illness. This fact is most clearly seen in table 9.3, which shows the treatment outcome of one study.[14] Either lithium, a placebo, or imipramine (a tricyclic) was given to hospitalized patients, who were later discharged and observed for a prolonged period. For patients diagnosed as unipolar, a relapse means an episode of depression, whereas for the bipolar patients relapse can mean either a depressed or a manic period.

The results are relatively clear: Lithium was very effective in preventing relapses in bipolar subjects, whereas imipramine treatment showed no clinical improvement compared with a placebo. With unipolar subjects imipramine was superior to lithium, but both drugs were superior to placebo treatment. It is of interest to note one major difference between the unipolar and bipolar patients: 55 percent of next-of-kin relatives of bipolar patients had some type of psychiatric illness, compared with only 28 percent of the unipolar patients. This suggests a stronger genetic component in bipolar mood disorders than in unipolar disorders.

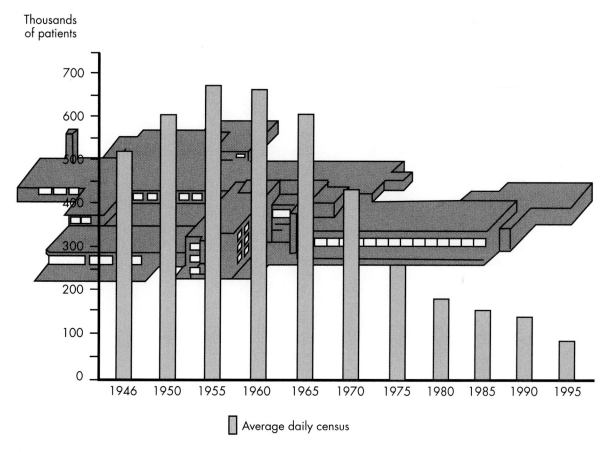

Figure 9.1 Number of patients in nonfederal psychiatric hospitals, 1946–1995

THE CONSEQUENCES OF DRUG TREATMENTS FOR MENTAL ILLNESS

There is no question that the use of modern psychopharmaceuticals, which began in the mid 1950s in the United States, has affected the lives of millions of Americans who have been treated with them. But the availability of these effective medications has also brought about revolutionary changes in our society's treatment of and relationship with our mentally ill citizens. Figure 9.1 depicts quite graphically what hap-

pened to the population of our large mental hospitals over the period from 1946 to 1995.[15] These hospitals had grown larger and larger and held a total of over half a million people in the peak years of the early 1950s. The year in which chlorpromazine was first introduced in the United States, 1955, was the last year in which the population of these hospitals increased. Since then the average population has continued to decline. Remember that the antipsychotics do not cure schizophrenia or other forms of psychosis, but they can control the symptoms to a

The homeless mentally ill are a topic of special concern today.

great degree, allowing the patients to leave the hospital, live at home, and often earn a living. These drugs began the liberation of mental patients from hospitals, where many of them had previously stayed year after year, committed for an indefinite time.

The movement out of mental hospitals was accelerated in the 1960s with the establishment of federally supported community mental health centers. The idea was to treat mental patients closer to home in a more natural environment, at lesser expense, and on an outpatient basis. Needless to say, the opportunity for such a program to work was greatly enhanced by the availability of potent, effective psychopharmaceuticals, especially the antipsychotics.

The mental health professions have been greatly affected by these drugs. It is probably safe to say that the majority of psychiatrists in practice today spend less time doing psychotherapy than did their colleagues in the 1950s. In fact, for many psychiatrists the first issue is to establish an appropriate drug regimen, and only after the initial symptoms are controlled will they engage in much talk therapy. For some psychiatrists the prescription pad has completely replaced the couch as their primary tool. This may be sensible in terms of overall cost effectiveness, but it has certainly altered the doctor/patient relationship.

Concomitant with the liberation of patients from hospitals and their return to the commu-

---

Catch-22 for the Mentally Ill

In an article in *Newsweek* magazine,[16] a 30-year old X-ray technician named Vickie described the tragedy of her mother's schizophrenia. In her terms, "Hospitals take her in, lock her up, inject her with drugs—and wait the legal amount of involuntary holding time and then send her back out on the streets." Vickie described the routine of filing a petition for an involuntary commitment against her own mother, the 72-hour holding period for observation, the court hearing, and the institutionalization. Her mother had made a dozen suicide attempts and had a dozen hospitalizations, and sometimes she "escaped." She was once found after six weeks, hundreds of miles away, sleeping on a park bench. She weighed 85 pounds and had spent some nights in jail. The mother believed this was all part of her job "for the CIA."

Vickie found it ironic that, in spite of her mother's obvious need for help, because her problem was mental and she didn't want help, there was no way for her to get treatment except through involuntary commitment.

Three weeks after the mother's last hospitalization, she took an overdose of her medication and died in Vickie's bed.

The most important ethical issue raised by this case and others like it has to do with a person's right to choose or refuse treatment when there is reason to believe that the individual's ability to make a rational choice is impaired. Can you think of a system for deciding when a patient should be compelled to accept treatment that would provide sufficient protection for the individual's rights?

---

nities came a concern with their civil rights. Indefinite commitment to a hospital had been declared unconstitutional, and all states have developed procedures to protect the rights of individual patients. Hearings are required before a person can be committed for treatment against his or her will, and it is usually necessary to demonstrate a clear and present danger to the patient's own person or to others. Periodic reviews of the patient's status are called for, and if at any time the immediate danger is not present, the patient must be released. No one would want to argue that mental patients should not have these rights, but the availability of psychoactive medications helps to create difficult situations. A patient who is dangerously psychotic might be admitted for treatment, and

after a few weeks on an antipsychotic drug might be sufficiently in control to be allowed to leave the hospital. However, if the patient remains suspicious or simply doesn't like to take the medication, he or she will eventually stop taking it and again become psychotic. Or patients might be released into the community, perhaps functioning with medication or perhaps not, too sick to really take care of themselves but not sick enough to present an immediate danger (see the Up for Debate box). About one third of all homeless people in the United States have some form of serious mental illness. The plight of our homeless, rootless, mentally ill citizens has been the subject of magazine and television reports, and efforts are being made to change the way these people are treated.

SUMMARY

▲ The "medical model" of mental illness has been widely criticized, yet psychotherapeutic drugs are often discussed in the context of this model.

▲ Diagnosis of mental disorders is difficult and controversial, but the DSM-IV provides a standard diagnostic approach for most purposes.

▲ The introduction of antipsychotics in the mid 1950s started a revolution in mental health care and increased interest in psychopharmacology.

▲ The antipsychotics are helpful for the majority of schizophrenics, but they often produce movement disorders, some of which resemble Parkinson's disease.

▲ The major groups of antidepressant drugs are the MAO inhibitors, the tricyclics, and the new SSRIs.

▲ Fluoxetine (Prozac) has quickly become the largest-selling antidepressant drug in history.

▲ Lithium is useful in treating mania and in preventing mood swings in bipolar disorder.

▲ The number of people occupying beds in mental hospitals has declined since 1955, largely because psychotherapeutic drugs allow people to be released after shorter stays.

REVIEW QUESTIONS

1. Give two examples of anxiety disorders.
2. Is schizophrenia a functional or an organic psychosis?
3. Besides sadness, what are some other indicators of a major depressive episode?
4. What type of drug is chlorpromazine, and where was it first tested on patients?
5. What is tardive dyskinesia, and how does it respond to a reduction in the dose of an antipsychotic drug?

6. Which type of drug was discovered while testing an antituberculosis agent?
7. How do the new SSRIs differ from the older tricyclics in terms of their actions in the brain?
8. What were two of the three reasons it took so long for lithium to be available for use in the United States?
9. If clozapine is so dangerous, why is it prescribed at all?
10. Why is Prozac the most widely prescribed antidepressant drug ever?

Related Internet Sites on Psychotherapeutic Drugs

Psychopharmacology Tips: http://uhs.bsd.uchicago.edu/~bhsiung/tips/tips.html

Experimental and Clinical Psychopharmacology: http://www.apa.org:80/journals/pha.html

And of course, find the latest links on our own *Drugs, Society, and Human Behavior* site: http://www.uwyo.edu/A&S/psyc/dshb.htm

REFERENCES

1. Feldman RS, Meyer JS, Quenzer LF: Principles of Neuropsychopharmacology. Sunderland, MA, Sinauer, 1997.
2. American Psychiatric Association: Diagnostic and statistical manual of mental disorders, ed 4, Washington DC, 1994, the Association.
3. Gitlin M: The Psychotherapist's Guide to Psychopharmacology. New York, The Free Press, 1996.
4. Goldman D: Treatment of psychotic states with chlorpromazine, JAMA 157:1274-1278, 1955.
5. Freyhan FA: The immediate and long-range effects of chlorpromazine on the mental hospital. In Smith, Kline and French Laboratories: Chlorpromazine and mental health, Philadelphia, 1955, Lea & Febiger.

6. Veterans Administration: Drug treatment in psychiatry, Washington, DC, 1970, US Government Printing Office.

7. Kessler KA, Waletzky JP: Clinical use of the antipsychotics, Am J Psychiatry 138:202, 1981.

8. Physician's desk reference, Oradell, NJ, 1998, Medical Economics.

9. Janssen launches new treatment for schizophrenia, Drug Topics, April 11, 1994.

10. Poling A and others: Drug therapy for behavior disorders, New York, 1991, Pergamon Press.

11. Bollini P and others: Antipsychotic drugs: is more worse? A meta-analysis of the published randomized control trials, Psychol Med 24:307, 1994.

12. Barondes SH: Molecules and mental illness, New York, 1993, WH Freeman.

13. Kathol RG, Carter JL: Use of HPA axis tests in patients with major depression. In: Pharmacotherapy of Depression, JD Amsterdam (Ed.), New York, Marcel Dekker, 1990.

14. Pokorny AD, Prein RF: Lithium in treatment and prevention of affective disorder, *Diseases of the Nervous System* 35:327, 1974.

15. American Hospital Association: Hospital Statistics, 1996-97 edition, Chicago, 1997, the Association.

16. Wish VR: Catch-22 for the mentally ill, *Newsweek*, Dec 9, 1985.

ASSESS YOURSELF!

Daily Mood Changes

Some days are better than others—we all experience that. Try using this psychological "instrument" to measure how your outlook on life changes on a day-to-day basis. Decide on a particular time to mark the scales and try to do them at the same time each day, because your mood also varies with time of day. Mark a spot on each vertical scale that corresponds to how you're feeling at the moment.

After you've finished the week, look back and see if you can relate the "highs" and "lows" to particular events or activities that happened at that time. Do all your scores tend to vary together, or are some areas unrelated to others?

1. **How optimistic do you feel about accomplishing something useful or meaningful in the next 24 hours?**

	Day 1	Day 2	Day 3	Day 4	Day 5	Day 6	Day 7
Quite certain I will							
Probably will							
Not sure							
Probably won't							
Quite certain I won't							

2. **How energetic do you feel at the moment?**

	Day 1	Day 2	Day 3	Day 4	Day 5	Day 6	Day 7
Have lots of energy							
Fairly energetic							
About average							
Not much energy							
Almost no energy							

3. How happy or sad are you today?

	Day 1	Day 2	Day 3	Day 4	Day 5	Day 6	Day 7
Very happy							
Happy							
Neither happy nor sad							
Sad							
Very sad							

4. How mentally sharp do you feel today (ability to remember things, ability to think)?

	Day 1	Day 2	Day 3	Day 4	Day 5	Day 6	Day 7
Quite sharp							
Pretty sharp							
Average							
A bit dull							
Very dull and slow							

5. How satisfied are you with yourself today?

	Day 1	Day 2	Day 3	Day 4	Day 5	Day 6	Day 7
Quite satisfied							
Fairly satisfied							
Not sure							
Fairly dissatisfied							
Quite dissatisfied							

Alcohol

Alcohol: social lubricant, adjunct to a fine meal, or demon rum? People today are no different from people throughout the centuries: many use alcohol, and many others condemn its use. This love-hate relationship with alcohol has been going on for a long time. The last two decades have brought a slight swing of the pendulum: health-conscious Americans are opting for low-alcohol or no-alcohol drinks, consumption of hard liquor is down, and we receive frequent reminders to use alcohol responsibly, not to drink and drive, and not to let our friends drive if they've been drinking. Let's take a closer look at the world's number one psychoactive substance.

10 Alcohol in the Body
What is alcohol and how does it affect the body and brain?

11 Alcohol and Society
How does alcohol affect the individual's relationships with others, and what is its impact on the society as a whole?

10

Alcohol in the Body

KEY TERMS	OBJECTIVES

After reading this chapter, you should be able to:

fermentation
distillation
proof
congeners
blood alcohol concentration
detoxification
delirium tremens
Wernicke-Korsakoff syndrome
cirrhosis
fetal alcohol syndrome
fetal alcohol effect

- Describe how alcohol is fermented and distilled, and how these processes are used to produce various alcoholic beverages.
- Discuss various types of beer, wine, and liquor and recent trends in the consumption of these beverages.
- Explain how alcohol is absorbed and broken down in the body and how blood alcohol concentration relates to changes in behavior.

- Explain why some alcoholic beverages are more likely to produce a hangover than others.
- Understand the role of alcohol toxicity and malnutrition in producing brain damage, heart disease, and liver damage.
- Know what is meant by FAS and FAE, and discuss the issue of a "safe" level of drinking during pregnancy.

Stops @ 15% - Fermentation

ALCOHOLIC BEVERAGES

Fermentation and Fermentation Products

Many thousands of years ago Neolithic humans discovered "booze." Beer and berry wine were known and used about 6400 B.C. and grape wine dates from 300 to 400 B.C. Mead, which is made from honey, might be the oldest alcoholic beverage; some authorities suggest it appeared in the Paleolithic Age, about 8000 B.C. Early use of alcohol seems to have been worldwide: beer was drunk by the Native Americans whom Columbus met.

Fermentation forms the basis for all alcoholic beverages. Certain yeasts act on sugar in the presence of water, and this chemical action

is fermentation. Yeast recombines the carbon, hydrogen, and oxygen of sugar into ethyl alcohol and carbon dioxide. Chemically, $C_6H_{12}O_6$ (glucose) is transformed to C_2H_5OH (ethyl alcohol) + CO_2 (carbon dioxide).

Most fruits, including grapes, contain sugar, and addition of the appropriate yeast (which is pervasive in the air wherever plants grow) to a mixture of crushed grapes and water will begin the fermentation process. The yeast has only a limited tolerance for alcohol; when the concentration reaches 15 percent, the yeast dies and fermentation ceases.

Cereal grains can also be used to produce alcoholic beverages. However, cereal grains contain starch rather than sugar, and before fer-

Examples of the many kinds of alcoholic beverages

mentation can begin, the starch must be converted to sugar. This is accomplished by means of enzymes formed during a process called *malting*. In American beer the primary grain is barley, which is malted by steeping it in water and allowing it to sprout. The sprouted grain is then slowly dried to kill the sprout but preserve the enzymes formed during the growth. This dried, sprouted barley is called malt, and when crushed and mixed with water, the enzymes convert the starch to sugar. Only yeast is needed then to start fermentation.

Distilled Products

To obtain alcohol concentrations above those that can be reached by fermentation, distillation must be used. **Distillation** is a process in which the solution containing alcohol is heated, and the vapors are collected and condensed into liquid form again. Alcohol has a lower boiling point than water, so there is a higher percentage of alcohol in the distillate (the condensed liquid) than there was in the original solution.

There is still debate over who discovered the distillation process and when the discovery was made, but many authorities place it in Arabia around A.D. 800. The term *alcohol* comes from an Arabic word meaning "finely divided spirit" and originally referred to that part of the wine collected through distillation—the essence of the

---

fermentation: (fer men *tay* shun) the production of alcohol from sugars through the action of yeasts.

distillation: (dis ti *lay* shun) the evaporation and condensing of alcohol vapors to produce beverages with higher alcohol content.

wine! In Europe, only fermented beverages were used until the tenth century, when the Italians first distilled wine, thereby introducing "spirits" to the Western world. These new products were studied and used in the treatment of many illnesses, including senility. The prevalent feeling about their medicinal value is best seen in the name given these condensed vapors by a thirteenth-century professor of medicine at the French University of Montpelier: *aqua vitae*, "the water of life." Around the end of the seventeenth century the more prosaic Dutch called the liquid *brandy*, meaning "burnt wine."

The name *whiskey* comes from the Irish-Gaelic equivalent of *aqua vitae* and was already commonplace around 1500. The distillation of whiskey in America started on a large scale toward the end of the eighteenth century. The chief product of the area just west of the Appalachian Mountains—western Pennsylvania, western Virginia, and eastern Kentucky—was grain. It was not profitable for the farmers to ship the grain or flour across the mountains to the markets along the eastern seaboard. But ten bushels of corn could be converted to one barrel of whiskey, which could be profitably shipped east, so distillation started on a grand scale.

In the United States the alcoholic content of distilled beverages is indicated by the term **proof**. The percentage of alcohol by volume is one-half of the proof number: for instance, 90-proof whiskey is 45 percent alcohol. The word *proof* developed from a British Army procedure to gauge the alcohol content of distilled spirits before there were modern techniques. The liquid was poured over gunpowder and ignited. If the alcohol content was high enough, the alcohol would burn and ignite the gunpowder, which would go "poof" and explode! That was proof that the beverage had an acceptable alcohol content, about 57 percent.

ALCOHOL AS A CONSUMER ITEM

Alcoholic beverages are of considerable economic importance in the United States, with Americans spending over $100 billion a year on alcoholic beverages.[1] The average American household reports spending about $3.00 per week for alcohol consumed at home and just over $2.00 per week for alcohol consumed away from home. Both the apparent frequency of drinking within the general population and the total per capita alcohol consumption reached a peak in about 1980 and have declined gradually since then.

Beer

Beer is made by adding barley malt to other cereal grains such as ground corn or rice. The enzymes in the malt change the starches in these grains into sugar, then the solids are filtered out before the yeast is added to the mash to start fermentation. Hops (dried blossoms from only the female hop plant) are added with the yeast to give beer its distinctive, pungent flavor. One-fourth pound of hops is enough to flavor a 31-gallon barrel of beer. Most of the beer sold today in America is *lager*, from the German word *lagern*, meaning "to store." To brew lager, a type of yeast is used that settles to the bottom of the mash to ferment. After fermentation and before packaging, the beer is stored for a period to age. In most commercial beers today, alcohol content

The leading brands of beer actually represent only a few brewers.

is a little over 4 percent. Because most American beer is sold in bottles or cans, the yeast must be removed to prevent it from spoiling after packaging. This is usually accomplished by heating it (pasteurization), but some brewers use microfilters to remove the yeasts while keeping the beer cold. The carbonation is added at the time of packaging.

Ale requires a top-fermentation yeast, warmer temperatures during fermentation, and more malt and hops, which produce a more flavorful beverage. *Malt liquor* is brewed much like lager but is aged longer, has less carbonation, more calories, and 1 percent to 3 percent more alcohol. If you were asked to produce a "light" beer, with fewer calories, a lighter taste, and less alcohol, what would you do—add water? That's only part of the answer, because light beers have about 10 percent less alcohol and 25 to 30 percent fewer calories. The mash is fermented at a cooler temperature for a longer time so that more of the sugars are converted to alcohol. *Then* the alcohol content is adjusted by adding water, resulting in a beverage with considerably less remaining sugar and only a bit less alcohol. The latest wrinkle is "ice" beer. After fermentation, the beer is slightly frozen and some ice crystals are removed. This results in a beer with slightly more alcohol and more overall taste. Although no-alcohol beer has been around since Prohibition, the introduction of several new brands by the major U.S. brewers has resulted in significant sales increases during the 1990s.

The beer-drinking, free-lunch saloon with nickel beer and bucket-of-suds-to-go disappeared forever with Prohibition. And so did a couple of thousand breweries. Two years after Prohibition ended there were 750 brewers, and by 1941 that had dwindled to 507. From 1960 to the mid 1970s about 10 beer makers vanished each year, until in 1976 there were fewer than 50. This declined to about 40 in the early 1980s and then began to increase again as small, local "boutique" breweries began to sprout up, especially on the West Coast. These were followed by the increasing popularity of *microbreweries*,

TABLE 10.1
Largest-Selling Beer Brands (1995)

Brand	Brewer
Budweiser	Anheuser-Busch
Bud Light	Anheuser-Busch
MillerLite	Miller
Coors Light	Adolph Coors
Busch	Anheuser-Busch
Natural Light	Anheuser-Busch
Genuine Draft	Miller
High Life	Miller
Milwaukee's Best	Miller
Busch Light Draft	Anheuser-Busch

or *brewpubs*, which make beer for sale only on the premises. These specialty brewers now capture 1 percent of the overall beer market in gallons, but presumably a larger share of the beer dollar because of their higher average sale price.

Table 10.1 points to a couple of sales trends. First, you might notice that the top ten brands are manufactured by only three brewers. As a result of mergers and consolidations during the 1980s, six major brewing companies now control over 90 percent of the beer market in the United States. The industry leader, Anheuser-Busch, controls over 40 percent of the total market. In fact, their top-selling beer, Budweiser, accounts for over 20 percent of all beer sales. The other trend to notice is that three of the top four beers are "light" beers, which have increased in popularity and now constitute 35 percent of the U.S. beer market.[2]

Imported beers have become increasingly popular in the past twenty years. The largest-selling imported beer is Corona, from Mexico. Overall, Mexican and Canadian beers are the

proof: a measure of a beverage's alcohol content; twice the alcohol percentage.

biggest imports. In spite of this increased appetite for foreign beers, imports still represent only about 5 percent of total U.S. sales. One way to look at what has happened to the beer market recently is that the craft beers produced by new, small breweries combined with an increased variety of imports and the new no-alcohol beers to add many new choices for the beer connoisseur, but Budweiser alone outsells all of these specialty beers combined.

Americans drink almost 25 gallons of beer for every man, woman, and child each year, and that hasn't changed much in the past decade. We're somewhat behind the Irish and Australians, at over 30 gallons, and the Germans and Czechs, who drink about 40 gallons per capita.

On a per capita basis, Mexicans and Japanese drink less than half of the amount of beer consumed by Americans.

Figure 10.1 shows the trends in consumption by Americans age 14 or older since 1970. The popularity of beer increased during the 1970s, and consumption has declined somewhat since the peak year of 1981. Overall, beer now accounts for 60 percent of the money Americans spend on alcoholic beverages.

Wine

Wine is one of humankind's oldest beverages, a drink that for generations has been praised as a gift from heaven and condemned as a work of

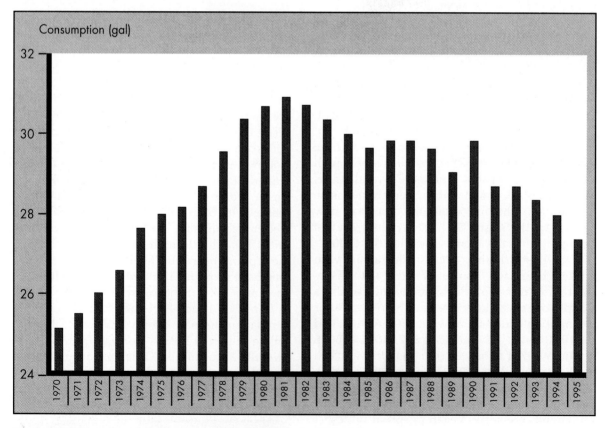

Figure 10.1 Annual per capita consumption of beer in the United States

Wine consumption has increased considerably during the past 30 years.

the devil. Although a large volume of wine is now produced in mechanized, sterilized wine "factories," there are many small wineries that operate alongside the industry giants, and the tradition continues that careful selection and cultivation of grapevines, good weather, precise timing of the harvest, and careful monitoring of fermentation and aging can result in wines of noticeably higher quality. An interesting ecological story resulted from the fact that most American wine grapes were originally transplanted from France and Spain. After a late-nineteenth-century disease destroyed almost all of the European vineyards, it became necessary to transplant American vines, which had been protected by isolation, back into Europe. Today most of the French, Italian, and Spanish wine grapes are grown from descendants of those American vines.

There are two basic types of American wines. *Generics* usually have names taken from European land areas where the original wines were produced: Chablis, Champagne, Burgundy, Bordeaux, and Rhine are examples. These are all blended wines, made from whatever grapes are available, and during processing they are made to taste something like the traditional European wines from those regions. However, there is little guarantee of quality in these generic names among American wines. *Varietals* are named after one variety of grape that by law must make up at least 51 percent of the grapes used in producing the wine. Chardonnay, pinot noir, and zinfandel are some examples. There are many varietal wines, and traditionally they have been sold in individual bottles and are more expensive than the generics. In some other countries the rules for naming wines are more restrictive. For example, in France the name *Chablis* is carefully protected by law. A French Chablis must come from the Chablis region and be made only from the chardonnay grape. In America, many inexpensive dry white wines are labeled Chablis, and they are likely to include a considerable amount of juice from table grapes such as the Thompson seedless. Thus it would be illegal to sell American "Chablis" wines in France without relabeling them. One varietal that seems to be uniquely Californian is zinfandel. This variety of red grape has been so widely planted that the wine is often packaged in large jugs or boxes and marketed more like a generic. Most white wines are made from white grapes, although it is possible to use red grapes if the skins are removed before fermentation. Red wines are made from red grapes by leaving the skins in the crushed grapes while they ferment. Rose (pronounced *rose-ay*) wines were traditionally made by leaving the skins in for only a day or two, but most inexpensive American rose wine is made by mixing generic red and white wines. During the 1980s, "blush" wines such as white zinfandel became quite popular. With the zinfandel grape, which is red, there might be enough staining of the juice because some of the grapes are crushed during transport, or the skins might be left in the crushed grapes for a short while, resulting in a wine that is just slightly pink.

Besides red versus white and generic versus varietal, another general distinction is dry versus sweet. Most table wines are relatively dry, but some are sweeter than others. Also, the sweeter wines are likely to have a "heavier" taste overall, with the sweetness balancing out flavors that might be considered harsh in a dry wine. As a general rule, lighter foods such as broiled fish call for a light, dry, white wine. With Thanksgiving turkey a Rhine or a blush wine would be appropriate, and red wine would be considered an appropriate accompaniment to a steak.

Because carbon dioxide is produced during fermentation, it is possible to produce naturally carbonated sparkling wines by adding a small amount of sugar as the wine is bottled and then keeping the bottle tightly corked. French champagnes are made in this way, as are the more expensive American champagnes, which might be labeled "naturally fermented in the bottle," or "methode Champagnoise." A less expensive way is to do the secondary fermentation in a large sealed tank and then maintain pressure while the wine is put in a bottle. A still cheaper method is used on inexpensive American champagnes and sparkling burgundies: carbon dioxide is injected into a generic wine during bottling. Champagnes vary in their sweetness, also, with brut being the driest (dry and extra dry are not as dry).

It was discovered many years ago in Spain that if enough brandy is added to a newly fermented wine, the fermentation will stop and the wine will not spoil (turn to vinegar). Sealing the wine in charred oak casks for aging further refined its taste, and soon *sherry* was in great demand throughout Europe. Other fortified wines, all of which have an alcohol content near 20 percent, include port, Madeira, and Mus-

catel. Dry sherry is typically consumed before dinner, whereas the sweeter fortified wines may be drunk as a dessert wine.

In the 1960s, Americans consumed less wine than they do now, and most of it consisted of dessert wines. Sales of the sweet wines have decreased, and sales of the drier table wines increased to several times their 1960 level, bringing total wine sales up with them. The trend to increased wine drinking continued until 1986, as Figure 10.2 demonstrates.[3] There has been a decline in per capita wine consumption during the 1990s.

Part of the increase in per capita wine consumption in the mid 1980s was due to the introduction of the *wine cooler*, a mixture of wine with various carbonated beverages. These sweet, bubbly drinks look and taste a lot like soda pop, a fact that has not been lost on the marketers. They've even been sold in two-liter plastic bottles resembling soft-drink bottles. Coolers are popular with young drinkers who might not be aware that they contain both more alcohol and more calories than a bottle of beer. Wine coolers were first introduced in 1981; by

Wine coolers account for an increasing share of total wine sales.

Figure 10.2 Annual per capita consumption of wine and distilled spirits in the United States

the end of the 1980s wine cooler sales represented 25 percent of the dollar sales for the American wine industry. It appears that these coolers have replaced beer as a common "gateway" alcoholic beverage for many beginning drinkers.

Distilled Spirits

Although brandy, distilled from wine, was probably the first type of "spirits" known to Europeans, the Celts of Ireland and the Scottish highlands were distilling a crude beverage known as *uisgebaugh*—"water of life"—before 1500. Today's Scotch whisky (without the *e*; it's

whiskey in the United States and in Ireland, *whisky* in Scotland and Canada) is the distillate of fermented malted barley. The distinctive smoky flavor comes from two sources: the malted barley is dried in kilns in which burning peat provides the heat, and some of the distinctive characteristics of peat are picked up by the malt. With so many casks of sherry wine being sent to the British Isles after the seventeenth century, the ever-frugal Scots began to use the empty casks to age their whisky, and current practice calls for this storage in old sherry casks for at least three years. Pure malt whisky of this type is more popular in the Highlands than elsewhere because of its strong flavors. Most commercial Scotch whisky is blended with lighter-tasting grain spirits to provide a more pleasing drink.

In America the economics of trade resulted in an expanding production of spirits distilled from grain just as our new federal government was forming. In 1789 one of the early distillers who established a good reputation was Elijah Craig, a Baptist minister living in what was then Bourbon County, Kentucky. He began storing his whiskey in charred new oak barrels, originating a manufacturing step still used with most American whiskeys.

By the seventeenth century, improved distillation techniques made possible the production of relatively pure alcohol. Today's standard product from many large commercial distilleries is 95 percent pure alcohol (190 proof). Into the process goes whatever grain is available at a cheap price and tank loads of corn syrup or other sources of sugars or starches. Out the other end comes *grain neutral spirits*, a clear liquid that is essentially tasteless (except for the strong alcohol taste), which might be sold in small quantities as Everclear or for use in medicine or research. More often, it is processed in bulk in various ways. For example, large quantities of grain neutral spirits are now being added to gasoline in some areas to produce a less polluting fuel that also helps out the American farmer. Besides other industrial uses for ethyl alcohol, such as in cleaners and solvents, bulk grain neutral spirits are also used in making various beverages. We have already mentioned its use in blended Scotch whiskys. One of the first beverages to be made from straight grain neutral spirits was gin. By filtering the distillate through juniper berries and then diluting it with water, a medicinal-tasting drink was produced. First called "jenever" by the Dutch and "genievre" by the French, the British shortened the name first to "geneva" and then to "gin." Gin became a popular beverage in England and now forms the basis for many an American martini.

Consumers have turned away from bourbon toward the lighter, more mixable vodka and blended whiskeys.

Another major use for bulk grain neutral spirits is in the production of *vodka*. All American vodkas, and most vodkas from other countries, are simply a mixture of grain neutral spirits and water, adjusted to the desired proof. You may wonder why vodkas of the same proof are priced differently if they are all identical— and they are. The best answer to that question was given by an official of Heublein's, a company that produces both the high-priced Smirnoff vodka and a medium-priced vodka. "That's a very embarrassing question. Shall we say it's a difference in pricing policy?" Yes, we shall say that—maybe one label costs more?

The proof at which distillation is carried out influences the taste and other characteristics of the liquor. When alcohol is formed, other related substances, known as **congeners**, are also formed. These may include alcohols other than ethanol, oils, and other organic matter. Luckily they are present only in small amounts, because some of them are quite toxic. Grain neutral spirits contain relatively few congeners and none of the flavor of the grains used in the mash. Whiskey is usually distilled at a lower proof, not more than 160, and thus the distillate contains more congeners and some of the flavor of the grain used. If 51 percent or more of the grain used was rye, then the product is labeled straight *rye whiskey*. When corn constitutes over 51 percent of the grain in the mash, the liquor is called *bourbon*. (To be called *corn whiskey* requires that the mash be 80 percent or more corn.) Both rye and bourbon are then diluted to 120 to 125 proof and aged in new, charred oak barrels for at least two years, and usually longer. Whiskey accumulates congeners during aging, at least for the first five years, and the congeners and the grain used provide the variation in taste among whiskeys.

Until Prohibition almost all whiskey consumed in the United States was straight rye or bourbon manufactured in the United States. Prohibition introduced smuggled Canadian and Scotch whisky to American drinkers, and they liked them. World War II sent American men around the world, further exposing them to this different type of liquor. Scotch and Canadian whiskys are lighter than American whiskey, which means lighter in color and less heavy in taste. They are lighter because Canadian and Scotch whiskys are typically *blended* whiskys, made from about two-thirds straight whisky and one-third grain neutral spirits. After World War II, U.S. manufacturers began selling more blended whiskey. Seagram's 7-Crown has been one of the most popular blended American whiskeys. If you were so inclined, you could make your own blended whiskey by mixing two bottles of straight bourbon with one bottle of vodka, which would soften the whiskey flavor and lighten the color.

Liqueurs, or cordials, are similar in some ways to the fortified wines. Originally the cordials were made from brandy, but rather than mixing the brandy with wine, it was mixed with other flavorings derived from herbs, berries, or nuts. After dilution with sugar and water, the beverages are highly flavored, sweet, and usually about 20 to 25 percent alcohol. Some of the old recipes are still closely guarded secrets of a particular group of European monks. The 1980s saw an increase in popularity for these drinks, which are usually consumed in small amounts and have only about half the alcohol content of vodka or whiskey. Many new types were introduced, from Bailey's Irish Cream to varieties of schnapps. Modern American peppermint, peach, and other types of schnapps are made from grain neutral spirits that is diluted, sweetened, and flavored with artificial or natural flavorings.

Americans have changed their tastes in distilled spirits. For many years domestic whiskey dominated sales, but the trend toward lighter taste and increased "mixability," which began with imported and domestic blended whiskeys, also led to increased sales of gin, vodka, and rum. In 1983, domestic vodka finally surpassed domestic whiskey to become the leading single type of distilled spirits consumed by Americans. Sales of imported whisky have declined more slowly, and 1983 also marked the first time in recent years that sales of domestic whiskey fell behind sales of imports. Sales of vodka, gin, and rum peaked in 1983 and have declined somewhat since then. The resulting trend in overall per capita consumption of distilled spirits was downward during the 1980s and 1990s, as shown in figure 10.2.

---

congeners: (*con* **je nurz**) other alcohols and oils contained in alcoholic beverages.

The physical consequences of long-term indulgence

ALCOHOL PHARMACOLOGY

Absorption

Some of the alcohol is absorbed from the stomach, but the small intestine is responsible for most absorption. In an empty stomach the overall rate of absorption depends primarily on the concentration of alcohol. Alcohol taken with or after a meal is absorbed more slowly. This is because the food remains in the stomach for digestive action, and the protein in the food retains the alcohol with it in the stomach. Plain water, by decreasing the concentration, slows the absorption of alcohol, but carbonated liquids speed it up. The carbon dioxide acts to move everything quite rapidly through the stomach to the small intestine. It is because of this emptying of the stomach and the more rapid ab-

sorption of alcohol in the intestine that champagne and sparkling burgundy have a faster onset of action than wine.

Metabolism

As a "food" item, alcohol has a couple of unusual characteristics. First, it requires no digestion and is absorbed unchanged into the bloodstream. Second, although alcohol does contain usable calories (it produces energy when it is metabolized), alcohol itself cannot be stored nor can it be converted into lipids or protein so that this energy can be stored for later use. You might think that this means that alcohol itself cannot contribute to weight gain, but that is not so. With alcohol in the system, other calories that might be burned are not. In

Symptoms of withdrawl

fact, a recent report indicated that alcohol actually decreases the rate at which humans "burn" fat for energy.[4]

A 1990 study attracted a great deal of attention when it was reported that compared to men, women absorb a greater proportion of the alcohol they drink. It seems that some metabolism of alcohol actually takes place in the stomach, where the enzyme alcohol dehydrogenase is present. Because this stomach enzyme is more active, on the average, in men than in women, women might be more susceptible to the effects of alcohol.[5]

Once absorbed, alcohol remains in the bloodstream and other body fluids until it is metabolized, and over 90 percent of this metabolism occurs in the liver. A small amount of alcohol, less than 2 percent, is normally excreted unchanged—some in the breath, some through the skin, and some in the urine.

The primary metabolic system is a simple one: the enzyme *alcohol dehydrogenase* converts alcohol to *acetaldehyde*. Acetaldehyde is then converted fairly rapidly by aldehyde dehydrogenase to acetic acid. With most drugs a constant *proportion* of the drug is removed in a given amount of time, so that with a high blood level the amount metabolized is high. With alcohol, the *amount* that can be metabolized is constant at about 0.25 to 0.3 ounces per hour, regardless of the blood alcohol concentration (BAC). The major factor determining the rate of alcohol metabolism is the activity of the enzyme alcohol dehydrogenase. Exercise, drinking coffee, and so on have no effect on this enzyme, so the sobering-up process is essentially a matter of waiting for this enzyme to do its job at its own speed.

Acetaldehyde might be more than just an intermediate step in the oxidation of alcohol. Acetaldehyde is quite toxic; though its blood levels are only one-thousandth of those of alcohol, this substance might cause some of the physiological effects now attributed to alcohol. One danger in heavy alcohol use might be in the

FYI   The "Flushing" Reaction and Alcohol Consumption in Asia

About half of all Asians carry a gene that renders their liver's aldehyde dehydrogenase much less effective, and each time they drink there is a buildup of acetaldehyde, a toxic by-product of alcohol metabolism. This leads to a variety of reactions, including a facial flush, sweating, and nausea.

In spite of this common reaction, alcohol use, and especially heavy drinking, is becoming increasingly accepted in Japan, Korea, and China. Mixed drinks are sold in vending machines on the streets in Japan, and Japanese and Korean businessmen are increasingly likely to pressure each other to go out drinking, often to the point of intoxication. Perhaps this is part of an attempt to adopt what are viewed as American practices, but the rapid increase in heavy drinking promises to lead to severe social problems for these nations. South Korea is now reported to have the highest per capita consumption of distilled spirits in the world.[7]

higher blood levels of acetaldehyde (see the FYI box).

The second enzyme system is much more complicated and at this time has many more known ramifications. The liver responds to chronic intake of alcohol by increasing the levels of liver microsomal enzymes (see chapter 6). This gives rise to some interesting situations. In a person who drinks alcohol heavily over a long period of time, there is an increase in the activity of the microsomal enzymes. As long as there is alcohol in the system, alcohol gets preferential treatment and the metabolism of other drugs is *slower* than normal. When heavy alcohol use stops and the alcohol has disappeared from the body, the high activity level of the enzymes continues for four to eight weeks. During this time other drugs are metabolized more *rapidly*. To obtain therapeutic levels of the drugs metabolized by this enzyme system (e.g., the benzodiazepines), it is necessary to administer less drug to the drinking alcoholic and more drug to the just-nondrinking alcoholic. Thus alcohol increases the activity of one of the two enzyme systems responsible for its own oxidation. The increased activity of this microsomal pathway might be a partial basis for the tolerance to alcohol that is shown by heavy users of alcohol.[6]

Central Nervous System Effects

Alcohol is like any other general anesthetic: it depresses the CNS. It was used as an anesthetic until the late nineteenth century, when nitrous oxide, ether, and chloroform became more widely used. However, it was not just new compounds that decreased alcohol's use as an anesthetic; alcohol itself has some major disadvantages. In contrast to the gaseous anesthetics, alcohol is almost completely metabolized in the body and the rate of oxidation is slow. This gives alcohol a long duration of action that cannot be controlled. A second disadvantage is that the dose effective in surgical anesthesia is not much lower than the dose that causes respiratory arrest and death. Finally, alcohol makes blood slower to clot.

The exact mechanism for the CNS effect of alcohol is not clear. Until the mid 1980s the most widely accepted theory was that alcohol acted on all neural membranes, perhaps altering their electrical excitability. However, with increased understanding of the role of the GABA receptor complex in the actions of other depressant drugs (see chapter 8), many scientists now believe that the same receptor complex might play a special role in the action of alcohol. The study of GABA

receptors led to the discovery of an experimental drug, RO 15-4513, that appeared to be a specific antidote or antagonist for many of the behavioral effects of alcohol. In a dramatic demonstration, intoxicated rats that had been unable to roll over and stand up appeared, within two minutes after an injection of RO 15-4513, to be "sober" and walking normally. This drug antagonizes alcohol's enhancement of GABA action and is able to overcome some (but not all) of the depressant actions of alcohol.[8] It is not likely that a "sober-up" pill will be on the market at any time soon. Even if such a drug were available, the company selling it would be potentially liable for accidents occurring when a person who is over the legal BAC limit used their product to "sober up."

At the lowest effective blood levels, complex, abstract, and poorly learned behaviors are disrupted. As the dose increases, better learned and simpler behaviors are also affected. Inhibitions can be reduced, with the result that the overall amount of behavior increases under certain conditions. Even though alcohol can result in an increase in activity, most scientists would not call alcohol a stimulant. Rather, the increased behavioral output is usually attributed to decreased inhibition of behavior.

If the alcohol intake is "just right," most people experience a "high," a happy feeling. Below a certain **blood alcohol concentration** (BAC) there are no mood changes, but at some point we become uninhibited enough to enjoy our own charming selves and uncritical enough to accept the clods around us. This point seems to be when the alcohol has disrupted social inhibitions and impaired good judgment but has not depressed most behavior. We become witty, clever, and quite sophisticated! Fortunately, those around us at this time might also have slightly impaired judgment, so they can't say any different!

Another factor contributing to the feeling of well-being is the reduction in anxieties as a result of the disruption of normal critical

---

UP FOR DEBATE

Should Beer Labels State Alcohol Content?

It might seem strange in the era of nutrition labels on everything, but what is perhaps the most important ingredient in beer has remained a mystery to most consumers. Since the Prohibition era, it has been illegal to put alcohol content on a beer's label. In 1992 a federal judge overthrew that regulation, apparently paving the way for alcohol-content labels. In 1993, Anheuser-Busch, the nation's largest brewer, announced that it would begin putting alcohol content on its beers. However, the Bureau of Alcohol, Tobacco and Firearms (ATF) wasn't so certain that this was a good idea.

What the ATF folks were concerned about was that people would begin picking beers for higher alcohol content, causing the manufacturers to increase their alcohol levels and to advertise their newer, "stronger" beer. The concerns seemed to be justified in 1993 when the Miller Brewing Company, owners and importers of Canada's Molson brand, began just such an advertising campaign for their new Molson Ice beer, which has a higher alcohol content than their regular beer. The ATF Bureau threatened action, and Miller backed

down in early 1994. Later in 1994 the Adolph Coors Company brought the issue of alcohol content on beer labels to the U.S. Supreme Court, leading to a 1995 ruling in favor of alcohol labeling.

There are really two intertwined issues: Should the companies be allowed or even required to put alcohol content on the labels in order to inform consumers? Should the companies be allowed to refer to higher alcohol content in their advertising? Although traditionally most of the major beer brands have had alcohol contents near 4 percent by volume, beers are available with both higher and lower content, and the consumer currently has no way of knowing. Several of the beer marketers seem ready to challenge tradition and make alcohol content an issue. But the prospect of rising alcohol content due to advertising and manufacturing pressures concerns other groups as well as the federal government. What do you think will happen if brewers begin advertising alcohol content? What is the proper role of the regulatory agency, in your opinion?

---

thinking. The reduction in concern and judgment can range from not worrying about who'll pay the bar bill to being sure that you can take that next curve at 60 mph.

These effects depend on the BAC—also called blood alcohol level (BAL). BAC is reported as the number of grams of alcohol in 100 ml of blood and is expressed as a percentage. For example, 100 g in 100 ml would be 100 percent, and 100 mg of alcohol in 100 ml of blood is reported as 0.10 percent.

Before suggesting relationships between BAC and behavioral change, two factors must be mentioned. One is that the rate at which the BAC rises is a factor in determining behavioral effects.

blood alcohol concentration: a measure of the concentration of alcohol in blood, expressed in grams per 100 ml (percentage).

The more rapid the increase, the greater the behavioral effects. Second, a classic study using a variety of simple visual, motor, and visual-motor tests showed disruption of performance at an average BAC of 0.05 percent in abstainers, 0.07 percent in moderate drinkers, and 0.1 percent in heavy drinkers.[9] These results show clearly that behavioral and CNS tolerance to alcohol does develop. They also indicate that the better performance of the heavy drinker compared with the moderate drinker after equal amounts of alcohol is not caused by the greater rate of alcohol metabolism in heavy drinkers. A higher BAC is necessary to impair the performance of a chronic heavy drinker than to impair a moderate drinker's performance!

A partial explanation might be that the heavy drinker is better motivated to conceal the alcohol-induced impairment and probably has had more practice. Performance differences might reflect only the extent to which the two groups have learned to overcome the disruption of nervous system functioning. Another explanation might be that the CNS in the heavy drinker develops a tolerance to alcohol that does not exist in the moderate drinker. It is established that neural tissue becomes tolerant to alcohol, and tolerance can apparently develop even when the alcohol intake is well spaced over time.

Table 10.2 describes some general behavioral effects of increasing doses of alcohol. These relationships are approximately correct for moderate drinkers. There are some reports that changes in nervous system function have been obtained at concentrations as low as 0.03 percent to 0.04 percent.

The vomiting reflex can be activated by alcohol at a BAC of about 0.12 percent or even lower, but only if that level is approached rapidly. With slow, steady drinking the BAC increases gradually, and at high concentrations the vomiting center is depressed. The individual can then continue drinking up to lethal concentrations if he or she remains conscious!

TABLE 10.2

Blood Alcohol Concentration and Behavioral Effects

Percent BAC	Behavioral effects
0.05	Lowered alertness, usually good feeling, release of inhibitions, impaired judgment
0.10	Slower reaction times and impaired motor function, less caution
0.15	Large, consistent increases in reaction time
0.20	Marked depression in sensory and motor capability, decidedly intoxicated
0.25	Severe motor disturbance, staggering, sensory perceptions greatly impaired, smashed!
0.30	Stuporous but conscious—no comprehension of what's going on
0.35	Surgical anesthesia; about LD_1, minimal level causing death
0.40	About LD_{50}

The surgical anesthesia level and the minimum lethal level are perhaps the two least precise points in the table. In any case, they are quite close, and the safety margin is less than 0.1 percent blood alcohol. Death resulting from acute alcohol intoxication usually is the result of respiratory failure when the medulla is depressed.

The relationship between BAC and behavior is similarly, but more enjoyably, described in the following, which is modified from Bogen:[10]

At less than 0.03%, the individual is dull and dignified.

At 0.05%, he is dashing and debonair.

At 0.1%, he may become dangerous and devilish.

At 0.2%, he is likely to be dizzy and disturbing.

At 0.25%, he may be disgusting and disheveled.

At 0.3%, he is delirious and disoriented and surely drunk.

At 0.35%, he is dead drunk.

At 0.6%, the chances are that he is dead.

The relationship between BAC and alcohol intake is relatively simple and reasonably well understood. Remember, alcohol is not appreciably excreted from, or stored anywhere in, the body before metabolism. When taken into the body, alcohol is distributed throughout the body fluids, including the blood. However, alcohol does not distribute much into fatty tissues, so a 180-pound lean person will have a lower BAC than a 180-pound fat person who drinks the same amount of alcohol.

Table 10.3 demonstrates the relationships among alcohol intake, BAC, and body weight for hypothetical *average* females and males. The chart distinguishes between the sexes because the average female has a higher proportion of body fat and therefore for a given weight has less volume in which to distribute the alcohol. It's worth spending a bit of time to try to understand this table because you can learn a lot about how much you can probably drink to avoid going above a specified BAC.

First, table 10.3 makes the simplifying assumption that all of the alcohol is absorbed quickly and "in one hour," so that there is little opportunity for metabolism. If the 150-pound female had a tank of about 100 pounds (12.5 gallons, or 45 liters) of water and just dumped 1 ounce (28.3 g) into it and stirred it up, the concentration would be about 0.6 g/liter, or 0.06 g/100 ml (0.06%). Figure 10.3 shows a schematic of such a tank. The 150-pound average male has a "tank" with more water in it, so his alcohol concentration after 1 ounce is about 0.05 percent. The major factor determining individual differences in BAC is the volume of distribution, so find your own weight on table 10.3 and estimate how many drinks could be poured into your "tank" to obtain a BAC of 0.05 percent.

TABLE 10.3
Relationships among Gender, Weight, Alcohol Consumption, and Blood Alcohol Concentration

Blood alcohol concentrations (g/100 ml)

Absolute alcohol (ounces)	Beverage intake*	Female (100 lb)	Male (100 lb)	Female (150 lb)	Male (150 lb)	Female (200 lb)	Male (200 lb)
½	1 oz spirits† / 1 glass wine / 1 can beer	0.045	0.037	0.03	0.025	0.022	0.019
1	2 oz spirits† / 2 glasses wine / 2 cans beer	0.090	0.075	0.06	0.050	0.045	0.037
2	4 oz spirits† / 4 glasses wine / 4 cans beer	0.180	0.150	0.12	0.100	0.090	0.070
3	6 oz spirits† / 6 glasses wine / 6 cans beer	0.270	0.220	0.18	0.150	0.130	0.110
4	8 oz spirits† / 8 glasses wine / 8 cans beer	0.360	0.300	0.24	0.200	0.180	0.150
5	10 oz spirits† / 10 glasses wine / 10 cans beer	0.450	0.370	0.30	0.250	0.220	0.180

*in one hour
†100 proof

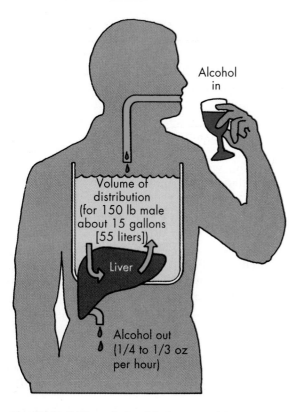

Alcohol
in

Volume of
distribution
(for 150 lb male
about 15 gallons
[55 liters])

Liver

Alcohol out
(1/4 to 1/3 oz
per hour)

Figure 10.3 The relationship between blood alcohol concentration and alcohol intake

Second, notice that several beverages are equated to ½ ounce of absolute alcohol. A 12-ounce can or bottle of beer at about 4.2 percent alcohol contains $12 \times 0.042 = \frac{1}{2}$ ounce of alcohol. This same amount is found in a glass of wine containing about 4 ounces of 12 percent alcohol, 1 ounce of 100-proof spirits, or 1.25 ounces of 80-proof spirits. Each of these can be equated as a standard "drink."

We have not yet taken metabolism into account, but we can do so with one more simple calculation. As we already know, alcohol is removed by the liver at essentially a constant rate of 0.25 to 0.3 ounce of ethanol per hour. There are some individual differences in this rate, but most people fall within this range no matter

what their body size or drinking experience, unless they have consumed so much alcohol that their liver is damaged. To be on the safe side, estimate that you can metabolize about 0.25 ounce per hour, and note that this is one-half of one of our standard drinks (one beer, one shot, or one glass of wine). Over the course of an evening, if your rate of intake equals your rate of metabolism, you will maintain a stable BAC. If you drink faster than one drink every 2 hours, your BAC will climb. The extra drinks, those over the one every 2 hours, will be added to your tank. Let's take an example from the chart: a 150-pound male goes to the bar at 8 P.M. and consumes six beers before midnight. During that 4 hours his liver metabolized the alcohol from two of the beers, so he still has four drinks, or 2 ounces of ethanol, in his system. His BAC at midnight should be about 0.10 percent, making him legally intoxicated and unfit to drive home. If he had had two fewer beers (four over the 4-hour period), his BAC would be about 0.05 percent. In other words, once the two drinks for 4 hours of metabolism are accounted for, you simply add up the extra drinks and look up the estimated BAC on the chart. If you want to do other calculations for yourself, follow these two steps: first, calculate the number of "drinks" metabolized at the rate of half a drink per hour. Second, pour the remaining drinks into the tank for a person of that size using table 10.3. A 100-pound female who had kept up with our six-pack-consuming friend would have metabolized the same two beers, but the four remaining ones would leave her in pretty bad shape at 0.18 percent. If he were driving home in a "dangerous and devilish" state, she might be too "dizzy and disturbed" to notice.

Let's take a brief look at some other-than-standard drinks. What if our male friend had been drinking "3.2" beer? Each 12-ounce beer at 3.2 percent has almost 0.4 ounce of alcohol instead of 0.5, so six of them contain 2.3 ounces. After metabolizing 1 ounce in 2 hours, his tank has 1.3 ounces, or enough to put him at about

0.065 percent. He's better off than when he drank the six regular beers, but it's wrong to say that 3.2 beer is not intoxicating. Alcohol is alcohol, no matter what beverage it comes from. As an exercise, figure out how many 3.2 beers it would take to put this guy over the 0.10 percent line. Wine coolers contain 12 ounces of about 5 percent alcohol, more than one of our standard drinks, so you might try some calculations with drinks containing 0.6 ounces.

What's a safe BAC? After we remember that nothing in this world is totally safe, let's say that if you are going to drink and want to remain in reasonable control of your faculties you should probably stay below 0.05 percent. Individuals differ considerably in their sensitivities to alcohol, however, so the best rule is to learn about your own sensitivity and not to feel compelled to keep up with anyone else's drinking. And alcohol-induced impairment is dose related and depends on what you're trying to do. Carrying on bar conversation places fewer demands on your nervous system than driving on a Los Angeles freeway during rush hour, where any alcohol at all might interfere.

BAC gives a good estimate of the alcohol concentration in the brain, and the concentration of alcohol in the breath gives a good estimate of the alcohol concentration in the blood. The concentration in the blood is almost exactly 2,100 times the concentration in air expired from the lungs, making breath samples accurate indicators of BAC. Such breath samples are easily collected by police and can be the basis for conviction as a drunk driver in most states.

Blackouts

Alcohol-induced blackouts are periods of time during alcohol use in which the drinking individual appears to function normally but later, when the individual is sober, the individual cannot recall any events that occurred during that period. The drinker might drive home or dance all night, interacting in the usual way with others. When the individual cannot remember the activities, the people, or anything else—that's a blackout. Most authorities include it as one of the danger signs suggesting excessive use of alcohol. The limited amount of recent research on this topic is probably related to ethical concerns about giving such high doses of alcohol to experimental subjects. An article from 1884 titled "Alcoholic Trance" referred to the syndrome:

> This trance state is a common condition in inebriety, where . . . a profound suspension of memory and consciousness and literal paralysis of certain brain-functions follow.
>
> This trance state may last from a few moments to several days, during which the person may appear and act rationally, and yet be actually a mere automaton, without consciousness or memory of his actual condition.[11]

Sexual Behavior

> Lechery, sir, it provokes, and unprovokes; it provokes the desire, but it takes away the performance.[12]

Alcohol, because it is a depressant drug, decreases inhibitions and at least makes the thought of sexual activity more likely. The amount of sexual behavior might increase after moderate alcohol intake, but there is considerable anecdotal evidence that the quality decreases.

Whether alcohol enhances sexual activity through pharmacological mechanisms or through attitudes and beliefs is not clear. Those who believe alcohol to be an aid to sexual pleasure are more likely to drink, and the act of drinking can provide a sort of "license" to be more relaxed and behave less responsibly. In fact, one clear finding is that alcohol use by adolescents is associated with increased "risky" sex (not using a condom, promiscuity).[8]

A sophisticated and well-designed study[13] using college women as subjects explored the relationships among the dose of alcohol ingested (0.05, 0.25, 0.50, and 0.75 alcohol per kg body weight), self-reports of sexual arousal, and vaginal vasocongestion. There were two experimental conditions—watching an erotic-pornographic film and watching a nonerotic film of a tour of a computer facility—and two sets of instructions, one suggesting that alcohol would increase sexual arousal and the other suggesting that alcohol would decrease sexual arousal. The subjects were tested about 40 minutes after alcohol intake. Each subject was tested under each alcohol dose, and in each session both the erotic and the nonerotic film were viewed.

Several results are worthy of note. The instructional set did not generally alter the expected effect of alcohol: most of the college women expected alcohol to increase sexual arousal. On the self-report measure, (1) sexual arousal increased with alcohol intake and (2) the percentage of subjects reporting arousal to the erotic film increased as the amount of alcohol ingested increased.

The erotic film elicited much greater vaginal vasocongestion than the computer film, providing some validity to vaginal vasocongestion as a measure of sexual arousal. Importantly, the amount of increase in vaginal vasocongestion decreased as the dose of alcohol increased. For women, increased alcohol intake results in self-reports of increased sexual arousal along with a decrease in a physiological measure of arousal.

A similar study[14] was carried out on college men by the same research team. The physiological measure of arousal was also vasocongestion—speed, amount, and duration of penile erection. The doses of alcohol ingested were 0.08, 0.4, 0.8, and 1.2 g/kg. All three measures of penile vasocongestion decreased as the dose of alcohol was increased. Self-reports of degree of arousal were highly correlated with the extent of vasocongestion.

Alcohol Withdrawal—Delirium Tremens

The physical dependence associated with prolonged heavy use of alcohol is revealed when alcohol intake is stopped. *The abstinence syndrome that develops is medically more severe and more likely to cause death than withdrawal from narcotic drugs.* In untreated advanced cases, mortality can be as high as one in seven. For that reason it has long been recommended that the initial period of **detoxification** (allowing the body to rid itself of the alcohol) be carried out in an inpatient medical setting, especially for those alcoholics who have been drinking very heavily or have other medical complications.

The progression of withdrawal, the abstinence syndrome, has been described in the following way:

- Stage 1: Tremors, excessively rapid heartbeat, hypertension, heavy sweating, loss of appetite, and insomnia
- Stage 2: Hallucinations—auditory, visual, tactile, or a combination of these; and, rarely, olfactory signs
- Stage 3: Delusions, disorientation, delirium, sometimes intermittent in nature and usually followed by amnesia
- Stage 4: Seizure activity

Medical treatment is usually sought in stage 1 or 2, and rapid intervention with a sedative drug such as chlordiazepoxide will prevent stage 3 or 4 from occurring. The old term **delirium tremens** is used to refer to severe cases including at least stage 3.

Tremors are one of the most common physical changes associated with alcohol withdrawal and can persist for a long period after alcohol intake has stopped. The classic drunk, bending over to sip from his cup, attests to the frequency of tremors. Anxiety, insomnia, feelings of unreality, nausea, vomiting, and many other symptoms can also occur.

The withdrawal symptoms do not develop all at the same time or immediately after abstinence begins. The initial signs (tremors, anxiety) might develop within a few hours, but the individual is relatively rational. Over the next day or two, hallucinations appear and gradually become more terrifying and real to the individual. Huckleberry Finn described these in his father quite vividly:[15]

> Pap took the jug, and said he had enough whisky there for two drunks and one delirium tremens. . . . He drank and drank. . . .
>
> I don't know how long I was asleep, but . . . there was an awful scream and I was up. There was pap looking wild, and skipping around every which way and yelling about snakes. He said they was crawling up on his legs; and then he would give a jump and scream, and say one had bit him on the cheek—but I couldn't see no snakes. He started and run round . . . hollering "Take him off! he's biting me on the neck!" I never see a man look so wild in the eyes. Pretty soon he was all fagged out, and fell down panting; then he rolled over . . . kicking things every which way, and striking and grabbing at the air with his hands, and screaming . . . there was devils a-hold of him. He wore out by and by . . . He says . . .
>
> "Tramp-tramp-tramp; that's the dead; tramp-tramp-tramp; they're coming after me; but I won't go. Oh, they're here; don't touch me—don't! hands off—they're cold; let go. . . ."
>
> Then he went down on all fours and crawled off, begging them to let him alone. . . .
>
> By and by he . . . jumped up on his feet looking wild . . . and went for me. He chased me round and round the place with a claspknife, calling me the Angel of Death, and saying he would kill me, and then I wouldn't come for him no more . . . Pretty soon he was all tired out . . . and said he would rest for a minute and then kill me.

The sensation of snakes or bugs crawling on the skin should ring a bell with you—this also occurs after high doses of stimulant drugs. In the context of alcohol withdrawal, it is an indication that the nervous system is rebounding from constant inhibition and is hyperexcitable.

Optimal treatment of patients during the early stages involves the administration of a benzodiazepine such as chlordiazepoxide or diazepam (see chapter 8). Because of the high degree of cross-dependence between alcohol and chlordiazepoxide, one drug can be substituted for the other and withdrawal continued at a safer rate.[16]

There is increasing recognition that some withdrawal symptoms can last for up to several weeks. Unstable blood pressure, irregular breathing, anxiety, panic attacks, insomnia, and depression are all reported during this period. These phenomena have been referred to as a protracted withdrawal syndrome, and they can trigger intense cravings for alcohol. Thus some alcoholics might benefit from residential or inpatient treatment for up to four to six weeks simply to prevent relapse during this critical period. To keep the alcoholic from resuming drinking for longer periods is a difficult task that is discussed in chapter 11.

Physiological Effects

Peripheral circulation

One effect of alcohol on the CNS is the dilation of the peripheral blood vessels. This increases heat loss from the body but makes the drinker feel warm. The heat loss and cooling of the interior of the body are enough to cause a slowdown in some biochemical processes. This dilation of the peripheral vessels argues against giving alcohol to individuals in shock or extreme cold. Under these conditions blood is needed in the central parts of the body, and heat loss must be diminished if the person is to survive.

---

detoxification: early treatment stage in which the body eliminates the alcohol or other substance.

delirium tremens: (de *leer* ee um *tree* mens) alcohol withdrawal syndrome that includes hallucinations and tremors.

Fluid balance

One of the actions of alcohol on the brain is to decrease the output of the antidiuretic hormone (ADH, also called vasopressin) responsible for retaining fluid in the body. It is this effect, rather than the actual fluid consumption, that increases the urine flow in response to alcohol. This diuretic effect can lower blood pressure in some individuals.

Hormone effects

Even single doses of alcohol can produce measurable effects on a variety of hormone systems: adrenal corticosteroids are released, as are catecholamines from the adrenal medulla, and the production of the male sex hormone testosterone is suppressed. It is not known what significance, if any, these effects might have for occasional, moderate drinkers. However, chronic alcoholics can develop a variety of hormone-related disorders, including testicular atrophy and impotence in men and impaired reproductive functioning in women.

ALCOHOL TOXICITY

Hangover

The Germans call it "wailing of cats" (*Katzenjammer*), the Italians "out of tune" (*stonato*), the French "woody mouth" (*gueule de boise*), the Norwegians "workmen in my head" (*jeg har tommeermenn*), and the Swedes "pain in the roots of the hair" (*hont i haret*).[17] Hangovers aren't much fun. And they aren't very well understood, either. Even moderate drinkers who only occasionally overindulge are well acquainted with the symptoms: upset stomach, fatigue,

The night before and the morning after

headache, thirst, depression, anxiety, and general malaise.

Some authorities believe that the symptoms of a hangover are the symptoms of withdrawal from a short- or long-term addiction to alcohol. The pattern certainly fits. Some alcoholics report continuing to drink just to escape the pain of the hangover. This behavior is not unknown to moderate drinkers, either: many believe that the only "cure" for a hangover is some of "the hair of the dog that bit you"—alcohol. And it might work to minimize symptoms, because it spreads them out over a longer period of time. There is no evidence that any of the "surefire-this'll-fix-you-up" remedies are effective. The only known "cures" are an analgesic for the headache, rest, and time. Some of the ways to reduce the probability and the severity of a hangover are evident from the following discussion.

A study titled "Experimental Induction of Hangover"[18] provided support for two factors as contributing to the hangover syndrome: (1) The higher your BAC, the more likely you are to have a hangover; and (2) with the *same* BAC, bourbon drinkers were more likely (two out of three) than vodka drinkers (one out of three) to have a hangover. This fits with the belief that some hangover symptoms are reactions to congeners. Congeners are natural products of the fermentation and preparation process, some of which are quite toxic. Congeners make the various alcoholic beverages different in smell, taste, color, and, possibly, hangover potential. Beer, with a 4 percent alcohol content, has only a 0.01 percent congener level, whereas wine has about 0.04 percent and distilled spirits between 0.1 and 0.2 percent congener level. Gin, being a mixture of almost pure alcohol and water, has a congener content about the same as wine, whereas a truly pure mixture of alcohol and water (vodka) has the same congener level as beer. Aging distilled spirits does not decrease the level of congeners—it increases their level about threefold.

Still other factors contribute to the trials and tribulations of the "morning after the night before." Thirst means that the body has excreted more fluid than was taken in with the alcoholic beverages. However, this does not seem to be the only basis for the thirst experienced the next day. Another cause might be that alcohol causes fluid inside cells to move outside the cells. This cellular dehydration, without a decrease in total body fluid, is known to be related to, and might be the basis of, an increase in thirst.

The nausea and upset stomach typically experienced can most likely be attributed to the fact that alcohol is a gastric irritant. Consuming even moderate amounts causes local irritation of the mucosa covering the stomach. It has been suggested that the accumulation of acetaldehyde, which is quite toxic even in small quantities, contributes to the nausea and headache. The headache can also be a reaction to fatigue. Fatigue sometimes results from a higher than normal level of activity while drinking. Increased activity frequently accompanies a decrease in inhibitions, a readily available source of energy, and a high blood sugar level. One of the effects of alcohol intake is to increase the blood sugar level for about an hour after ingestion. This can be followed several hours later by a low blood sugar level and an increased feeling of fatigue. Although hangover cures might be just around the corner, for now the only sure cure is time.

When alcohol intake occurs regularly and in large quantities over a period of years, physical dependence on the drug follows. Abrupt withdrawal from alcohol results in dangerous changes in body physiology. Before the addiction to alcohol reaches this point, physical symptoms sometimes develop, with facial appearance the first to be affected. The capillaries around the conjunctiva of the eyes become enlarged, and the skin of the face, forehead, and under the eyes becomes puffy and filled with fluid. In an individual with a fair complexion, the skin might appear continually flushed and, after prolonged use, a "whiskey nose" might develop. The frequent hoarseness of the alcoholic results from the accumulation of fluid in the mucous membranes of the nose, pharynx, larynx, and vocal cords. Continual ingestion of alcohol leads to an inflamed stomach associated with nausea and loss of appetite.

Chronic Disease States

The relationship of alcohol use to many diseases has been studied extensively and still continues. Let's review some of the major health concerns discussed in the National Institute on Alcohol Abuse and Alcoholism's (NIAAA's) 1993 report to Congress on alcohol and health.[8] As a general rule, we can say that heavy alcohol use, either directly or indirectly, affects every organ system in the body. The alcohol or its primary metabolite, acetaldehyde, can irritate and damage tissue directly. Because alcohol provides "empty" calories, many heavy drinkers do not eat well, and chronic malnutrition leads to tissue damage. Separating the effects of alcohol exposure from those of malnutrition relies to a great extent on experiments with animals, so that some animals can be fed adequate diets and exposed to high concentrations of alcohol, while other animals are fed diets deficient in certain vitamins or other nutrients.

Brain Damage

Perhaps the biggest concern is the damage to brain tissue that is seen in chronic alcoholics. It has been reported for years that the brains of deceased alcoholics demonstrate an obvious overall loss of brain tissue: the ventricles (internal spaces) in the brain are enlarged, and the fissures (sulci) in the cortex are widened. Modern imaging techniques, first CT scans and then MRI, have demonstrated this tissue loss in living alcoholics as well. This generalized loss of brain tissue is probably a result of direct alcohol toxicity rather than malnutrition and is associated with *alcoholic dementia*, a global decline of intellect. Patients with this type of organic brain syndrome might have difficulty swallowing in addition in impaired problem-solving, difficulty in manipulating objects, and abnormal electroencephalograms. Another classical alcohol-related organic brain syndrome has two parts that so often go together that the disorder is referred to as **Wernicke-Korsakoff syndrome**. *Wernicke's disease* is associated with a deficiency of thiamine (vitamin B_1) and can sometimes be corrected nutritionally. The symptoms include confusion, ataxia (impaired coordination while walking), and abnormal eye movements. Most patients with Wernicke's disease also exhibit *Korsakoff's psychosis*, characterized by an inability to remember recent events or to learn new information. Korsakoff's psychosis can appear by itself in patients who maintain adequate nutrition, and it appears to be mostly irreversible. There has been great controversy about the specific brain areas that are damaged in Wernicke-Korsakoff syndrome, and about the relationship between the two parts of the disorder.

Important practical questions include these: Exactly how much alcohol exposure is required before behavioral and/or anatomical evidence can be found indicating brain damage? And how much of the cognitive deficit seen in alcoholic dementia can be reversed when drinking is stopped and adequate nutrition is given? Both have been the subject of several recent experiments. As for the first question, there is no definitive answer. Some of the studies on "moderate" drinkers have included individuals who consume up to ten drinks per day! Most studies with lower cutoffs for moderate drinking have not found consistent evidence for anatomical changes in the brain. As for recovery, several studies have now reported both behavioral improvement and apparent regrowth of brain size in alcoholics after some months of abstinence. However, not all such studies find improvement, and some have found improvement in some types of mental tasks but not in others. There is some room for hope, especially in younger alcoholics.

Liver Disorders

Fatty acids are the usual fuel for the liver. When present, alcohol has higher priority and is used as fuel instead. As a result, fatty acids (lipids) accumulate in the liver and are stored as small droplets in liver cells. This condition is known as alcohol-related *fatty liver*, which for most drinkers is not a serious problem. If alcohol input ceases, the liver uses the stored fatty acids for energy. Sometimes the droplets increase in size until they rupture the cell membrane, causing death of the liver cells. Before the liver cells die, a fatty liver is completely reversible and usually of minor medical concern.

Sometimes, with prolonged or high-level alcohol intake, another phase of liver damage is observed. This is alcoholic hepatitis, which is a serious disease and includes both inflammation and impairment of liver function. Usually this occurs in areas of the liver where cells are dead and dying, but it is not known if an increasingly fatty liver leads to alcoholic hepatitis. It is known that you can have alcoholic hepatitis in the absence of a fatty liver, so this form of tissue damage might be due to direct toxic effects of alcohol.

Cirrhosis is the liver disease everyone knows is related to high and prolonged levels of alcohol consumption. It's not easy to get cirrhosis from drinking alcohol—you have to work at it. Usually it takes about ten years of steady drinking of the equivalent of a pint or more of whiskey a day. Not all cirrhosis is alcohol related, but a high percentage is, and cirrhosis is the seventh leading cause of death in the United States. In large urban areas it is the fourth or fifth leading cause of death in men ages 25 to 65. In cirrhosis, liver cells are replaced by fibrous tissue (collagen), which changes the structure of the liver (Figure 10.4). These changes decrease blood flow and, along with the loss of cells, result in a decreased ability of the liver to function. When the liver does not function properly, fluid accumulates in the body, jaundice develops, and other infections or cancers have a better oppor-

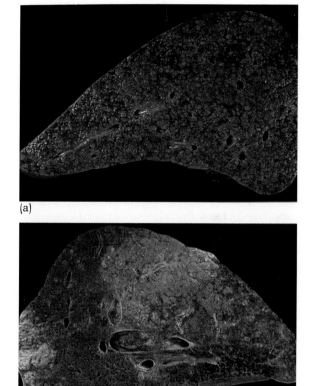

(a)

(b)

Figure 10.4 (a) Normal liver (b) cirrhotic liver

tunity to establish themselves in the liver. The yellow color of the jaundiced individual's skin (and in the whites of the eyes) is the result of bile pigment distributed throughout the body, but most importantly it is a sign that the liver is

> **Wernicke-Korsakoff syndrome:** (*wer* **nick ee core sa kof**) chronic mental impairments produced by heavy alcohol use over a long period of time.
>
> **cirrhosis:** (**sir** *oh* **sis**) irreversible, frequently deadly, liver disorder associated with heavy alcohol use.

not functioning properly and that toxins are beginning to accumulate in the blood. Cirrhosis is not reversible, but stopping the intake of alcohol will retard its development and decrease the serious medical effects. The liver has a large reserve capacity and is able to function adequately with mild cirrhosis. One of the important unanswered questions is why not all alcoholics develop cirrhosis. Also, when comparing different countries, there is an imperfect correlation between alcohol consumption and rates of cirrhosis. France, Portugal, Italy, and Spain, which are among the top per capita consumers of alcohol, also have the highest rates of cirrhosis. But Switzerland, which reports much lower per capita alcohol consumption than the United States, has a higher rate of cirrhosis than the United States. Differences in susceptibility to cirrhosis might reflect different drinking patterns, inherited susceptibilities, nutritional differences, or other factors.

In alcoholics with severely damaged livers, liver transplants have been quite successful—a 64 percent survival rate after two years. The success rate has no doubt been helped by the fact that most of these recipients do not resume drinking after the transplant.

Heart Disease

Another area of concern is the effect of alcohol on the heart and circulation. There is no doubt that heavy alcohol use is associated with increased mortality resulting from heart disease. Much of this is due to damage to the heart muscle (cardiomyopathy), but there is also an increased risk of the more typical heart attack resulting from coronary artery disease. Heavy drinkers are also more likely to suffer from high blood pressure and strokes. An interesting twist to this story is that several studies have found a *lower* incidence of heart attacks in moderate drinkers than in abstainers, and for several years there has been discussion about this "protective" effect of moderate alcohol consumption and the

possible mechanism for it. It has been pointed out that the "abstainers" in such studies might include both abstaining alcoholics who once drank heavily or others who quit on their doctor's advice because of poor health. However, a recent study separated those who never drank from the "quitters" and still reported fewer heart attacks and lower overall mortality in moderate drinkers, with increased mortality for both abstainers and heavy drinkers.[19] It has been proposed that alcohol increases high-density lipoproteins (HDL, sometimes called "good cholesterol"), some of which seem to protect against high blood pressure. The reduced blood clotting produced by alcohol could also play a role. There has been some speculation that red wine might have better effects than other forms of alcohol due to the presence of antioxidants in the grapes from which the wine is made. But the scientific evidence supports only a beneficial effect of alcohol on heart attacks, with an optimal effect occurring at about one drink per day.[20]

Cancer

Alcohol use is associated with cancers of the mouth, tongue, pharynx, larynx, esophagus, stomach, liver, lung, pancreas, colon, and rectum. There are many possible mechanisms for this, from direct tissue irritation to nutritional deficiencies to the induction of enzymes that activate other carcinogens. There is a particularly nasty interaction with cigarette smoking that increases the incidence of cancers of the oral cavity, pharynx, and larynx. Also, suppression of the immune system by alcohol, which occurs to some extent every time intoxicating doses are used, probably increases the rate of tumor growth.

The Immune System

The immune deficits seen in chronic alcoholics are associated with at least some increase in the frequency of various infectious diseases, including tuberculosis, pneumonia, yellow fever, cholera, and hepatitis B. Alcohol use might be a factor in AIDS, for several reasons: loss of behavioral inhibitions probably increases the likelihood of engaging in unprotected sex; alcohol could increase the risk of HIV infection in exposed individuals; and alcohol could suppress the immune system and therefore increase the chances of developing full-blown AIDS once an HIV infection is established. Although one epidemiological study did not find an acceleration of HIV-related disease in infected individuals who drank, heavy alcohol use is probably not a good idea for anyone who is HIV-positive.

After all is said and done, there is no evidence that occasional drinking of one or two drinks has overall negative effects on the physical health of most individuals. An important exception to this statement might be drinking during pregnancy.

FETAL ALCOHOL SYNDROME

The unfortunate condition of infants born to alcoholic mothers was noted in an 1834 report to the British Parliament: they have a "starved, shriveled, and imperfect look." Until fairly recently most scientists and physicians believed that any effects on the offspring of heavy alcohol users were the result of poor nutrition or poor prenatal care. Those beliefs changed, however, when a 1973 article reported the following:

> Eight unrelated children of three different ethnic groups, all born to mothers who were chronic alcoholics, have a pattern of craniofacial, limb, and cardiovascular defects associated with prenatal-onset growth deficiency and developmental delay. This seems to be the first reported association between maternal alcoholism and aberrant morphogenesis in the offspring. [21]

That publication signaled the recognition of **fetal alcohol syndrome** (FAS), a collection of physical and behavioral abnormalities that

Figure 10.5 Two girls born with fetal alcohol syndrome. Symptoms include small eyes, flattened bridge of the nose, and flattening of the vertical groove between the nose and mouth.

seems to be caused by the presence of alcohol during development of the fetus (Figure 10.5). There are three primary criteria for diagnosing FAS, at least one of which *must* be present:
1. Growth retardation occurring before and/or after birth
2. A pattern of abnormal features of the face and head, including small head circumference, small eyes, or evidence of retarded formation of the midfacial area, including a flattened bridge and short length of the nose and flattening of the vertical groove between the nose and mouth (the philtrum)
3. Evidence of CNS abnormality, including abnormal neonatal behavior, mental retardation, or other evidence of abnormal neurobehavioral development

Each of these features can be seen in the absence of alcohol exposure, and other features

---

fetal alcohol syndrome: facial and developmental abnormalities associated with the mother's alcohol use during pregnancy.

might also be present in FAS, such as eye and ear defects, heart murmurs, undescended testicles, birthmarks, and abnormal fingerprints or palmar creases. Recent research also found a high frequency of various abnormalities of the eyes, often associated with poor vision.[22] Thus the diagnosis of FAS is a matter of judgment, based on several symptoms and often on the physician's knowledge of the mother's drinking history.

A large number of animal studies have now been done in a variety of species, and they indicate rather clearly that FAS is related to peak BAC and to duration of alcohol exposure, even when malnutrition is not an issue. In mice and other animal models, with increasing amounts of alcohol there is an increase in mortality, a decrease in infant weight, and increased frequency of soft-tissue malformation. The different components of the complete FAS reflect damage occurring at different developmental stages, so heavy alcohol exposure throughout pregnancy is the most damaging situation, followed by intermittent high-level exposure designed to imitate "binge" drinking.

By no means do all infants born to drinking mothers show abnormal development. If they did, it would not have taken so long to recognize FAS as a problem. Estimates of the prevalence of FAS in the overall population have ranged from 0.4 per 1,000 births to 2.9 per 1,000. Estimating the prevalence among problem drinkers or alcohol abusers is more of a problem. There is the difficulty not only of diagnosing FAS but also of diagnosing alcohol abuse. If the physician knows that the mother is a heavy drinker, this can increase the probability of noticing or diagnosing FAS, thus inflating the prevalence statistics among drinking mothers. FAS itself seems to occur in 23 to 29 per 1,000 births among women who are problem drinkers. If all alcohol-related birth defects are counted (referred to as **fetal alcohol effect**, or FAE), the rate among heavy-drinking women is higher, from 80 to a few hundred per 1,000. Maternal alcohol abuse

might be the most frequent known environmental cause of mental retardation in the Western world.

In addition to the risk of FAS, the fetus of a mother who drinks heavily has a risk of not being born at all. Spontaneous abortion early in pregnancy is perhaps twice as likely among the 5 percent of women who are the heaviest drinkers. The data on later pregnancy loss (stillbirths) are not as clearly related to alcohol for either animals or humans.

An important question, and one that can never be answered in absolute terms, is whether there is an acceptable level of alcohol consumption for pregnant women. The data we do have on drinking during pregnancy rely on self-reports by the mothers, who are assumed to be at least as likely as everyone else to underreport their drinking. In addition, almost every study that has been done has used different definitions of heavy drinking, alcohol abuse, or problem drinking. It is clear that the heaviest drinkers in each study are the most at risk for alcohol-related problems with their children, but we don't really know if the large number of light or moderate drinkers are causing significant risks. Based on the dose-related nature of birth problems in animal studies, one might argue that any alcohol use at all produces some risk, but at low levels the increased risk is too small to be revealed except in a large-scale study. In 1981 the U.S. surgeon general recommended that "pregnant women should drink absolutely no alcohol because they may be endangering the health of their unborn children." Maybe that's going a bit too far. The bottom line is this: Scientific data do not demonstrate that occasional consumption of one or two drinks definitely causes FAS or other alcohol-related birth defects. On the other hand, neither do the data prove that low-level alcohol use is safe nor do they indicate a safe level of use. Remember from chapter 6 that it is not within the realm of science to declare something totally safe, so it will be impossible ever to set a safe limit on

Protecting the Unborn from Alcohol

Increased concern about fetal alcohol syndrome has led to some significant changes in the status of pregnant women, at least in certain instances and certain locations. Waiters have refused to serve wine to pregnant women, women have been arrested and charged with child abuse for being heavily intoxicated while pregnant, and others have been charged with endangerment for breastfeeding while drunk. These social interventions represent real concerns for the welfare of the child. However, to women already concerned about their own rights because of the issue of government regulation of abortion, such actions seem to be yet another infringement, yet another signal that the woman's rights are secondary to the child's.

We know that heavy alcohol consumption during pregnancy does increase the risk to the child of permanent disfigurement and mental retardation. We also know that even among the heaviest drinkers, the odds still favor a normal-appearing baby (less than 10 percent of the babies born to the heaviest-drinking 5 percent of mothers exhibit full-blown FAS).

Do you think that men are more likely than women to support limiting the rights of pregnant women to drink while they are pregnant? You might ask a group of both men and women to give you answers to the following questions:

How strongly do you agree (5 = strong agreement, 1 = strong disagreement) with these statements:

1. Women who repeatedly get drunk while they are pregnant should be kept in jail if necessary until the baby is born.
2. All bartenders should be trained not to serve any drinks at all to a woman who is obviously pregnant.
3. If a man and a woman are drinking together and both become intoxicated while the woman is pregnant, both the man and the woman should be arrested for child abuse.

alcohol use. It is good to know that most women decrease their alcohol use once they have become pregnant, and many decrease it further as pregnancy progresses.

SUMMARY

▲ Alcohol is made by yeasts in a process called fermentation. Distillation is used to increase the alcohol content of a beverage.
▲ Beer has the lowest alcohol content of the traditional beverages and is consumed in much greater volumes than wine or liquor. Beer consumption has not changed greatly in the past decade.
▲ Wine consumption increased until the mid 1980s and has declined somewhat since then.

---

fetal alcohol effect: individual developmental abnormalities associated with the mother's alcohol use during pregnancy.

- Consumption of distilled spirits, especially of the stronger-tasting whiskeys, has declined considerably over the past fifteen years.
- Alcohol is metabolized by the liver at a constant rate that is not much influenced by body size.
- The exact mechanism by which alcohol affects the nervous system is still not known but might involve the neurotransmitter GABA.
- By the use of simple calculations and table 10.3, it is possible to estimate a person's blood alcohol concentration if you know how many drinks he or she consumed over what period of time.
- Alcohol appears to enhance interest in sex but impair physiological arousal in both sexes.
- The alcohol withdrawal syndrome is referred to as delirium tremens.
- Chronic heavy drinking can lead to neurological damage, as well as damage to the heart and liver. However, light drinking has been associated with a decrease in heart attacks.
- Recognition of fetal alcohol syndrome and fetal alcohol effect since 1973 has led to educational and other programs aimed at preventing this important cause of mental retardation.

REVIEW QUESTIONS

1. What is fortified wine, and why was it invented?
2. Grain neutral spirits is 95 percent alcohol. What is its "proof"?
3. The largest-selling brand of beer has about what share of the overall domestic market?
4. The experimental drug RO 15-4513 has what effect on an intoxicated rat?
5. What is the typical behavior of a person with a BAC of 0.20 percent?
6. Describe the stages of alcohol withdrawal syndrome in a very heavy drinker.

7. Why does bourbon produce more hangover symptoms than vodka?
8. What are the behavioral characteristics of Korsakoff's psychosis?
9. How could alcohol play a role in contracting AIDS?
10. What are the three defining characteristics of FAS?

WEB WATCH

Related Internet Sites on Alcohol in the Body

The Beer Institute: http://beerinst.org/home.htm

The Wine Institute: http://wineinstitute.org/

Distilled Spirits Council: http://www.discus.health.org/

McKim's Blood Alcohol Calculator: http://dogsbody.psych.mun.ca/tools/BAL/

National Institute on Alcohol Abuse and Alcoholism: http://www.niaaa.nih.gov/

And our own site: http://www.uwyo.edu/a&s/psyc/dshb.htm

REFERENCES

1. Shaken and stirred: the state of the liquor industry, *Washington Post*, November 12, 1996.
2. Data courtesy of Beer Marketer's Insights, 1997, West Nyack, NY.
3. Williams GD and others: *NIAAA Surveillance Report #39: Apparent per capita alcohol consumption*, Bethesda, MD, USPHS, 1996.
4. Suter PM and others: The effect of ethanol on fat storage in healthy subjects, *New Engl J Med* 326:983, 1992.
5. Frezza M and others: High blood alcohol levels in women: the role of decreased gastric alcohol dehydrogenase activity and first-pass metabolism, *New Engl J Med* 322:95, 1990.
6. NIAAA: *Alcohol Alert*, Bethesda, MD, USPHS, January, 1997

7. Gibbons B: Alcohol, the legal drug, *National Geographic*, February, 1992.

8. *Eighth Special Report to the U.S. Congress on Alcohol and Health*, Bethesda, MD, USPHS, 1993.

9. Goldberg L: Quantitative studies on alcohol tolerance in man, *Acta Physiol Scand Suppl* 5(16): 1–128, 1943.

10. Bogen E: The human toxicology of alcohol. In Emerson H, editor: *Alcohol and man*, New York, 1932, Macmillan.

11. Crothers TD: Alcoholic trance, *Popular Science* 26:189, 191, 1884.

12. Shakespeare W: *Macbeth*, Act II, Scene 1.

13. Wilson GT, Lawson DM: Effects of alcohol on sexual arousal in women, *J Abnorm Psychol* 85(5):489–497, 1976.

14. Briddell DW, Wilson GT: Effects of alcohol and expectancy set on male sexual arousal, *J Abnorm Psychol* 85(2):225–234, 1976.

15. Twain M: *The adventures of Huckleberry Finn*, 1885.

16. Mayo-Smith ME: Pharmacological management of alcohol withdrawal: a meta-analysis and evidence-based practice guideline, *JAMA*, 278:144–151, 1997.

17. Brody J: Personal health, New York Times, December 27, 1976, p C13.

18. Chapman LF: Experimental induction of hangover, *Quarterly Studies on Alcohol* (Suppl 5), March 10, 1970, pp 67–86.

19. DeLabry LO and others: Alcohol consumption and mortality in an American male population: recovering the u-shaped curve—findings from the normative aging study, *J Stud Alcohol* 53:25–32, 1992.

20. Alcohol and the heart: consensus emerges, *Harvard Health Letter* 6(5), January, 1996.

21. Jones KL and others: Pattern of malformation in offspring of chronic alcoholic mothers, *Lancet* 1(7815): 1267–1271, 1973.

22. Stromland K, Hellstrom A: Fetal alcohol syndrome: an opthalmological and socioeducational prospective study, *Pediatrics* 97:845–850, 1996.

Alcohol and Society

KEY TERMS	OBJECTIVES

After reading this chapter, you should be able to:

temperance
Prohibition
expectancies
alcoholism
balanced placebo
genetic marker
Antabuse
controlled drinking
abstinence

- Discuss the history of alcohol use and its regulation in the United States.
- Understand the impact of alcohol Prohibition during the 1920s and the reasons for the repeal of Prohibition.
- Describe some cultural and regional influences on drinking patterns.
- Describe some of the important social problems related to alcohol use.

- Discuss the factors that go into describing an individual as an alcoholic.
- Discuss the issue of genetic determinants for alcoholism.
- Describe traditional alcoholism treatment approaches and how they are changing.

ALCOHOL USE AND "THE ALCOHOL PROBLEM"

Historians seem to agree that at the time of America's revolution against the English in the late 1700s, most Americans drank alcoholic beverages and most people valued these beverages compared to drinking water, which was often contaminated. The per capita consumption of alcohol was apparently much greater than current levels, and little public concern was expressed. Even the early Puritan ministers, who were quite moralistic about all kinds of behavior, referred to alcoholic drink as "the Good Creature of God." They denounced drunkenness as a sinful misuse of the "Good Creature," but the blame was clearly placed on the sinner, not on alcohol itself.[1]

Because American colonial history and American law evolved from English law, it is worth noting that England had tried to control drunkenness as early as 1327 by limiting the number of establishments that could sell alcoholic beverages. Drunkenness apparently continued, and this first law was repealed. Other regulations were passed over the years, but none of them attacked alcohol per se, nor did they attempt to prevent "normal," moderate use of alcoholic beverages.

A new view of alcohol as the *cause* of serious problems began to emerge in America soon after the Revolution. That view took root and still exists as a major influence in American culture today. It is so pervasive that some people have a hard time understanding what we mean by what has been called the "demonization" of alcohol (viewing alcohol as a demon, or devil). The concept is important, partly because alcohol was the first psychoactive substance to become "demonized" in American culture, leading the way for similar views of cocaine, heroin, and marijuana in this century. What we are referring to is a tendency to view a substance as an *active* (sometimes almost purposeful) source of *evil*, damaging everything it touches. Whenever harmful consequences result from the use of something (firearms and nuclear energy are other possible examples), there are those who find it easiest to simply view that thing as "bad" and avoid all contact with it. Such a view of alcohol might be personally convenient for an alcoholic if it helps him or her to stay sober, but it is too simple an explanation for the social scientist or policy maker who needs to understand the complex interplay between alcohol and human society. The danger is that alcohol (or marijuana, cocaine, or heroin) can become a scapegoat, thus causing us to ignore all the other factors contributing to whatever problem we might be concerned about. Later in this chapter we examine this social interplay in more detail. For now, let's ask how this "new" idea about alcohol as a demon developed about two hundred years ago.

The Temperance Movement in America

The first writings indicating a negative view of alcohol itself are attributed to a prominent Philadelphia physician named Benjamin Rush, one of the signers of the Declaration of Independence. Rush's 1784 pamphlet, "An Inquiry into the Effects of Ardent Spirits on the Mind and Body," was aimed particularly at distilled spirits (*ardent* means "burning or fiery"), not at

the weaker beverages such as beer and wine. As a physician, Rush had noticed a relationship between heavy drinking and jaundice (an indicator of liver disease), "madness" (perhaps the delirium tremens of withdrawal, perhaps what we now call Korsakoff's psychosis), and "epilepsy" (probably the seizures seen during withdrawal). All of those are currently accepted and well-documented consequences of heavy alcohol use and were reviewed in chapter 10. However, Rush also concluded that hard liquor damaged the drinker's morality, leading to a variety of antisocial, immoral, and criminal behaviors. Although the correlation between these types of behavior and alcohol use has been documented many times, Rush believed that this was a direct toxic action of distilled spirits on the part of the brain responsible for morality. Rush then introduced for the first time the concept of *addiction* to a psychoactive substance, describing the uncontrollable and overwhelming desires for alcohol experienced by some of his patients. For the first time this condition was referred to as a *disease* (caused by alcohol), and he recommended total abstinence from alcohol for those who were addicted.[1]

Other physicians readily recognized these symptoms in their own patients, and physicians became the first leaders of the **temperance** movement. What Rush proposed, and most early followers supported, was that everyone should avoid distilled spirits entirely, because they were considered to be toxic, and consume beer and wine in a *temperate*, or moderate, manner. Temperance societies were formed in many parts of the country, at first among the upper classes of physicians, ministers, and

---

temperance: (*temp* a rance) the idea that people should drink beer or wine in moderation, but drink no hard liquor.

Carrie Nation became a symbol of the temperance movement with her
"hachetations," which also led to her being arrested more than 30 times.

businessmen. In the early 1800s it became possible, and fashionable, for the middle classes to join the elite in this movement, and hundreds of thousands of American businessmen, farmers, lawyers, teachers, and their wives and daughters "took the pledge" to avoid spirits and to be temperate in their use of beer or wine.

In the second half of the nineteenth century things changed. Up to this time there had been little consumption of commercial beer in the United States. It was only with the advent of artificial refrigeration and the addition of hops, which helped to preserve the beer, that there was an increase in the number of breweries. The waves of immigrants who entered the country in this period provided the necessary beer-drinking consumers. At first, encouraged by temperance groups who preferred beer consumption to the use of liquor, breweries were constructed everywhere. However, alcohol-related problems did not disappear. Instead, disruptive, drunken behavior became increasingly associated in the public's mind with the new wave of immigrants: Irish, Italians, and eastern Europeans, more often Catholic than Protestant, and they drank beer and wine. Temperance workers now advocated total abstinence from all alcoholic beverages, and pressure grew to prohibit the sale of alcohol altogether.

Prohibition

The first state **prohibition** period began in 1851 when Maine passed its prohibition law. Between 1851 and 1855, thirteen states passed statewide prohibition laws, but by 1868 nine had repealed them. The National Prohibition Party, organized in 1874, provided the impetus for the second wave of statewide prohibition that developed in the 1880s. From 1880 to 1889 seven states adopted prohibition laws, but by 1896 four had repealed them.

In 1899 a group of educators, lawyers, and clergymen described the saloon as the "working-man's club, in which many of his leisure hours are spent, and in which he finds more of the things that approximate luxury than in his home. . . ." They went on to say: "It is a centre of learning, books, papers, and lecture hall to them. It is the clearinghouse for common intelligence, the place where their philosophy of life is worked out, and their political and social beliefs take their beginnings."[2]

Truth lay somewhere between those statements and the sentiments expressed in a sermon:

> The liquor traffic is the most fiendish, corrupt and hell-soaked institution that ever crawled out of the slime of the eternal pit. It is the open sore of this land. . . . It takes the kind, loving husband and father, smothers every spark of love in his bosom, and transforms him into a heartless wretch, and makes him steal the shoes from his starving babe's feet to find the price for a glass of liquor. It takes your sweet innocent daughter, robs her of her virtue and transforms her into a brazen, wanton harlot. . . .
>
> The open saloon as an institution has its origin in hell, and it is manufacturing subjects to be sent back to hell.[3]

Prohibition was not just a matter of "wets" versus "drys," or a matter of political conviction or health concerns. Intricately interwoven with these factors was a middle-class, rural, Protestant, evangelical concern that the good and true life was being undermined by ethnic groups with a different religion and a lower standard of living and morality. One way to strike back at these groups was through prohibition.

Between 1907 and 1919, thirty-four states enacted legislation enforcing statewide prohibition, whereas only two states repealed their prohibition laws. By 1917, 64 percent of the population lived in dry territory, and between 1908 and 1917 over 100,000 licensed bars were closed.

It should also be remembered that the fact that there was a state prohibition law did not mean that the residents did not drink. They did, both legally and illegally. They drank illegally in speakeasies and other private clubs. They drank legally from a variety of the many patent medicines that were freely available. A few of the more interesting ones were Whisko, "a nonintoxicating stimulant" at 55 proof; Golden's Liquid Beef Tonic, "recommended for treatment of alcohol habit" with 53 proof; and Kaufman's Sulfur Bitters, which "contains no alcohol" but was in fact 20 percent alcohol (40 proof) and contained no sulfur!

In August 1917 the U.S. Senate adopted a resolution, authored by Andrew Volstead, that submitted the national prohibition amendment to the states. The U.S. House of Representatives concurred in December, and 21 days later, on January 8, 1918, Mississippi became the first state to ratify the Eighteenth Amendment. A year later, January 16, 1919, Nebraska was the thirty-sixth state to ratify the amendment, and the deed was done!

As stated in the amendment, a year after the thirty-sixth state ratified it, national prohibition came into effect: on January 16, 1920. The amendment was simple, with only two operational parts:

> Section 1. After one year from the ratification of this article the manufacture, sale or transportation of intoxicating liquors within, the importation thereof into, or the exportation thereof from the United States and all territory subject to the jurisdiction thereof for beverage purposes is hereby prohibited.

Prohibition: laws prohibiting all sales of alcoholic beverages in the United States in the period 1920–1933.

Section 2. The Congress and the several States shall have concurrent power to enforce this article by appropriate legislation.

The beginning of Prohibition was hailed in a radio sermon by the popular preacher Billy Sunday:

The reign of tears is over. The slums will soon be a memory. We will turn our prisons into factories and our jails into storehouses and corncribs. Men will walk upright now, women will smile, and the children will laugh. Hell will be forever for rent.[1]

The law did not result in an alcohol-free society, and this came as quite a surprise to many people. Apparently the assumption was that Prohibition would be so widely accepted that little enforcement would be necessary. Along with saloons, breweries, and distilleries, hospitals that had specialized in the treatment of alcoholics closed their doors, presumably because there would no longer be a need for them.[4]

It soon became clear that people were buying and selling alcohol illegally and that enforcement of Prohibition was not going to be easy. The majority of the population might have supported the idea of Prohibition, but such a large minority insisted on continuing to drink that *speakeasies*, *hip flasks*, and *bathtub gin* became household words. Organized crime became both more organized and vastly more profitable as a result of Prohibition.

The popular conception is that Prohibition was a total failure, leading to its repeal. That is not the whole picture. Prohibition did have the apparent effect of reducing overall alcohol intake. Hospital admissions for alcoholism and deaths from alcoholism declined sharply at the beginning of Prohibition. During the decade of the 1920s it appears that the Prohibition laws were increasingly violated, particularly in large eastern cities like New York, and the rates of alcoholism and alcohol-related deaths began to increase.[5] But even toward the end of the "noble experiment," as Prohibition was called by its detractors, alcoholism and alcohol-related deaths were still lower than before Prohibition.

If Prohibition did reduce alcohol-related problems, why was it repealed? In 1926 the Association Against Prohibition was founded by a small group of America's wealthiest men, including the heads of many of the largest corporations in America. Their primary concern seems to have been the income taxes they were paying. Historically, taxes on alcohol had been one of the primary sources of revenue for the federal government. Indeed, the federal government relied heavily on alcohol taxes before the income tax was initiated in 1913. A major hope of the repeal supporters was that income taxes could be reduced. There was also fear that the widespread and highly publicized disrespect for the Prohibition law encouraged a sense of "lawlessness," not just among the bootleggers and gangsters but in the public at large. The Depression, which began in 1929, not only made more people consider the value of tax revenues but also increased fears of a generalized revolt. If Prohibition weakened respect for law and order, it had to go.[1]

The Eighteenth Amendment was repealed by the Twenty-First Amendment proposed in Congress on February 20, 1933, and ratified by thirty-six states by December 5 of that year. So ended an era. The Twenty-First Amendment was also short and sweet:

Section 1. The eighteenth article of amendment of the Constitution of the United States is hereby repealed.
Section 2. The transportation or importation into any State, Territory, or possession of the United States for delivery or use therein of intoxicating liquors, in violation of the laws thereof, is hereby prohibited.

When national Prohibition ended, America did not return overnight to the pre-1920s levels of alcohol consumption. Sales increased until after World War II, at which point per capita consumption was approximately what it had been before Prohibition. Thus prohibition of alcohol, much like the current prohibitions of marijuana and heroin, did work in that it reduced alcohol availability, use, and related problems. On the other hand, even at its best it did not allow us to close all the jails and mental hospitals, and it encouraged organized crime and created expensive enforcement efforts.

Regulation after 1933

After national Prohibition, control over alcohol was returned to the states. Each state has since had its own means of regulating alcohol. Although a few states remained totally "dry" after national Prohibition, most allowed at least beer sales. Thus the temperance sentiment that beer was a safer beverage continued to influence policy. In many cases, beer containing no more than 3.2 percent alcohol by weight was allowed as a "nonintoxicating" beverage. Even states that remained dry, like Kansas and Oklahoma, allowed 3.2 percent beer. As we saw in chapter 10, alcohol is alcohol, and 3.2 percent beer *is* intoxicating.

Over the years the general trend was for a relaxation of laws: states that did not allow sales of liquor became fewer until in 1966 the last dry state, Mississippi, became wet. The minimum age to purchase alcoholic beverages was set at 21 in all states except New York and Louisiana before 1970, when the national voting age was lowered to 18. During the 1970s, thirty states lowered the drinking age to 18 or 19. Per capita consumption rates, which were relatively stable during the 1950s, increased steadily from 1965 through 1980. However, times have changed; pushed by concerns over young people dying in alcohol-related traffic accidents, in the 1980s Congress authorized the Transportation Department to withhold a portion of the federal highway funds for any state that did not raise its minimum drinking age to 21. In 1988 the final state raised its drinking age, making 21 the uniform drinking age all across the United States.

UP FOR DEBATE   Advertising Alcohol

After Prohibition, purveyors of distilled spirits did not advertise on radio, and later, on television. This was a voluntary ban by the radio and television and liquor industries. Seagram was the first liquor manufacturer to break the voluntary ban in 1996, and other companies followed suit. The ads are shown on local TV stations in several large cities, but the big networks have not accepted them.

Rep. Joseph Kennedy has introduced a bill to force the Federal Communications Commission to begin a formal inquiry into TV liquor ads.

Involved are the constitutional issues of freedom of speech (limited in the area of "commercial" speech, and further limited by FCC licensing of broadcasters), as well as the practical issues: Would lifting the ban increase alcohol use or not? What would the economic effects be on broadcasters, print media, and liquor producers?

Taxation

Federal taxes on alcoholic beverages are a significant means of gathering money for the federal government. Although most of the federal revenue comes from individual income taxes, taxes on alcohol produce about 1 percent of the total collections by the Internal Revenue Service ($7.6 billion in 1994). The states also collect over $3 billion each year in excise taxes and license fees for alcoholic beverages. When all these are added up, over half the consumer's cost for an average bottle of distilled spirits is taxes. In 1991, after hearing arguments that taxes on alcoholic beverages had not kept up with inflation, Congress initiated a significant tax increase: the beer tax doubled to $18 per barrel, the tax on bottled wine increased sixfold to about 22 cents per bottle, and the tax on distilled spirits rose less than 10 percent to $13.50 per gallon of 100-proof liquor.[6] There was some controversy about how much such an increase would affect sales, especially because at the same time most producers increased their own prices by about 5 percent. The total increase in cost to the consumer (averaging about 10 percent more) did result in about a 2 percent decrease in sales of beer and liquor during the first half of the year. Domestic wine sales decreased even more, almost 9 percent. That such large price increases resulted in fairly modest declines in purchases might indicate that very large tax increases would be needed if part of the goal is to reduce alcohol intake significantly.

problems relating to culture

WHO DRINKS? AND WHY?

Cultural Influences on Drinking

Comparing alcohol use in various cultures around the world gives us a chance to look at ethnic and social factors that lead to differences in patterns of alcohol use. For example, both the Irish and the Russian cultures are associated with heavy drinking, especially of distilled spirits. This has been attributed to several factors, including early invasions by the hard-drinking Vikings at a time when each of these regions was beginning to develop a national identity. Also, both regions experienced frequent famine, and they were not exposed to the notion of individual potential that characterized the Renaissance or to the notions of individual responsibility and sobriety that came with the Protestant Reformation.[7] Americans of Irish descent have been studied and found to have higher rates of alcohol-related problems than other ethnic groups. A comparison of Irish-Americans with Italian-Americans is of interest: the Irish forbid children and adolescents from learning to drink, but they seem to expect adult men to drink large quantities. They value hard liquor more than beer and promote drinking in pubs, away from family influences. By contrast, Italian families give their children wine from an early age in a family setting but disapprove of intoxication at any age.[8]

The French drink primarily wine and consume it in the family setting and with meals, so it might be expected that they would not have many heavy drinkers or drinking-related problems. Unfortunately, the French consume more alcohol per capita than any other nation and also have the highest rates of alcoholism, suicide, and deaths from cirrhosis of the liver.[9] The French associate wine drinking with virility, and French working men have traditionally consumed large amounts of wine during the work day (it was not unusual for a French laborer to consume a liter of wine with lunch). The French government has had campaigns to promote responsible drinking of wine and the drinking of alternative beverages. That, combined with a greater tendency to stay home and watch television instead of going to a bistro in the evenings, has led to a decrease in wine consumption, but it is still high relative to other countries.

Regional Differences in the United States

In the United States it has been true for many years that about one-third of the adult population label themselves as abstainers. The two-thirds who use alcohol consume an amount that averages out to about three drinks per day. Most of us don't drink anything near that amount—in fact, another consistent finding is that half the alcohol is consumed by about 10 percent of the drinkers.

Whites are more likely to drink than blacks, Northerners more than Southerners, younger adults more likely than older, Catholics and Jews more than Protestants, nonreligious more than religious, urban more than rural, large-city dwellers more than small-city residents, and college-educated people more than those with only a high school or grade school education.

Figure 11.1 shows estimated overall alcohol consumption combining beer, wine, and distilled spirits (about half the total U.S. alcohol consumption comes from beer) for each state, based on sales.[10] Nevada and New Hampshire have the highest per capita sales, followed by the District of Columbia. The District of Columbia is the leader in consumption of wine, whereas Nevada consumes the most beer. Note the generally low consumption in the southern states and the generally higher consumption in the western states, with the notable exception of Utah, which has a large Mormon population. These differences in per capita sales reflect differences in the proportion of drinkers in various parts of the country. If the sales figures are divided by the estimated number of drinkers rather than by the total population, it appears that southern drinkers might consume at higher levels than northern drinkers.[11]

One theory about heavy drinking proposes that those populations of people who experience a great deal of social stress and tension (as in

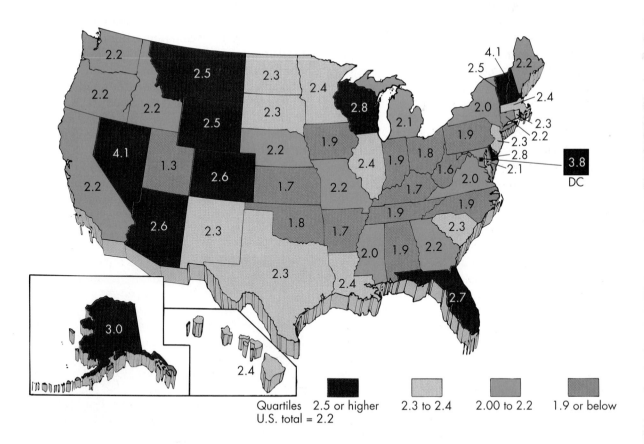

Quartiles   2.5 or higher   2.3 to 2.4   2.00 to 2.2   1.9 or below
U.S. total = 2.2

Figure 11.1 Total estimated U.S. per capita consumption of beer, wine, and distilled spirits, by state, 1994, based on sales

cities) and approve of the use of alcohol to release tension and relieve stress will drink more and have more drinking problems. One study compared the various states with regard to such stress indicators as business failures, unemployment, divorces, abortions, disasters, percentage of new residents, and high school dropout rates. On the overall state stress index, Nevada and Alaska scored the highest, Iowa and Nebraska the lowest. Alcohol norms were rated based on the percentage of fundamentalist or Mormon church members, the percentage of dry areas in the state, the number of liquor outlets per capita, and the number of hours per week allowed for drinking in bars. On this scale Mississippi and Utah were the most restricted, Nevada and Wisconsin the least. Overall, both the stress index and the drinking norms were significantly correlated with indicators of heavy drinking and alcohol-related arrests.[12]

Gender Differences

Looking at individual people, efforts to relate personality factors to drinking have not been terribly enlightening. Recently people have been studying the learned **expectancies** each of us has about what alcohol is for and what it does. We learn much of what we expect alcohol to do even before we take our first drink, from books, movies, and other people. One study reported that men who have strong expectations that alcohol will lead to increased social and physical pleasure and to sexual enhancement are most likely to drink heavily, whereas among women the heaviest drinkers are those who believe that alcohol will reduce tension.[13] You can see how these different expectancies might lead to different types of drinking in different situations, thus complicating attempts to predict simply who drinks and how much. Combining those differences in beliefs about alcohol with a greater pharmacological effect of alcohol on the average woman, as reviewed in chapter 10, means that men and women differ with re-

spect to predictions of problem drinking and alcoholism.

Drinking among College Students

The college years have traditionally been associated with alcohol use, and in 1994 the proportion of "drinkers" was indeed about 10 percent higher among 18- to 22-year-old college students than among the general population of that age (e.g., about 70 percent of college students reported drinking within the past month, compared with about 61 percent of all 18- to 25-year-olds in the NIDA household survey described in chapter 1).[14] Colleges and universities have followed the lead established by the federal government's mandating a uniform 21-year-old drinking age, and many campuses have banned the sale or advertising of alcohol. Many fraternities have banned keg parties and the use of alcohol during "rush," partly out of concern for legal liability for the consequences if a guest becomes intoxicated and has an accident. In spite of the changes in laws and rules, drinking behavior itself has not changed much in the past few years. In fact, there is some evidence that among college drinkers, there might be a slightly increased incidence of some alcohol-related

Drinking, especially of beer, sometimes begins at a young age.

problems such as fighting, vandalism, poor grades, getting into trouble with the police, and missing class because of hangovers.[15] These adverse consequences might result from more students drinking off campus in less controlled and less friendly environments. One ray of hope is that today's college students are less likely than those of the early 1980s to drive after drinking.

"Time-Out" and Alcohol "Myopia"

It has been pointed out that many of the effects experienced by drinkers are based on what they expect to happen, which interacts somewhat with the pharmacological effects of alcohol. One important component of alcohol use is that drinking serves as a social signal, to the drinker and others, indicating a "time-out" from responsibilities, work, and seriousness. Sitting down with a drink indicates "I'm off duty now" and "Don't take anything I may say too seriously." Steele and Josephs have proposed[16] that alcohol serves to induce a kind of social and behavioral "myopia," or nearsightedness. After drinking, people tend to focus more on the here and now and to pay less attention to long-term consequences. That might be why some people are more violent after drinking, whereas others become more helpful to others even if there is some possible personal risk or cost involved. The idea is that alcohol releases people from their inhibitions, largely because the inhibitions represent concerns about what might happen, whereas the intoxicated individual focuses on the immediate irritant or the person who needs help right now.

SOCIAL PROBLEMS

Driving under the Influence

Attention was focused in the early 1980s on the large number of traffic fatalities involving alcohol. The total number of traffic fatalities in 1980 was over 50,000, but by 1983 that had dropped to nearer 40,000, where it has remained

since.[17] It is difficult to estimate exactly how many of those fatalities are *caused* by alcohol, but we can obtain some relevant information. Many states mandate that the coroner measure blood alcohol in all fatally injured drivers. Based on those measurements, estimates have been made of the number of alcohol-related traffic crash fatalities. Figure 11.2 shows the downward trend in the percentage of all traffic fatalities that are alcohol related. From the peak of over 42 percent in 1982, by 1994 the percentage had declined to under 34 percent.[18]

Several studies have demonstrated that the danger of combining alcohol with automobiles is dose related. At a BAC of 0.08 percent the relative risk of being involved in a fatal crash is about three times as great as for a sober driver, and about fifteen times as great at 0.12 percent. (Note how close these figures are to the commonly used value for legal intoxication of 0.10 percent.) Similarly, the risk of involvement in a personal injury crash increases with BAC, as does the risk of involvement in a fatal pedestrian accident. As with other dose-response curves, these data provide strong evidence that the relationship between drinking and accidents is causal and not merely related to the lifestyles of individuals who drink.

Some other interesting facts have emerged from studies of alcohol and accidents. Alcohol-related traffic fatalities are not a random sample of all fatalities. Single-vehicle fatalities are more likely to involve alcohol than are multiple-vehicle fatalities in which the fatally injured person was driving the striking vehicle. The probability of alcohol involvement is lower if the fatally injured individual was driving a vehicle that was struck by another driver. Alcohol-related fatalities are a greater proportion of the

---

expectancies: learned beliefs about the effects of alcohol or another drug.

Figure 11.2 Percentage of traffic fatalities that were alcohol related

fatalities occurring during dark hours than of those occurring in daylight and are a greater proportion of fatalities occurring on the weekend than of those occurring during the week. In fact, if someone is killed in a struck vehicle during daylight hours on Monday through Thursday, the odds are less than 1 in 10 that the victim was impaired by alcohol. The odds are more like 9 in 10 for a single-vehicle accident occurring in the early morning hours on a weekend.[19]

When you hear that about 85 percent of all the fatally injured drivers who had been drinking were male, that sounds like a big difference, and it is. But it is important to remember that 75 percent of all fatally injured drivers are male, whether or not drinking is involved. That men are more likely to be involved in alcohol-related traffic fatalities reflects three important facts:

Any given car is more likely to have a male than a female driver, men might take more chances when driving even when they're sober, and male drivers are more likely than female drivers to have been drinking.

Who is responsible for all these alcohol-related traffic accidents? One question is whether there are certain individuals, such as problem drinkers, responsible for much of the drunk driving. In one study of drivers involved in fatal crashes who had BACs of 0.10 percent or more, 11 percent had previous convictions for driving under the influence (DUI).[19] Problem drinkers, although a relatively small fraction of the drinking population, are more likely on a given day to be driving around with a high BAC. On the other hand, almost 90 percent of those intoxicated drivers involved in fatal crashes had never been convicted of DUI in the past. There-

FYI | Alcohol and Violence

One of the interesting things about alcohol's involvement in accidents or violence is that it is so common it is not newsworthy. For example, a local newspaper article reported an incident that occurred in the wee hours of a Saturday morning in which one man stabbed another over a piece of leftover meatloaf. The article didn't mention alcohol involvement, but it seemed so likely that someone was drunk that the example was used in class. One of the class members happened to be a sheriff's deputy and was able to get a copy of the arrest report. Sure enough, both men had high BACs (one was over 0.20%).

Such incidents are more common than you might think. Another example was a man in Los Angeles who was being taunted by bystanders because he was having trouble parking his car in front of a nightclub. He proceeded to shoot one of the taunters. The news account didn't mention that he was drunk, but what do you think?

Check the Saturday and Sunday morning newspapers for two or three weeks and see how many reports you can find for which it seems likely that alcohol was involved. Does the news article state or imply that drinking was involved or avoid the issue entirely?

fore, whereas individual problem drinkers cause more than their share of traffic accidents, the majority of alcohol-related traffic accidents are caused by individuals who have not been identified as problem drinkers. Anyone who drinks and drives is a potential threat.

Younger drivers have more than their share of alcohol-related accidents. In 1994, persons aged 16 to 24 made up 14 percent of the U.S. population yet were involved in 28 percent of the alcohol-related traffic accidents.[18]

What can be done about this problem? Current efforts focus mainly on three fronts: identifying repeat offenders and keeping them off the roads, publicizing in the mass media the dangers of drinking and driving, and targeting younger drinkers for special prevention efforts. Although it is impossible to determine the effectiveness of any one of these measures, figure 11.2 indicates that the total effort has worked to reduce alcohol-related fatalities.

Crime and Violence

Homicide

The correlation between alcohol use and homicides is well known to police and judicial systems all around the world. Based on several studies of police and court records, the proportion of murderers who had been drinking before the crime ranged from 36 percent in Baltimore to 70 percent in Sweden.[20] It is also interesting that across all these studies, about 50 percent of the murder victims had been drinking. These data certainly imply that homicide is more likely to occur in situations in which drinking also occurs, but they leave open the question as to whether alcohol plays a causal role in homicides.

Assault and other crimes of violence

As with homicide, studies of assault, spousal abuse, and child abuse all reveal correlations with drinking: heavier drinkers are more likely to engage in such behaviors, and self-reports by offenders indicate a high likelihood that they had been consuming alcohol before the violent act.[21] However, scientists are still cautious in trying to determine how much of a causal role alcohol plays in such activity. For example, if fights are likely to occur when men get together in groups at night and drinking is also likely to occur when men get together in groups at night, how much of a role does alcohol itself play in increasing the chances of violence? Similarly, if both heavy drinking and violent arguments are characteristics of dysfunctional family situations, how much of the ensuing family violence can be "blamed" on the use of alcohol? Unfortunately, it has proven difficult to perform controlled experimental studies on these complex problems, and so the answers remain unclear.[22]

Suicide

Most studies show that alcohol is involved in about one-third of all suicides. Suicide attempts seem to have a different background than actual suicides, but alcoholism is second only to depression as the diagnosis in suicide attempters. The relationship between alcoholism and depression is a strong one and has been the subject of many studies. One interesting finding is that people who were alcoholics first and probably became depressed as a result of their repeated failures and shortcomings have a better prognosis than those who showed clear signs of clinical depression before they became alcoholics.[21]

WHO IS AN ALCOHOLIC?

Defining **alcoholism** is not an easy thing to do. The term has different meanings to different authorities, so picking any one of them gets you into a discussion right away. How one defines alcoholism has important implications for the approaches that are taken in treatment, the treatment goals, and how one measures success. Our immediate concern is how many and what types of people will be included in the group defined as alcoholics.

When we see a man who drinks to the point of drunkenness every day, who has lost his job and family, who has a damaged liver, and who will suffer from delirium tremens if he doesn't drink for a day, then everyone can agree that we have an alcoholic. Some definitions have focused on the *physiological* aspects of this model alcoholic and define alcoholism on the basis of

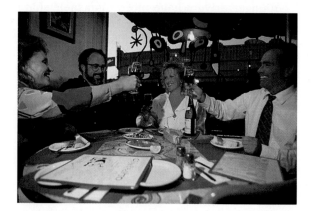

The street wino fits our idea of an alcoholic, but most alcoholics are not so easy to spot.

obvious liver or brain damage, tolerance, or withdrawal symptoms. Other definitions have focused on the *psychosocial* aspects, using criteria such as daily use or interference with personal, social, or occupational behavior. The problem arises when we leave the stereotypical, model alcoholic and start looking at ourselves and our friends and neighbors. There are lots of people who do not have obvious symptoms of liver or brain damage and who don't get the "shakes" if they don't drink on a given day but who drink regularly, depend on drinking at least as an important aspect of their individual and social lives, and who suffer some level of interference with their personal, social, or occupational life. In fact, it is probably true that almost anyone who drinks at all will occasionally drink too much and have a hangover at work, be embarrassed socially, or fail to accomplish some personal goal on that day. How do we decide when such a person becomes an alcoholic? As far as this text is concerned, we don't think it is possible to develop a universal decision rule. The term has too many meanings to too many people for us to be at all specific in our definition and still do justice to this important topic. What we will do is describe several of the ways in which this issue has been addressed.

Probably the most significant influence on American attitudes about alcoholism was a fifty-year-old book called *Alcoholics Anonymous*. This book described the experiences of a small group of people who formed a society whose "only requirement for membership is a desire to stop drinking." That society has now grown to include more than 1.5 million members in over a hundred countries. A central part of their belief system is that alcoholism is a progressive disease characterized by a loss of control over drinking and that alcoholism can never be cured. People who do not have the disease might drink and even become intoxicated, but they do not "lose control over alcohol." There is a suspicion that the alcoholic might be different even before the first drink is taken. The only

treatment is to arrest the disease by abstaining from drinking. This *disease model* of alcoholism has received support from many medical practitioners and has been endorsed by the American Medical Association and other professional groups. In one sense, this description of alcoholism as a disease is a reaction against long-held notions that excessive drinking is only a symptom of some other underlying pathology such as depression or some type of personality defect. Traditional psychoanalysts practicing many years ago might have treated the alcoholic by trying to discover the unconscious conflicts or personality deficiencies that caused the person to drink. One important consequence of defining alcoholism as a *primary* disease is to recognize that the drinking itself could be the problem and that treatment and prevention should be aimed directly at alcoholism.

However, there are many scientific critics of the disease concept. If alcoholism is a disease, what is its cause? How are "alcoholics" different from "nonalcoholics," except that they tend to drink a lot and have many alcohol-related problems? Let's accept for the purpose of discussion that those who go into hospitals or treatment programs with a primary diagnosis of alcoholism are alcoholics. What are their characteristics? Although sequential stages have been described for this "progressive disease," most individual alcoholics don't seem to fit any single set of descriptors. Some don't drink alone, some don't drink in the morning, some don't go on binges, some don't drink every day, and some don't report strong cravings for alcohol. Experiments have shown that alcoholics do retain considerable control over their drinking, even while drinking—it's not that they completely lose control when they start drinking, but they might

---

alcoholism: a term for alcohol dependence or addiction.

have either less ability or less desire to limit their drinking because they do drink excessively. Although an "alcoholic personality" has been defined that characterizes many alcoholics who enter treatment, the current belief is that these personality factors (impulsive, anxious, depressed, passive, dependent) reflect the years of intoxication and the critical events that led to the decision to enter treatment rather than being preexisting abnormalities that caused the alcoholism.

The American Psychiatric Association's *Diagnostic and Statistical Manual of Mental Disorders*, fourth edition (*DSM-IV*, 1994)[23] is probably the closest thing we have to a single official, widely accepted set of labels for behavior disorders, including substance abuse and dependence (see chapter 3). The *DSM-IV* does not separately define these for alcohol but includes alcohol as one of the psychoactive substances. This manual implies, but does not directly state, that the term *alcoholism* may refer either to alcohol abuse, which is defined in psychosocial terms (a maladaptive pattern of use indicated by either continued use despite knowledge of having persistent problems caused by alcohol), or alcohol dependence, which involves more serious psychosocial characteristics and includes the physiological factors of tolerance and withdrawal among the possible symptoms.

In 1989 it may have appeared that the U.S. Supreme Court had finally decided the issue of whether alcoholism is or is not a disease. Two veterans of the armed services had filed for educational benefits after the ten-year eligibility period after their service had elapsed. The Veterans Administration denied their benefits, even though extensions of the eligibility period can be granted if the individual was delayed in education by physical or mental disorders "not the result of their own willful misconduct." These individuals argued that they were alcoholics and that because alcoholism is a disease over which they had no control, they should be allowed the extension. Newspapers, magazines,

and television commentators widely touted the case as deciding once and for all whether alcoholism is "truly" a disease or whether it should be considered more akin to misbehavior (willful misconduct).[24] On one side were legions of treatment professionals and alcoholics (or exalcoholics, if there can be such a thing) who believe very strongly in the disease model on which most programs of treatment and recovery are based. On the other side were a smaller number of professionals and academics who argued that we have gone too far in the "medicalization" of alcohol, with every wife-beater and criminal claiming the illness and being sent off for treatment. They argued that people must be held accountable for their behavior and misbehavior regarding alcohol. The Supreme Court ruled in favor of the Veterans Administration, but we cannot conclude from that that alcoholism is not "truly" a disease. We should recognize by now that alcoholism is one of those complex concepts that means different things to different people in different contexts, not something that can be defined perfectly and absolutely. "Disease" is the same kind of concept. We could pick an official definition of alcoholism, which we should recognize as being somewhat arbitrary, and an official definition of disease, similarly somewhat arbitrary, and then match them up to see if alcoholism is "truly" a disease. A more sensible conclusion would be that there are probably contexts in which it makes sense to think of alcoholism as a disease, other contexts in which it probably does not make sense to think that way, and perhaps many contexts in which it is not at all clear.

Factors Predisposing to Alcoholism

Why are some people able to drink in moderation all their lives, whereas others repeatedly become intoxicated, suffer from alcohol-related problems, and continue to drink excessively? So far, no single factor and no combination of multiple factors has been presented that allows us to predict which individuals will become alcoholics. Multiple theories exist, including biochemical, psychoanalytic, and cultural approaches. At this period of scientific history, probably the most attention is being focused on understanding two types of factors: cognitive and genetic. The importance of cognitive factors with regard to alcohol's effects is perhaps best demonstrated by a series of experiments conducted by Marlatt and his colleagues on "loss of control" in alcoholics and social drinkers.[25] The experimental subjects are given drinks that either do or do not contain alcohol, and half of each group are told that the drinks do contain alcohol, whereas the other half of each group are told that the drinks do not have alcohol in them (this is referred to as a **balanced placebo** design). Of course, there's a limit to how much alcohol you can give a person before they will be able to detect it with no doubt, but the most interesting results from these studies are when people have not actually had any alcohol but believe that they have. Both alcoholics and social drinkers report more intoxication and consume more drinks when they are told the drinks have alcohol, regardless of the actual alcohol content. It is important that alcoholics actually given small amounts of alcohol (equivalent to one or two drinks) did not report becoming intoxicated and did not increase their drinking if they were led to expect that the drink contained no alcohol. Therefore, it would seem that if alcoholics do lose control when they begin drinking, it might be because they have come to *believe* that they will lose control if they drink (this is sometimes referred to as the *abstinence violation effect*). These balanced placebo experiments have been replicated several times by others. In such experiments, which contrast the pharmacological effects of alcohol with the cognitive effects of expecting to drink alcohol, typically alcohol itself can be shown to impair information-processing ability and motor performance regardless of expectation. Expectancy of alcohol increases alcohol consumption, sexual arousal,

and aggressiveness.[26] The most obvious interpretation of such results is that alcohol use provides a social excuse for behaving in certain ways that would otherwise be considered inappropriate, and it is enough for one to believe that he or she has drunk alcohol for such behaviors to be released.

There is considerable evidence in support of the idea that some degree of vulnerability to alcoholism might be inherited. Alcoholism does tend to "run in families," but some of that could be due to similar expectancies developed through similar cultural influences and children learning from their parents. Studies on twins provide one way around this problem. Monozygotic (one-egg, or identical) twins share the same genetic material, whereas dizygotic (two-egg, or fraternal) twins are no more genetically related than any two nontwin siblings. Both types of twins are likely to share very similar cultural and family learning experiences. If one adult twin is diagnosed as alcoholic, what is the likelihood that the other twin will also receive that diagnosis (are the twins concordant for the trait of alcoholism)? Almost all such studies report that the concordance rate for monozygotic twins is higher than that for dizygotic twins, and in some studies it is as high as 50 percent. These results imply that inheritance plays a strong role but is far from a complete determinant of alcoholism. Another important type of study looks at adopted sons whose biological fathers were alcoholics. These reports consistently find that such adoptees have a much greater than average chance of becoming alcoholics, even though they are raised by nonalcoholic parents. Although these studies again provide clear evidence for a genetic influence, it

---

balanced placebo: a research design in which alcohol is compared with a placebo beverage, and subjects either believe they are drinking alcohol or believe they are not.

is important to remember that most children of alcoholics do not become alcoholics—they simply have a statistically greater risk of doing so. For example, in one study 18 percent of adopted-away sons of alcoholics became alcoholic, compared with 5 percent of adopted-away sons whose parents had not received the diagnosis of alcoholism.

Further evidence for an inherited risk factor in alcoholism comes from experiments on young men (because alcoholism is more common in men) who are drinking but have not yet demonstrated alcoholism. If these young men had an alcoholic parent, they were less affected by a dose of alcohol than were control subjects with no family history of alcoholism. The argument is that these vulnerable individuals might drink more alcohol because they are less able to detect the initial effects of alcohol. Another type of study examined electrical brain-wave responses recorded from the scalp in response to repeated auditory stimuli. Alcoholic men as a group have a smaller response at a particular time point after the stimulus (the P300 wave). In addition, young men who have never themselves drunk alcohol, but whose fathers are alcoholics, as a group show a similarly reduced P300 wave.[27]

In 1990, national attention was focused on a report that a possible **genetic marker** had been found for alcoholism. Studying brain tissue obtained from 35 people who had died from complications of alcoholism, with 35 nonalcoholic brains as controls, researchers found that an unusual form of one type of dopamine receptor was present in 69 percent of the alcoholic brains and only 20 percent of the nonalcoholics. The genetic code for this dopamine receptor is located on chromosome 11 in humans. Could this be the long-sought key to an alcoholism gene?[28] The research that has emerged since then does not give a clear answer—some studies have continued to find a relationship between this dopamine receptor type and alcoholism, whereas others have not.[29] Of course, alcoholism is a complicated feature of human be-

havior, and even if genetic influences are critical, there could be more than one genetic factor involved. Probably it is too much to hope that a single genetic marker will ever be found to be a reliable indicator of alcoholism in all individuals.

TREATING ALCOHOLISM

Excessive alcohol consumption is an age-old human problem, and one that exacts enormous costs from contemporary society, both in dollars and in wasted human potential. Where do we place the blame for this difficulty? If we believe that the fault is a moral defect in the alcoholic, then we might "treat" the problem by using the same sort of approach we use with other social transgressions such as stealing. Historically, these have consisted of social ostracism, imprisonment, or other forms of punishment. If we believe that the fault lies with alcohol itself ("demon rum"), then our treatment consists of attempts to control the availability of alcohol. If we believe that alcoholism is a disease, then we seek medical treatment.

Historically, all these ideas and all these approaches have coexisted. For example, at the turn of the century it was common to view drunkards as social outcasts and to throw them in jail. At the same time the temperance movement was rapidly gaining ground in its rush toward the eventual prohibition of alcohol. Meanwhile, some physicians were advocating the use of morphine, cocaine, or other drugs as preferable substitutes for alcohol.

Alcoholics Anonymous

The formation of Alcoholics Anonymous (AA) in 1935 can now be seen as an important milestone in treatment. This group, which has total abstinence as a goal, has given support to the disease model of alcoholism. One of the basic tenets of this group is that the alcoholic is biologically different from the nonalcoholic person

FYI The Twelve Steps of Alcoholics Anonymous

1. We admitted we were powerless over alcohol—that our lives had become unmanageable.
2. Came to believe that a Power greater than ourselves could restore us to sanity.
3. Made a decision to turn our will and our lives over to the care of God *as we understood Him.*
4. Made a searching and fearless moral inventory of ourselves.
5. Admitted to God, to ourselves, and to another human being the exact nature of our wrongs.
6. Were entirely ready to have God remove all these defects of character.
7. Humbly asked Him to remove our shortcomings.
8. Made a list of all persons we had harmed and became willing to make amends to them all.
9. Made direct amends to such people wherever possible, except when to do so would injure them or others.
10. Continued to take moral inventory and when we were wrong promptly admitted it.
11. Sought through prayer and meditation to improve our conscious contact with God *as we understood Him,* praying only for knowledge of His will for us and the power to carry that out.
12. Having had a spiritual awakening as the result of these steps, we tried to carry this message to alcoholics, and to practice these principles in all our affairs.

The Twelve Steps are reprinted with permission of Alcoholics Anonymous World Services, Inc. Permission to reprint the Twelve Steps does not mean that A.A. has reviewed or approved the contents of this publication, nor that A.A. agrees with the views expressed herein. A.A. is a program of recovery from alcoholism *only* - use of the Twelve Steps in connection with programs and activities which are patterned after A.A., but which address other problems, or in any other non-A.A. context, does not imply otherwise.

and therefore can never safely drink any alcohol at all. Central to this disease model is the idea that the disease takes away the person's control of his own drinking behavior and therefore removes the blame for the problem. AA members are quick to point out that removing blame for the disease does not remove responsibility for dealing with it. By analogy, we would not blame diabetics for being diabetic, but we do expect diabetics to control their diets, take their medication, and so on. Thus the alcoholic is seen as having the responsibility for managing the "disease" on a day-by-day basis but need not feel guilty about being different. The major approach used by AA has been group support and a "buddy system." The members of AA help each other through difficult periods and encourage each other in their sobriety.

Although AA has been described as a loose affiliation of local groups, each with its own character, they have in common adherence to a twelve-step program of recovery from alcoholism (see the FYI box).

Everyone agrees that AA has been helpful for many people and, because it has reached more individuals than any other approach, has undoubtedly helped more people than any other method. Nevertheless, formal evaluations of the success of AA have been few and have not been very positive. For example, studies of court-ordered referrals to AA or to other types of interventions have not shown AA to be more effective. However, AA was developed by and for people who have made a personal decision to stop drinking and who want to affiliate with others who have made that decision, and it might not be the most appropriate approach for individuals who are coerced into attending

genetic marker: a chemical or physiological characteristic that is known to be caused by a particular gene and that is highly correlated with some disease state.

meetings as an alternative to jail. More appropriate (and more difficult and expensive) evaluations of AA should be done to determine which types of alcoholics are most likely to benefit from this organization's program.

Medical Approaches

One of the most influential contributors to the disease concept of alcoholism was E. M. Jellinek, who portrayed alcoholism as a progressive disease leading characteristically through several stages.[30] In the final and most severe stage, which he called *gamma alcoholism*, the individual has suffered liver and nervous system damage and has a profound physical dependence so that dangerous withdrawal symptoms appear when alcohol intake is stopped. More recent studies have discounted the notion that all, or even most, alcoholics go through such a consistent set of stages. However, a large number of alcoholics come into treatment with liver and nervous system damage and will suffer withdrawal symptoms. In fact, thousands of people die each year under these circumstances. In such severe cases, it is clear that medical intervention is called for.

Detoxification

The first problem is to get the individual over the immediate crisis. There is some danger of death from respiratory depression at first, simply from alcohol overdose. Clearing the stomach and supporting respiration will hopefully get the individual through this first threat. The next hurdle is to allow the alcohol to clear the system (detoxification), while preventing convulsions and delirium tremens because of withdrawal. Intravenous administration of diazepam or another benzodiazepine sedative is an accepted method for controlling these potentially dangerous symptoms.

Treatment

Regardless of which approach is taken to try to alter drinking behavior, the next stage of medical treatment is based on the fact that many alcoholics are malnourished and that at least some of the alcohol-related brain damage could be a result of a vitamin (thiamine) deficiency. Thus an important part of treating chronic alcoholics is providing a nutritious diet supplemented by extra vitamins. There might be other physical problems associated with liver occlusion and altered blood circulation, and these also require symptomatic medical treatment.

Aftercare

Once an individual has been "dried out" and has received the primary treatment, it can be appropriate to provide some long-term medical support. A common approach, which might be considered part of the treatment itself, is the prescribing of disulfiram (**Antabuse**). Alcohol is normally metabolized in the liver through two enzymatic steps. Disulfiram inhibits the enzyme aldehyde dehydrogenase, the second of these steps. Alcohol is then converted into acetaldehyde, but further conversion is prevented and acetaldehyde builds up in the system. High levels of acetaldehyde usually produce a severe reaction: headache, nausea, vomiting, throbbing of the head and neck, breathing difficulties, and a host of other unpleasant symptoms. Therefore a person taking Antabuse can't take a drink without becoming ill, and this threat can be sufficient to help many people avoid the impulse to drink. It takes two or three days after a person stops taking disulfiram before a drink can be taken safely, so a person on this treatment must make a decision to stop taking Antabuse for that length of time if he or she wants to drink.

Antabuse treatment has been employed in court-ordered treatment programs, but there is considerable doubt as to its long-term usefulness when employed in that way. If Antabuse does help, it is by helping those who want to avoid drinking by making it impossible for them to give in to a momentary impulse or to social pressure.

Naltrexone is a drug that was originally developed as a narcotic antagonist and has been used in the treatment of narcotic addiction (see chapter 15). Research in the early 1990s found that naltrexone given in conjunction with outpatient rehabilitation treatment for alcoholism reduced reported cravings for alcohol, and in the first three months after treatment only about one-fourth of the naltrexone-treated patients relapsed, compared with about 50 percent of the placebo control group.[31] Based on such research, the FDA in 1994 approved naltrexone for use in the treatment of alcoholism. Although great fanfare accompanied this approval and no doubt many alcoholics will receive naltrexone, it is too early to tell what the long-term impact of this treatment will be.

Behavioral Approaches   *Violence*

One behavioral approach involves teaching coping skills. Some of the same behaviors that are taught in prevention programs are used, such as recognizing peer pressure and practicing ways to deal with it. In addition, therapists often get the patients to pay special attention to high-risk situations and teach alternative behaviors that can be used to get through those difficult times. For example, if the individual is accustomed to having a drink or two before dinner, it might be suggested that a nonalcoholic drink be substituted, that the person assist with the dinner preparations, or even that the dinner hour be moved up to eliminate the difficult time gap. The idea is to help the client to manage her or his behavior to decrease the probability of drinking. Some studies have reported positive results from such treatment approaches, whereas others have not.

Some behavior-management approaches have accepted **controlled drinking** as a desirable outcome and have attempted to teach methods that will limit alcohol intake. Such strategies as switching to drinks with lower alcohol content, keeping track of each drink taken, or even learning to recognize a target BAC have been tried. A number of such experiments have reported success in producing a higher percentage of improved patients (both abstaining and "controlled") than with traditional abstinence-oriented approaches. However, there is enormous controversy about both the success and the desirability of controlled-drinking approaches.

Is Controlled Drinking a Realistic Goal?

The notion that alcoholism is a disease that produces a loss of control over drinking seems to be inconsistent with AA's belief that alcoholics do have the responsibility to decide to remain sober. This apparent dilemma is resolved by the commonly used saying, "One drink is too much and a thousand not enough." In other words, the belief is that the alcoholic does have control over that first drink and can choose not to take it, but once alcohol has entered her system she is helpless and her drinking is out of control. This seems to be descriptive of binge drinking, in which a problem drinker might not drink at all for days or weeks and then really "tie one on." But does this notion of loss of control have any further merit? Does it describe the behavior of all alcoholics all of the time? A number of experimental studies have been done with hospitalized alcoholics, and virtually all of them report that alcoholics do not differ fundamentally in the types of events that control drinking, although they do drink more than control subjects. Other descriptive studies of the drinking patterns of large numbers of active alcoholics show a great variety of patterns. Some drink in this binge fashion, whereas others have extended periods of what can be described only as controlled drinking. Also, a surprisingly large number of alcoholics who have been through

---

Antabuse: (disulfiram) a drug that alters alcohol metabolism and is used in treating alcoholism.

controlled drinking: the idea that alcohol abusers might be able to drink limited amounts of alcohol.

abstention-oriented treatment programs are found on later follow-ups to be drinking, but in a controlled manner.[32]

Just about everyone can agree that anyone who has drinking problems would be best advised to stop drinking and to abstain completely. But there are arguments against having abstention as the only treatment goal. First, problem drinkers might be reluctant to enter treatment if they are required to accept the label *alcoholic* and the goal of total **abstinence**. Second, about two-thirds of adult Americans are drinkers (and even more among urban, college-educated adults). Thus, assuming that the alcoholic has been part of a social group that accepts or even expects drinking, we are in a sense trying to promote a "deviant" behavior. Third, if abstention has been tried several times with no success, why not try controlled drinking as a treatment goal? Those opposed to such approaches believe that they are doomed to failure because their definition of alcoholism includes the individual's powerlessness to control drinking. Any apparent successes can be argued away either by agreeing that alcoholics might appear to be under control for a few weeks or months or by saying that the controlled-drinking successes were not really alcoholics when they entered treatment. These experts are concerned that even discussing the possibility might just encourage alcoholics to drink. After all, they've probably been telling themselves and others for years that they could "handle it." Do we really need scientists providing support for such self-delusion?

A widely publicized Rand Corporation report added fuel to this controversy. This study, funded by the NIAAA, examined treatment effectiveness in eight large treatment centers. After establishing clearly that the alcoholics in these programs were seriously impaired (they drank nine times more than the average person), they found that about 70 percent of them were improved eighteen months after treatment. Their controversial conclusion was this:

It is important to stress that the improved clients include only a relatively small number who are long-term abstainers. . . . The majority of improved clients are either drinking moderate amounts of alcohol—but at levels far below what could be described as alcoholic drinking—or engaging in alternating periods of drinking and abstention.[33]

You should be aware that these programs had abstention as their primary goal, yet controlled drinking seemed to have been the result for a large number of the clients. This report came under immediate and highly emotional attack, as did the Rand Corporation itself and the NIAAA for funding such a study.

The traditional view was vindicated to some extent by the four-year follow-up of these clients. Of those who had been drinking without symptoms at eighteen months, 41 percent had relapsed by the four-year follow-up, compared with 30 percent of those who had been abstaining at eighteen months.[34] This was widely hailed as indicating that abstention was a more desirable treatment outcome than controlled drinking. However, we should not ignore the fact that the *majority* of those who were drinking in a controlled fashion at eighteen months did not relapse and were found to be either controlled drinkers or abstainers at four years. At this point it seems reasonable to conclude that abstention is the preferred goal and the one adopted by the vast majority of programs, but that controlled drinking is a realistic option for some alcoholics.

Although research continues on disulfiram, naltrexone, controlled drinking, and other approaches, the mainstay of alcoholism treatment in the United States has been a four- to six-week visit to a residential (inpatient) treatment facility. Most of these programs adopt the AA model of alcoholism as a disease and use individual counseling, group counseling, and family therapy approaches to help the alcoholic "work the steps" (the twelve steps of AA). Because health insurance companies were willing to pay for such treatment, these residential facilities became a growth industry during the 1980s. As health insurance companies began to limit coverage to shorter stays and to fewer clients, most of the treatment facilities that opened during the 1980s were closed during the 1990s.

Is Alcoholism Treatment Effective?

Are the insurance companies getting anything for their money when they pay for someone to go to treatment? The answers to these questions about alcoholism treatment aren't necessarily simple, but we can start by saying a qualified yes. If an individual receives the diagnosis of alcoholism (or alcohol dependence disorder), the prognosis is not good. Most such individuals can be expected to drink again, drink heavily, and have further alcohol-related problems. But it is clear that those who enter treatment do better than those who do not. Thus, statistically, alcoholism treatment is effective. However, the same studies show over and over that most of the people who go through treatment will drink again, with typical first-year relapse rates running about 65 percent to 75 percent.[21] Therefore it might seem that treatment is not effective for most of the individuals. A further complication has been hinted at: how do we define relapse? If the goal is 100 percent abstinence, then even one drink at any time after treatment would be considered a relapse and therefore a treatment failure. It is quite possible for someone to go through a treatment program, spend a couple of months going to AA meetings and not drinking, think they have the problem licked, try drinking again, drink too much for a month or two, and then go back to AA and quit drinking. Neither recovery nor relapse should be viewed as a permanent condition.

Many studies over the years have examined the characteristics of the treatment programs and the characteristics of the clients to determine whether one type of treatment is better than another, which clients do better than

others, and whether certain types of clients do better in certain types of programs. Because of the difficulties in measuring relapse and other indicators of success, this type of research is difficult to do and individual reports can often be criticized on procedural grounds. But several large-scale studies agree that differences among treatment approaches are less important in predicting success than differences among the clients when they enter treatment.

Those clients who have jobs, stable family relationships, minimal psychopathology, no history of past treatment failures, and minimal involvement with other drugs tend to do better than the clients with no jobs, no meaningful relationships, and so on. What is surprising is that the type of treatment program seems to make little or no difference: residential versus outpatient, shorter versus longer, intensity of therapy, and theoretical approach are all factors that have not consistently influenced outcome. This seems to imply that insurance companies could save money by providing for shorter term, less intense, outpatient treatment and still have about the same success rate. The companies paid attention and have placed further restrictions on long-term residential treatment.

One important new approach might have some value in reducing the frequency of severe alcoholism. Medical patients in primary care settings are given a screening survey, and those who are found to be heavy drinkers then are counseled by a physician that their drinking is much higher than average and they should cut down. Surprisingly, several studies have shown this type of intervention to be effective. In one report, two brief counseling sessions with a primary care physician resulted in an average 37 percent reduction in average number of drinks in men and a 47 percent reduction in women, twelve months after the counseling sessions.[35]

---

abstinence: no alcohol or drug use at all.

SUMMARY

▲ In colonial America alcohol use was widespread and drunkenness was frowned on, but alcohol itself was not seen as a cause of major social and medical ills.

▲ Reformers first proposed temperate use of alcoholic beverages, and it was not until the late 1800s that proposals to prohibit alcohol were instituted in several states.

▲ National prohibition of alcohol did not achieve the results expected by its proponents, but it was successful in reducing total consumption and alcohol-related problems.

▲ Alcohol use and alcohol-related problems vary widely among different cultural groups and in different regions of the United States.

▲ Alcohol use is associated with thousands of traffic fatalities and has been correlated with homicide, assault, family violence, and suicide.

▲ The concept of alcoholism is complex. No single definition or theory is adequate to cover all the people who are called or who call themselves alcoholic.

▲ One continuing controversy is whether every alcoholic should have abstinence as the only goal or whether controlled drinking is also a worthwhile treatment outcome.

▲ Although many alcoholics relapse after treatment, not all do, and treatment programs are statistically effective.

REVIEW QUESTIONS

1. What important concepts regarding alcohol's social and medical effects were first introduced by Benjamin Rush in 1784?
2. What were the effects on American society of Prohibition of alcohol during the 1920s?
3. What was the impact on sales of the 1991 increase in U.S. alcohol taxes?

4. What are some differences between Irish-American and Italian-American cultures relating to alcohol use?
5. Which state has the highest apparent per capita alcohol consumption and which the lowest?
6. What are some effects of restrictive campus drinking policies on college student drinking and alcohol-related problems?
7. What is meant by "alcohol myopia"?
8. What has been the trend since 1980 in alcohol-related traffic fatalities?
9. Describe the balanced placebo research design and what types of alcohol effects might be due to the belief that alcohol has been consumed, rather than the actual alcohol itself.
10. What is the role of God in the twelve steps of AA?
11. What three arguments have been given in favor of controlled drinking as a treatment outcome?
12. What are some individual client characteristics that predict success in alcoholism treatment?

 Related Internet Sites on Alcohol and Society

Alcoholics Anonymous: http://www.alcoholics-anonymous.org/index.html

National Institute on Alcohol Abuse and Alcoholism: http://www.niaaa.nih.gov

National Commission Against Drunk Driving: http://www.ncadd.com/

And see our *Drugs, Society, and Human Behavior* site for more links: http://www.uwyo.edu/A&S/psyc/dshb.htm

REFERENCES

1. The alcohol problem in America: from temperance to alcoholism, *British Addiction* 79:109–119, 1984.
2. Koren J: *Economic aspects of the liquor problem*, New York, 1899, Houghton Mifflin.
3. Clark NH: *The dry years: prohibition and social change in Washington*, Seattle, 1965, University of Washington Press.
4. Keller M: Alcohol problems and policies in historical perspective. In Kyvig DE, editor: *Law, alcohol and order*, Westport, CT, 1985, Greenwood Press.
5. Emerson H: *Alcohol and man*, New York, 1932, MacMillan, reprinted 1981, New York, Arno Press.
6. *U.S. industrial outlook 1992*, Washington, DC, 1992, US Department of Commerce.
7. Segal BM: *The Soviet heavy-drinking culture and the American heavy-drinking subculture*. In Babor TF, editor: *Alcohol and culture: comparative perspectives from Europe and America*, New York, 1986, New York Academy of Sciences.
8. Vaillant G: *Cultural factors in the etiology of alcoholism: a prospective study*. In Babor TF, editor: *Alcohol and culture: comparative perspectives from Europe and America*, New York, 1986, New York Academy of Sciences.
9. Geddes D: France sets records in suicide, alcoholism and anxiety, *The Times* (London), June 14, 1986, p 9.
10. Williams GD and others: *NIAAA Surveillance Report #39: Apparent per capita alcohol consumption*. Bethesda, MD, USPHS, 1996.
11. *Sixth special report on alcohol and health*, DHHS Pub No (ADM) 87-1519, Washington, DC, 1987, US Government Printing Office.
12. Linsky AS and others: Social stress, normative constraints and alcohol problems in American states, *Social Science and Medicine* 24:875–883, 1987.
13. Mooney DK and others: Correlates of alcohol consumption: sex, age, and expectancies relate differentially to quantity and frequency, *Addict Behav* 12:235–240, 1987.
14. Johnston LD, O'Malley PM, Bachman JG: *Results from the monitoring the future study, 1975–1994. Volume 2: College students and young adults*. Bethesda MD, USPHS, 1995.
15. Wet or dry: schools ponder variety of strategies to curb alcohol problems, *The Bottom Line* 18(3) 68–72, 1997.
16. Steele CM, Josephs RA: Alcohol myopia, *Am Psychol* 45:921–933, 1990.
17. Update: Alcohol-related traffic fatalities—United States, 1982–1993, *JAMA*, 272:1892, 1994.
18. Campbell KE and others: *NIAAA Surveillance Report #38: Trends in alcohol-related fatal traffic crashes*. Bethesda MD, USPHS, 1996.
19. Insurance Institute for Highway Safety: *Fatality facts 1991*, Washington, DC, 1991, IIHS.
20. Pernanen K: *Alcohol in human violence*, New York, 1991, Guilford Press.
21. *Eighth special report on alcohol and health*, NIH Pub No 94-3699, Washington, DC, 1993, US Public Health Service.
22. Bushman BJ, Cooper HM: Effects of alcohol on human aggression: an integrative research review, *Psychol Bull* 107:341–354, 1990.
23. *Diagnostic and statistical manual of mental disorders*, ed 4, Washington, DC, 1994, American Psychiatric Association.
24. Alcoholism a disease or foible? *Denver Post*, December, 1988.
25. Wilson GT: Cognitive studies in alcoholism, *J Consult Clin Psychol* 55:325–331, 1987.
26. Hull JG, Bond CF: Social and behavioral consequences of alcohol consumption and expectancy: a meta-analysis, *Psychol Bull* 99:347–360, 1986.
27. Schuckit MA: Biological vulnerability to alcoholism, *J Consult Clin Psychol* 55:301–309, 1987.
28. Cowley G: The gene and the bottle, *Newsweek*, April 30, 1990.
29. Ackerman SJ: Research on the genetics of alcoholism is still in ferment, *The Journal of NIH Research* 4:61–65, 1992.
30. Jellinek EM: *The disease concept of alcoholism*, New Brunswick, NJ, 1960, Hillhouse Press.
31. Volpicelli JR and others: Naltrexone in the treatment of alcohol dependence, *Arch Gen Psychiatry* 49:876, 1992.
32. Pomerleau O, Pertschuk M, Stinnet J: A critical examination of some current assumptions in the treatment of alcoholism, *J Stud Alcohol* 37:849–867, 1976.
33. Armor DJ, Polich JM, Stambul HB: *Alcoholism and treatment*, NIAAA Pub No R-1739, Washington, DC, 1976, US Government Printing Office.
34. Polich JM, Armor DJ, Braiker HB: *The course of alcoholism: four years after treatment*, New York, 1981, Wiley.
35. Fleming MF and others: *Brief physician advice for problem alcohol drinkers: A randomized controlled trial in community-based primary care practices. JAMA*, 277: 1039–1045, 1997.

ASSESS YOURSELF!

How Can You Tell if You Have a Drinking Problem?

There have been many self-tests published for people to use to determine if they are alcoholics or if they have a drinking problem. None of them should be taken as an absolute test or as providing a definite answer to that question, because in most cases it is a complex, subjective judgment as to whether someone should seek help. One of the best popularly printed self-tests appeared in a "Dear Abby" column, and it is offered here as a possible guide. If these questions seem to indicate that you or a friend need to seek help, we recommend a visit to a counselor, psychologist, or physician who is experienced in the assessment of chemical dependence. An assessment would probably include the use of a more professional questionnaire such as the Michigan Alcoholism Screening Test (MAST) or the Alcohol Dependency Scale (ADS).

Check those that apply to you:

( ) 1. Have you ever decided to stop drinking for a week or so, but lasted for only a couple of days?
( ) 2. Do you wish people would stop nagging you about your drinking?
( ) 3. Have you ever switched from one kind of drink to another in the hope that this would keep you from getting drunk?
( ) 4. Have you had a drink in the morning in the past year?
( ) 5. Do you envy people who can drink without getting into trouble?
( ) 6. Have you had problems connected with drinking during the past year?
( ) 7. Has your drinking caused problems at home?
( ) 8. Do you ever try to get "extra" drinks at a party because you did not get enough to drink?
( ) 9. Do you tell yourself you can stop drinking anytime you want to, even though you keep getting drunk when you don't mean to?
( ) 10. Have you missed days at work (or school) because of drinking?
( ) 11. Do you have "blackouts"?
( ) 12. Have you ever felt that your life would be better if you did not drink?

If you checked four or more of these, it would be a good idea to seek the guidance of a specialist in chemical dependence or to seek help directly through Alcoholics Anonymous or a similar organization. It's perfectly acceptable to go to an open AA meeting, listen to what is being said, and decide for yourself if their program would be useful to you.

Familiar Drugs

Some drugs are seen so often that they don't seem to be drugs at all, at least not in the same sense as cocaine or marijuana. However, tobacco and its ingredient nicotine, as well as caffeine in its various forms, are psychoactive drugs meeting any reasonable definition of the term *drug*. Certainly the drugs sold over-the-counter (OTC) in pharmacies are drugs, and many of them have their primary effects on the brain and behavior. In section 5, we learn about the psychological effects of all these familiar drugs, partly because they are so commonly used. Also, they provide several interesting points for comparison with the less well known, more frightening drugs.

12 Tobacco
Why do people smoke, and why do they have such a hard time quitting?

13 Caffeine
How much of an effect does caffeine really produce?
What are the relative strengths of coffee, tea, and soft drinks?

14 Over-the-Counter Drugs
Which of the common drugstore drugs are psychoactive?

12

Tobacco

KEY TERMS	OBJECTIVES

After reading this chapter, you should be able to:

Nicotiana tobacum
Nicotiana rustica
smokeless tobacco
moist snuff
quid
nitrosamines
leukoplakia
passive smoking
sidestream smoke
emphysema

- Describe the history of tobacco and the spread of tobacco use around the world.
- Describe how cigarettes are made and how they have changed over the years.
- Discuss the increased use of smokeless tobacco and cigars.
- List facts about the consequences of smoking for cancer, heart disease, obstructive lung disease, and pregnancy.

- Describe the pharmacology of nicotine and evidence indicating that it is the dependence-producing agent in tobacco.
- Describe drug and nondrug approaches to smoking cessation.

Long before Columbus stumbled onto the Western Hemisphere, the Indians here were using tobacco. It was one of the many contributions of the New World to Europe: tobacco, corn, sweet potatoes, white potatoes, chocolate, and—so you could lie back and enjoy it all—the hammock. Christopher Columbus recorded that the natives of San Salvador presented him with tobacco leaves on October 12, 1492. A fitting birthday present.

In 1497 a monk who had accompanied Columbus on his second trip wrote a book on native customs that contained the first printed report of tobacco smoking. It wasn't called to-

bacco, and it wasn't called smoking. Inhaling smoke was called drinking. In that period you either "took" (used snuff) or "drank" (smoked) tobacco.

The word *tobacco* came from one of two sources. *Tobaco* referred to a two-pronged tube used by natives to take snuff. But some early reports confused the issue by applying the name to the plant they incorrectly thought was being used. Another idea is that the word developed its current usage from the province of Tobacos in Mexico where everyone used the herb. Be that as it may, in 1598 an Italian-English dictionary published in London translated the

[handwritten margin notes: "why gained prominence & what was it used for"]

[handwritten margin notes: "drugs alcohol tobacco opposition to legal marij."]

Italian *Nicosiana* as the herb *Tobacco*, and that spelling and usage gradually became dominant.

One member of Columbus's party was the poor fellow who introduced tobacco drinking to Europe. He was also the first European to touch Cuba and possibly the first to smoke tobacco. When he continued his habit in Portugal, his friends were convinced the devil had possessed him as they saw the smoke coming out his mouth and nose. The priest agreed, and Rodrigo spent the next several years in jail, only to find on his release that people were doing the same thing for which he had been jailed!

TOBACCO

Early Medical Uses ✗

Tobacco was formally introduced to Europe as an herb useful for treating almost anything. A 1529 report[1] indicated that tobacco was used for "persistant headaches," "cold or catarrh," and "abscesses and sores on the head." Between 1537 and 1559, fourteen books mentioned the medicinal value of tobacco.

Jean Nicot was sent to Lisbon, Portugal, in 1559 to arrange a royal marriage. The marriage never took place, but Nicot became enamored with the medical uses of tobacco. He tried it on enough people to convince himself of its value and sent glowing reports of the herb's effectiveness to the French court. He was successful in "curing" the migraine headaches of Catherine de Medicis, Queen of Henry II of France, which made tobacco use very much "in." It was called the *herbe sainte*, "holy plant", and *the herbe à tous les maux,* "the plant against all evils." The French loved it and, although tobacco had been introduced earlier to Paris, Nicot received the credit. By 1565 the plant had been called nicotiane, and Linnaeus sanctified it in 1753 by naming the genus *Nicotiana*. When a pair of French chemists isolated the active ingredient in 1828, they acted like true nationalists and called it nicotine.

In the late sixteenth century:

it was more likely than not that . . . the doctor would prescribe tobacco. . . . Did the patient suffer from flatulence? The remedy was a tobacco emetic. . . . A heavy cough? Smoke of tobacco, deeply inhaled. Pains accompanying gestation or labor? Place a leaf of tobacco, very hot, on the navel. If a form of delirium ensued, blow smoke up the nostrils.[2]

In this period Sir Anthony Chute[1] summarized much of the earlier material and said, "Anything that harms a man inwardly from his girdle upward might be removed by a moderate use of the herb." Others, however, felt differently: "If taken after meals the herb would infect the brain and liver," and "Tobacco should be avoided by (among others) women with child and husbands who desired to have children."[1]

A few years later in 1617, Dr. William Vaughn phrased the last thought a little more poetically:

Tobacco that outlandish weede
It spends the braine and spoiles the seede
It dulls the spirite, it dims the sight
It robs a woman of her right.[3]

Dr. Vaughn may have been ahead of his time: a December 1994 report indicated that smokers are 50 percent more likely than nonsmokers to be impotent.[4]

Special note must be made of a series of experiments reported in 1805 by Dr. D. Legare, because his work pushed back the boundaries of ignorance and clearly disproved an old folk remedy. Beyond the shadow of a doubt, Dr. Legare personally proved that, contrary to general opinion, blowing tobacco smoke into the intestinal canal did *not* resuscitate drowned animals or people! The slow advance of medical science through the eighteenth and nineteenth centuries gradually removed tobacco from the doctor's black bag, and nicotine was dropped from *The United States Pharmacopeia* in the 1890s.

Tobacco Use Spreads

To fully appreciate the history of tobacco, you must know that there are over sixty species of Nicotiana, but only two major ones. **Nicotiana tobacum**, the major species grown today in more than a hundred countries, is large-leaf. Most importantly, *tobacum* was indigenous only to South America, so the Spanish had a monopoly on its production for over a hundred years. **Nicotiana rustica** is a small-leaf species and was the plant existing in the West Indies and eastern North America when Columbus arrived.

The Spanish monopoly on tobacco sales to Europe was a thorn in the side of the British. When settlers returned to England in 1586 after failing to colonize Virginia, they brought with them seeds of the *rustica* species and planted them in England, but this species never grew well. The English crown again attempted to establish a tobacco colony in 1610 when they sent John Rolfe as leader of a group to Virginia. From 1610 to 1612, Rolfe tried to cultivate *rustica,* but the small-leaf plant was weak and poor in flavor, and had a sharp taste.

In 1612, Rolfe somehow got hold of some seeds of the Spanish *tobacum* species. This species grew beautifully and sold well in 1613. The colony was saved, and every available plot of land was planted with *tobacum.* By 1619 as much Virginia tobacco was sold in London as Spanish tobacco. That was also the year that King James prohibited the cultivation of any tobacco in England and declared the tobacco trade a royal monopoly.

Tobacco became one of the major exports of the American colonies to England. The Thirty Years' War spread smoking throughout central Europe, and nothing stopped its use. Measures such as one in Bavaria in 1652 probably slowed tobacco use, but only momentarily. This law said that "tobacco-drinking was strictly forbidden to the peasants and other common people" and made tobacco available to others only on a doctor's prescription from a druggist.[5]

During the eighteenth century, smoking gradually diminished, but the use of tobacco did not. Snuff replaced the pipe in England. At the beginning of that century the upper class was already committed to snuff. The middle and lower classes only gradually changed over, but by 1770 very few people smoked. The reign of King George III (1760–1820) was the time of the big snuff. His wife Charlotte was so addicted to the powder that she was called "Snuffy Charlotte," although for obvious reasons not to her face. On the continent Napoleon had tried smoking once, gagged horribly, and returned to his seven pounds of snuff per month.

Tobacco in Early America

Trouble developed in the colonies, which, being democratic, made the richest man in Virginia (perhaps the richest in the colonies) commander in chief of the Revolutionary Army. In 1776, George Washington said in one of his appeals, "if you can't send money, send tobacco."[6] Tobacco played an important role in the Revolutionary War, because it was one of the major products for which France would lend the colonies money. Knowing the importance of tobacco to the colonies, one of Cornwallis's major campaign goals in 1780 and 1781 was the destruction of the Virginia tobacco plantations.

After the war ordinary Americans rejoiced and rejected snuff as well as tea and all other things British. The aristocrats who organized the republic were not as emotional, though, and installed a communal snuff box for members of Congress. Only in the mid 1930s did this remembrance of things past disappear. However, to emphasize the fact that snuff was a nonessential, the new Congress put a luxury tax on it in 1794.

Chewing Tobacco

If you don't smoke and you don't snuff
How can you possibly get enough?

gross income from farmers from tobacco 4,000

You can get enough, of course, by chewing, which gradually increased in the United States. Chewing was a suitable activity for a country on the go; it freed the hands, and the wide-open spaces made an adequate spittoon. There were also other considerations: Boston, for example, passed an ordinance in 1798 forbidding anyone from being in possession of a lighted pipe or "segar" in public streets. The original impetus was a concern for the fire hazard involved in smoking, not the individual's health, and the ordinance was finally repealed in 1880. Today it is difficult to appreciate how much of a chewing country we were in the nineteenth century. In 1860 only 7 of 348 tobacco factories in Virginia and North Carolina manufactured smoking tobacco. The amount of tobacco for smoking did not equal the amount for chewing until 1911 and did not surpass it until the 1920s.

The high level of chewing-tobacco production during the Industrial Age led to occasional accidents, as suggested by a quote from a 1918 decision of the Mississippi Supreme Court:

> We can imagine no reason why, with ordinary care, human toes could not be left out of chewing tobacco, and if toes are found in chewing tobacco, it seems to us that somebody has been very careless.[2]

The turn of the century was the approximate high point for chewing tobacco, the sales of which slowly declined through the early part of the century as other tobacco products became more popular. In 1945, cuspidors were removed from all federal buildings.

Cigars and Cigarettes

The transition from chewing to cigarettes had a middle point, a combination of both smoking and chewing: cigars. Cigarette smoking was coming, and the cigar manufacturers did their best to keep cigarettes under control. They suggested that cigarettes were drugged with opium so you could not stop using them and that the

People smoking cigars at a "cigar aficionado" smoke-in.

paper was bleached with arsenic and thus was harmful to you. They had some help from Thomas Edison in 1914:

> The injurious agent in Cigarettes comes principally from the burning paper wrapper. . . . It has a violent action in the nerve centers, producing degeneration of the cells of the brain, which is quite rapid among boys. Unlike most narcotics, this degeneration is permanent and uncontrollable. I employ no person who smokes cigarettes.[2]

Most cigars had been hand rolled or at least made by hand shaping in a mold, but as sales increased, machines had to be used. Today, a good worker hand rolls about two hundred cigars in an eight- to-nine-hour day. There was an

> ***Nicotiana tobacum:*** (ni co she *ann* a toe *back* um) species of tobacco widely cultivated for smoking and chewing products.
>
> ***Nicotiana rustica:*** (*russ* tick a) less desirable species of tobacco not widely grown in the United States.

aversion to machine-made cigars, so some advertising was educational in nature. As an example of the high level of advertising before television and Madison Avenue:

> Spit is a horrid word, but it's worse on the end of your cigar. Why run the risk of cigars made by dirty yellowed fingers and tipped in spit?[2]

The efforts of the cigar manufacturers worked for a while, and cigar sales reached their highest level in 1920, when 8 billion were sold. As sales increased, though, so did the cost of the product. The whole world knows that "what this country *needs* is a really good five-cent cigar," but how many know that this statement was made by a vice president of the United States as an aside in the Senate when one of the members was going on at great length about the needs of the country?

Thin reeds filled with tobacco had been seen by the Spanish in Yucatan in 1518. In 1844 the French were using them, and the Crimean War circulated the cigarette habit throughout Europe. The first British cigarette factory was started in 1856 by a returning veteran of the Crimean War, and in the late 1850s an English tobacco merchant, Phillip Morris, began producing handmade cigarettes. On the continent the use of this new dose form must have developed fairly rapidly. One company in Austria began making double cigarettes in 1865—both ends had a mouthpiece, and the consumer cut them in two—and sold 16 million in 1866.

In the United States, cigarettes were being produced during the same period (14 million in 1870), but it was in the 1880s that their popularity increased rapidly. The date of the first patent on a cigarette-making machine was 1881, and by 1885 over a billion cigarettes a year were being sold. Not even that great he-man, boxer John L. Sullivan, could stem the tide, though in 1905 his opinion of cigarette smokers was pretty clear:

> Smoke cigarettes? Not on your tut-tut. . . . You can't suck coffin-nails and be a ring-champion. . . .

You never heard of . . . a bank burglar using a cigarette, did you? They couldn't do it and attend to biz. Why, even drunkards don't use the things. . . . Who smokes 'em? Dudes and college stiffs—fellows who'd be wiped out by a single jab or a quick undercut. It isn't natural to smoke cigarettes. An American ought to smoke cigars. . . . It's the Dutchmen, Italians, Russians, Turks and Egyptians who smoke cigarettes and they're no good anyhow.[2]

By the turn of the century there was a preference for cigarettes with an aromatic component, that is, Turkish tobacco. A new cigarette in 1913 capitalized on the lure of the Near East while rejecting it in actuality. Camels were a blend of burley and bright with just a hint of Turkish tobacco—you had the camel and pyramid on the package, what more could you want? Besides, eliminating most of the imported tobacco made the price lower. Low price was combined with a big advertising campaign: "The Camels are coming. Tomorrow there'll be more CAMELS in town than in all of Asia and Africa combined." By 1918 Camels had 40 percent of the market, and they stayed in front until after World War II.

The year 1919 was marked by the first ad showing a woman smoking. To make the ad easier to accept, the woman was pictured as Asian and the ad was for a Turkish type of cigarettes. King-size cigarettes appeared in 1939 in the form of Pall Mall, which became the number-one seller. Filter cigarettes as filter cigarettes, not cigarettes that happen to have filters along with a mouthpiece, appeared in 1954 with Winston, which rapidly took over the market and continued to be number one until the mid 1970s. Filter cigarettes captured an increasing share of the market and now constitute over 90 percent of all U.S. cigarette sales.

CURRENT TOBACCO PRODUCTS

Tobacco is grown on about 125,000 American farms, most with only a few acres devoted to tobacco. There's a lot of hand labor involved, requiring about 250 man-hours for each harvested acre (compared with about 3 man-hours per acre for wheat). Tobacco seeds are started in seed beds and transplanted, 5,000 to 10,000 plants to an acre, when they are 6 to 8 inches high. In two to three months, when the tobacco is ready to harvest, the leaves will be 1 to 2½ feet long, and a typical burley tobacco plant will have ten leaves. The nicotine content of a raw tobacco leaf ranges from 0.3 to 7 percent and varies with the variety, climatic conditions, fertilizer used, and many other factors. Nicotine levels can be manipulated during processing to any desired level.

Burley is one of the major tobaccos used in cigarettes. It is harvested by cutting the stalk close to the ground, then hanging the entire stalk in a curing barn for four to six weeks. The plant uses its stored food, dies, and loses about 80 percent of its weight through moisture loss. This is "air-curing," the method used for most cigarette tobacco grown west of the Appalachians. East of the mountains, "flue-curing" is used to produce *bright* tobacco. Tobacco that is to be flue-cured has the leaves separated from the stalks during harvesting, and heat is added to the curing barn so that the process is complete in less than a week.

After curing, the burley leaves are removed from the stalk and sorted on the basis of color, size, and stalk position. Almost all tobacco is still sold at one of the 136 auction houses in this country. The farmer's hard work is well rewarded, with an average gross income of almost $4,000 per acre (compared with less than $100 per acre for wheat). Overall, tobacco is America's seventh largest legal cash crop.[7]

When the tobacco reaches the buyer's processing plant, modern technology takes over. Here the tobacco leaves are shredded, dried, picked, blown clean of foreign matter and stems, remoistened to a particular level, and packed in huge wooden barrels called hogsheads. The hogsheads are placed in store-

Although labor-intensive, tobacco farming is more profitable per acre than other crops.

houses, where the tobacco ages for two to three years.

Proper aging is one of the secrets to good tobacco. Aging allows fermentation to occur so that the tobacco gets darker and loses moisture, as well as nicotine (probably about one-third of its original level) and other volatile substances. When the aging is complete, moisture is again added, and various types of tobacco are blended. During the blending process (top secret!), other substances are also added. Glycerine is used to stabilize the moisture content, and a variety of flavorants are included. A 1972 publication by the Reynolds Tobacco Company listed 1,290 flavorants that could be added to tobacco, including such common tastes as chocolate, licorice, and sugar. The blended material is compressed and then cut into hangnail-size strips to prepare it for the cigarette machine.

In the 1870s James Buchanan Duke thought his cigarette girls were doing very well if they could consistently roll four cigarettes a minute. In 1881 he started the cigarette revolution by using a machine that had just been patented. It produced 200 cigarettes a minute! He would love today's machine. It starts with a roll of cigarette paper 3½ miles (5.6 km) long, makes a continuous clothesline-like tube filled with tobacco, cuts it to length, weighs the cigarette, rejecting those over or under the correct weight, and checks it for uniformity. It does everything but salute and still turns out 3,600 cigarettes a minute. Filter cigarettes are made by adding a machine that attaches a double-size filter between two cigarettes and then cuts them apart at the same rapid rate.

Toward a Less Hazardous Cigarette

The cigarette of the 1950s was quite different from the cigarette of the 1990s. For one thing, in the 1950s, it required 2¾ pounds (1.2 kg) of leaf tobacco to produce 1,000 cigarettes. Now only about 1¾ pounds (0.8 kg) are required to produce the same number. Besides the addition of filters, two other technological changes have decreased the amount of leaf tobacco per cigarette. One is the use of reconstituted sheets of tobacco. Parts of the tobacco leaf and stems that had been discarded in earlier years are now ground up, combined with various ingredients, and then rolled out as a flat sheet of tobacco. After shredding, this material is combined with normally processed leaf tobacco. Today about 20 percent of all cigarette tobacco is reconstituted sheet.

The second development that reduced the need for tobacco in cigarettes is "fluffing." Tobacco is freeze-dried, and an inert gas such as Freon is used to expand the tobacco cells so that they take up more space and absorb more additives. One low-tar cigarette introduced in the early 1970s was able to reduce by 35 percent the tobacco in each cigarette because of its process to "fluff" the tobacco. Fluffing, of course, reduces the tar, nicotine, and carbon monoxide content of a cigarette, but it also reduces smoking time, perhaps by 15 percent. Carbon monoxide is important because it decreases the oxygen-carrying capacity of the blood, putting more strain on the heart and reducing oxygenation of all the tissues.

For many years the Federal Trade Commission (FTC) measured the tar and nicotine content of cigarettes and published a listing of the results by brand name and type. These were measured by standardized smoking machines. The machine contained a filter, and the word *tar* refers to a complex mixture that remains on the filter after moisture and nicotine have been removed. This tar mixture contains most of the cancer-causing chemicals in tobacco smoke. As you might suspect, cigarettes with less tobacco have less tar and less nicotine, and measurements across brands found very high correlations between the two. Thus it is possible to speak of the tar and nicotine (T/N) content of a cigarette. Because of the previously mentioned changes in cigarette manufacturing, T/N levels declined regularly from the 1950s to the 1980s. The average 1950s cigarette delivered about 2.5 mg of nicotine, whereas the average cigarette now delivers about 1 mg of nicotine. Average tar yield has dropped from over 40 mg to under 20 mg per cigarette.

Low T/N cigarettes are associated with a lower health risk, and low T/N became a significant factor in advertising and in brand selection. However, there are a few things you should know about low T/N cigarettes. First is that the measurements are made by a machine that smokes each cigarette in a standard manner (e.g., to within 3 mm of the filter "overwrap"). Manufacturers were able to reduce T/N content by manipulations such as using a longer overwrap or putting airholes around the filter. Smokers could and did smoke differently from the machine (for instance, covering some or all of the air holes while puffing), thus obtaining more tar and nicotine. It seems that smokers aim for a certain nicotine input, and when switched to a low T/N brand they take more puffs and inhale more deeply so as to largely compensate for the change in cigarettes.[8] Obviously, if a smoker compensates in this manner, there might be little value in switching. Also, there is a limit to how low a T/N level the consumer will accept because there is a decrease in satisfaction. At some point (about 8 mg tar and 0.3 mg nicotine) smokers begin to lose interest.

Trends in Smoking Behavior

The health warnings and the educational programs certainly had an effect (figure 12.1). After World War II cigarette sales increased, both on a per capita basis and in total sales. The peak year for per capita sales was 1963. In 1964 the

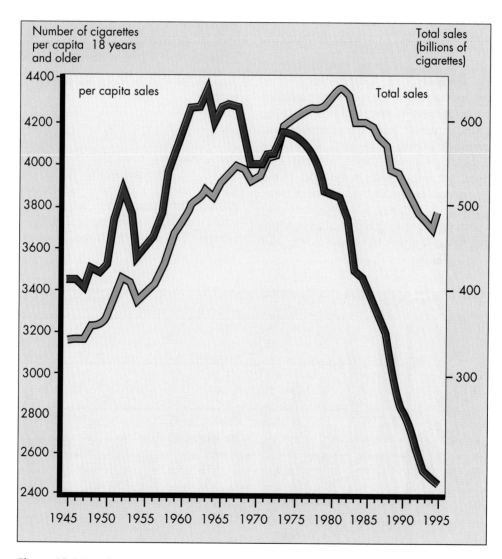

Figure 12.1 Trends in cigarette sales since 1945

Surgeon General's Report on Smoking and Health declared that smoking is a health hazard. For the next several years per capita sales decreased, with a more rapid decrease after 1973. Because of the expanding adult population, total cigarette sales continued to climb slowly even while per capita sales dropped. This trend continued until 1981, when the peak was reached with sales of over 640 billion cigarettes. For the past several years both total and per capita sales have declined. Per capita sales are now lower than at any time since World War II.

For many years a much greater percentage of adult men smoked than adult women. The 1970s saw an alarming increase in smoking among young females: for the first time, in 1976, more female than male high school seniors reported smoking (figure 12.2, data from the annual high school senior survey described in chapter 1). From then through the mid 1980s fewer high school seniors of both genders were smoking, but girls retained a higher smoking rate than boys throughout this period of decline. In the mid-1980s the decline leveled off, and

Workers on a cigarette break outside a smoke-free building.

then smoking rates for high school seniors began to increase again. Slightly greater increases among boys have led to essentially no gender difference in the latest reports. Among adult smokers, men still slightly outnumber women; however, the trend is toward equality.

Figure 12.2 Percentage of high school seniors reporting daily use of cigarettes

Women are also moving toward equality with men in lung cancer, heart disease, and overall life expectancy.

Smokeless Tobacco

In the early 1970s many cigarette smokers apparently began to look for alternatives that would reduce the risk of lung cancer. Pipe and cigar smoking enjoyed a brief, small increase followed by a long period of decline. Sales of **smokeless tobacco** products—specifically different kinds of chewing tobacco, began to increase. Once limited to western movies and the baseball field as far as public awareness was concerned, smokeless tobacco use grew to become a matter of public concern.

The most common types of oral smokeless tobacco in the United States are loose leaf (Red Man, Levi Garrett, Beech Nut), which is sold in a pouch, and **moist snuff** (Copenhagen, Skoal), which is sold in a can. When you see a baseball player on TV with a big wad in his cheek, it is probably composed of loose-leaf tobacco. Sales of loose-leaf tobacco, growing from a traditional base in the Southeast and Midwest, increased by about 50 percent during the decade of the 1970s and then remained stable or declined slightly through the 1980s. Moist snuff is not "snuffed" into the nose in the European manner; a small pinch is dipped out of the can and placed beside the gum, often behind the lower lip. One form of moist snuff also comes in a little teabag type of packet, so that loose tobacco fragments don't stray out onto the teeth. Moist snuff, which has its traditional popularity base in the rural West, continued to show large sales gains into the late 1980s. With all forms of oral smokeless tobacco, nicotine is absorbed through the mucous membranes of the mouth into the bloodstream, and users achieve blood nicotine levels comparable to those of smokers.

Smokeless tobacco enjoys many competitive advantages over smoking. First, it is unlikely to cause lung cancer. Smokeless tobacco is less expensive than cigarettes, with an average user spending only a few dollars a week. In spite of the Marlboro advertisements, a cowboy or anyone else who is working outdoors finds it more convenient to keep some tobacco in his mouth than to try to light cigarettes in the wind and then have ashes blowing in his face. And, believe it or not, chewing might be more socially acceptable than smoking under most circumstances. After all, the user doesn't blow smoke all around, and most people don't even notice when someone is chewing, unless the chewer has one of those huge wads in his mouth or spits frequently. Many users can control the amount of tobacco they put in their mouths so that they don't have to spit very often. What they do with the leftover **quid** of tobacco is a different story and often not a pretty sight.

The use of chewing tobacco had never completely died out in rural areas, and its resurgence was strongest there. It is primarily a male phenomenon, and surveys of high school students in Oregon, Colorado, and Louisiana have found 20 percent to 25 percent of the boys reporting smokeless tobacco use. In one survey of Wyoming junior high school students, about 25 percent of the boys reported being current users of smokeless tobacco, compared with only 1.2 percent of the girls. For the boys, the median reported age of first use was 11 years.[9] Although these studies indicate high rates of regional use, increased sales of smokeless tobacco were not limited to the rural West and South. Promoted by sport celebrities, increased advertising budgets, and sponsorship of auto racing, college

---

smokeless tobacco: term used for chewing tobacco during the 1980s.

moist snuff: finely chopped tobacco, held in the mouth rather than "snuffed" into the nose.

quid: a piece of chewing tobacco.

rodeo, and skiing, smokeless tobacco use increased among young men in many parts of the country. The high school senior class of 1993 reported that 6.4 percent of boys and less than 1 percent of girls were daily users of smokeless tobacco.[10]

Chewing tobacco might not be as unhealthy as smoking it. However, smokeless tobacco is not without its hazards. The one of most concern is the increased risk of cancer of the mouth, pharynx, and esophagus. In spite of the fact that snuff and chewing tobacco are not burned during use, they do contain potent carcinogens, including high levels of tobacco-specific **nitrosamines**. Many users experience tissue changes in the mouth, with **leukoplakia** (a whitening, thickening, and hardening of the tissue) a relatively frequent finding. Leukoplakia is considered to be a precancerous lesion (a tissue change that can develop into cancer). The irritation of the gums can cause them to become inflamed or to recede, exposing the teeth to disease. The enamel of the teeth can also be worn down by the abrasive action of the tobacco. In short, dentists are also becoming more aware of the destructive effects of oral tobacco.

Concerns about these oral diseases led the Surgeon General's office to sponsor a conference and produce a report on that conference, *The Health Consequences of Using Smokeless Tobacco.*[11] This report went into some depth in reviewing epidemiological, experimental, and clinical data, and concluded, "the oral use of smokeless tobacco represents a significant health risk. It is not a safe substitute for smoking cigarettes. It can cause cancer and a number of noncancerous oral conditions and can lead to nicotine addiction and dependence." Packages of smokeless tobacco now carry a series of rotating warning labels describing these dangers.

Cigars Are Back?

After may years of declining popularity, for some unknown reason cigar smoking reap-

peared on the cultural scene in the mid 1990s. Yuppies, businessmen, and celebrities of both sexes began lighting up large, expensive cigars, many of which are made in Florida from tobacco supposedly grown using Cuban seeds. Magazines devoted to cigars, "cigar bars," and radio talk-show discussions of the merits of various $25 "stogies" all point to the trendiness of this phenomenon.[36] Perhaps it's a reaction against the abstinent '80s, with a slight hope that cigars are safer than cigarettes. All the same, it is another example of the unpredicatable faddishness of people's recreational use of psychoactive substances.

A SOCIAL AND ECONOMIC DILEMMA

It is now clear that cigarette smoking is deadly. People have been slow to accept this fact, perhaps partly because tobacco, like alcohol and other substances, has long been the subject of emotional diatribes. In 1604, King James of England (the same one who had the Bible translated) wrote and published a strong antitobacco pamphlet stating that tobacco was "harmefull to the braine, dangerous to the lungs." Never one to let morality or health concerns interfere with business, he also supported the growing of tobacco in Virginia in 1610, and when the crop prospered, he declared the tobacco trade a royal monopoly.

New York City made it illegal in 1908 for a woman to use tobacco in public, and in the Roaring Twenties women were expelled from schools and dismissed from jobs for smoking. These concerns were partly for society and partly to "protect women from themselves." Those sensitive to feminist issues will find an analogy to 1990s America's reactions to drug and alcohol use by pregnant women:

> Smoking by women and even young girls must be considered from a far different stand point than smoking by men, for not only is the female organism by virtue of its much more frail structure

Would tougher laws or enforcement of laws against selling tobacco to minors prevent kids like this from getting cigarettes?

and its more delicate tissues much less able to resist the poisonous action of tobacco than that of men, and thus, like many a delicate flower, apt to fade and wither more quickly in consequence, but the fecundity of woman is greatly impaired by it. Authorities cannot be expected to look on unmoved while a generation of sterile women, rendered incapable of fulfilling their sublime function of motherhood, is being produced on account of the immoderate smoking of foolish young girls.[12]

And those familiar with the 1930s "Reefer Madness" arguments might find it interesting that earlier in the same decade a weed other than marijuana had been blamed for the same ills once laid at alcohol's door:

> Fifty percent of our insanity is inherited from parents who were users of tobacco. . . . Thirty-three percent of insanity cases are caused direct from cigarette smoking and the use of tobacco. . . .
>
> Judge Gimmill, of the court of Domestic Relations of Chicago, declared that, without exception, every boy appearing before him that had lost the faculty of blushing was a cigarette fiend. The poison in cigarettes has the same effect upon girls: it perverts the morals and deadens the sense of shame and refinement. . . .

The bathing beaches have become resorts for women smokers, where they go to show off with a cigarette in their mouths. The bathing apparel in the last ten years has been reduced from knee skirts to a thin tight-fitting veil that scarcely covers two-thirds of their hips. Many of the girl bathers never put their feet in the water, but sit on the shore, show their legs and smoke cigarettes.[13]

Besides people's tendency to be suspicious of anticigarette claims, there are other potent forces that work to keep billions of cigarettes going up in smoke. Everyone knows that the tobacco industry has a lot of clout. Tobacco founded the English colonies and funded the American Revolution. But more significant is the continued economic importance of these products. Recent downturns in total sales have largely been offset by increased prices and reduced manufacturing costs, so that making and selling tobacco products is still a highly profitable business, with net income representing about 18 percent of sales.[14] It is perhaps not surprising that these companies were involved in some of the largest corporate mergers and leveraged buyouts of the 1980s. The large profits made by tobacco companies have made them the targets of an increasing number of lawsuits during the 1990s, and have allowed them to make multi-million dollar settlements with several states to offset increased medical costs.

A lot of people make their living, either directly or indirectly, from tobacco. Tobacco products are sold in 625,000 retail outlets, and total sales are almost $50 billion. Grocery stores sell more cigarettes than any other outlet, and

nitrosamines: (nye *troh* sa meens) a type of chemical that is carcinogenic; several are found in tobacco.

leukoplakia: (luke o *plake* ee ah) a whitening and thickening of the mucous tissue in the mouth, considered to be a precancerous tissue change.

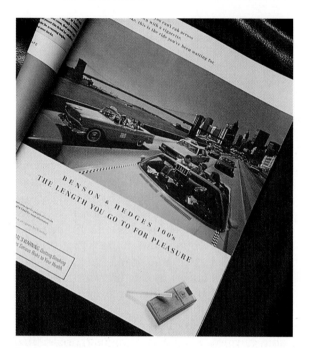

Is cigarette smoking compatible with a health-conscious lifestyle?

recently cigarette sales in gasoline stations have been increasing, whereas the number of vending machines has been cut in half in the past ten years. Cigarette companies were the largest advertisers on television and radio until such ads were banned in 1971. Now they spend their advertising money on magazine and newspaper ads. It has been pointed out that most magazines need those revenues to survive, and they are therefore not likely to print many articles about the dangers of smoking.[15]

Governments, too, derive significant income from tobacco taxes, with almost $6 billion per year going to the federal government and about another $7.5 billion going to the states. Also, at a time in which the trade deficit is of such concern, it is important to remember that the value of tobacco exports exceeds imports by over $5 billion.[7]

CAUSES FOR CONCERN

Although the first clear scientific evidence linking smoking and lung cancer appeared in the 1950s, acceptance of the evidence was slow to come. Each decade brought clearer evidence and more forceful warnings from the Surgeon General. The tobacco industry fought back by establishing in 1954 the Council for Tobacco Research to provide funds to independent scientists to study the health effects of tobacco use. A 1993 expose in the *Wall Street Journal*[16] detailed the manipulation of this "independent" research by tobacco industry lawyers who arranged direct funding for research casting doubt on smoking-related health problems, and who suppressed publication of findings that threatened the industry. In spite of tobacco industry efforts, by now it is abundantly clear that tobacco is America's true "killer weed" and is a bigger public health threat than all the other drug substances combined, including alcohol. It was not until the late 1990s, however, that a tobacco manufacturer admitted that cigarettes have seriously adverse effects on health. These admissions have come as a part of various state-by-state settlements in which the companies reimburse states for increased health-care costs associated with smoking.

Adverse Health Effects

There have been so many government and other reports detailing the health hazards of tobacco use that the smoke has now cleared and we can see the overall picture. If we add it all up it comes out like this: although lung cancer is not common, about 85 percent of all lung cancers occur in smokers. Among deaths resulting from all types of cancer, smoking is estimated to be related to 30 percent, or about 150,000 premature deaths per year. However, cancer is only the second leading cause of death in the United States. It now appears that

Figure 12.3 Mortality ratios (total deaths, mean ages, 55 to 64) as a function of the age at which smoking started and the number of cigarettes smoked per day

smoking might also be related to about 30 percent of deaths from the leading killer, cardio-vascular disease, or about 180,000 premature deaths per year. In addition, cigarette smoking is the cause of 80 to 90 percent of deaths resulting from chronic obstructive lung disease—another 80,000 cigarette-related premature deaths per year. The total "smoking attributed mortality" is over 400,000 premature deaths per year in the United States, representing about 20 percent of all U.S. deaths.[17] No wonder these reports keep saying that "cigarette smoking is the chief,

single, avoidable cause of death in our society and the most important public health issue of our time."

One final comment: think of anything related to good physical health; what the research says is that cigarette smoking will impair it! The earlier the age at which you start smoking and the more smoking you do, and the longer you do it—the greater the impairment (figure 12.3). Smoking doesn't do any part of the body any good, at any time, under any conditions (figure 12.4).

SURGEON GENERAL'S WARNING: Smoking Causes Lung Cancer, Heart Disease, Emphysema, And May Complicate Pregnancy.

SURGEON GENERAL'S WARNING: Quitting Smoking Now Greatly Reduces Serious Risks to Your Health.

SURGEON GENERAL'S WARNING: Smoking By Pregnant Women May Result in Fetal Injury, Premature Birth, And Low Birth Weight.

SURGEON GENERAL'S WARNING: Cigarette Smoke Contains Carbon Monoxide.

Figure 12.4 Cigarette packages and advertisements are required to "rotate" among different warning labels.

In 1990 the U.S. Surgeon General's office released a report on the health benefits of smoking cessation (quitting). This 600-plus page report not only points out once again the increased risk of mortality resulting from smoking but makes it clear that quitting smoking has an immediate impact on a person's chances of living to a ripe old age. For example, a 35-year-old man who quits smoking will on the average increase his life expectancy by 5.1 years. Even a 65-year-old can add an extra year or more of life by quitting smoking.[18]

Passive Smoking

There has been a great deal said and written about **passive smoking**—that is—the inhaling of cigarette smoke from the environment by nonsmokers. The importance of this issue can best be demonstrated by a couple of court cases. In 1976 the Superior Court of New Jersey ruled in favor of a Mrs. Shimp, a telephone company employee who was allergic to cigarette smoke and who worked in a small office along with some smokers. The judge's opinion established several principles:

The evidence is clear and overwhelming. Cigarette smoke contaminates and pollutes the air creating a health hazard not merely to the smoker but to all those around her who must rely upon the same air supply. The right of an individual to risk his or her own health does not include the right to jeopardize the health of those who must remain around him or her in order to properly perform the duties of their jobs. The portion of the population which is especially sensitive to cigarette smoke is so significant that it is reasonable to expect an employer to foresee health consequences and to impose upon him a duty to abate the hazard which causes the discomfort.

In determining the extent to which smoking must be restricted the rights and interests of smoking and nonsmoking employees alike must be considered. The employees' rights to a safe working environment makes it clear that smoking must be forbidden in the work area. The employee who desires to smoke on his own time, during coffee breaks and lunch hours should have a reasonably accessible area in which to smoke.[19]

It is obvious that cigarette smoke can be irritating to others, but is it damaging? Besides the cases of individuals who have lung disorders or are allergic to smoke, is there evidence that cigarette smoke is harmful to exposed nonsmokers? Research is complicated; the smoke rising from the ash of the cigarette (**sidestream smoke**) is higher in many carcinogens than is the mainstream smoke delivered to the smoker's lungs. Of course, it is also more diluted. How many smokers in the room? How much do they smoke? How good is the ventilation? How much time does the nonsmoker spend in this room? These variables have made definitive research difficult, but enough studies have produced consistent enough findings that the Environmental Protection Agency in 1993 declared secondhand smoke to be a known carcinogen and estimated that passive smoking is responsible for several thousand lung cancer deaths each year. The tobacco companies countered with full-page newspaper ads attacking the methods used by the EPA, but a review of the issue by an independent consumer group found that the EPA had used accepted techniques and that the tobacco company objections were based on the opinions of a few industry-funded scientists.[20]

Concerns about the effects of secondhand smoke have led to many more restrictions on smoking in the workplace and in public. Most states and municipalities now have laws prohibiting smoking in public conveyances and requiring the establishment of smoking and nonsmoking areas in public buildings and restaurants, and some communities have banned smoking in all restaurants. A few employers have gone so far as to either encourage or attempt to force their employees to quit smoking both on the job and elsewhere, citing health statistics indicating more sick days and greater health insurance costs associated with smoking. This conflict between smoker and nonsmoker seems destined to get worse before it gets better. Although to some this battle might seem silly, it represents a very basic conflict between individual freedom and public health.

Smoking and Health in Other Countries

Cigarette smoking is a social and medical problem worldwide. A 1994 international report estimated that, worldwide, smoking is killing 3 million people a year and that by the year 2020 the rate might be as high as 10 million per year.[21] As sales level and decline in developed countries, advertising and promotions in Third World countries (touting cigarettes as delivering "the great taste of America") resulted in large increases in exports of American cigarettes throughout the 1970s and 1980s. Asians in particular seem to want American cigarettes, and one of the major efforts has been to open Japanese, Taiwanese, and Korean cigarette markets to U.S. imports.[22] There are *no* warnings printed on the packs we sell to them!

(Shades of patent medicines in the late nineteenth century.) Most of the countries U.S. cigarette manufacturers are exporting to are underdeveloped countries with lots of preventable disease and high infant mortality. According to the World Health Organization, "the control of cigarette smoking could do more to improve health and prolong life in these countries than any single action in the whole field of preventive medicine."[23]

Smoking and Pregnancy

The nicotine, hydrogen cyanide, and carbon monoxide in a smoking mother's blood also reach the developing fetus and have significant negative consequences there. On the average, infants born to smokers are about half a pound lighter than infants born to nonsmokers. This basic fact has been known for almost thirty years and has been confirmed in almost fifty studies.[24] There is a dose-response relationship: the more the woman smokes during pregnancy, the greater the reduction in birth weight. Is the reduced birth weight the result of an increased frequency of premature births or of retarded growth of the fetus? Smoking shortens the gestation period by an average of only two days, and when gestation length is accounted for, the smokers still have smaller infants. Ultrasonic measurements taken at various intervals during pregnancy show smaller fetuses in smoking women for at least the last 2 months of pregnancy. The infants of smokers are normally proportioned, are shorter and smaller than the infants of nonsmokers, and have smaller head circumference. The reduced birth

---

passive smoking: inhalation of tobacco smoke by individuals other than the smoker.

sidestream smoke: smoke arising from the ash of the cigarette or cigar.

How damaging is cigarette smoking to a child's health?

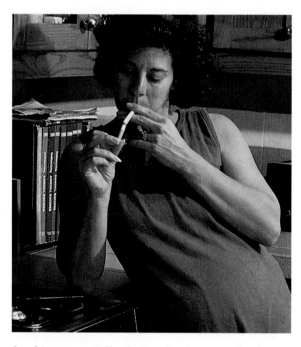

Smoking, especially during the last month of pregnancy, is likely to result in retardation of growth in the fetus.

weight in infants of women smokers is not related to how much weight the mother gains during pregnancy, and the consensus is that reduced availability of oxygen is responsible for the diminished growth rate. Women who give up smoking early in pregnancy (by the fourth month) have infants of similar weight to those of nonsmokers.

Besides the developmental effects evident at birth, several studies indicate small but consistent differences in body size, neurological problems, reading and mathematical skills, and hyperactivity at various ages. It therefore appears that smoking during pregnancy can have long-lasting effects on both the intellectual and the physical development of the child. Several studies have also found an increased risk of sudden infant death syndrome (SIDS) if the mother smokes, but it is not clear if this is related more to the mother's smoking during pregnancy or to passive smoking (the infant's breathing smoke) after birth.

So far we have been talking about normal deliveries of babies. Spontaneous abortion (miscarriage) has also been studied many times in relation to smoking and with consistent results: smokers have more spontaneous abortions than nonsmokers (perhaps 1.5 to 2 times as many). As for congenital malformations, the evidence for a relationship to maternal smoking is not as clear. If there is a small effect here, it could be either related to or obscured by the fact that many smokers also drink alcohol and coffee. One study indicated an increased risk of facial malformations associated with the father's

carbon

nitrogen

Figure 12.5 Nicotine (1-methyl-2 [3-pyridyl] pyrrolidone)

smoking. Neonatal death rates are higher among children of smoking mothers, and this effect is much greater among older women of low socioeconomic status who have had more than three pregnancies.

The overall message is very, very clear. There are definite, serious risks associated with smoking during pregnancy. In fact, the demonstrated effects of cigarette smoking on the developing child are of the same magnitude and type as those reported for the infamous "crack babies," and there are many more pregnant women smoking cigarettes than using cocaine. If a woman smoker discovers herself to be pregnant, that should be a clear signal to her to quit smoking.

PHARMACOLOGY OF NICOTINE

Nicotine is a naturally occurring liquid alkaloid that is colorless and volatile. On oxidation it turns brown and smells much like burning tobacco. Tolerance to its effects develops, along with the dependency that led Mark Twain to remark how easy it was to stop smoking—he'd done it several times!

Nicotine was isolated in 1828 and has been studied irregularly since then. It has no therapeutic actions, so no drug company has exhaustively looked at its effects. Because it has proved to be a valuable pharmacological tool for studying synaptic functions, as well as being the active ingredient in tobacco, there is some relevant information. The structure of nicotine is shown in figure 12.5; it should be noted that there are both *d* and *l* forms, but they are equipotent. It is of some importance that nicotine in smoke has two forms, one with a positive charge and one that is electrically neutral. The neutral form is more easily absorbed through the mucous membranes of the mouth, nose, and lungs.

Absorption and Metabolism

Inhalation is a very effective drug-delivery system; 90 percent of inhaled nicotine is absorbed. The physiological effects of smoking one cigarette have been mimicked by injecting about 1 mg of nicotine intravenously.

Acting with almost as much speed as cyanide, nicotine is well established as one of the most toxic drugs known. In humans, 60 mg is a lethal dose, and death follows intake within a few minutes. A cigar contains enough nicotine for two lethal doses (who needs to take a second one?), but not all of the nicotine is delivered to the smoker or absorbed in a short enough period of time to kill a person.

Nicotine is primarily deactivated in the liver, with 80 to 90 percent being modified before excretion through the kidneys. Part of the tolerance that develops to nicotine might result from the fact that either nicotine or the tars increase the activity of the liver microsomal enzymes that are responsible for the deactivation of drugs. These enzymes increase the rate of deactivation and thus decrease the clinical effects of the benzodiazepines and some antidepressants and analgesics. The final step in eliminating deactivated nicotine from the body may be somewhat slowed by nicotine itself, since it acts on the hypothalamus to cause a release of the hormone that acts to reduce the loss of body fluids.

Physiological Effects

The effect of nicotine on areas outside the CNS has been studied extensively. Nicotine mimics acetylcholine by acting at the nicotinic type of cholinergic receptor site and stimulating the dendrite. Nicotine is not rapidly deactivated, and continued occupation of the receptor prevents incoming impulses from having an effect, thereby blocking transmission of information at the synapse. Thus nicotine first stimulates and then blocks the synapse. This blockage of cholinergic synapses is responsible for some of nicotine's effects, but others seem to be the result of a second action.

Nicotine also causes a release of adrenaline from the adrenal glands and other sympathetic sites and thus has in part a sympathomimetic action. Additionally, it stimulates and then blocks some sensory receptors, including the chemical receptors found in some large arteries and the thermal pain receptors found in the skin and tongue.

The symptoms of low-level nicotine poisoning are well known to beginning smokers

FYI Possible New Painkiller?

One of the early uses of tobacco was as a painkiller. Nicotine itself does have some analgesic properties, but its toxicity limits its usefulness for this. The discovery of a substance in the skin of Ecuadorian "poison-arrow" frogs that binds strongly to nicotinic acetylcholine receptors led in 1997 to the development of a synthetic analgesic with a novel mechanism. Animal testing with ABT-594 indicates that it may be a potent pain reliever with fewer side effects and less addiction potential than morphine and other opiate analgesics.[35] As the drug begins to be tested for safety and then effectiveness in humans, we will learn whether this potentially revolutionary new type of powerful painkiller will live up to its promise.

and small children behind barns and in alleys: nausea, dizziness, and a general weakness. In acute poisoning, nicotine causes tremors that develop into convulsions, terminated frequently by death. The cause of death is suffocation resulting from paralysis of the muscles used in respiration. This paralysis stems from the blocking effect of nicotine on the cholinergic system that normally activates the muscles. With lower doses there is actually an increase in respiration rate because the nicotine stimulates oxygen-need receptors in the carotid artery. At these lower doses of 6 to 8 mg there is also a considerable effect on the cardiovascular system as a result of the release of adrenaline. Such release leads to an increase in coronary blood flow, along with vasoconstriction in the skin and increased heart rate and blood pressure. The increased heart rate and blood pressure increase the oxygen need of the heart but not the oxygen supply. Another action of nicotine with negative health effects is that it increases platelet adhesiveness, which increases the tendency to clot. Within the CNS, nicotine seems to act at the level of the cortex to increase somewhat the frequency of the electrical activity, that is, to shift the EEG toward an arousal pattern.

Smoking

Many effects of nicotine are easily discernible in the smoking individual. The heat releases the nicotine from the tobacco into the smoke. Inhaling while smoking one cigarette has been shown to inhibit hunger contractions of the stomach for up to an hour. That finding, along with a very slight increase in blood sugar level and a deadening of the taste buds, might be the basis for a decrease in hunger after smoking.

In line with the last possibility, it has long been folk lore that a person who stops smoking begins to nibble food and thus gains weight. Some studies support such a finding, but one recent study reported that nicotine might actually increase eating behavior![25] In addition, there is evidence that smoking may increase metabolism rate, so that a weight gain on quitting might be partially due to a decreasing metabolism rate or less energy utilization by the body.

In a regular smoker, smoking results in a constriction of the blood vessels in the skin along with a decrease in skin temperature and an increase in blood pressure. The blood supply to the skeletal muscles does not change with smoking, but in regular smokers the amount of carboxyhemoglobin in the blood is usually abnormally high (up to 10 percent of all hemoglobin). All smoke contains carbon monoxide; cigarette smoke is about 1 percent carbon monoxide, pipe smoke 2 percent, and cigar smoke 6 percent. The carbon monoxide combines with the hemoglobin in the blood so that it can no longer carry oxygen. It is this effect of smoking, a decrease in the oxygen-carrying ability of the blood, that probably explains the shortness of breath

smokers experience when they exert themselves.

The decrease in oxygen-carrying ability of the blood and the decrease in placental blood flow probably are related to the many results showing that pregnant women who smoke greatly endanger their unborn children.

Behavioral Effects

In spite of all the protests and the cautionary statements you might read or hear, the evidence is overwhelming that nicotine is the primary, if not the only, reinforcing substance in tobacco. Monkeys will work very hard when their only reward consists of regular intravenous injections of nicotine. The more nicotine in a cigarette, the lower the level of smoking. Intravenous injections and oral administration of nicotine will decrease smoking under some conditions—but not all.

An ongoing debate—in smokers as well as researchers—is whether nicotine acts to arouse and activate the smoker or whether it calms and tranquilizes the drug user. One review of the literature pointed very nicely to the paradoxical effects of nicotine: "a substantial number of studies have shown that nicotine increases heart rate, blood pressure, and numerous other indices of autonomic arousal; yet rather than producing expected increases of emotional behavior and feelings, it usually decreases emotions."[26]

Most people smoke in a fairly consistent way, averaging one to two puffs per minute, with each puff lasting about two seconds with a volume of 25 ml. This rate delivers to the individual about 1 to 2 μg of nicotine per kg of body weight with each puff. There must be something unique about this dose, because smokers could increase the dose by increasing the volume of smoke with each puff or puffing more often. This dose appears to be optimal for producing stimulation of the cerebral cortex.

Several recent British studies have shown that smokers are able to sustain their attention to a task requiring rapid processing of information from a computer screen much better if they are allowed to smoke before beginning the task. This could be either because the nicotine produces a beneficial effect on this performance or because when the smokers were not allowed to smoke they were suffering from some sort of withdrawal symptom. Subsequent experiments on both smokers and nonsmokers using an oral nicotine tablet established that nicotine improved performance in both groups, at least for a few minutes.[27]

Addiction to Nicotine

Evidence that nicotine is a reinforcing substance in nonhumans, and that most people who smoke want to stop and can't, and that when people do stop smoking they gain weight and exhibit other withdrawal signs, and that people who chew tobacco also have trouble stopping,

led to a need for a thorough look at the addicting properties of nicotine. The 1988 Surgeon General's report provided it, in the form of a 600-page tome.[28] This had been a traditionally difficult subject: not that many years ago psychiatrists were arguing that smoking fulfilled unmet needs for oral gratification and therefore represented a personality defect. It has recently come to light that the cigarette manufacturing company Philip Morris obtained evidence of the addicting nature of nicotine with rats in the early 1980s, but instead of publishing the results they fired the researchers and closed the laboratory.[29] Industry executives in 1994 congressional hearings unanimously testified that nicotine was not addicting, still arguing that smoking is simply a matter of personal choice and that many people have been able to quit. As we should know by now, one can theoretically choose to stop using a drug but have a very difficult time doing so because of the potent rein-

---

UP FOR DEBATE

Should the Federal Government Arrange a Settlement with the Tobacco Companies?

After years of successfully fighting lawsuits brought against them for illness and death among smokers, a series of expensive court judgments in the late 1990s led to proposals for federal legislation that would limit the companies' future liability in exchange for their funding over several years a $350 billion, federal effort to fund research, treatment, and youth-oriented smoking prevention programs. Former FDA Commissioner David Kessler and former Surgeon General C. Everett Koop argued against the proposed settlement, feeling that the companies were being let off with too few concessions. They argued that tobacco taxes should be increased

substantially, which should reduce use somewhat and provide funding for prevention efforts without allowing the companies to avoid big lawsuits. Others recognized that it would be extremely difficult to pass such high taxes and instead have focused on the beneficial programs that could be funded with the tobacco money. As of this writing, the "deal" remained in limbo. Even if the federal government reaches a settlement, several states have sued the tobacco companies to recover the state's share of Medicare costs for treating smoking-related illnesses. This issue is likely to be debated in legislature, courts, and the news media for some time to come.

forcing properties of the substance. That is the case with nicotine. The following conclusions of the 1988 report were pretty strong medicine:

1. Cigarettes and other forms of tobacco are addicting.
2. Nicotine is the drug in tobacco that causes addiction.
3. The pharmacological and behavioral processes that determine tobacco addiction are similar to those that determine addiction to drugs such as heroin and cocaine.

Obviously this statement, although based on an exhaustive review of scientific data, was at one level a political message. It said to Congress and the American people that heroin and cocaine are not in some fundamental way more evil than tobacco. That message met with some predictably negative reactions from the tobacco industry and from some tobacco-state politicians, and the debate continued through the 1994 congressional hearings. Successful lawsuits by former smokers or their survivors finally convinced the tobacco companies that they were going to have to take seriously the issues of toxicity and addictiveness of tobacco products. In 1998 one company even faced criminal charges for growing a high-nicotine strain of tobacco with the presumed intent of manipulating nicotine levels to "hook" more smokers.

For the past several years, research into the mechanism of nicotine dependence has focused on the fact that nicotine produces a release of dopamine in the nucleus accumbens, a major target of the mesolimbic dopamine system described in chapter 5.[30] A recent finding is that the brains of chronic nicotine smokers also show a large reduction in one type of monamine oxidase (MAO), the enzyme that breaks down dopamine and some other neurotransmitters.[31] This slowing of the breakdown of dopamine in chronic smokers might therefore enhance the effect of the dopamine released by each acute dose of nicotine, perhaps contributing to the strength of the dependence on nicotine experienced by most smokers.

SMOKING—HOW NOT TO

When you're young and healthy, it's difficult, if not impossible, to imagine dying, being chronically ill, or having such bad **emphysema** that you can't get enough oxygen to walk across the room without having to stop to catch your breath. By the time you're old enough to worry about those things, it's difficult to change your health habits.

Think about this. If you smoke about a pack a day, you increase your probability of dying of lung cancer by about 1100 percent, of any other cancer by about 200 percent, of respiratory disease by about 400 percent, and of other causes by about 200 percent. Looked at another way, smoking two packs of cigarettes a day decreases the remaining years of your life by 20 percent if you're 35, by 24 percent if you're 45, 29 percent at 55, and 35 percent at 65.[32]

A lot of people want to stop smoking. A lot of people have already stopped. Are there ways to efficiently and effectively help those individuals who want to stop smoking to stop? With any form of pleasurable drug use it is easier to keep people from starting to use the drug than it is to get them to stop once they have started. All the educational programs have had an effect on our society and on our behavior. There are now over 40 million former smokers in the United States, and about 90 percent of them report that they quit smoking without formal treatment programs. There is some indication that those who quit on their own do better than those who have been in a treatment program, but then those who quit on their own also tend not to have been smoking as much or for as long.

One reason it is so hard for people to stop is that a pack-a-day smoker puffs at least 50,000

---

emphysema: (em fah *see* mah) a chronic lung disease characterized by difficulty breathing and shortness of breath.

FYI   Young Children and Cigarette Advertising

In 1992 a flurry of editorial writing and reactions from advertising agencies and cigarette companies were generated by an interesting and unusual experiment. A sample of 229 children, aged three through six, were shown various advertising logos, including the Disney Channel's mouse ears, the Chevrolet and Ford symbols, and the Nike athletic shoe symbol. They were then allowed to match the logos with product symbols—a car, shoe, television, etc. Camel cigarettes' Old Joe the Camel was included, and 30 percent of the three-year-olds and 91 percent of the six-year-olds correctly matched Old Joe with a cigarette. This indicated that cigarette advertising, perhaps especially if it includes a "cartoon" character such as Old Joe, does have a major impact on young children. Such evidence led to federal regulations prohibiting the association of tobacco products with cartoon-like characters, and limiting other forms of advertising such as children's caps and T-shirts with cigarette logos. In 1998 it was revealed that Reynolds tobacco executives had discussed in the 1970s the importance of smokers as young as thirteen or fourteen to their future marketing plans.

how tobacco industry has influenced & society legislation

times a year. That's a lot of individual nicotine "hits" reinforcing the smoking behavior. There are a variety of behavioral treatment approaches to assist smokers who want to quit, and hundreds of research articles have been published on them. Although most of these programs are able to get almost everyone to quit for a few days, by six months 70 to 80 percent of them are smoking again. Some of the programs that combine multiple approaches seem to have better success, with up to 40 percent remaining abstinent for one year.[33]

If nicotine is the critical thing, why not provide nicotine without the tars and carbon monoxide? Prescription nicotine chewing gum became available in 1984, after carefully controlled studies showed it to be a useful adjunct to smoking cessation programs. This gum is now available over the counter. In 1991, several companies marketed nicotine skin patches that allow slow release of nicotine to be absorbed through the wearer's skin.[34] Within a few weeks of their introduction, the producers were unable to keep up with the demand and pharmacies had waiting lists of customers. There have been efforts to introduce smokeless cigarettes, as much for the convenience of a smoker who can't light up as an aid to cutting down or quitting. However, various technical problems have led to these smokeless cigarette products being withdrawn.

There is money to be made helping people quit smoking, especially if it can apparently be done painlessly with a substitute. One problem is that the controlled studies done to demonstrate the usefulness of gum or skin patches have been carried out under fairly strict conditions, with a prescribed quitting period, several visits to the clinic to assess progress, and the usual trappings of a clinical research study, often including the collection of saliva or other samples to detect tobacco use. That's a far cry from buying nicotine gum or a patch off the shelf, with no plan for quitting, no follow-up interviews, and no monitoring. No wonder that some people have found themselves, in spite of warnings, wearing a nicotine patch and smoking at the same time!

Is there an effective nondrug program for quitting smoking? Yes and no. A review of programs and techniques, "Behavioral Treatment of Smoking Behavior,"[33] made a point that is relevant here: There is a lot of variability in the effect of any given program—some people do very well, some very poorly, and if one program won't work for an individual, maybe another one will. The fact is, we don't know enough yet to know which program will be best for any particular individual. If you want to stop smoking, keep trying programs; odds are you'll find one that works . . . eventually.

SUMMARY

- ▲ Tobacco was introduced to Europe and the East after Columbus's voyage to the Americas.
- ▲ As with most other "new" drugs, Europeans either loved tobacco and prescribed it for all ailments or hated it and considered it responsible for many ills.
- ▲ The predominant style of tobacco use went from pipes to snuff to chewing to cigars to cigarettes.
- ▲ The typical modern cigarette is about half as "strong" in tar and nicotine content as a cigarette of forty years ago.
- ▲ Cigarette smoking declined considerably during the 1960s and 1970s, but about 20 percent of young people still become regular smokers.
- ▲ The use of smokeless tobacco increased during the 1980s, causing concerns about increases in oral cancer.
- ▲ Although tobacco continues to be an important economic factor in American society, it is also responsible for more annual deaths than all other drugs combined, including alcohol.

▲ Cigarette smoking is clearly linked to increased risk of heart disease, lung and other cancers, emphysema, and stroke.

▲ There is increased concern about the health consequences of passive smoking.

▲ Smoking cessation leads to immediate improvements in mortality statistics, and new products, including nicotine skin patches, are being widely used by those who wish to quit.

REVIEW QUESTIONS

1. Why was nicotine named after Jean Nicot?

2. Which was the desired species of tobacco that saved the English colonies in Virginia?

3. What techniques have been used to lower the tar and nicotine content of modern cigarettes?

4. Who smokes more, men or women? What effect does age have on this?

5. What is the significance of tobacco-specific nitrosamines?

6. What are the major causes of death associated with cigarette smoking?

7. What evidence is there that passive smoking can harm nonsmokers?

8. What are the effects of smoking during pregnancy?

9. Nicotine acts through which neurotransmitter in the brain? How does it interact with this neurotransmitter?

10. What is the evidence as to why cigarette smoking is so addictive?

Related Internet Sites on Tobacco

NicNet: http://tobacco.arizona.edu/

Action on Smoking and Health: http://ash.org/

Smoking Control Advocacy: http://www.scarcnet.org/

Friends of Tobacco: http://www.fuji-pub.com/fot/

American Cancer Society: http://www.cancer.org/frames.html

And see our *Drugs, Society, and Human Behavior* site for additional links: http://www.uwyo.edu/a&s/psyc/dshb.htm

REFERENCES

1. Stewart GG: A history of the medicinal use of tobacco, 1492–1860, *Med Hist* 11:228–268, 1967.
2. Brooks JE: *The mighty leaf*, Boston, 1952, Little, Brown.
3. Vaughn W, Quoted in Dunphy EB: Alcohol and tobacco amblyopia: a historical survey, *Am J Ophthalmol* 68:573, 1969.
4. Mannino DM and others: Cigarette smoking: an independent risk factor for impotence? *Am J Epidemiol* 140:1003, 1994.
5. Corti: *A history of smoking*, London, 1931, George G Harrap.
6. Heimann RK: *Tobacco and Americans*, New York, 1960, McGraw-Hill.
7. *Tobacco Industry Profile*, Washington, DC, 1996, The Tobacco Institute.

8. Russell MAH: Nicotine intake and its regulation by smokers. In Martin WR and others, editors: *Tobacco smoking and nicotine: a neurobiological approach*, New York, 1988, Plenum Press.

9. Gritz ER, Ksir C, McCarthy WJ: Smokeless tobacco use in the United States: present and future trends, *Ann Behav Med* 7:2, 24–27, 1985.

10. Johnston LD and others: National survey results on drug use from the Monitoring the Future study, 1975–1993. NIH Pub No 94-3809, Washington, DC, 1994, US Government Printing Office.

11. *The health consequences of using smokeless tobacco: a report of the advisory committee to the Surgeon General*, NIH Pub No 86-2874, Washington, DC, 1986, US Government Printing Office.

12. Lorand A: *Life shortening habits and rejuvenation*, Philadelphia, 1927, FA Davis.

13. Eaglin J: The CC cough-fin brand cigarettes, Cincinnati, 1931, Raisbeck.

14. US Public Health Service Office on Smoking and Health: *Smoking, tobacco and health: a fact book*. Washington, DC, 1987, US Government Printing Office.

15. Okie S: The press and cigarette ads: smoke gets in their eyes, New York, 1987, HealthLink, National Center for Health Education.

16. Smoke and mirrors: How cigarette makers keep health question "open" year after year, *Wall Street Journal,* Feb 11, 1993.

17. Bartecchi CE and others: The human costs of tobacco use, *N Engl J Med* 330:907, 1994.

18. *The health benefits of smoking cessation: a report of the Surgeon General*, DHHS Pub No (CDC) 90-8416, Washington, DC, 1990, US Government Printing Office.

19. *Shimp v. New Jersey Bell Telephone Company*, Superior Court of New Jersey, Chancery Division, Salem County, Docket No C-2904-75, filed December 22, 1976.

20. Secondhand smoke: is it a hazard? *Consumer Reports,* Jan 1995.

21. *Mortality from smoking in developed countries*, World Health Organization, 1994.

22. Jain M: Foreign tobacco firms puffing way into Asian market, Associated Press newspaper report, Jan 17, 1988.

23. Broady JE: Personal health, *New York Times,* July 8, 1981.

24. *The health consequences of smoking for women: a report of the Surgeon General*, Washington, DC, 1981, US Government Printing Office.

25. Perkins KA and others: Effects of nicotine on hunger and eating in male and female smokers, *Psychopharmacology* (Berl) 106:53–59, 1992.

26. Gilbert OG: Paradoxical tranquilizing and emotion reducing effects of nicotine, *Psychol Bull* 86(4): 643–662.

27. Wesnes K: Nicotine increases mental efficiency: but how? In Martin WR and others, editors: *Tobacco smoking and nicotine: a neurobiological approach,* New York, 1988, Plenum Press.

`28. *The health consequences of smoking: nicotine addiction, a report of the Surgeon General*, DHHS Pub No (CDC)88-8406. Washington, DC, 1988, US Government Printing Office.

29. Tobacco company suppressed study on nicotine addiction, Associated Press newspaper report, April 1, 1994.

30. Ksir C: Behavioral neuropharmacology of nicotine. In Watson RR, editor: *Drugs of Abuse and Neurobiology.* New York, Raven Press, 1994

31. Fowler JS and others: Inhibition of manoamine oxidase B in the brains of smokers. *Nature* 379: 733, 1996.

32. Rogot E: Smoking and life expectancy among US veterans, Public Health Briefs, *Am J Public Health* 68(10):1023–1025, 1978.

33. Glasgow RE, Bernstein DA: Behavioral treatment of smoking behavior. In Prokop CK, Bradley LA, editors: *Medical psychology,* New York, 1981, Academic Press.

34. Transdermal nicotine study group: transdermal nicotine for smoking cessation, *JAMA* 266:3133–3138, 1991.

35. Strauss E: New nonopioid painkiller shows promise in animal tests, *Science* 279: 32, 1998.

36. Hamiton K: Blowing smoke, *Newsweek,* July 27, 1997

13

Caffeine

KEY TERMS	OBJECTIVES

After reading this chapter, you should be able to:

xanthines
theophylline
theobromine
adenosine
caffeinism

- Describe three plant sources and several other dietary and medical sources for caffeine.
- Discuss the time course of caffeine's action in the body and on behavior.
- Describe the mechanism by which caffeine acts in the brain.
- Describe several physiological and behavioral effects of caffeine.

- Explain the concerns that have been expressed about caffeinism and the potential toxicity of caffeine.
- Identify the potential effects of excessive caffeine use during pregnancy.

THE WORLD'S MOST COMMON PSYCHOSTIMULANT

On a daily basis, more people use caffeine than any other psychoactive drug. Many use it regularly, and there is evidence for dependence and some evidence that regular use can interfere with the very activities people believe that it helps them with. It is now so domesticated that most modern kitchens contain a specialized device for extracting the chemical from plant products (a coffeemaker), but Western societies were not always so accepting of this drug.

How many drugs can lay claim to divine intervention in their introduction to humankind? The **xanthines,** of which caffeine is the best known, have three such legends, and that fact

alone tells you that this has been an important class of drugs throughout the ages.

Coffee

The legends surrounding the origin of coffee are at least geographically correct. The best one concerns an Arabian goatherd named Kaldi who couldn't understand why his goats were bounding around the hillside so playfully. One day he followed them up the mountain and ate some of the red berries the goats were munching. "The results were amazing. Kaldi became a happy goatherd. Whenever his goats danced, he danced and whirled and leaped and rolled about on the ground." Kaldi had taken the first human coffee trip! A holy man took in the scene, and "that night he danced with Kaldi and the goats."

Historic facts of caffeine

de-cafinating coffee

Caffeine in a variety of products

A veritable orgy. The legend continues with Muhammad telling the holy man to boil the berries in water and have the brothers in the monastery drink the liquid so they could keep awake and continue their prayers.[1]

Around A.D. 900 an Arabian medical book suggested that coffee was good for just about everything, including measles and reducing lust. Once something gets into the literature, it's very difficult to change people's minds about it. Women in England argued against the use of coffee over 700 years later, in a 1674 pamphlet titled "The Women's Petition Against Coffee," representing to public consideration the grand inconveniences accruing to their sex from the excessive use of the drying and enfeebling liquor." The women claimed men used too much coffee, and as a result the men were as "unfruitful as those *Desarts* whence that unhappy *Berry* is said to be brought." The women were *really* unhappy, and the pamphlet continued:

> Our Countrymens pallates are become as *Fanatical* as their Brains; how else is't possible they should *Apostatize* from the good old primitive way of Ale-drinking, to run a *Whoreing* after such va-

riety of distructive Foreign Liquors, to trifle away their time, scald their *Chops*, and spend their *Money*, all for a little *base, black, thick, nasty bitter stinking, nauseous* Puddle water.[2]

Some men probably sat long hours in one of the many coffeehouses composing "The Men's Answer to the Women's Petition Against Coffee," which said in part:

> Why must innocent COFFEE be the object of your Spleen? That harmless and healing Liquor, which Indulgent Providence first sent amongst us. . . . Tis not this incomparable fettle Brain that shortens Natures standard, or makes us less Active in the Sports of Venus, and we wonder you should take these Exceptions.[2]

We can all rest easier today and discuss over a cup of coffee the fact that gradually became clear: there is no truth to the idea that coffee diminishes sexual excitability or reduces lust. It is doubtful that the Arabians believed it either, because the use of coffee spread throughout the Muslim world. In Mecca, people spent so much time in coffeehouses that the use of coffee was outlawed and all supplies of the coffee bean were burned. Prohibition rarely works, and coffee speakeasies began to open. Wiser heads prevailed, and the prohibition was lifted.

The middle of the seventeenth century saw the same play enacted but with a new cast of characters and a different locale. Coffeehouses began appearing in England (1650) and France (1671), and a new era began. Coffeehouses were all things to all people: a place to relax, to learn the news of the day, to seal bargains, to plot! This last possibility made Charles II of England so nervous that he outlawed coffeehouses, labeling them "hotbeds of seditious talk and slanderous attacks upon persons in high stations."

---

xanthines: (*zan theens*) the class of chemicals to which caffeine belongs.

King Charles was no more successful than the women. In only eleven days the ruling was withdrawn, and the coffeehouses developed into the "penny universities" of the early eighteenth century. For a penny a cup you could listen to and learn from most of the great literary and political figures of the period. Lloyds of London, the insurance house, started in Edward Lloyd's coffeehouse around 1700.

Across the channel, cheap wine made the need for another social drink less essential in France than in England, but French coffeehouses made at least one contribution to Western culture—the cancan! French cabaret owners were not ready to turn the other cheek, and they fought back: one owner was able to persuade his cancan girls to perform without any bloomers! In spite of this, coffeehouses survived, and coffee consumption increased.

Across the Atlantic, coffee drinking increased in the English colonies, although tea was still their thing. Cheaper and more available than coffee, tea had everything, including, beginning in 1765, a 3-pence-a-pound tax on its importation.

The British Act that taxed tea helped fan the fire that lit the musket that fired the shot heard around the world. That story is better told in connection with tea, but the final outcome was that to be a tea drinker was to be a Tory. Coffee became the new country's national drink.

Coffee use expanded as the West was won, and per capita consumption steadily increased. Some experts became worried about the tendency to "have another cup of coffee," although they believed they could explain it. One wrote:

> The absolute coercion which is imposed on the Americans of the United States by the Prohibition Act with respect to alcohol has necessarily had the result of greatly increasing the use of other excitants and also narcotics. . . . The consumption of coffee has also developed in an undreamt-of manner. In 1919, 929.2 million pounds were consumed and in 1920 as many as 1,360 million pounds. The consumption therefore increased

from 9 to 12.9 pounds per head per year, and is approaching the threshold of abuse.[3]

Funny thing: Prohibition went away, coffee consumption continued to rise. We must have been well over the "threshold of abuse" in 1946 when annual per capita coffee consumption reached an all-time high of twenty pounds. The overall trend has been basically downhill since then, in spite of an upsurge of interest in espresso and specialty coffees in the late 1990s.

Some of the decrease can be attributed to changing lifestyles—sun and fun and convenient canned drinks seem to fit together better, and soft drinks seem to go with fast food. In 1970, Americans still drank more gallons of coffee per capita than of any other nonalcoholic beverage product, but by 1995 Americans consumed over fifty gallons of soft drinks per person, compared to about twenty gallons of coffee.[4]

If the national drink is not as national as it once was, neither is it as simple. Kaldi and his friends were content to simply munch on the coffee beans or put them in hot water. Somewhere in the dark past, probably when the warehouses were burned down, the Middle East discovered that roasting the green coffee bean did not ruin it but, in fact, improved the flavor, aroma, and color of the drink made from the bean. For years housewives, storekeepers, and coffeehouse owners bought the green bean, then roasted and ground it just before use. Commercial roasting started in 1790 in New York City, and the process gradually spread through the country. One problem is that, although the green bean can be stored indefinitely, the roasted bean deteriorates seriously within a month. Ground coffee can be maintained at its peak level in the home only for a week or two, and then only if it is in a closed container and refrigerated. Vacuum packing of ground coffee was introduced in 1900, a process that maintains the quality until the seal is broken.

Coffee growing spread worldwide when the Dutch began cultivation in the East Indies in

Different Stimulants

1696. Latin America had an ideal climate for coffee growing, and with the world's greatest coffee-drinking nation just up the road several thousand miles, it became the world's largest producer. Different varieties of the coffee tree and different growing and processing conditions provide many opportunities for varying the characteristics of coffee.

No one really went commercial with a combination of different coffee beans until J. O. Cheek developed a blend in 1892 and introduced it through a famous Nashville hotel: Maxwell House. The coffee was so well received that the hotel owners let the coffee be named after the hotel.

In the early 1950s about 94 percent of American coffee was from Latin America, but that percentage has steadily declined; today less than half is grown in this hemisphere. Brazil is the principal exporter to the United States, with Colombia second. Both countries grow *arabica*, which has a caffeine content of about 1 percent. *Robusta*, with a caffeine level at 2 percent, is the variety grown in Africa and is usually of a lower grade and price.

The economics of coffee (it is number two in international trade, far behind oil) have as much to do with coffee consumption as does our changing lifestyle. A price increase in the early fifties—to a dollar a pound!—shifted us from being a 40-cups-per-pound nation to being a 60-cups-per-pound nation. This dilution reduced the cost but also the quality of the beverage. Two things happen when prices go up: the quality of the coffee decreases and people drink less coffee.

Instant coffee has been around since before the turn of the century, but sales began their marked increase in the hustle and bustle after World War II: another decrease in the quality of the beverage, but an increase in the convenience. Interestingly, Brazil imports many inexpensive African coffee beans to use in manufacturing instant coffee, because they believe that their coffee is too good to be used in that way.

Variety of caffeine-free products (coffee, tea, pop, weight loss pills, etc.)

In the 1980s, health-conscious Americans began to drink more decaffeinated coffee and less regular coffee. There are several ways of removing caffeine from the coffee bean. In the process used by most American companies, the unroasted beans are soaked in an organic solvent, and there have been concerns about residues of the solvent that might remain in the coffee. The most widely used solvent has been methylene chloride, and studies have shown that high doses of that solvent can cause cancer in laboratory mice. In 1985 the FDA banned the use of methylene chloride in hair sprays, which can be inhaled during use, but allowed the solvent to be used in decaffeination as long as residues did not exceed ten parts per million. Because the solvent residue evaporates during roasting, decaffeinated coffees contain considerably lower amounts than that, so the assumption is that the risk is minimal. The Swiss water process, which is not used on a large commercial scale in the United States, removes more of the coffee's flavor. By the way, the caffeine that is taken out of the coffee is used mostly in soft drinks. One of the largest decaffeinating companies is owned by Coca-Cola.

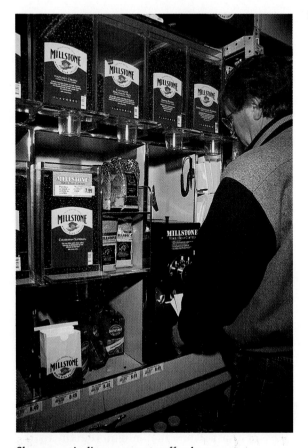

Shopper grinding gourmet coffee beans

Today's supermarket shelves are filled with an amazing variety of products derived from this simple bean—pure Colombian, French Roast, decaf, half-caf, flavored coffees, instants, mixes, and even cold coffee beverages. The competition for the consumer's coffee dollar has never been greater, it seems. And Americans are lining up in record numbers at espresso bars to buy cappuccinos, lattes, and other exotic-sounding mixtures of strong coffee, milk, and flavorings. The number of these specialty coffee shops increased from fewer than 200 in 1989 to more than 5,000 by 1994 and has continued to climb.[5]

Tea

Tea and coffee are not like day and night, but their differences are reflected in the legends surrounding their origins. The bouncing goatherd of Arabia suggests that coffee is a boisterous, blue-collar drink. Tea is a different story: much softer, quieter, more delicate. According to one legend, Daruma, the founder of Zen Buddhism, fell asleep one day while meditating. Resolving that it would never happen again, he cut off both eyelids. From the spot where his eyelids touched the earth grew a new plant. From its leaves a brew could be made that would keep a person awake. Appropriately, the tea tree, *Thea sinensis* (now classed as *Camellia sinensis*), is an evergreen, and *sinensis* is the Latin word for "Chinese."

The first report of tea that seems reliable is in a Chinese manuscript from around A.D. 350, when it was primarily seen as a medicinal plant. The nonmedical use of tea is suggested by an A.D. 780 book on the cultivation of tea, but the real proof that it was in wide use in China is that a tax was levied on it in the same year. Before this time Buddhist monks had carried the cultivation and use of tea to Japan.

Europe had to wait eight centuries to savor the herb that was "good for tumors or abscesses that come from the head, or for ailments of the bladder . . . it quenches thirst. It lessens the desire for sleep. It gladdens and cheers the heart." The first European record of tea, in 1559, says "One or two cups of this decoction taken on an empty stomach removes fever, headache, stomach-ache, pain in the side or in the joints. . . ." Fifty years later, in 1610, the Dutch delivered the first tea to the continent of Europe.

An event that occurred ten years before had tremendous impact on the history of the world and on present patterns of drug use. In 1600 the English East India Company was formed, and Queen Elizabeth gave the company a monopoly on everything from the east coast of Africa across the Pacific to the west coast of South America. In this period the primary imports from the Far East were spices, and the company prospered. A major conflict developed between Dutch and English trade interests over who belonged where in the East. In 1623 a resolution "gave" the Dutch East India Company the islands (the Dutch East Indies), and the English East India Company had to be content with India and other countries on the continent.

The English East India Company concentrated on importing spices, so the first tea was brought to England by the Dutch. As the market for tea increased, the English East India Company expanded its imports of tea from China. Coffee had arrived first, so most tea was sold in coffeehouses. Even as tea's use as a popular social drink expanded in Europe, there were some prophets of doom. A 1635 publication by a physician claimed that, at the very least, using tea would speed the death of those over forty years old. The use of tea was not slowed, however, and by 1657 tea was being sold to the public in England. This was no more than ten years after the English had developed the present word for it: *tea*. Although spelled *tea*, it was pronounced *tay* until the nineteenth century. Before this period the Chinese name *ch'a* had been used, anglicized to either *chia* or *chaw*.

With the patrons of taverns off at coffeehouses living it up with tea, coffee, and chocolate, tax revenues from alcoholic beverages declined. To offset this loss, coffeehouses were licensed, and a tax of 8 pence was levied on each gallon of tea and chocolate sold. To keep at home the profits from the expanding tea trade, Britain banned Dutch imports of tea in 1669, which gave the English East India Company a monopoly. Profit from the China tea trade colonized India, brought about the Opium Wars between China and Britain, and induced the English to switch from coffee to tea. In the last half of the eighteenth century the East India Company carried out a "Drink Tea" campaign

unlike anything ever seen before that time. Advertising, patriotism, low cost on tea, and high taxes on alcohol made Britain a nation of tea drinkers.

It was the same profit motive that led to the American Revolution. Because the English East India Company had a monopoly on importing tea to England and thence to the American colonies, the British government imposed high duties on tea when it was taken from warehouses and offered for sale. But, as frequently happens, when taxes went up, smuggling increased. It reached the point in Britain where more smuggled tea than legal tea was being consumed. The American colonies, ever loyal to the king, had become big tea drinkers, which helped the king and the East India Company stay solvent. The Stamp Act of 1765, which included a tax on tea, changed everything. Even though the Stamp Act was repealed in 1766, it was replaced by the Trade and Revenue Act of 1767, which did the same thing.

These measures made the colonists unhappy over paying taxes they had not helped formulate (taxation without representation), and in 1767 this resulted in a general boycott on the consumption of English tea. Coffee use increased, but the primary increase was in the smuggling of tea. The drop in legal tea sales filled the tea warehouses and put the East India Company in financial trouble. To save the company, in 1773 Parliament gave the East India Company the right to sell tea in the American colonies without paying the tea taxes. The company was also allowed to sell the tea through its own agents, and this would eliminate the profits of the merchants in the colonies.

Several boatloads of this tea, which would be sold cheaper than any before, sailed toward various parts in the colonies. The American merchants would not have made any profit on this tea, and they were the primary ones who rebelled at the cheap tea. Some ships were just turned away from port, but the beginning of the end came with the 342 chests of tea that turned

THE DESTRUCTION OF TEA IN BOSTON HARBOR.

Boston Tea Party

the Boston harbor into a teapot on the night of December 16, 1773.

The revolution in America and the colonists' rejection of tea helped tea sales in Great Britain—to be a tea drinker was to be loyal to the Crown. Many factors contributed to change the English from coffee drinkers to tea drinkers, and the preference for tea persists today. Although their use of coffee increases yearly and that of tea declines, the English are still tea drinkers. The annual per capita consumption of tea in the United Kingdom is about eight pounds, second in the world only to Ireland. In comparison, Americans consume less than one pound of tea per person per year.

From Plant to Pot

Most of the tea (about 70 percent) that comes to America starts life on a 4- to 5-foot bush high in the mountains of Sri Lanka (Ceylon), India, or Indonesia. Unpruned, the bush would grow into a 15- to 30-foot tree, which would be difficult to pluck, as picking tea leaves is called. The pluckers select only the bud-leaf and the first two leaves at each new growth. The bud-leaf is called flowering orange pekoe, the second leaf is larger and called orange pekoe, and the third and largest is pekoe (pekoe is pronounced "peck-ho," not "peak-o"). Thus, orange pekoe is not a variety of tea plant but rather a size and quality of tea leaf; generally the bud-leaf is of the highest quality and the third leaf of lowest quality.

In one day a plucker will pluck enough leaves to make ten pounds of tea as sold in the grocery store. Plucking is done every six to ten days in warm weather as new growth develops on the many branches. The leaves are dried, rolled to crush the cells in the leaf, and placed in a cool, damp place for fermentation (oxidation) to occur. This oxidation turns the green leaves to a bright copper color. Nonoxidized leaves are packaged and sold as green tea, the type used in Chinese restaurants in this country. Oxidized tea is called black tea and accounts for about 98 percent of the tea Americans consume. Oolong tea is greenish-brown, consisting of partially oxidized leaves.

Until 1904 the only choices available were sugar, cream, and lemon with your hot tea. At the Louisiana Purchase Exposition in St. Louis in 1904, iced tea was sold for the first time. It now accounts for 75 percent of all tea consumed in America. Tea lovers found 1904 to be a very good year. Fifteen hundred miles east of the fair, a New York City tea merchant decided to send out his samples in handsewn silk bags rather than tin containers. Back came the orders—send

Tea can be found in many forms—bags, instant powder, and bottled.

us tea, and send it in the same little bags you used to send the samples. From that inauspicious beginning evolved the modern tea bag machinery that cuts the filter paper, weighs the tea, and attaches the tag: all this at a rate of 150 to 180 tea bags per minute.

Pound for pound, loose black tea contains a higher concentration of caffeine than coffee beans. However, because about 200 cups of tea can be made from each pound of dry tea leaves, compared with 50 or 60 cups of coffee per pound, a typical cup of tea has less caffeine than a typical cup of coffee. The caffeine content of teas varies widely, depending on brand and the strength of the brew. Most instant teas have 50 to 60 mg of caffeine per cup.[6]

Most tea is sold in tea bags these days, and the market has been flooded with a variety of tea products. Instant teas, some containing flavorings and sweeteners, are popular for convenience. Flavored teas, which contain mint or spices or other substances along with tea, offer other options. The biggest boom in recent years has been in so-called herbal teas, which mostly contain no real "tea" at all. These teas are made

up of mixtures of other plant leaves and flowers for both flavor and color and have become quite popular among people who avoid caffeine.

It can only gladden and cheer the hearts of tea drinkers to know that the largest seller of tea in America is a company named after a man, born in Scotland of Irish parents, who emigrated to America, became rich and famous in England, and believed in ships with sails right up to the end: Sir Thomas Lipton (1850–1931).

Although tea contains another chemical that derived its name from the tea plant, **theophylline** ("divine leaf") is present only in very small, nonpharmacological amounts in the beverage. Theophylline is very effective at relaxing the bronchial passages and is widely prescribed for use by asthmatics.

Chocolate

Now we come to the third legend, concerning the origin of the third xanthine-containing plant. Long before Columbus landed on San Salvador, Quetzalcoatl, Aztec god of the air, gave humans a gift from paradise: the chocolate tree. Linnaeus was to remember this legend when he named the cocoa tree *Theobroma*, "food of the gods." The Aztecs treated it as such, and the cacao bean was an important part of their economy, with the cacao bush being cultivated widely. Montezuma, emperor of Mexico in the early sixteenth century, is said to have consumed nothing other than fifty goblets of *chocolatl* every day. The *chocolatl*—from the Mayan words *choco* ("warm") and *latl* ("beverage")—was flavored with vanilla but was far from the chocolate of today. It was a thick liquid like honey that was sometimes frothy and had to be eaten with a spoon. The major difference

---

theophylline: (thee *off* a lin) a xanthine found in tea.

was that it was bitter; the Aztecs didn't know about sugarcane.

Cortez introduced sugarcane plantations to Mexico in the early 1520s and supported the continued cultivation of the *Theobroma cacao* bush. When he returned to Spain in 1528, Cortez carried with him cakes of processed cocoa. The cakes were eaten, as well as being ground up and mixed with water for a drink. Although chocolate was introduced to Europe almost a century before coffee and tea, its use spread very slowly. Primarily this was because the Spanish kept the method of preparing chocolate from the cacao bean a secret until the early seventeenth century. When knowledge of the technique spread, so did the use of chocolate.

During the seventeenth century chocolate drinking reached all parts of Europe, primarily among the wealthy. Maria Theresa, wife of France's Louis XIV, had a "thing" about chocolate, and this furthered its use among the wealthy and fashionable. Gradually it became more of a social drink, and by the 1650s chocolate houses were open in England, although usually chocolate was sold alongside coffee and tea in the established coffeehouses.

In the early eighteenth century there were health warnings in England against the use of chocolate, but use expanded. Its use and importance is well reflected in a 1783 proposal in the U.S. Congress that the United States raise revenue by taxing chocolate as well as coffee, tea, liquor, sugar, molasses, and pepper.

Although the cultivation of chocolate never became a matter to fight over, it too has spread around the world. The New World plantations were almost destroyed by disease at the beginning of the eighteenth century, but cultivation had already begun in Asia, and today a large part of the crop comes from Africa.

Until 1828 all chocolate sold was a relatively indigestible substance obtained by grinding the cacao kernels after processing. The preparation had become more refined over the years, but it still followed the Aztec procedure of letting the

Chocolate candy, etc.

pods dry in the sun, then roasting them before removing the husks to get to the kernel of the plant. The result of grinding the kernels is a thick liquid called chocolate liquor. This is baking chocolate. In 1828 a Dutch patent was issued for the manufacture of "chocolate powder" by removing about two-thirds of the fat from the chocolate liquor. The chocolate powder was the forerunner of today's breakfast cocoa.

The fat that was removed, cocoa butter, became important when someone found that if it was mixed with sugar and some of the chocolate powder, it could easily be formed into slabs or bars. In 1847 the first chocolate bars appeared, but it was not until 1876 that the Swiss made their contribution to the chocolate industry by inventing milk chocolate, which was first sold under the Nestlé label. By FDA standards, milk chocolate today must contain at least 12 percent milk solids, although better grades contain almost twice that amount.

When chocolate turns white, it might still be all right to eat, but it is probably old, because the white color comes from the separation of the cocoa butter. Someday when you have the time, you can check on whether your piece of chocolate is all chocolate and properly manufactured. Put it on your tongue: it should melt at body temperature. But be careful! One chocolate lover has said, "Each of us has known such moments of orgastic anticipation, our senses focused at their finest, when control is irrevocably abandoned. Then the tongue possesses, is possessed by, what it most desires; the warm, liquid melting of thick, dark chocolate."[7]

The unique xanthine in chocolate is **theobromine.** It has physiological actions that closely parallel those of caffeine but is much less potent in its effects on the central nervous system. The average cup of cocoa contains about 200 mg of theobromine but only 4 mg of caffeine. Table 13.1 compares the caffeine contents of various forms of coffee, tea, and chocolate.

TABLE 13.1
Caffeine in Beverages and Foods

Item	Caffeine (mg)	
	Average	Range
Coffee (5 oz cup)		
Brewed, drip method	115	60–180
Brewed, percolater	80	40–170
Instant	65	30–120
Decaffeinated, brewed	3	2–5
Decaffeinated, instant	2	1–5
Tea (5 oz cup)		
Brewed, major U.S. brands	40	20–90
Brewed, imported brands	60	25–110
Instant	30	25–50
Iced (12 oz glass)	70	67–76
Cocoa beverage (5 oz cup)	4	2–20
Chocolate milk beverage (8 oz glass)	5	2–7
Milk chocolate (1 oz)	6	1–15
Dark chocolate, semi-sweet (1 oz)	20	5–35
Baker's chocolate (1 oz)	26	26
Chocolate-flavored syrup (1 oz)	4	4

OTHER SOURCES OF CAFFEINE

Soft Drinks

The early history of cola drinks is not shrouded in the mists that veil the origins of the other xanthine drinks, so there is no problem in selecting the correct legend. And that's what the story of Coca-Cola is: a true legend in our time. From a green nerve tonic in 1886 in Atlanta, Georgia, that did not sell well at all, Coca-Cola has grown into . . . but you *know* what it is— everyone does everywhere! Unbelievable, it must be "the real thing" and provide "the pause that refreshes," or else it couldn't sell over two billion cases a year worldwide. And that includes mainland China, where it's called "Ke Koy Ke Le"—which translated means "tasty happiness."[8] Yes, "Coke is it!"

Dr. J. C. Pemberton's tonic contained caramel, fruit flavoring, phosphoric acid, caffeine, and a secret mixture called Merchandise No. 5. A friend, F. M. Robinson, suggested the name by which it is still known: *Coca-Cola.* The unique character of Coca-Cola and its later imitators comes from a blend of fruit flavors that makes it impossible to identify any of its parts. An early ad for Coca-Cola suggests its varied uses:

> The "INTELLECTUAL BEVERAGE" and TEMPERANCE DRINK contains the valuable TONIC and NERVE STIMULANT properties of the Coca plant and Cola (or Kola) nuts, and makes not only a delicious, exhilarating, refreshing and invigorating Beverage, (dispensed from the soda water fountain or in other carbonated beverages), but a valuable Brain Tonic, and a cure for all nervous affections—SICK HEADACHE, NEURALGIA, HYSTERIA, MELANCHOLY, &c.[9]

Coca-Cola was touted as "the new and popular fountain drink, containing the tonic

> **theobromine:** (thee oh *broh* meen) a xanthine found in chocolate.

properties of the wonderful coca plant and the famous cola nut." You must remember that this was the period of Sherlock Holmes, Sigmund Freud, and patent medicine—all saying very good things about the product of the coca plant: cocaine. In 1903 the company admitted that there were small amounts of cocaine in its beverage, but soon after that they quietly removed it all; a government analysis of Coca-Cola in 1906 did not find any.

The name *Coca-Cola* was originally conceived to indicate the nature of its two ingredients with tonic properties. The suggestion of the presence of extracts of coca leaves and cola (kola) nuts in the beverage was supposed to be furthered by the use on each bottle of a pictorial representation of the leaves and nuts. Unfortunately the artist-glass blower didn't know that the coca and cacao plants were different, so the bottle had kola leaves and cacao pods! In 1909 the FDA seized a supply of Coca-Cola syrup and made

two charges against the company. One was that it was misbranded because it contained "no coca and little if any cola" and second, that it contained an "added poisonous ingredient," caffeine.

Before the 1911 trial in Chattanooga, Tennessee, the company paid for some research into the physiological effects of caffeine, and when all the information was in, the company won. The government appealed the decision. In 1916 the U.S. Supreme Court upheld the lower court by rejecting the charge of misbranding, stating that the company has repeatedly said that "certain extracts from the leaves of the coca shrub and the nut kernels of the cola tree were used for the purpose of obtaining a flavor" and that "the ingredients containing these extracts" with the cocaine eliminated is called Merchandise No. 5. The way this is done today is that coca leaves are imported by a pharmaceutical company in New Jersey. The cocaine is extracted for medical use and the decocainized leaves are

Soft-drink manufacturers each offer a wide variety of products these days to take advantage of every corner of the market.

shipped to the Coca-Cola plant in Atlanta, where Merchandise No. 5 is produced. A 1931 report indicated that Merchandise No. 5 contained an extract of three parts coca leaves and one part cola nuts, but to this day it remains a secret formula. Then there was the problem of the caffeine:

> It is clear that the only question arising under section 7 is whether the caffeine in the Coca Cola is an "added poisonous or other added deleterious ingredient which may render such article injurious to health."[10]

The question of whether caffeine was an "added poisonous ingredient" was not so readily resolved. Caffeine was added, but it was an essential part of the Coca-Cola formula. In that respect it was not added above and beyond the essential ingredients; it was one of them. The Supreme Court said that the lower courts should decide whether the caffeine made the drink injurious to health. At that time the company substantially reduced the amount of caffeine in its syrup, and the government never felt it had a case worth pursuing beyond that point.

In 1981 the FDA changed its rules so that a "cola" no longer has to contain caffeine. If it does contain caffeine, it may not be more than 0.02 percent, which is 0.2 mg/ml, or a little less than 6 mg per ounce. Some consumer and scientist groups believe that all cola manufacturers should indicate on the label the amount of caffeine the beverage contains. This has not happened, even though soft drinks, as with other food products, must now list nutrition information such as calories, fat, sodium, and protein content.

Table 13.2 lists some popular soft drinks along with their caffeine content in a twelve-ounce serving. Diet soft drinks, now mostly sweetened with aspartame, and caffeine-free colas are commanding a larger share of the market, but regular colas are still the single most popular type of soft drink. As with beers and some other products, the modern marketing

TABLE 13.2
Caffeine in Popular Soft Drinks

Brand	Caffeine* (mg)
Sugar-Free Mr. Pibb	58.8
Mountain Dew	54.0
Mello Yello	52.8
Tab	46.8
Coca-Cola	45.6
Diet Coke	45.6
Shasta Cola	44.4
Mr. Pibb	40.8
Dr. Pepper	39.6
Big Red	38.4
Pepsi-Cola	38.4
Diet Pepsi	36.0
Pepsi Light	36.0
RC Cola	36.0
Diet Rite	36.0
Canada Dry Jamaica Cola	30.0
Canada Dry Diet Cola	1.2

*Per 12-oz serving.

strategy seems to be for each company to try to offer products of every type, in order to cover the market. Also as with beers, the large companies are buying up their competitors: In 1990 the Coca-Cola and PepsiCo companies represented more than 70 percent of total shipments. Coca-Cola Classic remains the most popular single brand, with almost 20 percent of the total market. We saw earlier that soft drinks have become increasingly popular. Per capita consumption of soft drinks has continued to edge upward and is now over fifty gallons per year.

"Extreme" Beverages

Spurred by the huge marketing success of Mountain Dew among young consumers, in the late 1990s several companies introduced high-caffeine drinks with frankly suggestive advertising: "high energy"; "feed the rush"; "blow your mind"; and "raw, primal power."[11] Some of these drinks are no more than caffeine and water; others resemble soft drinks or fruit drinks, adorned with symbols such as lightning bolts. Although the overall market for these

TABLE 13.3

Caffeine Content of OTC Drugs

Drug	Caffeine (mg)
Stimulants	
No Doz	100
Vivarin	200
Analgesics	
Anacin	32
Excedrin	65
Goody's Headache Powders	32.5
Midol	32.4
Vanquish	33
Cold remedies	
Coryban-D	30
Triaminicin	30
Diuretics	
Aqua-Ban	100
Maximum-strength Aqua-Ban plus	200

products is not yet clear, they have become very popular among young children and teenagers, causing concern about the potential for behavioral disturbance and for dependence.

Over-the-Counter Drugs

Few people realize that many nonprescription drugs also include caffeine, some in quite large amounts. Table 13.3 lists the caffeine content of some of these drugs. Presumably many people who buy "alertness tablets" such as No Doz are aware that they are buying caffeine. But many buyers of such things as Excedrin might not realize how much caffeine they are getting. Imagine the condition of someone who took a nonprescription water-loss pill, a headache tablet, and a cold tablet all containing caffeine, and who then drank a couple of cups of coffee!

A 1985 report[12] described a study in which 400 men and women were asked to report on their consumption over a three-day period of all foods, beverages, and medications that might contain caffeine. Only 11 of the 400 did not take in any caffeine at all, and the total intake averaged around 400 mg per day. The sources of this intake in both men and women are reported in table 13.4.

CAFFEINE PHARMACOLOGY

Xanthines are the oldest stimulants known. *Xanthine* is a Greek word meaning "yellow." Yellow is the color of the residue that remains after xanthines are heated with nitric acid until dry. The three xanthines of primary importance are caffeine, theophylline, and theobromine. These three chemicals are methylated xanthines and are closely related alkaloids. Most alkaloids are insoluble in water, but these are unique, because they are slightly water soluble.

These three xanthines have similar effects on the body. Caffeine has the greatest effect. Theobromine has almost no stimulant effect on the central nervous system and the skeletal muscles. Theophylline is the most potent, and caffeine the least potent, agent on the cardiovascular system. Caffeine, so named because it was isolated from coffee in 1820, has been the most extensively studied and, unless otherwise indicated, is the drug under discussion here.

Time Course

In humans, absorption of caffeine is rapid after oral intake; peak blood levels are reached 30 minutes after ingestion. Although maximal CNS effects are not reached for about two hours, the onset of effects can begin within half an hour after intake. The half-life of caffeine in humans is about three hours, and no more than 10 percent is excreted unchanged.

Cross-tolerance exists among the methylated xanthines; loss of tolerance can take more than two months of abstinence. The tolerance, however, is low grade, and, by increasing the dose two to four times, an effect can be obtained even in the tolerant individual. There is less tolerance

TABLE 13.4

Caffeine Consumption during a 72-Hour Period among 173 Men and 228 Women

Source	Men Caffeine consumption (mg)	% of total caffeine intake	Reported use during study period (%)	Women Caffeine consumption (mg)	% of total caffeine intake	Reported use during study period (%)
Coffee	914.86	79.2	79.29	970.07	76.2	83.8
Tea	111.75	9.7	34.7	125.58	9.9	40.8
Soft drinks	65.79	5.7	28.9	75.82	6.0	28.1
Chocolate beverages	2.43	0.2	10.4	4.32	0.3	18.0
Bar chocolate	7.19	0.6	23.7	5.73	0.5	22.4
OTC drugs	48.32	4.2	21.4	92.17	7.2	26.8
TOTAL	1150.34			1273.69		

to the CNS stimulation effect of caffeine than to most of its other effects. The direct action on the kidneys, to increase urine output, and the increase of salivary flow do show tolerance.

Dependence on caffeine is real (see the Up for Debate box on p. 305. People who are not coffee drinkers or who have been drinking only decaffeinated coffee often report unpleasant effects (nervousness, anxiety) after being given caffeinated coffee, but those who regularly consume caffeine report mostly pleasant mood states after drinking coffee. Various experiments have reported on the reinforcing properties of caffeine in regular coffee drinkers; one of the most clear-cut allowed patients on a research ward to choose between two coded instant coffees, identical except that one contained caffeine. Subjects had to choose at the beginning of each day which coffee they would drink for the rest of that day. Subjects who had been drinking caffeine-containing coffee before this experiment almost always chose the caffeine-containing coffee.[13] Thus the reinforcing effect of caffeine probably contributes to psychological dependence.

There has long been clear evidence of physical dependence on caffeine as well. The most reliable withdrawal sign is a headache, which occurs an average of 18 to 19 hours after the most recent caffeine intake. Other symptoms include increased fatigue and decreased sense of vigor. These withdrawal symptoms are strongest during the first two days of withdrawal, then decline over the next five or six days.[14]

Mechanism of Action

For years no one really knew the mechanism whereby the methylxanthines had their effects on the CNS. In the early 1980s, evidence was presented that caffeine and the other xanthines block the brain's receptors for a substance known as adenosine, which is a neurotransmitter or neuromodulator. Adenosine normally acts in several areas of the brain to produce behavioral sedation by inhibiting the release of other neurotransmitters. Caffeine's stimulant action results from blocking the receptors for this inhibitory effect.[15] Now that this mechanism

> **adenosine:** (a *den* o sen) an inhibitory neurotransmitter through which caffeine acts.

is understood, it may lead to the development of new chemicals having similar but perhaps more potent effects.

Physiological Effects

The pharmacological effects on the CNS and the skeletal muscles are probably the basis for the wide use of caffeine-containing beverages.

With two cups of coffee taken close together (about 200 mg of caffeine), the cortex is activated, the EEG shows an arousal pattern, and drowsiness and fatigue decrease. This CNS stimulation is also the basis for "coffee nerves," which can occur at low doses in sensitive individuals and in others when they have consumed large amounts of caffeine. In the absence of tolerance, even 200 mg will increase the time it takes to fall asleep and will cause sleep disturbances. There is a strong relationship between the mood-elevating effect of caffeine and the extent to which it will keep the individual awake.

Higher dose levels (about 500 mg) are needed to affect the autonomic centers of the brain, and heart rate and respiration can increase at this dose. The direct effect on the cardiovascular system is in opposition to the effects mediated by the autonomic centers. Caffeine acts directly on the vascular muscles to cause dilation, whereas stimulation of the autonomic centers results in constriction of blood vessels. Usually dilation occurs, but in the brain the blood vessels are constricted, and this constriction might be the basis for caffeine's ability to reduce migraine headaches.

The opposing effects of caffeine, directly on the heart and indirectly through effects on the medulla, make it very difficult to predict the results of normal (that is, less than 500 mg) caffeine intake. At higher levels there is an increase in heart rate, and continued use of large amounts of caffeine can produce an irregular heartbeat in some individuals.

The basal metabolic rate might be increased slightly (10 percent) in chronic caffeine users, because 500 mg has frequently been shown to have this effect. This action probably combines with the stimulant effects on skeletal muscles to increase physical work output and decrease fatigue after use of caffeine.

Behavioral Effects

Stimulation

A hundred years ago the French essayist Balzac spoke with feeling when describing the effects of coffee:

> It causes an admirable fever. It enters the brain like a bacchante. Upon its attack, imagination runs wild, bares itself, twists like a pythoness and in this paroxysm a poet enjoys the supreme possession of his faculties; but this is a drunkenness of thought as wine brings about a drunkenness of the body.[16]

In the original French the description is even more stimulating and erotic. Unfortunately it does not refer to the effect most people receive from their morning cup of coffee. The hard research data are not so uniformly positive—the effects of caffeine depend on the difficulty of the task, the time of day, and to a great extent on how much caffeine the subject normally consumes. When regular users of "high" amounts of caffeine (more than 300 mg/day, only the equivalent of three cups of brewed coffee) were tested on a variety of study-related mental tasks without caffeine, they performed more poorly than users of low amounts, perhaps because of withdrawal effects. Although their performance was improved after being given caffeine, they still performed more poorly on several of the tasks than users of low amounts. It seems as though the beneficial short-term effects can be offset by the effects of tolerance and dependence in regular users.[17] There has been a report that high

UP FOR DEBATE

Caffeine Dependence Syndrome?

As reviewed in chapter 3, the American Psychiatric Association's *DSM-IV* lists the criteria for substance abuse, substance dependence, substance withdrawal, and substance intoxication. The team that developed this latest revision did not iclude caffeine among the substances that would be considered to produce substance dependence. However, in 1994 a group of researchers reported the cases of 16 individuals who they considered to meet the general criteria for a *DSM-IV* diagnosis of substance disorder.[33]

Of 99 subjects who responded to newspaper notices asking for volunteers who believed they were psychologically or physically dependent on caffeine, 27 were asked to undergo further testing, which included a psychiatric interview to assess caffeine dependence. Although the *DSM-IV* requires that only 3 of 7 criteria be met for a diagnosis of dependence, this study was more conservative in that they required 3 of the 4 most serious criteria (tolerance, withdrawal, persistent desire or efforts to cut down, and continued use despite knowledge of a persistent or recurrent problem caused by use). Sixteen of the 27 were diagnosed as having caffeine dependence using these criteria.

Of those 16, 11 agreed to participate in a double-blind caffeine withdrawal experiment. All were placed on a restricted diet during two 2-day study periods and were given capsules to take at various times of the day to match their normal caffeine intake. During one of the two sessions, each subject was given caffeine, and during the other session the capsules contained a placebo. Neither the subjects nor the interviewers were told on which session they were getting the caffeine. Withdrawal symptoms found during the placebo session included headaches, fatigue, decreased vigor, and increased depression scores. Several of the subjects were unable to go to or stay at work, went to bed several hours early, or needed their spouse to take over child-care responsibilities.

A decision to accept caffeine dependence syndrome as an official diagnosis would have several implications—some feel that it might trivialize the diagnosis for "serious" drug dependence or complicate questions of insurance payment for treatment of substance dependence. Others feel that this syndrome can be a serious dependence disorder for some coffee drinkers and deserves to be recognized as such.

---

levels of caffeine consumption among college students are associated with lower academic performance.[18]

There is considerable evidence that 200 to 300 mg of caffeine will partially offset fatigue-induced decrement in the performance of motor tasks. Like the amphetamines, but to a much smaller degree, caffeine prolongs the amount of time an individual can perform physically exhausting work.

Headache

It has already been mentioned that caffeine's vasoconstricitve effects are considered to be responsible for the drug's ability to relieve migraine headaches. However, a recent study of nonmigraine headache pain found that caffeine reduced headache pain, even in individuals who normally consume little or no caffeine (in other words, not only headaches resulting from caffeine withdrawal).[19] As for migraine headaches, in 1998 the FDA allowed the relabeling of extra-strength Excedrine, which contains 65 mg caffeine, for over-the-counter use as "Excedrine Migraine."

Hyperactivity

Many studies have looked at the effect of caffeine on the behavior of hyperkinetic children (see chapter 6) and most have not shown any therapeutic effect. One report[20] of the effects of 3 and 10 mg/kg of caffeine on normal 8- to 13-year-old boys showed decreased reaction times and increased vigilance along with increased motor activity. That's pretty much what might be expected from a mild stimulant.

Sobering Up

Even the television ads tell you—make that "one last drink for the road" coffee. There is not a lot of evidence to support the value of this. Caffeine will not lower blood alcohol concentration, but it might arouse the drinker. As they say—put coffee in a sleepy drunk and you get a wide-awake drunk. You can easily imagine that this might be more dangerous than if the drunk had been left to sleep it off.

CAUSES FOR CONCERN

Caffeine is one of those drugs that seem to always be in trouble. It's always suspected of doing bad things. Because it is probably the most widely used psychoactive drug in the world (it's acceptable to those in the Judeo-Christian as well as Islamic traditions), it is understandable that it would elicit both good and bad reports. Although it is important to point out that there is not yet clear evidence that moderate caffeine consumption is dangerous, the scientific literature has investigated the possible effects of caffeine in cancer, benign breast disease, reproduction, and heart disease. Part of the problem in knowing for certain about some of these things is that epidemiological research on caffeine consumption is difficult to do well. Coffee drinkers also tend to smoke more, for example, so the statistics have to correct for smoking behavior. Also, some studies have asked only how many cups of coffee people drink per day, without correcting for decaffeinated coffee, tea, colas, or other sources of caffeine, or without correcting for differences between weekend and weekday coffee drinking.[21]

Cancer

In the early 1980s there was a report that coffee drinkers have an increased risk of pancreatic cancers. However, the studies since then have criticized procedural flaws in that report and have found no evidence of such a link. The 1984 American Cancer Society nutritional guidelines indicated that there is no reason to consider caffeine a risk factor in human cancer.

Benign Breast Disease

A relationship has been suggested between use of the methylxanthines and *fibrocystic breast disease*. This is not a form of breast cancer, but a condition in which benign lumps form in a woman's breasts. The condition can also be quite painful. The early studies have been criticized for not having proper controls, and in 1984 the AMA's Council on Scientific Affairs concluded that "there is currently no scientific basis for associating methylxanthine consumption with fibrocystic disease of the breast."

A large study[22] of all types of benign breast diseases found no significant relationship to caffeine use. This study, which appeared in 1985, was widely cited as indicating that there might be no such risk associated with caffeine. The author who originally reported the positive relationship continued to maintain that patients with fibrocystic disease who stop the use of coffee and other methylxanthines will improve.[23] However, a controlled clinical trial found no such improvement when patients were put on a caffeine-free diet.[24] The bottom line? As of yet, there is no clear evidence that anyone should not drink coffee or colas in moderation. However, anyone who has received a diagnosis of sensitive benign breast disease might want to consider stopping consumption of all coffee, tea, colas, and other sources of methylxanthines to see if this will help to improve the condition.

Reproductive Effects

Although studies in pregnant mice have indicated that large doses of caffeine can produce skeletal abnormalities in the pups, studies on humans have not found a relationship between caffeine and birth defects.[25] Recent studies do strongly suggest that caffeine consumption by a woman can reduce her chances of becoming pregnant,[26] increase the chances of spontaneous abortion (miscarriage), and slow the growth of the fetus so that the baby weighs less than normal at birth.[27] The most controversial of these findings has been the reported increase in spontaneous abortion, which is found in some studies,[28] but not in others.[29] This is an issue of obvious importance, so for now the best advice for a woman who wants to become pregnant, stay pregnant, and produce a strong, healthy baby, is to avoid caffeine, alcohol, tobacco, and any other drug that is not absolutely necessary for her health.

Heart Disease

There are many reasons for believing that caffeine might increase the risk of heart attacks, including the fact that it increases heart rate and blood pressure. Until recently, there were about as many studies that found no relationship between caffeine use and heart attacks as there were studies that found such a relationship. One very interesting report used a somewhat different approach. Rather than ask people who had just had heart attacks about their prior caffeine consumption and compare them with people who were hospitalized for some other ailment (the typical retrospective study), this study began in 1948 to track male medical students enrolled in the Johns Hopkins Medical School.[30] More than 1,000 of these subjects were followed for twenty years or more after graduation and were periodically asked about various habits, including drinking, smoking, and coffee consumption. Thus this was a prospective study, to see which of these habits might predict future health problems. Those who drank five or more cups per day were about 2.5 times as likely as nondrinkers to suffer from coronary heart disease. This result and recent indications that coffee drinking can increase blood cholesterol levels have stimulated more research, including a large-scale retrospective study that reported that the incidence of nonfatal heart attacks in men under 55 years old was directly related to the amount of coffee consumed, among both smokers and nonsmokers. Those drinking five or more cups per day were about twice as likely to suffer a heart attack as those who drank no coffee.[31]

The best research, then, gives a strong suggestion that caffeine can increase the risk of heart attacks. This would be of special concern to those with other risk factors (e.g., smoking, family history of heart disease, overweight, high blood pressure, high cholesterol levels).

Caffeinism

Caffeine is not terribly toxic, and overdose deaths are extremely rare. It is estimated that over 10 g (equivalent to 100 cups of coffee) would be required to cause death from oral caffeine taken by mouth. Death is produced by convulsions, which lead to respiratory arrest.

How Much Caffeine Do You Use?

How many different products do you use that contain caffeine (see tables 13.1 to 13.3)? Keep a complete record of your own intake of coffee, tea, soft drinks, and so on for a typical three-day period (72 hours). From that record, estimate as closely as you can your total caffeine intake in milligrams. If you regularly consume 300 mg or more per day, you might ask yourself if caffeine is interfering with your sleep, work, or studying.

However, **caffeinism** (high intake of caffeine) can cause a variety of unpleasant symptoms, and because of caffeine's domesticated social status it might be overlooked as the cause. For example, nervousness, irritability, tremulousness, muscle twitching, insomnia, flushed appearance, and elevated temperature can all result from excessive caffeine use. There can also be palpitations, heart arrhythmias, and gastrointestinal disturbances. In several cases in which serious disease has been suspected, the symptoms have miraculously improved when coffee was restricted.

SUMMARY

- ▲ The ancient plants coffee, tea, and cacao all contain caffeine and two related xanthines.
- ▲ Caffeine is also contained in soft drinks and nonprescription medicines.
- ▲ Caffeine has a longer-lasting effect than many people realize.

---

caffeinism: excessive use of caffeine.

▲ Caffeine exerts a stimulating action in several brain regions by blocking inhibitory receptors for adenosine.

▲ In regular caffeine users, headache, fatigue, or depression can develop if caffeine use is stopped.

▲ Caffeine is capable of reversing the effects of fatigue on both mental and physical tasks, but it might not be able to improve the performance of a well-rested individual, particularly on complex tasks.

▲ Excessive caffeine consumption, referred to as *caffeinism,* can produce a panic reaction.

▲ Daily use of large amounts of caffeine increases the risk of heart attack.

▲ Caffeine use during pregnancy is not advisable.

Related Internet Sites on Caffeine

The Caffeine Archive: http://www.austinlinks.com/General/caffeine.html

Caffeine FAQ: http://www.seas.upenn.edu/~cpage/caffeine/FAQmain.html

And, our own highly stimulating *Drugs, Society, and Human Behavior* site: http://www.uwyo.edu/A&S/psyc/dshb.htm

REVIEW QUESTIONS

1. What role did the American Revolution and alcohol prohibition play in influencing American coffee consumption?

2. What are the differences among black tea, green tea, and oolong?

3. What are the two xanthines contained in tea and chocolate, besides caffeine?

4. Rank the caffeine content of a cup of brewed coffee, a cup of tea, a chocolate bar, and a twelve-ounce Coca-Cola.

5. How does caffeine interact with adenosine receptors?

6. What are some of the behavioral and physiological effects of excessive caffeine consumption?

7. Describe the effects of caffeine on migraine headaches, caffeine-withdrawal headaches, and other headaches.

8. Give an informed reaction to the statement that caffeine increases the risk of breast cancer.

9. What are three possible ways in which caffeine use by a woman might interfere with reproduction?

10. What is the relationship between caffeine and panic attacks?

REFERENCES

1. Uribe Compuzano A: *Brown gold,* New York, 1954, Random House.

2. Meyer H: *Old English coffee houses,* Emmaus, PA, 1954, Rodale Press.

3. Lewin L: *Phantastica, narcotic, and stimulating drugs,* New York, 1931, EP Dutton.

4. *Statistical abstract of the United States,* US Department of Commerce, Washington, DC, 1997, US Government Printing Office.

5. A business built on beans, *Consumer Reports,* Oct 1994.

6. Groisser DS: A study of caffeine in tea, *Am J Clin Nutr* 31(10):1727–1731, Oct 1978.

7. Prial FJ: Secrets of a chocoholic, *New York Times,* May 16, 1979.

8. Sterba JP: Coke brings "tasty happiness" to China, *New York Times,* April 16, 1981.

9. Huisking CL: *Herbs to hormones,* Essex, CT, 1968, Pequot Press.

10. Sixth Circuit Court of Appeals, 1914: 215 *Federal Reporter* 539, June 13, 1914.

11. Barboza D: Caffeine-loaded "extreme beverages" go after the youth market, *New York Times,* August 22, 1997.

12. Weidner G, Istvan J: Dietary sources of caffeine, *N Engl J Med* 313:1421, 1985.

13. Griffiths RR and others: Human coffee drinking: reinforcing and physical dependence producing effects of caffeine, *J Pharmacol Exp Ther* 239:416–425, 1986.

14. Hughes JR and others: Should caffeine abuse, dependence, or withdrawal be added to DSM-IV and ICD-10? *Am J Psychiatry* 149:33, 1992.

15. Feldman RS, Meyer JS, Quenzer LF: Principles of Neuropsychopharmacology, Sunderland, MA, 1997, Sinauer.

16. Mickel EJ: *The artificial paradises in French literature,* Chapel Hill, NC, 1969, University of North Carolina Press (Free translation from French).
17. Mitchell PJ, Redman Jr: Effects of caffeine, time of day, and user history on study-related performance. *Psychopharmacology (Berl)* 109:121, 1992.
18. Gilliland K, Andress D: Ad lib caffeine consumption, symptoms of caffeinism, and academic performance, *Am J Psychiatry* 138(4):512–514, 1981.
19. Ward N and others: The analgesic effects of caffeine in headache, *Pain* 44:151–155, 1991.
20. Elkins RN and others: Acute effects of caffeine in normal prepubertal boys, *Am J Psychiatry* 138(2):178–183, 1981.
21. Schreiber GB and others: Measurement of coffee and caffeine intake: implications for epidemiological research, *Prev Med* 17:280–294, 1988.
22. Lubin F and others: A case-control study of caffeine and methylxanthines in benign breast disease, *JAMA* 253:2388–2392, 1985.
23. Minton JP: Caffeine and benign breast disease, *JAMA* 254:2408, 1985.
24. Allen SS, Froberg DG: The effect of decreased caffeine consumption on benign proliferative breast disease: a randomized clinical trial, *Surgery* 101:720–730, 1987.
25. Dews P and others: Report of Fourth International Caffeine Workshop, *Food Chemistry and Toxicology* 22:163–169, 1984.
26. Wilcox A and others: Caffeinated beverages and decreased fertility, *Lancet* 1:1453–1455, 1988.
27. Vlajinac HD and others: Effect of caffeine intake during pregnancy on birth weight, *Am J Epidemiol* 145:335–338, 1997.
28. Infante-Rivard C and others: Fetal loss associated with caffeine intake before and during pregnancy, *JAMA,* 270:2940, 1993.
29. Mills JL and others: Moderate caffeine use and the risk of spontaneous abortion and intrauterine growth retardation, *JAMA,* 269:593, 1993.
30. LaCroix AZ and others: Coffee consumption and the incidence of coronary heart disease, *N Engl J Med* 315:977–982, 1986.
31. Rosenberg L and others: Coffee drinking and nonfatal myocardial infarction in men under 55 years of age, *Am J Epidemiol* 128:570–578, 1988.
32. Stewart SA: Caffeine can push the panic button, *USA Today,* Oct 23, 1985.
33. Strain EC and others: Caffeine dependence syndrome, *JAMA,* 272:1043, 1994.

Over-the-Counter Drugs

KEY TERMS	OBJECTIVES

After reading this chapter, you should be able to:

GRAS
phenylpropanolamine
antihistamine
acetylsalicylic acid
antipyretic
antiinflammatory
Reye's syndrome
acetaminophen
ibuprofen
NSAID
chlorpheniramine maleate
pseudoephedrine
dextromethorphan

- Describe the process by which the FDA reviews OTC products for safety and effectiveness.
- Discuss the effects of three types of OTC psychoactive drugs: stimulants, weight-control products, and sedatives.
- Explain how aspirin and related products work to relieve pain.

- Describe the causes of colds and which symptoms are treated with which type of ingredient.
- List eight chemicals that are the main active ingredients in all the OTC products covered in this chapter.

Over-the-counter (OTC) drugs are those that are self-prescribed and self-administered for the relief of symptoms of self-diagnosed illnesses. The Food and Drug Administration (FDA) estimates that consumers self-treat four times more health problems than doctors treat, often using OTC drugs.

Americans spend over $18 billion a year on OTC products.[1] That's not as much as we spend on prescription drugs or booze or cigarettes or illicit cocaine, but it's enough to keep several OTC drug manufacturers locked in fierce competition for those sales. The two biggest markets are for aspirin-like analgesics and for the collection of cough, cold, and flu products. Do we really need all these nonprescription tablets, capsules, liquids, and creams? How much of what we buy is based on advertising "hype," and how much is based on sound decisions about our health? How are we as consumers to know the difference? The FDA is in the process of trying to help us with these decisions.

FDA REGULATION OF OTC PRODUCTS

The 1962 Kefauver-Harris amendment required that all drugs be evaluated for both safety and efficacy. The FDA was not only to set up criteria for new drugs entering the market but also to establish a procedure for reviewing all the OTC drugs already on the market. At first glance this seemed an impossible task, because there were somewhere between 250,000 and 300,000 different products already being sold (no one knew for sure how many). In addition, each product was likely to change its ingredients without warning, just like the "new" and "improved" soaps and toothpastes do. The FDA made the decision not to study individual products but to review each active ingredient. The reason for this decision is that then, as now, many of the competing brands contain the same ingredients, so there are many fewer ingredients than products. The FDA divided OTC products into 26 classes and appointed an advisory panel for each class. Each panel was to look at the active ingredients contained in the products in its class, to decide for each ingredient whether there was evidence indicating that it was safe and effective for its purpose, and also to decide what sorts of claims could be made for that ingredient on the label.

Several of the 26 classes of OTC drugs to be reviewed by the FDA included psychoactive ingredients: sedatives and sleep aids, analgesics, cold remedies and antitussives, antihistamines and allergy products, and stimulants.

Before the panel could begin work, some rules had to be laid down about what was meant by such terms as *safe* and *effective*, keeping in mind that no drug is entirely safe and that many might have only limited effectiveness. The FDA uses the acronym **GRAS** ("generally recognized as safe") to mean that, given the currently available information, people who are informed and qualified would agree that the ingredient should be considered safe. "Safe" means "a low incidence of adverse reactions or significant side effects under adequate directions for use and warnings against unsafe use as well as low potential for harm which may result from abuse." Similar acronyms are used for two other important concepts: *GRAE* ("generally recognized as effective") and *GRAHL* ("generally recognized as honestly labeled").

Effectiveness means a reasonable expectation that, in a significant proportion of the target population, the pharmacological effect of the drug, when used under adequate directions for use and warnings against unsafe use, will provide clinically significant relief of the type claimed.

The advisory panel was to rule on each active ingredient and decide whether the evidence indicates that the ingredient is both GRAS and GRAE, or failed on one or both criteria, or if further information was needed.

You'd think that because they simplified the approach and began appointing panels in 1972, this work would be about done. Well, not quite yet. The FDA began to publish "Tentative Final Monographs" on each class in 1985. The idea was to solicit comments from the public and the drug companies before publishing Final Monographs, but the amount of comment was so great that revised Tentative Final Monographs are still appearing. By 1992, twenty years after the process began, only 34 of the proposed 71 monographs had become finalized. It's not clear whether the remaining Tentative Final Monographs are becoming more final or more tentative as the process continues. They are certainly becoming longer, as they include more comments and responses to comments. This does not mean that there has been no regulation at all during this time; far from it. As advisory panels made tentative decisions, those were communicated to the manufacturers, who were encouraged to change their formulations. Because the process was taking so long, in 1980 the FDA commissioner acted to speed up both the reviews and the effects of those reviews. Thus the FDA began publishing some brief advisory opinions banning certain products or combinations and sent letters to manufacturers and distributors of the products ordering that the products be removed from the market immediately. In spite of the progress that has been made in reviewing ingredients and removing many products from the market, in 1992 the

U.S. General Accounting Office released a critical report claiming that the FDA still didn't know exactly how many OTC products are being marketed and still couldn't guarantee that everything being sold is both safe and effective.[2] By the late 1990s the list of therapeutic classes had grown from 26 to over 80. The exact number of OTC products on the market is still not known because they still come and go and change, but we do know that there are more than 100,000, and they contain fewer than 1,000 total active ingredients. Most of those are old ingredients, which were being sold prior to 1972 and have survived the review process.[3]

The overall result of this procedure can be seen by taking a trip to your neighborhood drugstore and looking at the lists of ingredients on medications of a given type. You should be struck that all the competing brands contain much the same few ingredients. In some classes, there might be only one approved active ingredient, meaning that all competing brands will be essentially identical. The differences among them often are in the long list of other (inactive) ingredients (colorings, flavorings, etc.).

SIMPLIFYING LABELS

Both the safety and the effectiveness of OTC drugs depend greatly upon their being used according to the directions and warnings on the label. To reduce confusion and make it more likely that consumers will be able to understand the labels, the FDA proposed in 1997 to create uniform standards for labels, with minimum print size, topics in a consistent order (active ingredients, directions for use, warnings), with bold, bulleted headings. One important proposal was to make the language clearer and more concise, avoiding medical terminology (e.g., "pulmonary" will be replaced by "lung").[4] Look for this new, consistent approach to labeling to show up in drugstores and supermarkets soon.

OVER-THE-COUNTER VERSUS PRESCRIPTION DRUGS

You might remember that it was the 1938 Food, Drug, and Cosmetic Act that established a classification of drugs that would be available only by prescription. The rule is that a drug is supposed to be permitted for OTC sale unless, because of potential toxicity or for other reasons (e.g., if it must be injected), it may be safely sold and used only under a prescription.

Sometimes the only difference between an OTC product and a prescription product is the greater amount of active ingredient in each prescription dose. More often, however, prescription drugs are chemicals that are unavailable OTC. Until the FDA began its OTC Drug Review process, once a new drug was approved for prescription sale it almost never became available OTC. Neither the FDA nor the manufacturers seemed to have much interest in switching drugs to OTC status. However, the FDA advisory panels that reviewed products in a given OTC category sometimes did more than was required of them. In some cases, they recommended that higher doses be allowed in OTC preparations—and as a result we can now buy higher-strength OTC antihistamines. And in several cases the suggestion was that previous prescription-only ingredients such as ibuprofen be sold OTC.

Between 1972 and 1992 a total of twenty ingredients were switched to OTC status. Then the FDA established the Nonprescription Drug Advisory Committee, which has an advisory role regarding all the different drug categories and has helped to move more drugs from prescription to OTC. Drugs recently switched to OTC status include nicotine chewing gum and patches and the hair-growing drug minoxidil.[3] Several drug manufacturers have now seen the

---

GRAS: "generally recognized as safe."

Should There Be a Third Class of "Pharmacist-Recommended" Drugs?

Professional pharmacists may feel that they "get no respect" from some drug purchasers. Pharmacists are trained to be familiar with not only the prescription orders they fill but also with the ingredients and indications for OTC products. Most feel that consumers should take advantage of their advice on decisions to purchase and use OTC drugs. However, increasing numbers of people are purchasing their OTC medications in grocery and "convenience" stores rather than in pharmacies. In addition, there is concern that as more and more former prescription products are allowed for OTC sale, many people will simply assume that the

drugs are "safe" and will use them carelessly. Pharmacists' organizations have proposed the establishment of "pharmacist-legend" drugs in the United States, similar to programs that have been used in England and Australia and that are being studied in Canada. Ibuprofen is one drug that Australian pharmacists keep "behind the counter"—no physician's prescription is required, but the pharmacist will dispense it only after giving some advice on its safe use. With such a system, perhaps other drugs (including oral contraceptives?) could become available without a physician's order.

potential for greater markets for some of their products, and it is expected that more and more OTC switches will be based on revised New Drug Applications (NDAs) from the manufacturers.

SOME PSYCHOACTIVE OTC PRODUCTS

Stimulants

Stimulants, one of the original FDA categories, turns out to be one of the simplest categories. The FDA allows stimulants to be sold to "help restore mental alertness or wakefulness when experiencing fatigue or drowsiness." If it sounds like caffeine could do this, you're right! No Doz, a well-known product that has been around for years, has the tried-and-true formula: 100 mg of caffeine (about the equivalent of an average cup of brewed coffee). The recommended dose is

two tablets initially, then one every three hours. Another well-known product, Vivarin, contains 200 mg of caffeine, and the initial dose is one tablet. Thus, although the packages look different and different companies make them, a smart consumer would choose between these two based on the price per milligram of caffeine. Or they could choose a less expensive "store" brand, or buy coffee (usually more expensive), or just get enough rest and save their money. The labels warn against using these caffeine tablets with coffee, tea, or cola drinks. The only active ingredient the FDA allows in OTC stimulants is caffeine.[5]

Look-alikes

There is a reasonably brisk business in the semilegal field of selling caffeine tablets manufactured in either tablet or capsule form to resemble prescription stimulants, such as amphetamine. In fact, many street purchases of "speed" these days turn out to contain caffeine as their major ingredient. Some states have tried to ban the sale of these look-alikes, and the FDA has tried to regulate them, but doing so is tough, because caffeine itself is legal. Mail-order advertisements for these products can be found in the backs of various magazines. It is, however, a violation of the controlled substances act to sell something that is represented to be a controlled substance. Although they no longer use such suggestive names as "speed" for the products, one does claim the brand name "Amphetrazine." Some companies have manufactured combinations of caffeine with either *ephedrine* or **phenylpropanolamine** (**PPA**). You may remember from chapter 7 that ephedrine is a sympathomimetic derived from a Chinese herbal tea and sold as a bronchodilator. The amphetamine molecule was derived from it. PPA has a structure similar to that of amphetamine and ephedrine and is sold in weight-control preparations. Each of these has mild stimulant properties of its own. The FDA has ruled that products labeled as stimulants that contain anything other than caffeine as an active ingredient may not be sold OTC. They also outlawed OTC products labeled for any purpose that contained combinations of caffeine and ephedrine, and have taken legal action against several mail-order distributors of such combination products.

OTC products containing only ephedrine have come under recent scrutiny. Although these are allowed for sale as a bronchodilator for asthma, some people are apparently buying them to use as "pep" or "energy" pills. In addition, Oregon has switched ephedrine to prescription-only status over concern that illicit laboratories are using ephedrine as a precursor for making methamphetamine.

Weight-Control Products

The original FDA list of OTC drug categories did not include "appetite suppressants" or a

OTC weight loss products all have a single active ingredient

similar term. Apparently the FDA didn't think they would be dealing with such a product, because at the time the use of the prescription amphetamines for this purpose was under widespread attack. However, data were presented indicating that PPA was safe and effective, and by the late 1970s several products were being sold that contained PPA as their only active ingredient. Some studies indicated that caffeine could potentiate the appetite-suppressing effect of PPA, and for a brief period

---

phenylpropanolamine (PPA): (fen il pro pa *nole a meen*) the active ingredient in OTC weight-control products.

during the early 1980s several of the products included both PPA and caffeine. After the 1983 FDA ruling prohibiting such combinations on the grounds that they might not be safe, all products returned to PPA only. The recommended dose for appetite suppression is 75 mg per day. There is some concern about the safety even of 75 mg doses, with the threat being increased blood pressure resulting from sympathetic stimulation. There is also some controversy about the effectiveness of PPA, given that its effect, as with most appetite suppressant drugs, is small and rather short-lived. For now, those various competing weight-control products in the drugstore are essentially the same: 75 mg PPA. (Many proudly proclaim that they are caffeine free!) Some have only 25 or 37.5 mg and recommend taking them two or three times per day, some are in sustained-release capsules, and some include vitamin supplements (not considered an active ingredient by the FDA). An interesting aspect of this apparent competition can be seen in the fact that Appedrine, Control, Dexatrim, and Prolamine—all of them competing products containing PPA—are all made by the same company. These include tablets and capsules, with and without vitamin supplements, and have varying amounts of PPA per tablet. The point of these different packages and products is obviously to cover the market, but as far as the consumer is concerned the bottom line is the same for all of them: 75 mg PPA.

The FDA has reviewed and ruled against several other products that have been advertised for weight control. Benzocaine-containing candies and gums were supposed to numb the tongue, reducing the sense of taste, but it was never shown that this is an effective way to reduce food intake. Starch blockers, which were supposed to interfere with the absorption of carbohydrates from starchy foods, have never been proved to do so. The FDA asked for all sales to stop until safety and effectiveness could be established, and the government

seized the products after promoters failed to comply. Cholecystokinin (CCK) is a hormone that does decrease food intake when injected directly into the brains of experimental animals, but the chemical is quickly destroyed in the digestive tract if taken by mouth. Nevertheless, products claiming to include CCK have been advertised and sold, and the FDA has ordered this practice discontinued. Other unapproved products for weight reduction that have come under FDA scrutiny in recent years include DHEA, arginine and ornithine, spirulina, and glucomannan. None of these products has been demonstrated to be effective in weight loss, despite claims of "burning fat," "natural" weight loss, "Oriental weight-loss secret," and so on.

Sedatives and Sleep Aids

A few years ago the shelves contained a number of OTC sedative, or "calmative," preparations, including Quiet World and Compoz, which contained very small amounts of the acetylcholine receptor blocker *scopolamine* combined with the **antihistamine** methapy-

OTC sleep aids with antihistimines

rilene. At the same time, sleep aids, such as Sleep-Eze and Sominex, contained just a bit more of the same two ingredients. The rationale for the scopolamine, particularly at these low doses, was under FDA investigation, but scopolamine had traditionally been included in many such medications in the past. It is quite clear that some antihistamines do produce a kind of sedated state and might produce drowsiness. The FDA advisory panel accepted methapyrilene but eventually rejected scopolamine. For a while all of these medications contained only methapyrilene. Then in 1979 it was reported that methapyrilene caused cancer in laboratory animals, so it was no longer GRAS. Next came pyrilamine maleate, then doxylamine succinate, and then *diphenhydramine,* all antihistamines. The interesting thing about this whole process was that if you bought the same brand from one year to the next to the next, you would get a different formulation each time. But if you bought several different brands at the same time, you stood a good chance of getting the same formulation in all of them!

The "sedative" category no longer exists for OTC products. One product, Miles Nervine, which went from being a sedative containing bromide salts to a calmative containing whatever they all contained each year, is now Miles Nervine Nighttime Sleep-Aid, containing 25 mg of diphenhydramine. Nytol is also a nighttime sleep aid containing the same ingredient. Sominex and Sleep-Eze are still around, and both also contain diphenhydramine.

As we said in chapter 8, insomnia is perceived to be a bigger problem than it actually is for most people, and it is rare that medication is really required. These antihistamines can induce drowsiness, but not very quickly. If you do feel the need to use these to get you to sleep more rapidly, take them at least twenty minutes before retiring. Their sedative effects are potentiated by alcohol, so it is not a good idea to take them after drinking.

The Medicine Chest

The family medicine chest is often a treasure trove of old tablets, capsules, liquids, and lozenges. Start digging around and see how many different OTC drugs you can find in yours. How old do you think some of them might be? If any of them have expiration dates, have the dates passed?

Because formulations change from year to year, there's a good chance the medicines you now have are not the same as the ones being sold in the drugstore. Write down the formulations for a few of your medicine chest drugs. Then go to the drugstore and compare them with the current formulation for that same brand of product. Do you wonder if some of the old ingredients were removed because the FDA no longer considers them safe?

ANALGESICS

People and Pain

Pain is such a little word for such a big experience. Most people have experienced pain of varying intensities, from mild to moderate to severe to excruciating! Two major classes of drugs are used to reduce pain or the awareness of pain. Anesthetics (meaning "without sensibility") have this effect by reducing all types of sensation or by blocking consciousness completely. The local anesthetics used in dentistry and the general anesthetics used in major

---

antihistamine: active ingredients in OTC sleep aids and cough/cold products.

surgery are examples of this class of agent. The other major class, the analgesics (meaning "without pain"), are compounds that reduce pain selectively without causing a loss of other sensations. The analgesics are divided into two groups. Opiates (see chapter 15) are one group of analgesics, but this chapter primarily discusses the OTC internal analgesics, such as aspirin, acetaminophen, and ibuprofen.

Although pain itself is a complex psychological phenomenon, there have been attempts to classify different types of pain to develop a rational approach to its treatment. One classification divides pain into two types, depending on its place of origin. Visceral pain, such as intestinal cramps, arises from nonskeletal portions of the body; narcotics are effective in reducing pain of this type. Somatic pain, arising from muscle or bone and typified by sprains, headaches, and arthritis, is reduced by salicylates (aspirin) and related products.

Pain is unlike other sensations in many ways, mostly because of nonspecific factors. The experience of pain varies with personality, gender, and time of day and is increased with fatigue, anxiety, fear, boredom, and anticipation of more pain. Because pain is very susceptible to nonspecific factors, a brief comment is required on the effectiveness of a placebo in reducing pain. Classic studies were done by Beecher, who summarized reports of many investigators on the effectiveness of placebos in the reduction of pain.[6] These were real situations with a variety of clinical causes ranging from postoperative pain to the aches associated with the common cold. About 35 percent of the patients in these studies had their pain "satisfactorily relieved" by placebos. That is, when individuals in pain were given an inactive substance along with the suggestion that it would reduce the pain, 35 percent of the patients obtained relief.

This 35 percent proportion is quite high, considering that morphine provides satisfactory relief of pain in only about 75 percent of patients. It was also found that placebos are most effective in reducing pain in stressful situations, whereas mor-

Aspirin products on store shelves

phine has its smallest effect in these stressful situations. As might be expected from the last statement, placebos are more effective in real-life pain than in experimental pain. The internal analgesics mentioned in the next section have been repeatedly shown to be more effective at therapeutic doses than placebos for certain kinds of pain.

Aspirin

Salicylates are the most widely used class of internal analgesics. The word itself suggests their long heritage, coming from the Latin *salix*, meaning "willow". Over 2,400 years ago the Greeks used extracts of willow and poplar bark in the treatment of pain, gout, and other illnesses. Aristotle commented on some of the clinical effects of similar preparations, and Galen also made good use of these formulations. These remedies fell into disrepute, however, when St. Augustine declared that all diseases of Christians were the work of demons and thus a punishment from God. American Indians, unhampered by this enlightened attitude, used a tea brewed from willow bark to reduce fever. The salicylates were not rediscovered in Europe until about 200 years ago when an Englishman, the Reverend Edward Stone, combined two bits of the best information then available and put the result to a clinical test. The two pieces of data he combined were these: (1) listen to old folk lore tales, and (2) plants acquire the characteristics of the place where they grow. The old folk lore kept saying willow bark is good for pain and whatever else ails you! Stone phrased the second attitude nicely:

> As this tree delights in a moist or wet soil where aches chiefly abound, the general maxim that many natural maladies carry their cures along with them, or that their remedies lie not far from their causes, was so very apposite to this particular case that I could not help applying it. That this might be the intention of Providence had some little weight with me.[7]

Stone prepared an extract of the bark and gave the same dose to fifty patients with varying illnesses and found the results to be "uniformly excellent."

In the nineteenth century the active ingredient in these preparations was isolated and identified as salicylic acid. In 1838, salicylic acid was synthesized, and in 1859 procedures were developed that made bulk production feasible. Salicylic acid and sodium salicylate were then used for many ills, especially arthritis.

In the giant Bayer Laboratories in Germany in the 1890s, there worked a chemist named Hoffmann. His father had a severe case of rheumatoid arthritis, and only salicylic acid seemed to help. The major difficulty then, as today, was that the drug caused great gastric discomfort. So great was the stomach upset and nausea that Hoffmann's father frequently preferred the pain of the arthritis. Hoffmann studied the salicylates to see if he could find one with the same therapeutic effect as salicylic acid but without the side effects.

In 1898, he synthesized **acetylsalicylic acid** and tried it on his father, who reported relief from pain without stomach upset. The compound was tested, patented, and released for sale in 1899 as *Aspirin*. Aspirin was a trademark name derived from the name *acetyl and spiralic acid* (the old name for salicylic acid). It is interesting that the two famous compounds that the Bayer Laboratories in Germany were instrumental in introducing to the world are rapidly transformed to their original form after absorption. Both heroin and aspirin were first synthesized in the Bayer Laboratories. Aspirin, either in the gastrointestinal tract or in the bloodstream, is converted to salicylic acid. Taken orally, aspirin is a more potent analgesic than salicylic acid, because aspirin irritates the stomach less and is thus absorbed more rapidly.

Aspirin was marketed for physicians and sold as a white powder in individual dosage packets, available only on prescription. It was immediately popular worldwide, and the U.S. market became large enough that it was very soon manufactured in this country. In 1915 the 5 gram (325 mg) white tablet stamped "Bayer" first appeared, and, also for the first time, Aspirin became a nonprescription item. The Bayer Company was on its way. It had an effective drug that could be sold to the public and was known by one name—Aspirin. And they had the name trademarked! Before February 1917, when the patent on Aspirin was to expire, Bayer started an advertising campaign to make it clear that there was only one Aspirin, and its first name was Bayer. Several companies started manufacturing and selling Aspirin as aspirin, and Bayer sued. What happened after this is a long story, but you know who lost; aspirin is aspirin—or is it?

Therapeutic use

Say what you will, aspirin is truly a magnificent drug. It is also a drug with some serious side effects. Aspirin has three effects that are the

---

acetylsalicylic acid: (a *see* till sal i *sill* ick) the chemical known as aspirin.

primary basis for its clinical use. It is an analgesic that effectively blocks somatic pain in the mild-to-moderate range. Aspirin is also **antipyretic**: it reduces fever. Last but not least, aspirin is an **antiinflammatory** agent: it reduces the inflammation and soreness in an injured area. This action is the basis for its extensive use in arthritis. It is difficult to find another drug that has this span of effects coupled with a relatively low toxicity. It does, however, have side effects that pose problems for some people.

Aspirin is readily absorbed from the stomach but even faster from the intestine. Thus anything that delays movement of the aspirin from the stomach should affect absorption time. The evidence is mixed on whether taking aspirin with a meal, which delays emptying of the stomach, increases the time before onset of action. It should, however, reduce the stomach irritation that sometimes accompanies aspirin use.

For many years, some aspirin preparations have been *buffered* with additional ingredients meant to neutralize the acidity of aspirin. This is intended to have two effects: first, to reduce stomach irritation; second, by moving the aspirin more rapidly into the intestine, to produce faster relief. There is ample evidence that buffered aspirin does reach the blood somewhat more rapidly, but no one has ever been able to show that this results in faster or stronger pain relief.

The *therapeutic* dose for aspirin is generally considered to be in the range of 600 to 1,000 mg. Most reports suggest that 300 mg is usually more effective than a placebo, whereas 600 mg is clearly even more effective. Many studies indicate that increasing the dose above that level does not increase aspirin's analgesic action, but some research indicates that 1,200 mg of aspirin provides greater relief than 600 mg. In one study,[12] after ingestion of a 650 mg tablet of aspirin, headache and postpartum pain were not reduced significantly from placebo until 45 minutes had elapsed; maximum relief was obtained

after 60 minutes. At four hours after intake, pain levels were equivalent in the drug and placebo groups; that is, the analgesia was gone. These reports agree with the salicylate blood levels measured in the same patients.

At therapeutic doses aspirin does have analgesic actions that are fairly specific. First, and in marked contrast to narcotic analgesics, aspirin does not affect the impact of the anticipation of pain. It seems probable also that aspirin has its primary effect on the ability to withstand continuing pain. This no doubt is the basis for much of the self-medication with aspirin, because moderate, protracted pain is fairly common. The salicylates do not block all types of pain. They are especially effective against headache and musculoskeletal aches and pains, less effective for toothache and sore throat, and almost valueless in visceral pain, as well as in traumatic (acute) pain.

The antipyretic (fever-reducing) action of aspirin does not lower temperature in an individual with normal body temperature. It has this effect only if the person has a fever. The mechanism by which the salicylates decrease body temperature is fairly well understood. They act on the temperature-regulating area of the hypothalamus to increase heat loss through peripheral mechanisms. Heat loss is primarily increased by vasodilation of peripheral blood vessels and by increased perspiration. Heat production is not changed, but heat loss is facilitated so that body temperature can go down.

More aspirin has probably been used for its third major therapeutic use than for either of the other two. The antiinflammatory action of the salicylates is the major basis for its use after muscle strains and in rheumatoid arthritis.

Most tablets, including aspirin, develop a harder external shell the longer they sit. This hardening effect does not change the amount of the active ingredient, but it does make the active ingredient less effective because disintegration time is increased by the hard exterior coating. Along the same line, moisture and heat speed the decomposition of acetylsalicylic acid into two other compounds: salicylic acid, which causes gastric distress, and acetic acid—vinegar. When the smell of vinegar is strong in your aspirin bottle, discard it!

Aspirin Effects: Adverse and Otherwise

1. **Aspirin increases bleeding time by inhibiting blood platelet aggregation**. This is not an insignificant effect. Two or three aspirins can double bleeding time, the time it takes for blood to clot, and the effect can last for four to seven days. There's good and bad in the anticoagulant effect of aspirin. Its use before surgery can help prevent blood clots from appearing in patients at high risk for clot formation. For many surgical patients, however, facilitation of blood clotting is desirable, and the general rule is no aspirin or other salicylates for seven to ten days before surgery. The same principle—no aspirin—should hold for women in their last trimester of pregnancy. This might be particularly important, because aspirin does cross the placental barrier, and neither the short- nor the long-term effects on the fetus are known.

Two possibly big advantages of the anticoagulant effect are of particular interest to men. A *transient ischemic attack* (TIA) results when a tiny clot forms in the brain or the retina, temporarily cutting off the blood supply to a small region. This can be the precursor of a stroke, in which the loss of blood to a brain region results in permanent damage. You won't find this mentioned on aspirin bottles in the store, because the FDA doesn't want people self-diagnosing and self-treating TIAs or strokes, but the professional labeling (for physicians and pharmacists to read), says:

> For reducing the risk of recurrent transient ischemic attacks (TIA's) or stroke in men who have transient ischemia of the brain due to fibrin platelet emboli. There is inadequate evidence that aspirin or buffered aspirin is effective in reducing TIA's in women at the recommended dosage.

There is no evidence that aspirin or buffered aspirin is of benefit in the treatment of completed strokes in men or women.[8]

Perhaps even more importantly, evidence has been building for some time that men who have had one heart attack (myocardial infarction) and who take an aspirin tablet every other day have a reduced risk of a second heart attack. The Canadian government approved aspirin to prevent second heart attacks in 1982, and the FDA tentatively approved this use in 1985. Two large-scale 1988 experiments, one British and one American, make it very clear that this is a real effect. The FDA will include in the professional labeling only, and not to the general public, an indication for aspirin "to reduce the risk of death and/or non-fatal myocardial infarction in patients with a previous myocardial infarction or unstable angina pectoris (chest pain)."[8] Again, the FDA doesn't want people self-diagnosing and self-treating heart attacks. What we don't know, because the study hasn't been done, is whether it would make sense for people who have not experienced angina or a heart attack but who have other risk factors (overweight, high incidence of heart disease in the family) to use aspirin to prevent heart attacks. Such studies, as well as studies on women, are currently under way. The aspirin makers would probably like it if everyone over the age of 40 started taking an aspirin every other day, and the television ads have become rather suggestive that you should "ask your doctor" about this.

2. **Aspirin will induce gastrointestinal bleeding in about 70 percent of normal subjects**. In most cases, this is only about 5 ml per

---

antipyretic: (an tee pie *reh* tick) fever-reducing.

antiinflammatory: reducing swelling and inflammation.

day, but that is five times the normal loss. In some people the blood loss can be great enough to cause anemia. The basis for this effect is not clear but is believed to be a direct eroding by the aspirin tablets of the gastric mucosa. The rule is clear: drink lots of water when you take aspirin, or, better yet, crush the tablets and drink them in orange juice or other liquid.

3. Reye's syndrome. In the early 1980s there was increasing concern about the relationship of aspirin use to **Reye's syndrome**. This is a rare disease (fewer than 200 cases per year in the United States). Almost all of the cases occur in people under the age of twenty, usually after they have had a viral infection such as influenza or chicken pox. The children begin vomiting continuously, then they might become disoriented, undergo personality changes, shout, or become lethargic. Some enter comas, and some of those will either die or suffer permanent brain damage. The overall mortality rate from Reye's syndrome is about 25 percent.

No one knows what causes Reye's, and it isn't believed to be caused by aspirin. However, there are data that suggest the disease is more likely to occur in children who have been given aspirin during a preceding illness. In late 1984 the results of a Centers for Disease Control and Prevention pilot study were released, indicating that the use of aspirin can increase the risk of Reye's syndrome as much as 25 times. In 1985, makers of all aspirin products were asked to put warning labels on their packages. These labels recommend that you consult a physician before giving aspirin to children or teenagers with chicken pox or flu.

In early 1986, it was reported that fewer parents in Michigan were giving aspirin to children for colds or influenza, and the incidence of Reye's syndrome had also decreased in Michigan.[9] The Michigan study lends further strength to the relationship between aspirin use and Reye's syndrome. Our advice is that no one under the age of twenty use aspirin in treating chicken pox, influenza, or even what might be suspected to be a common cold.

4. Overdose poisonings. Aspirin has long been associated with a large number of accidental poisonings of children and also with suicide attempts. Although it has now been joined on the DAWN lists (see chapter 2) by its relatives acetaminophen and ibuprofen, aspirin remains a major cause of emergency room visits and was mentioned in 113 drug-related deaths in the 1993 DAWN data.

Mechanism of action

Aspirin is now believed to have both a central and a peripheral analgesic effect. The central effect is not clear, but the peripheral effect is well on its way to being understood; it is now known that aspirin modifies the *cause* of pain.

Prostaglandins are local hormones that are manufactured and released when cell membranes are distorted or damaged, that is, injured. The prostaglandins then act on the endings of the neurons that mediate pain in the injured areas. The prostaglandins sensitize the neurons to mechanical stimulation and to stimulation by two other local hormones, histamine and bradykinin, which are more slowly released from the damaged tissue. Aspirin blocks the synthesis of the prostaglandins.

There is now abundant evidence to support this rough outline of the mechanism of the action of aspirin. For one thing, aspirin does not block the pain induced by injections of prostaglandins. Aspirin also has an analgesic effect only in tissues where prostaglandin formation is taking place. A similar explanation seems most reasonable as the basis for the antiinflammatory action of aspirin.

The antipyretic action has also been spelled out: a specific prostaglandin acts on the anterior hypothalamus to decrease heat dissipation through the normal procedures of sweating and dilation of peripheral blood vessels. Aspirin blocks the synthesis of this prostaglandin in the anterior hypothalamus, and this is followed by increased heat loss.

Acetaminophen

There are two related analgesic compounds: *phenacetin* and **acetaminophen**. Phenacetin was sold for many years in combination with aspirin and caffeine in the "APC" tablets that fought headache pain "three ways." Phenacetin has been around since 1887 and had long been suspected of causing kidney lesions and dysfunction. In 1964 the FDA required a warning on all products containing phenacetin, which limited their use to ten days because the phenacetin might damage the kidneys. Phenacetin has now gone to the land of dead drugs: the review panel considered it not to be GRAS.

The only real question is why everything took so long to get off the market. Phenacetin was known to be rapidly converted to acetaminophen, which was the primary active agent. Acetaminophen is equipotent with aspirin in its analgesic and antipyretic effects. The antipyretic mechanism is similar to that of aspirin, but the analgesic effect might be additive to that produced by aspirin. Acetaminophen is not an antiinflammatory and thus is of minimal value in arthritis, gout, and the like.

Acetaminophen has been marketed as an OTC analgesic since 1955, but it was the big advertising pushes in the 1970s for two brand name products, Tylenol and Datril, that brought acetaminophen into the big time. It is usually advertised as having most of the good points of "that other pain reliever" and many fewer disadvantages. To a degree this is probably true: if only analgesia and fever reduction are desired, acetaminophen might be safer than aspirin *as long as dosage limits are carefully observed*. Overuse of acetaminophen can cause serious liver disorders.

That prediction came true in the 1980s, as more and more reports of acetaminophen-induced liver damage and deaths came in. Acetaminophen has now surpassed aspirin as far as both drug-related emergency-room visits and drug-related deaths, according to the DAWN statistics (see chapter 2). The FDA doesn't want to advertise on the package that acetaminophen can be lethal, for fear of attracting suicide attempts. So they require a warning against overdose and include the statement "Prompt medical attention is critical for adults as well as for children even if you do not notice any signs or symptoms." This statement reflects the fact that damage to the liver might not be noticed until 24 to 48 hours later, when the symptoms of impaired liver function finally emerge. You should remember that acetaminophen is not necessarily "safer" than aspirin, especially if the recommended dose is exceeded.

Ibuprofen and Other NSAIDs

Since the discovery that aspirin and similar drugs work by inhibiting the synthesis of prostaglandins, the drug companies have been able to use that information to design new and sometimes more potent analgesics, most of which have been available only as prescription products. **Ibuprofen**, which originally was available only by prescription, is now found in several OTC analgesics. In addition to its analgesic potency, ibuprofen is a potent antiinflammatory and has received wide use in the treatment of arthritis. The most common side

Reye's syndrome: a rare and potentially lethal disease associated with aspirin use by children.

acetaminophen: (a seet a *min* o fen) aspirin-like analgesic and antipyretic.

ibuprofen: (eye bu *pro* fen) aspirin-like analgesic and antiinflammatory.

TABLE 14.1

Ingredients in OTC Analgesics

Brand	Aspirin	Acetaminophen	Ibuprofen	Caffeine	Other
Anacin	400	—	—	32	—
Advil	—	—	200	—	—
Bufferin	325	—	—	—	Magnesium carbonate, calcium carbonate, magnesium oxide
Empirin	325	—	—	—	—
Excedrin	250	250	—	65	—
Mediprin	—	—	200	—	—
Nuprin	—	—	200	—	—
Vanquish	227	194	—	33	Magnesium hydroxide, aluminum hydroxide gel

effects of ibuprofen are gastrointestinal: nausea, stomach pain, and cramping. There have been reports of fatal liver damage with overdoses of ibuprofen, so again it is wise not to exceed the recommended dose.

Ibuprofen was the first of several new drugs that are now collectively referred to as "nonsteroidal antiinflammatory drugs" (**NSAIDs**). The newer ones, such as naproxyn and ketoprofen, are available only by prescription.

Table 14.1 contains a list of several OTC internal analgesics along with the amounts of each ingredient they contain. The FDA has been discussing whether or not to exclude products that contain both aspirin and acetaminophen. Products containing ibuprofen warn against combining them with aspirin, because that mixture hasn't been thoroughly studied.

Given the large potential market for OTC analgesics and antiinflammatory agents such as ibuprofen, we may expect requests to move other NSAIDs such as naproxen to OTC status in the future.

COLD AND ALLERGY PRODUCTS

The All-Too-Common Common Cold

There has to be something good about an illness that Charles Dickens could be lyrical about:

> I am at this moment
> Deaf in the ears,
> Hoarse in the throat,
> Red in the nose,
> Green in the gills,
> Damp in the eyes,
> Twitchy in the joints,
> And fractious in temper
> From a most intolerable
> And oppressive cold.[10]

The common cold is caused by a virus—well, viruses: over a hundred have been identified—but in 40 to 60 percent of individuals with colds, researchers cannot connect the infection to a specific virus. That makes it tough to find a cure. Two groups of viruses are known to be associated with colds—the *rhinoviruses* and the more recently identified *coronaviruses*. These viruses are clearly distinct from those that cause influenza, measles, and pneumonia. Success in developing vaccines against other diseases has made some experts optimistic about finding a vaccine for the common cold. Others are pessimistic because of the great variety of viruses and the fact that the rhinoviruses can apparently change their immunologic reactivity very readily.

Viruses damage or kill the cells they attack. The rhinoviruses zero in on the upper respiratory tract, at first causing irritation that can lead to reflex coughing and sneezing. Increased irritation inflames the tissue and is followed by soreness and swelling of the mucous membranes. As a defense against infection, the mucous membranes release considerable fluid, which causes the runny nose amd postnasal "drip" that irritates the throat.

Although the incubation period can be a week in some cases, the more common interval between infection and respiratory tract symptoms is two to four days. Before the onset of respiratory symptoms, the individual might just "feel bad" and develop joint aches and headaches. When fever does occur, it almost always develops early in the cold.

Most of us grew up believing that colds are passed by airborne particles jet-propelled usually through unobstructed sneezing. ("Cover your mouth! Cover your face!") The old folk lore—and the scientists—were wrong. You need to know four things so you can avoid the cold viruses of others—and avoid reinfecting yourself:

1. Up to 100 times as many viruses are produced and shed from the nasal mucosa as from the throat.
2. There are few viruses in the saliva of a person with a cold, probably no viruses at all in about half of these individuals.
3. Dried viruses survive on dry skin and nonporous surfaces—plastic, wood, and so on— for over three hours.
4. Most cold viruses enter the body through the nostrils and eyes.

Usually colds start by the fingers picking up viruses and then the individual rubs the eyes or picks the nose. In one study of adults with colds, 40 percent had viruses on their hands but only 8 percent expelled viruses in coughs or sneezes.[11] The moral of the story is clear. To avoid colds: wash your hands frequently, and you may kiss but not hold hands with your cold-infected sweetheart! You don't have to worry about your pets—only humans and some apes are susceptible to colds.

The experimental animal of choice for studying colds has to be the human. In many studies with human volunteers, three types of findings seem to recur. First, not all who are directly exposed to a cold virus develop cold symptoms. In fact, only about 50 percent do. Second, in individuals with already existing antibodies to the virus, there might be only preliminary signs of a developing cold. These signs might last for a brief period (12 to 24 hours) and then disappear. The last finding crosses swords with the old folk lore, so it is best to quote:

> Chilling experiments with volunteers did not show any particular influence on susceptibility to colds. Some volunteers were given an inoculation followed by a hot bath and made to stand in a draft in wet bathing suits. Some took walks in the rain and sat around in wet clothes. Other subjects were given the same chilling treatments with inoculations which contained no virus. No significant differences were found in these various well-controlled groups.[12]

Theoretically, it is possible to prevent rhinovirus infections by pretreating the individual with interferon or other antiviral drugs. This will be of little practical value, however, because most of us don't know when or where we picked up the virus, or if it's going to infect us at all, until it's too late.

Treating Cold Symptoms

There's no practical way to prevent colds and no way to cure the infection once it starts. So why do Americans spend billions each year on cold "remedies"? Apparently, it's in an effort to reduce those miserable symptoms described by Dickens. Cold symptoms are fairly complex, so most cold remedies have traditionally included several active ingredients, each aimed at a particular type of symptom. In some ways, the

---

NSAID: nonsteroidal antiinflammatory drugs, such as ibuprofen.

FYI   ## Cold Medications and Kids

In a 1991 article in the *Journal of Pediatrics,* Nancy Hutton and her colleagues reported the results of an experiment on 96 children ranging in age from six months to five years. As the children were brought in to be treated for colds, one-third were randomly assigned to receive a placebo, one-third received no drug at all, and one-third received a liquid cold medication containing brompheniramine maleate, phenylephrine, and phenylpropanolamine (one antihistamine and two decongestants). Two days later the parents were asked to rate improvement in the cold symptoms. Two thirds of those receiving placebo were considered to be improved, as were 57 percent of those receiving no drug! Although 71 percent of the drug-treated group were rated as improved, that was not statistically different from either the placebo or the no-drug group.

An experiment like this can't prove that cold medications don't do any good at all, but several such studies make us question the value of treating children with these drugs that may make them drowsy and in rare cases can have more serious side effects.

FDA's Cold, Cough, Allergy, Bronchodilator, and Antiasthmatic Advisory Review Panel probably had the most difficult job: multiple symptoms, many ingredients for each symptom, and rapid changes in scientific evidence during the time they have been studying these products. In the preliminary report, issued in 1976, the panel approved less than half of the 119 ingredients it reviewed. The Tentative Final Monograph was published in 1985,[13] and several ingredients were recommended for approval or for shifting to OTC status that had not been available when the panel started its job. There are three common types of ingredients in modern cold remedies: *antihistamines*, for the temporary relief of runny nose and sneezing; *nasal decongestants*, for temporary relief of swollen membranes in the nasal passages; and *analgesic-antipyretics*, for the temporary relief of aches and pains and to reduce fever. The FDA list included ten approved antihistamines, but by far the most common antihistamine to be found on the shelves is **chlorpheniramine maleate**. The 1985 list had thirteen approved nasal decongestants. These are primarily sympathomimetics, including our old friend ephedrine and **pseudoephedrine**. The FDA deferred a decision on PPA, which is also found in OTC weight-control products, until a later date. The most common nasal decongestants in cold remedies are now pseudoephedrine and PPA. The analgesic-antipyretic is usually acetaminophen.

Table 14.2 gives recent formulations for five popular OTC cold remedies. Note that three of them also contain the cough suppressant **dextromethorphan**, which is the most common active ingredient in OTC cough medicines.

It is ironic that the one type of ingredient found in almost every cold remedy since before the FDA began its review continues to be under attack. The FDA advisory panel had serious questions about the data supporting the effectiveness of antihistamines in treating colds. Although some studies have since reported that chlorpheniramine maleate is better than placebo at reducing runny noses, prompting the FDA to approve several antihistamines, more recent controlled experiments have not found any benefit. A 1987 symposium of specialists concluded that ". . . antihistamines do not have a place in the management of upper respiratory infection, though they continue to be useful for allergy." Still more studies have been done that question the effectiveness of antihistamines, and congressional hearings were held in 1992 asking

TABLE 14.2

Ingredients in Selected Brand Name OTC Cold and Allergy Products

Brand	Sympathomimetic	Antihistamine	Analgesic	Cough suppressant	Other
Comtrex*	30 pseudoephedrine HCl	2 chlorpheniramine maleate	325 acetaminophen	10 dextromethorphan hydrobromide	—
Contac*	75 phenylpropa-nolamine HCl	8 chlorpheniramine maleate	—	—	—
	30 pseudoephed-rine HCl	2 chlorpheniramine maleate	325 acetaminophen	15 dextromethor-phan hydrobromide	— —
Tylenol Cold*	5 phenylephrine HCl	2 chlorpheniramine maleate	325 acetaminophen	—	—
Dristan (capsules*)	60 pseudoephed-rine HCl)	7.5 doxylamine succinate	1000 aceta-minophen	30 dextromethor-phan hydrobromide	25% alcohol

*mg/tablet.

†mg/adult dose (1 ounce)

why the FDA still allowed antihistamines in cough and cold remedies.[14]

Allergy and Sinus Medications

There are other related products on your pharmacists' shelves. In addition to the cough medicines, there are *allergy* relief pills that rely mainly on the same antihistamine, chlorpheniramine maleate, to slow down the runny nose. There are sinus medicines that use one of the sympathomimetic nasal decongestants (PPA or pseudoephedrine), often combined with an analgesic, to reduce swollen sinus passages and treat sinus headache.

CHOOSING AN OTC PRODUCT

By now you should be getting the idea that, thanks to the FDA's decision to review ingredients rather than individual formulations, you as a consumer can now review and choose among the great variety of products by knowing just a few ingredients and what they are intended to accomplish. Table 14.3 lists only eight ingredients. Those eight are the major active ingredients to be found in different combinations in OTC stimulants, sleep aids, weight-control

products, analgesics, cold, cough, allergy, and sinus medications!

Want to treat your cold without buying a combination cold remedy? If you have aches and pains, take your favorite analgesic. For the vast majority of colds, the slight elevation in temperature should probably not be treated, because it is not dangerous and can even help fight the infection. Unless body temperature remains at 103°F or above or reaches 105°F, fever is not considered dangerous. If you have a runny nose, you might or might not get relief from an antihistamine. Generic chlorpheniramine maleate or a store-brand allergy tablet is an inexpensive source. These will probably give you a dry mouth and might produce some sedation or drowsiness (which, of course, is why some of the more

---

chlorpheniramine maleate: (clor fen *eer* a meen mal i ate) a common antihistamine in cold products.

pseudoephedrine: (soo doh eh *fed* rin) a common decongestant in cold products.

dextromethorphan: (dex tro meh *thor* fan) OTC antitussive (cough control) ingredient.

FYI   Abuse of OTC Dextromethorphan

High school and college students have been "getting high" with large doses of OTC cough suppressants containing dextromethorphan (DM). Possibly, students first came on the effects of DM by drinking large quantities of Robitussin or similar cough syrups containing alcohol. However, the effects reported by those using 4 to 8 oz of Robitussin (up to 720 mg DM) could not be due to the less than one-half ounce of alcohol in them and include visual and auditory hallucinations and in some cases seizures.[16] The altered psychological state may last for several hours. The few cases reported in the literature and individual reports from college students indicate that habitual use (e.g., twice per week or more) is common.

DM has been the standard ingredient in OTC cough suppressants for many years and was originally developed as a nonopiate relative to codeine. DM is not an opiate-like narcotic, produces no pain relief, and does not produce an opiate-like abstinence syndrome. More recent evidence indicates that it may interact with a specific receptor from the opiate family known as the sigma receptor. This apparently safe and simple drug, which is contained in over fifty OTC products, has more complicated effects when taken in the large doses used by some recreational users.

It's not clear how recent this phenomenon really is. The Swedish government restricted DM to prescription-only use in 1986 as a result of abuse of OTC preparations, and there were two later reports of DM-caused fatalities in Sweden. In the United States, this has remained a mostly underground activity, apparently spread by word-of-mouth.

One 1995 posting to the alt.psychoactives newsgroup on the Internet described a user's first DM experience, after taking twenty capsules of an OTC cough remedy (600 mg DM):

> . . . 45 minutes worth of itching and for ten seconds it stopped. During one of the most weirdest and stupidest visions, I flew quickly over a mountain. As I did this in that second the itching seemed to go away and it seemed like I wasn't in my body anymore. I flew from one side of a rainbow to another. Then I was flying quickly towards the head of an ostrich and when I got close it only showed the silhouette of the head and I flew into the black nothingness. All that craziness in ten seconds made me laugh out loud as I tried to look at it all soberly. Then the itching came back into my body. No matter how hard I tried the itching never went away.

The itching feeling reported by this user has been reported by others, along with nausea and other unpleasant side effects. In spite of such unpleasantness, some users find it difficult to stop using DM once they have tried it a few times.

sedating antihistamines are used in sleep aids). Stuffed-up nose? Pseudoephedrine nose drops will shrink swollen membranes for a time. Although oral sympathomimetics will work, nose drops are more effective. You can find these ingredients in sinus preparations (or weight-control products!). However, these sympathomimetics should be used cautiously. There is a rapid tolerance to their effects, and, if they are used repeatedly, a rebound stuffiness can develop when they are stopped. Cough? Dextromethorphan can be obtained in cough medications.

TABLE 14.3
Common OTC Ingredients

Ingredient	Action	Source
Acetylsalicylic acid (ASA; aspirin)	Analgesic-antipyretic	Headache remedies, arthritis formulas, cold and sinus remedies
Acetaminophen	Analgesic-antipyretic	Headache remedies, cold and sinus remedies
Caffeine	Stimulant	"Alertness" medications
Chlorpheniramine maleate	Antihistamine	Cold remedies, allergy products
Dextromethorphan	Antitussive	Cough suppressants, cold remedies
Diphenhydramine	Antihistamine	Sleep aids, some cold remedies
Phenylpropanolamine (PPA)	Sympathomimetic	Weight-control products, cold and sinus remedies
Pseudoephedrine	Sympathomimetic	Cold and sinus remedies

Why not buy all this in one tablet or capsule? That's a common approach. But why treat symptoms you don't have? During the course of a cold, a runny nose might occur at one time, congestion at another, and coughing not at all. By using just the ingredients you need, when you need them, you might save money, and you would have the satisfaction of being a connoisseur of colds. Then again, given the state of research on the effectiveness of these "remedies," why buy them at all? It's easy for a skeptic to conclude that there's little or no real value in cold remedies. The experts say to rest and drink fluids. But when they actually have a cold, most people are less inclined to be skeptical and more inclined to be hopeful that something will help.

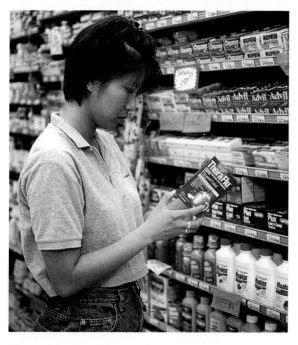

Shopper reading label on OTC medication

SUMMARY

- A drug may be sold OTC only if it can be used safely when following the label directions.
- The FDA began reviewing OTC ingredients for safety and efficacy in 1972, with the result that most of the various brands of medicines sold for a given use contain the same few ingredients.
- OTC stimulants are based on caffeine.
- OTC sleep aids are based on antihistamines.
- The main ingredient in OTC weight-control products is phenylpropanolamine (PPA).
- Aspirin has analgesic, antipyretic, and antiinflammatory actions. Acetaminophen and ibuprofen are related analgesics.
- Cold remedies usually contain an antihistamine, an analgesic, and a decongestant.
- An informed consumer can understand a large fraction of OTC medicines by knowing only eight ingredients.

REVIEW QUESTIONS

1. What do the acronyms GRAS, GRAE, and GRAHL stand for?
2. What is the process that is producing "tentative final monographs" on OTC products?
3. What are the criteria for deciding whether a drug should be sold OTC or by prescription?
4. What is the main ingredient found in "look-alike" pills for "speed"?
5. How safe and effective is PPA as a weight-control ingredient?
6. Diphenhydramine is found in what three brand-name sleep aids?
7. What effect of aspirin might be involved in its use to prevent TIAs and heart attacks?
8. What are the differences in the therapeutic effects of acetaminophen and ibuprofen?
9. What is the most common route for a cold virus to enter a person's system?
10. Which cold symptoms are supposed to be relieved by chlorpheniramine maleate and which by pseudoephedrine?

WEB WATCH

Related Internet Sites on OTC Drugs

The FDA OTC drug page: http://www.fda.gov/cder/otc/index.htm

Label Literacy for OTC Drugs: http://www.fda.gov/fdac/features/1997/497_otc.html

Nonprescription medicines: What's right for you? http://www.pueblo.gsa.gov/cic_text/health/nonmeds.txt

And our own "home remedy" for readers of *Drugs, Society, and Human Behavior*: http://www.uwyo.edu/A&S/psyc/dshb.htm

REFERENCES

1. FDA Proposes new, easy to understand labeling for OTC drugs, *Doctor's Guide to Medical and Other News*, Feb 26, 1997.
2. Conlan MF: FDA can't keep track of OTCs, GAO charges in report, *Drug Topics*, pp 58-50, Mar 23, 1992.
3. Rheinstein PH: FDA perspective: Prescription to over-the-counter drug switches, *American Family Physician*, Sept 15, 1997.
4. Farley D: Label literacy for OTC drugs, *FDA Consumer*, May–June, 1997.
5. FDA: OTC stimulant drug products, final monograph, *Federal Register*, Feb 29, 1988.
6. Beecher HK: Placebo effects of situations, attitudes and drugs: a quantitative study of suggestibility. In Rickels K, editor: *Non-specific factors in drug therapy*, Springfield, Ill, 1968, Charles C Thomas.
7. Smith LH Jr, Chairman, Medical Staff Conference: The clinical pharmacology of salicylates, *California Medicine* 110:411, 413, 1969.
8. FDA: Internal analgesic, antipyretic, and antirheumatic drug products for OTC human use: tentative final monograph, *Federal Register*, Nov 16, 1988.
9. Remington PL and others: Decreasing trends in Reye's syndrome and aspirin use in Michigan—1979 to 1984, *Pediatrics* 77:93-98, 1986.
10. Dickens C: *The collected letters of Charles Dickens*, 1880, Chapman & Hall.
11. Klumpp TG: The common cold—new concepts of transmission and prevention, *Medical Times* 108(11):98, 1s-3s, Nov 1980.
12. Adams JM: *Viruses and colds, the modern plague*, New York, 1967, American Elsevier.
13. *Federal Register* 50:10, Jan 15, 1985.
14. Conlan MF: House probes antihistamines in OTC cold medications, *Drug Topics*, p 59, May 4, 1992.
15. *FDA Consumer* 19(9):16, Nov 1985.
16. Murray S, Brewerton T: Abuse of over-the-counter dextromethorphan by teenagers, *South Med J* 86:1151, 1993.

ASSESS YOURSELF!

OTC Products

The following "product labels" include the actual list of ingredients from some OTC products. Your job is to figure out what each product is used for (hint: none of them is a laxative, acne medication, or contraceptive).

Use for:

Use for:

Use for:

Use for:

Use for:

Use for:

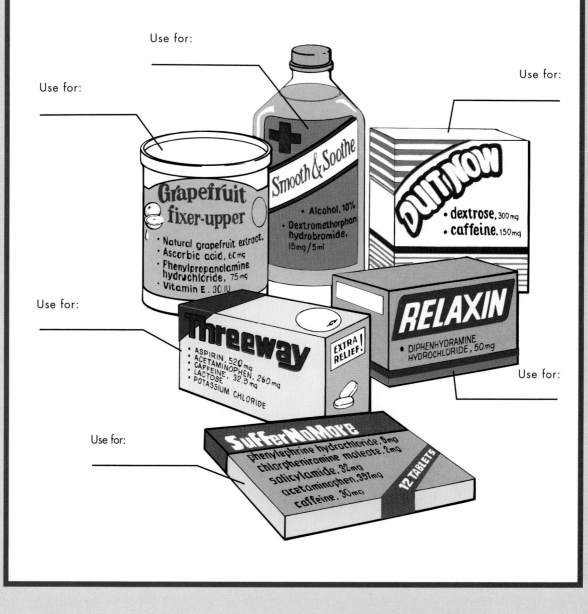

Grapefruit fixer-upper
• Natural grapefruit extract.
• Ascorbic acid, 60 mg
• Phenylpropanolamine hydrochloride, 75 mg
• Vitamin E, 30 IU

Smooth & Soothe
• Alcohol, 10%
• Dextromethorphan hydrobromide, 15 mg/5 ml

QUIT NOW
• dextrose, 300 mg
• caffeine, 150 mg

Threeway
• ASPIRIN, 520 mg
• ACETAMINOPHEN, 260 mg
• CAFFEINE, 32.5 mg
• LACTOSE
• POTASSIUM CHLORIDE
EXTRA! RELIEF!

RELAXIN
• DIPHENHYDRAMINE HYDROCHLORIDE, 50 mg

SufferNoMore
phenylephrine hydrochloride, 5 mg
chlorpheniramine maleate, 2 mg
salicylamide, 32 mg
acetaminophen, 357 mg
caffeine, 30 mg
12 TABLETS

6

Restricted Drugs

In contrast to the everyday drugs such as nicotine and caffeine, the drugs discussed in this section include some of the least familiar and most feared substances: heroin, LSD, and marijuana. More recently, the anabolic steroids used by some athletes have also become widely feared by the public, most of whom have no direct contact with the drugs. These substances, along with the stimulants cocaine and amphetamine, are commonly viewed as evil, "devil drugs."

15 Opiates

The opiates, or narcotics, include some of the oldest useful medicines. Why did they also become the most important illicit drugs of this century?

16 Hallucinogens

Are some drugs really capable of enhancing intellectual experience? Of producing madness?

17 Marijuana and Hashish

Why has a lowly and common weed become such an important symbol of the struggle between lifestyles?

18 Steroids and Other Drugs in Sport

What improvements can athletes obtain by resorting to drugs? What are the associated dangers?

15

Opiates

KEY TERMS	OBJECTIVES

After reading this chapter, you should be able to:

KEY TERMS

opium
morphine
codeine
heroin
black tar
narcotic antagonists
naloxone
enkephalins
endorphins
methadone
LAAM

OBJECTIVES

- Discuss the opium poppy as the original source of narcotic drugs and describe the history of this important plant substance.
- Describe how opiate addiction has changed over the years up to the present.
- Explain how the opiates work in the nervous system and what their effects are.
- List the ways in which opiates have been used to benefit human health and well-being.
- Discuss the dependence characteristics and the toxic properties of the opiates.
- Describe some of the behavioral patterns of narcotic abusers.
- Be able to discuss opiate antagonists and maintenance as chemical approaches to treating narcotic addiction.

And soon they found themselves in the midst of a great meadow of poppies. Now it is well known that when there are many of these flowers together their odor is so powerful that anyone who breathes it falls asleep, and if the sleeper is not carried away from the scent of the flowers he sleeps on and on forever. But Dorothy did not know this, nor could she get away from the bright red flowers that were everywhere about; so presently her eyes grew heavy and she felt she must sit down to rest and to sleep. . . . Her eyes closed in spite of herself and she forgot where she was and fell among the poppies, fast asleep. . . . They carried the sleeping girl to a pretty spot beside the river, far enough from the poppy field to prevent her breathing any more of the poison of the flowers, and here they laid her gently on the soft grass and waited for the fresh breeze to waken her.[1]

From the land of Oz to the streets of Harlem, the poppy has caused much grief—and much joy. **Opium** is a truly unique substance. This juice from the plant *Papaver somniferum* has a history of medical use perhaps 6,000 years long. Except for the last century and a half, opium stood alone as the one agent from which physicians could obtain sure results. Compounds containing opium solved several of the recurring problems for medical science wherever used. Opium relieved pain and suffering magnificently. Just as important in the years gone by was its ability to reduce the diarrhea and subsequent dehydration caused by dysentery, which is still a leading cause of death in underdeveloped countries.

Parallel with the medical use of opium was its use as a deliverer of pleasure and relief from anxiety. Because of these effects, extensive recreational use of opium has also occurred throughout history. Through all those years, many of its users experienced dependence.

HISTORY

Opium

Early history

The most likely origin of opium is in a hot, dry, Middle Eastern country several millennia ago when some unknown native discovered that for seven to ten days of its yearlong life *Papaver somniferum* produced a substance that, when eaten, would ease pain and suffering. The opium poppy is an annual plant three to four feet high with large flowers four to five inches in diameter. The flowers can be white, pink, red, purple, or violet.

Opium is produced and available for collection for only a few days of the plant's life, between the time the petals drop and before the seed pod matures. Today, as before, opium harvesters move through the fields in the early evening and use a sharp clawed tool to make shallow cuts into, but not through, the unripe seed pod. During the night a white substance oozes from the cuts, oxidizes to a red-brown color, and becomes gummy. In the morning the resinous substance is carefully scraped from the pod and collected in small balls. This raw opium forms the basis for the opium medicines used throughout history and is the substance from which morphine is extracted and then heroin is derived.

The importance and extent of use of the opium poppy in the early Egyptian and Greek cultures are still under debate, but in the Ebers papyrus (circa 1500 B.C.) a remedy is mentioned "to prevent the excessive crying of children." Because a later Egyptian remedy for the same purpose clearly contained opium (as well as fly ex- crement), many writers report the first specific medical use of opium as dating from the Ebers papyrus.

Homer's *Odyssey* (1000 B.C.) contains a passage that some authors believe refers to the use of opium. A party was about to become a real drag because everyone was sad thinking about Ulysses and the deaths of their friends, when:

> Helen, daughter of Zeus, poured into the wine they were drinking a drug, nepenthes, which gave forgetfulness of evil. Those who had drunk of this mixture did not shed a tear the whole day long, even though their mother or father were dead, even though a brother or beloved son had been killed before their eyes.[2]

The drug could only have been opium.

Opium was important in Greek medicine. Galen, the last of the great Greek physicians, emphasized caution in the use of opium but felt that it was almost a cure-all, saying that it

> resists poison and venomous bites, cures chronic headache, vertigo, deafness, epilepsy, apoplexy, dimness of sight, loss of voice, asthma, coughs of all kinds, spitting of blood, tightness of breath, colic, the iliac poison, jaundice, hardness of the spleen, stone, urinary complaints, fevers, dropsies, leprosies, the troubles to which women are subject, melancholy and all pestilences.[2]

Recreational use even then must have been extensive. Galen commented on the opium cakes and candies that were being sold everywhere in the streets.

Greek and Roman knowledge of opium use in medicine languished during the Dark Ages and thus had little influence on the world's use of opium for the next thousand years. The Arabic world, however, clutched opium to its breast,

---

opium: a raw plant substance containing morphine and codeine.

Left, Incised seedpod of the poppy plant. *Right,* Opium, the milky fluid of the seedpods, has been extracted from the poppy for thousands of years.

because the Koran forbade the use of alcohol in any form. Opium and hashish became the primary social drugs wherever the Islamic culture moved, and it did move. The Mohammadans were active fighters, explorers, and traders. While Europe rested through the Dark Ages, the Arabian world reached out and made contact with India and China. Opium was one of the products they traded, but they also sold the seeds of the opium poppy, and cultivation began in these countries. By the tenth century A.D., opium was referred to in Chinese medical writings.

During this period when the Arabic civilization flourished, two Arabic physicians made substantial contributions to medicine and to the history of opium. Shortly after A.D. 1000, Biruni composed a pharmacology book. His descriptions of opium contain what some believe to be the first written description of addiction.[3] In this same period the best-known Arabic physician, Avicenna, was using opium preparations very effectively and extensively in his medical practice. His writings, along with those of Galen, formed the basis of medical education in Europe

as the Renaissance dawned, and thus the glories of opium were advanced. (It is strange but true that a physician as knowledgeable as Avicenna, and a believer in the tenets of Islam, should die as a result of drinking too much of a mixture of opium and wine.)

Early in the sixteenth century lived a European medical phenomenon. Paracelsus apparently was a successful clinician and accomplished some wondrous cures for the day. One of his secrets was a potion called laudanum. Paracelsus was one of the early Renaissance supporters of opium as a panacea and referred to it as the "stone of immortality."

Due to Paracelsus and his followers, there was an increasing awareness of the broad effectiveness of opium, and new opium preparations were developed in the sixteenth, seventeenth, and eighteenth centuries. One of these was laudanum as prepared by Dr. Thomas Sydenham, the father of clinical medicine. Sydenham's general contributions to English medicine are so great that he has been called the English Hippocrates. He spoke more highly of opium than did Paracelsus, saying that "without opium the healing art would cease to exist." His laudanum contained 2 ounces of strained opium, 1 ounce of saffron, a dram of cinnamon, and a dram of cloves dissolved in 1 pint of Canary wine and taken in small quantities.

Writers and opium: the keys of paradise

In a momentous year for opium, 1805, Thomas De Quincey, a twenty-year-old English youth who had run away from home at seventeen, purchased some laudanum for a toothache and received change for his shilling from the apothecary. Here is his description of his response to this dose:

> I took it: and in an hour, O heavens! what a revulsion! what a resurrection, from its lowest depths, of the inner spirit! what an apocalypse of the world within me! That my pains had vanished was now a trifle in my eyes; this negative effect was swallowed up in the immensity of those positive effects which had opened before me, in the abyss of divine enjoyment thus suddenly revealed. Here was a panacea . . . for all human woes; here was the secret of happiness, about which philosophers had disputed for so many ages, at once discovered; happiness might now be bought for a penny, and carried in the waistcoat-pocket; portable ecstasies might be had corked up in a pint-bottle; and peace of mind could be sent down by the mail.[4]

For the rest of his life De Quincey used laudanum. He did not try to conceal the extent of his addiction. Rather, his writings are replete with insight into the opiate-hazed world, particularly his article "The Confessions of an English Opium-Eater," which was published in 1821 (and in book form in 1823). (Throughout this period, *opium eating* was the phrase generally used to refer to laudanum drinking.)

Several other famous English authors were also addicted to laudanum, including Elizabeth Barrett Browning and Samuel Taylor Coleridge. Coleridge's magnificently beautiful "Kubla Khan" was probably conceived and composed in

an opium reverie and then written down as best as he could remember it. However, De Quincey is of primary interest here. His emphasis was on understanding the effects that opium has on consciousness, experience, and feeling, and as such he provided some of the most vivid accounts of the power of opium.

Opium does not produce new worlds for the user:

> If a man, "whose talk is of oxen," should become an opium-eater, the probability is, that (if he is not too dull to dream at all)—he will dream about oxen; whereas, in the case before him [De Quincey], the reader will find that the opium-eater boasteth himself to be a philosopher; and accordingly, that the phantasmagoria of his dreams (waking or sleeping, day-dreams or night-dreams) is suitable to one of that character.[5]

Opium does, however, change the way the user perceives the world. For example, "an opium eater is too happy to observe the motion of time."[5]

De Quincey pointed out the sharp contrast between the effects of alcohol and those of opium:

> crude opium . . . is incapable of producing any state of body at all resembling that which is produced by alcohol. . . . It is not in the quantity of its effects merely, but in the quality, that it differs altogether. The pleasure given by wine is always rapidly mounting, and tending to a crisis, after which as rapidly it declines; that from opium, when once generated, is stationary for eight or ten hours. . . . The one is a flickering flame, the other a steady and equable glow. But the main distinction lies in this—that, whereas wine disorders the mental faculties, opium, on the contrary (if taken in a proper manner), introduces amongst them the most exquisite order, legislation, and harmony. Wine robs a man of his self-possession; opium sustains and reinforces it. Wine unsettles the judgment. . . . Opium, on the contrary, communicates serenity and equipoise to all the faculties.[5]

In spite of all the good things De Quincey said about opium and the effects it had on him, he suffered from its use. For long periods in his life he was unable to write as a result of his addiction. As with most things: "Opium gives and takes away. It defeats the steady habit of exertion; but it creates spasms of irregular exertion. It ruins the natural power of life; but it develops preternatural paroxysms of intermitting power."[6]

The publication of De Quincey's book in 1823 and its first translation into French in 1828 spurred the French Romantic writers to explore opium and hashish in the 1840s and later. The only associated American article of note in this period, "An Opium-Eater in America,"[7] appeared in an American magazine in 1842.

The Opium Wars

Although opium and the opium poppy had been introduced to China well before the year 1000, there was only a moderate level of use there by a select, elite group. Tobacco smoking spread much more rapidly after its introduction. It is not clear when tobacco was introduced to the Chinese, but its use had spread and become so offensive that in 1644 the emperor forbade tobacco smoking in China. The edict did not last long (as is to be expected), but it was in part responsible for the increase in opium smoking.

Up to this period the smoking of tobacco and the eating of opium had existed side by side. The restriction on the use of tobacco and the population's appreciation of the pleasures of smoking led to the combining of opium and tobacco for smoking. Presumably the addition of opium took the edge off the craving for tobacco. The amount of tobacco used was gradually reduced and soon omitted altogether. Although opium eating had never been very attractive to most Chinese, opium smoking spread rapidly, perhaps, at least partly, because smoking results in a rapid effect compared with oral use of opium.

In 1729, China's first law against opium smoking mandated that opium shop owners were to be strangled. Once opium for non-medical purposes was outlawed, it was necessary for the drug to be smuggled in from India,

where poppy plantations were abundant. Smuggling opium was so profitable for everyone—the growers, the shippers, and the customs officers—that unofficial rules were gradually developed for the game.[2] The background to the Opium Wars is too lengthy and complex to even attempt to sketch it adequately. However, some points must be made to explain why the British went to war so they could continue pouring opium into China against the wishes of the Chinese national government.

Since before 1557, when the Portuguese were allowed to develop the small trading post of Macao, pressure had been increasing on the Chinese emperors to open the country up to trade with the "barbarians from the West." Not only the Portuguese but the Dutch and the English repeatedly knocked on the closed door of China. Near the end of the seventeenth century the port of Canton was opened under very strict rules to foreigners. Tea was the major export, and the British shipped out huge amounts. There was little that the Chinese were interested in importing from the "barbarians," but opium could be smuggled so profitably that it soon became the primary import. The profit the British made from selling opium paid for the tea they shipped to England.[8] In the early nineteenth century the government of India was actually the British East India Company. As such it had a monopoly on opium, which was legal in India. However, smuggling it into China was not. The East India Company auctioned chests of opium cakes to private merchants, who gave the chests to selected British firms, who sold it for a commission to Chinese merchants. In this way the British were able to have the Chinese "smuggle" the opium into China! The number of chests of opium, each with about 120 pounds of smokable opium, that were annually imported to China increased from 200 in 1729 to about 5,000 at the century's end to 25,000 chests in 1838.

In the following year, 1839, the emperor of China made a fatal mistake—he sent an honest man to Canton to suppress the opium smuggling. Commissioner Lin demanded that the barbarians deliver all their opium supplies to him and subjected the dealers to confinement in their houses. After some haggling, the representative of the British government ordered the merchants to deliver the opium—20,000 chests worth about $6 million—which was then destroyed and everyone was set free. Pressures mounted, however, and an incident involving drunken American and British sailors killing a Chinese citizen started the Opium Wars in 1839. The British army arrived ten months later, and in two years, largely by avoiding land battles and by using the superior artillery of the royal navy ships, they won a victory over a country of more than 350 million citizens. As victors, the British were given the island of Hong Kong, broad trading rights, and $6 million to reimburse the merchants whose opium had been destroyed.

The Chinese opium trade posed a great moral dilemma for Britain. The East India Company protested until its end that it was not smuggling opium into China, and technically it was not. From 1870 to 1893, motions in Parliament to end the extremely profitable opium commerce failed to pass but did cause a decline in the opium trade. In 1893 a moral protest against the trade was supported, but not until 1906 did the government support and pass a bill that eventually ended the opium trade by 1913.

Morphine

In 1805 in London, twenty-year-old De Quincey eased a toothache and fell into the abyss of divine enjoyment. In Hanover, Germany, another twenty-year-old worked on experiments that were to have great impact on science, medicine, and the pleasure seekers. In 1806 this German youth, Frederich Sertürner, published his report of over fifty experiments, which clearly showed that he had isolated the primary active ingredient in opium. The active

agent was ten times as potent as opium. Sertürner named it *morphium* after Morpheus, the god of dreams. Use of the new agent developed slowly, but by 1831 the implications of his chemical work and the medical value of **morphine** were so overwhelming that this pharmacist's assistant was given the French equivalent of the Nobel Prize. Later work into the mysteries of opium found over thirty different alkaloids, with the second most important one being isolated in 1832 and named **codeine**, the Greek word for "poppy head."

The availability of a clinically useful, pure chemical of known potency is always capitalized on in medicine. The major increase in the use of morphine came as a result of two nondrug developments, one technological and one political. The technological development was the perfection of the hypodermic syringe in 1853 by Dr. Alexander Wood. This made it possible to deliver morphine directly into the blood or tissue rather than by the much slower process of eating opium or morphine and waiting for absorption to occur from the gastrointestinal tract. A further advantage of injecting morphine was thought to exist. Originally it was felt that morphine by injection would not be as addicting as the oral use of the drug. This belief was later found to be false.

The political events that sped the drug of sleep and dreams into the veins of people worldwide were the American Civil War (1861–1865), the Prussian-Austrian War (1866), and the Franco-Prussian War (1870). Military medicine was, and to some extent still is, characterized by the dictum "first provide relief." Morphine given by injection did work rapidly and well, and it was administered regularly in

---

morphine: active narcotic agent in opium

codeine: active narcotic agent in opium.

large doses to many soldiers for the reduction of pain and relief from dysentery. The percentage of veterans returning from these wars who were addicted to morphine was high enough that the illness was later called "soldier's disease" or the "army disease."

Heroin

Toward the end of the nineteenth century, a small but important chemical transformation was made to the morphine molecule. In 1874, two acetyl groups were attached to morphine, yielding diacetylmorphine, which was given the brand name Heroin and placed on the market in 1898 by Bayer Laboratories. The chemical change was important because **heroin** is about three times as potent as morphine. The pharmacology of heroin and morphine is identical except that the two acetyl groups increase the lipid solubility of the heroin molecule, and thus the molecule enters the brain more rapidly. The additional groups are then detached, yielding morphine. Therefore, the effects of morphine and heroin are identical except that heroin is more potent and acts faster.

Heroin was originally marketed as a nonaddicting substitute for codeine.[9] It seemed to be the perfect drug, more potent yet less harmful. Although not introduced commercially until 1898, heroin had been studied, and many of its pharmacological actions were reported in 1890.[10] By January 1900 a comprehensive review article concluded that tolerance and addiction (habituation) to heroin were only minor problems.

> Habituation has been noted in a small percentage . . . of the cases. . . . All observers are agreed, however, that none of the patients suffer in any way from this habituation, and that none of the symptoms which are so characteristic of chronic morphinism have ever been observed. On the other hand, a large number of the reports refer to the fact that the same dose may be used for a long time without any habituation.[11]

The basis for the failure to find addiction probably was the fact that heroin was initially used as a substitute for codeine, which meant oral doses of 3 to 5 mg used for brief periods of time. Slowly the situation changed, and a 1905 text *Pharmacology and Therapeutics* took a middle ground on heroin by saying that it "is stated not to give rise to habituation. A more extended knowledge of the drug, however, would seem to indicate that the latter assertion is not entirely correct."[12] In a few more years everyone knew that heroin could be very addicting when injected in higher doses.

Opiate Addiction before the Harrison Act

In the second half of the nineteenth century, three forms of opiate addiction were developing in the United States. The long-useful oral intake of opium, and then morphine, increased greatly as patent medicines became a standard form of self-medication. After 1850 Chinese laborers were imported in large numbers to the West Coast, and they introduced opium smoking to this country. The last form, medically the most dangerous and ultimately the most disruptive socially, was the injection of morphine.

Around the turn of the century the percentage (and perhaps the absolute number) of Americans addicted to one of the opiates was very probably greater than at any other time before or since. Several authorities, both then and more recently, agree that no less than 1 percent of the population was addicted to opium, although accurate statistics are not available. In spite of the high level of addiction, it was not a major social problem. In this period:

> The public then had an altogether different conception of drug addiction from that which prevails today. The habit was not approved, but neither was it regarded as criminal or monstrous. It was usually looked upon as a vice or personal misfortune, or much as alcoholism is viewed today. Narcotics users were pitied rather than loathed as criminals or degenerates.[13]

The opium smoking the Chinese brought to this country never became widely popular, although around the turn of the century about one-fourth of the opium imported was smoking opium. Perhaps it was because the smoking itself occupies only about a minute and is then followed by a dreamlike state of reverie that can last two or three hours—hardly conducive to a continuation of daily activities or consonant with the outward, active orientation of most Americans in that period. Another reason why opium smoking did not spread was that it originated with Asians, who were scorned by whites. Similarly, the opium smoking that did occur among whites was found within the asocial and antisocial elements of the culture. Amusingly, even the underworld has its standards of morality, and opium smokers looked down on those who used their drugs by injection. In a New York opium-smoking den early in this century, "one of the smokers discovered a hypodermic user in the bathroom giving himself an injection. He immediately reported to the proprietor that there was a 'God-damned dope fiend in the can.' The offender was promptly ejected."[13]

The growth of the patent medicine industry after the Civil War has been well documented. Everything seemed to be favorable for the industry, and it took advantage of each opportunity. There were few government regulations on the industry, and as a result addicting drugs were an important part of many tonics and remedies, although this fact did not have to be indicated on the label. Because labeling of ingredients was not required, a user who had become aware that he was addicted and who wanted to purchase a cure could be sold a remedy labeled as a cure that contained almost as much of the addicting drug as he had been receiving in the original tonic.

The generally poor level of health care in the country and a large number of maimed and diseased veterans created a need for considerable medical treatment. Patent medicines

promised, and in part delivered, the perfect self-medication. They were easily available, not too expensive, socially acceptable, and, miracle of miracles, they did work. The amount of alcohol and/or opiates in many of the nostrums was certain to relieve the user's aches, pains, and anxieties.

Gradually some medical concern developed over the number of people who were addicted to opiates, and this concern was a part of the motivation that led to the passage of the 1906 Pure Food and Drugs Act. In 1910 a government expert in this area made clear that this law was only a beginning:

> The thoughtful and foremost medical men have been and are cautioning against the free use of morphine and opium, particularly in recurring pain. The amount they are using is decreasing yearly. Notwithstanding this fact, and the fact that legislation, federal, state and territorial, adverse to the indiscriminate use and sale of opium and morphine, their derivatives and preparations, has been enacted during the past few decades, the amount of opium per capita imported and consumed in the United States has doubled during the last forty years. . . . It is well known that there are many factors at work tending to drug enslavement, among them being the host of soothing syrups, medicated soft drinks containing cocaine, asthma remedies, catarrh remedies, consumption remedies, cough and cold remedies, and the more notorious so-called "drug addiction cures." It is often stated that medical men are frequently the chief factors in causing drug addiction.[14]

Data were presented in this paper that tended to support the belief that medical use of opiates initiated by a physician was one, if not the, major cause of addiction in this country at that time. A 1918 government report clearly indicted

---

heroin: diacetylmorphine, a more potent derivative of morphine.

the physician as the major cause of addiction in addicts of "good social standing."

That physicians widely used opiates as drugs in treatment is understandable in light of articles that had been published, such as one in 1889 titled "Advantages of Substituting the Morphia Habit for the Incurably Alcoholic." The author stated:

> In this way I have been able to bring peacefulness and quiet to many disturbed and distracted homes, to keep the head of a family out of the gutter and out of the lock-up, to keep him from scandalous misbehavior and neglect of his affairs, to keep him from the verges and actualities of delirium tremens horrors, and above all, to save him from committing, as I veritably believe, some terrible crime.[15]

Besides all those good things, morphine addiction was cheap: by one estimate it was ten times as expensive to be an alcoholic—costing 25 cents a day. The article concluded:

> I might, had I time and space, enlarge by statistics to prove the law-abiding qualities of opium-eating peoples, but of this any one can perceive somewhat for himself, if he carefully watches and reflects on the quiet, introspective gaze of the morphine habitue, and compares it to the riotous, devil-may-care leer of the drunkard.[15]

This middle history period, 1806 to 1914, is rich in material on the use of opiates that gives background to the thesis that if drugs are widely used, it is because they meet the needs of a culture. An 1880 report called addiction a "vice of middle life." The typical opiate addict of this period was a thirty- to fifty-year-old white woman who functioned well and was adjusted to her life as a wife and mother. She bought opium or morphine legally at the local store, used it orally, and caused few, if any, social problems. She might have ordered her "family remedy" through the mail from Sears, Roebuck—two ounces of laudanum for 18 cents or $1\frac{1}{2}$ pints for $2. Of course there were problems associated with addiction during this period. There are

always individuals who are unable to control their drug intake, whether the drug is used for self-medication or recreation. Because of the high opiate content of patent medicines and the ready availability of addicting drugs for drinking and/or injecting, very high levels of drug were frequently used. As a result, the symptoms of withdrawal were very severe—much worse than today—and the only relief to be found was by taking more of the drug.

After the Harrison Act

The complex reasons for the passage of the 1914 Harrison Act were discussed in detail in chapter 4. Remember that this was a fairly simple revenue measure. However, as is true of most laws, it is not the law itself that becomes important in the ensuing years, but the court decisions and enforcement practices that evolve as the law interacts with the people it affects.

Eliminating Legal Sources

> The passing of the Harrison Act in 1914 left the status of the addict almost completely indeterminate. The act did not make addiction illegal and it neither authorized nor forbade doctors to prescribe drugs regularly for addicts. All that it clearly and unequivocally did require was that whatever drugs addicts obtained were to be secured from physicians registered under the act and that the fact of securing drugs be made a matter of record. While some drug users had obtained supplies from physicians before 1914, it was not necessary for them to do so since drugs were available for purchase in pharmacies and even from mail-order houses.[16]

In 1915 the United States Supreme Court decided that possession of smuggled opiates was a crime, and thus users not obtaining the drug from a physician became criminals with the stroke of a pen. Addicts could still obtain their supply of drugs on a prescription from a physician, until this avenue was removed by

---

UP FOR DEBATE

Should Heroin be Made Available for Medical Purposes?

Since the 1920s, heroin has been unavailable to physicians for any purpose. It was the first such drug to be so restricted, and its status has now been codified along with that of LSD and marijuana under the status of Schedule I controlled substances—those with "no medical use."

However, heroin has been available all along in most countries as a potent pain reliever. It has repeatedly been proposed over the years that heroin should be moved to Schedule II and thus become available for medical use by prescription. Whether heroin is actually a better pain reliever than morphine has been argued for many years—it is more potent, in that less is required for the same effect, but since heroin is converted to morphine in the brain, morphine should be just as effective if given in a higher dose. Regardless of the limited amount of evidence on either side, some physicians believe that heroin should be available in the United States for pain relief. Under some of the proposals heroin would only be available under restricted circumstances, such as the failure of other potent narcotics to control the pain.

As the situation now stands, according to one prominent proponent[45] of medical heroin, the drug is more readily available to a 16-year-old kid on the street than it is to a terminally ill cancer patient in constant pain.

Supreme Court decisions in 1920 and 1922 (see chapter 4). Even though the Lindner case in 1925 reversed these earlier decisions and stated that a physician could prescribe drugs to non-hospitalized addicts just to maintain them, the doctors had been harassed and arrested enough. Even though it was legal again to prescribe drugs to an addict, few physicians would do so. Clinics for the treatment of opiate addicts were closed during the 1920s under pressure from federal officials.

The number of oral opiate users began to decline in response to these pressures, and the primary remaining group were those who injected morphine or heroin. By 1922 about the only source of opiates for a nonhospitalized addict was an illegal dealer. Because heroin was the most potent opiate available, it was the easiest to conceal and therefore became the illegal dealer's choice. The cost through this source was thirty to fifty times the price of the same drug through legitimate sources, which no longer were available to the addict. Because of this cost, addicts wanted to be certain to get the most "bang for their buck," so intravenous injection became more and more common. To maintain a supply of the drug in this way was expensive. Many addicts resorted to criminal activity, primarily burglary and other crimes against property, to finance their addiction.

During this period, law enforcement agencies and the popular press brought about a change in the attitudes of society toward the addict. Thus sometime during the 1920s,

the addict was no longer seen as a victim of drugs, an unfortunate with no place to turn and deserving of society's sympathy and help. He became instead a base, vile, degenerate who was weak and self-indulgent, who contaminated all he came in contact with and who deserved nothing short of condemnation and society's moral outrage and legal sanction. The law enforcement approach was accepted as the only workable solution to the problem of addiction.[17]

The changing addict population

After the Harrison Act there almost certainly was a decline in the number of addicts using opiates orally and thus a drop in white middle-aged users. One paper commented that between World War I and World War II heroin received little publicity and was primarily used by "people in *the life*—show people, entertainers and musicians; racketeers and gangsters; thieves and pickpockets; prostitutes and pimps."[18] The transition from the 1930s to the 1950s in the United States has been best described by an internationally recognized expert who worked in the area of drug addiction through this period.

If you go back to 1935 the other problems, apart from alcohol, were primarily the opiates and cocaine, usually taken together in the form of the so-called "speed-ball" and then as now . . . drug use was multiple. These individuals that I know used morphine, cocaine, heroin, bromides, phenobarbital or whatever happened to come along but they preferred the opiates and cocaine. The people of those days were really predominately white individuals, they were on the whole members of various criminal trades, pickpockets and so on, and in fact most of them had been involved in these criminal trades either before or after their onset of their career of using drugs. These people more or less disappeared during the Second World War which practically made these drugs unavailable . . . the old fashioned addict, the expert pickpocket, the short change artist couldn't get drugs. This group was succeeded, after the war was over, by a new kind of opiate taker. These were primarily individuals from the minority groups in the big city slums and in contrast to the older addicts who got good drugs, who knew good stuff when they got it, this new group were getting drugs extremely diluted, full of all kinds of other poisons and were a very different kind of people. They were not expert thieves, in fact very inexpert.[19]

In the early years after World War II, heroin use slowly increased in the lower-class, slum areas of the large cities. Heroin was inexpensive in this period; a dollar would buy enough for a good high for three to six people; $2-a-day habits were real and not uncommon. As the 1950s passed by, heroin use spread rapidly. As demand increased, so did both the price and the amount of adulteration.

The 1960s

A brief summary of heroin use from 1940 to 1970 suggests that all the rules changed in late 1961.[18] A critical shortage of heroin developed, prices tripled, and adulteration was carried to new heights. Because this increased profits, the price and adulteration level stayed the same when heroin was again in good supply. It appears that it might have been the large increase in price that disrupted the previous social cohesiveness among addicts, increased the amount of crime, and contributed to the general social disorganization of the ghettos, where most addicts lived.

In the 1960s the use of heroin and other drugs skyrocketed. Flower children, hippies, Tim Leary, and LSD received most of the media attention, but within the central core of the large American cities the number of regular and irregular heroin users increased daily. As you might expect, mainstream USA gradually became concerned with the heroin problem of the large cities. The increase in crime was the key, and because the most visible addicts were black or Latino, the white majority saw little relevance of the addiction to their own personal, family, and social problems.

Vietnam

The attitude of people in the street toward the relevance of addiction to their personal lives changed rapidly with the reports that began to filter out of Southeast Asia toward the end of the 1960s. Public anxiety increased dramatically with the possibility that the Vietnam conflict might produce thousands of addicts among the military personnel stationed there.

The Department of Defense established a Task Force on Drug Abuse in 1967; its initial reports emphasized concern over the widespread use of marijuana by troops in combat zones, as well as in rest and rehabilitation areas. In 1970, public and federal concern began to focus on the problem of heroin addiction among service personnel stationed in Southeast Asia.[20]

Heroin was about 95 percent pure and almost openly sold in South Vietnam, whereas purity in the United States was about 5 percent in 1969. Not only was the Southeast Asia heroin undiluted, it was inexpensive. Ten dollars would buy about 250 mg, an amount that would cost over $500 in the United States. The high purity of the heroin made it possible to obtain psychological effects by smoking or sniffing the drug. This fact, coupled with the completely wrong belief that addiction occurs only when the drug is used intravenously, resulted in about 40 percent of the users sniffing, about half smoking, and only 10 percent mainlining their heroin.[21]

Some early 1971 reports estimated that 10 to 15 percent of the American troops in Vietnam were addicted to heroin. As a result of the increased magnitude and visibility of the heroin problem, the U.S. government took several rapid steps in mid 1971. One step was to initiate Operation Golden Flow, a urine testing program for opiates in service personnel ready to leave Vietnam. The testing program, which tested *only* for opiates, was later expanded to include nonmilitary personnel.

In October 1971 the Pentagon released figures for the first three months of testing, which showed that 5.1 percent of the 100,000 personnel tested showed traces of opiates in their urine. Most of the opiate users were in the lower ranks.

In retrospect the Vietnam drug-use situation was "making a mountain out of a molehill," but much was learned. An excellent follow-up study[22] of veterans who returned from Vietnam

in September 1971 showed that most of the Vietnam heroin users did not continue heroin use in this country. Only 1 to 2 percent were using narcotics eight to twelve months after returning from Vietnam and being released from the service, approximately the same percentage of individuals found to be using narcotics when examined for induction into the service.

One of the important things learned from this experience is that narcotic addiction and compulsive use are not inevitable among occasional users. The pattern of drug use in Vietnam also supports the belief that under certain conditions—availability and low cost of the drug, boredom, unhappiness—a relatively high percentage of individuals will use narcotic drugs recreationally.

The 1970s and 1980s

Beginning in the late 1960s the federal government made several efforts to estimate the number of heroin users in the United States. As we learned in chapter 1, this is an impossible task to perform with much accuracy, given that heroin use is conducted in great secrecy and is not uniformly distributed across the country. Nevertheless, several sophisticated statistical techniques were brought to bear, combining various sources of information. Different groups of researchers estimated the number of heroin addicts from 1970 to the mid 1980s, and the estimates mostly ranged between 400,000 and 500,000.[23] Perhaps because of considerable variability in the estimates, no particular trends or patterns can be seen in these data, and one might argue that heroin addiction didn't really change much over that period.

In 1972 the major source of U.S. heroin was opium grown in Turkey and converted into heroin in southern French port cities, such as Marseilles. This "French connection" accounted for as much as 80 percent of U.S. heroin before 1973. In 1972, Turkey banned all opium cultivation and production in return for $35 million the United States provided to make up for the

Skull and heroin paraphenalia

financial losses to farmers and to help them develop new cash crops. This action, combined with a cooperative effort with the French (also partially funded by the United States), did lead to a reduction in the supply of heroin on the streets of New York in 1973.

This relative shortage did not last for long. In Mexico, opium is processed into morphine by a different process, and the resulting pure heroin has a brown or black color. By 1975 the Drug Enforcement Administration (DEA) estimated that 80 percent or more of all U.S. heroin was from Mexico (depending on its appearance, either called *Mexican brown* or **black tar**). The supply was plentiful, the price low, and the purity high. In 1974 the United States began to finance opium eradication programs in Mexico.

Although it is a hopeless task to try to eliminate all such production, these monumental and expensive efforts did slow the importation from Mexico to some extent, and the "epidemic" of the 1970s began to decline.

In the mid 1980s, about half of the U.S. heroin supply apparently originated in Southwest Asia (Afghanistan, Pakistan, Iran). Mexico was the next biggest contributor, with the Golden Triangle area of Southeast Asia (Burma, Laos, and Thailand) producing about 15 to 20 percent of the total. Production of opium and availability of refined heroin from all three of these regions increased during the second half of the 1980s, but the biggest increase came from Southeast Asia, which by 1990 was estimated to be producing 56 percent of the U.S. supply (figure 15.1).[24]

Current use of heroin

It seems as though every few years the media rediscover a new "heroin epidemic" among young, upper-class, or middle-class Americans. And every generation does have its few who dare. Also in every generation a few well-known musicians or entertainers either die from heroin overdoses or make a public announcement of their "kicking the habit." One new twist in the 1990s was the popularity of models who were very thin, with sunken eyes and the overall appearance of addicts—"heroin chic" as it was known in the fashion industry.[25] Many expressed fear that glamorizing addicts in this way would attract new users, and self-reported experimental heroin use did increase in the 1990s among high school seniors.

For many years the DEA has used informants to purchase heroin in various regions of the country and arrived at an estimated average "street" price and purity. From the mid 1970s through the mid 1980s the average purity varied from 4 to 6 percent heroin (yes, that means that over 90 percent was something else that the dealers had used to "cut" the heroin). However, in the late 1980s increased shipments of increas-

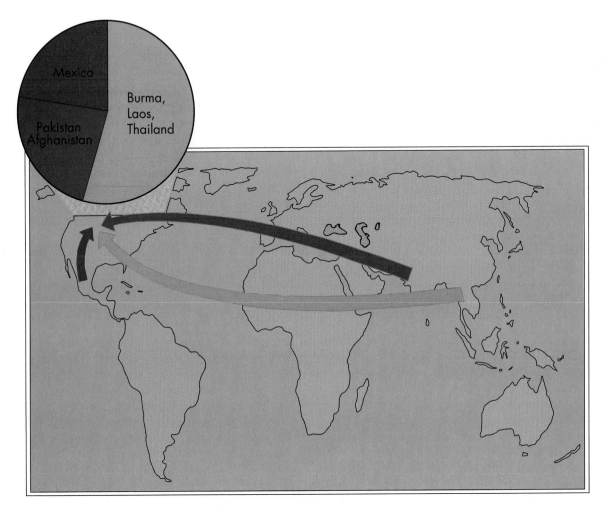

Figure 15.1 Sources of illicit heroin for the United States

ingly pure heroin began to arrive, and in 1990 the average street purity was estimated to be 18.2 percent, at least three times as strong as in years past.   By 1995 the estimated average purity had increased further, to over 50 percent. The price of a "bag" did not change much, so the price per milligram of actual heroin was down considerably.

One big change in the 1990s was that smoking opiates was back, although in a slightly different form than the old opium den. Piggybacking on the smoking of crack cocaine, inner-city users were either mixing the new high-potency heroin with crack or simply

black tar: a type of illicit heroin usually imported from Mexico.

In the 1990s, there has been an increase in the number of Nigerians and other West Africans arrested for smuggling heroin.[24] Although West Africa is not a major growing or manufacturing area, Nigerians have become increasingly involved in the worldwide traffic in cocaine and heroin, bound not only for the U.S. market but also for Europe.

Typical Nigerian "mules" might each swallow 80 or 100 condoms filled with heroin totaling a pound or more, then take a regular airline flight to New York, Paris, or wherever

the buyers are waiting. On arrival, if they are not caught, they wait for the condoms to pass through their intestine, hand them over, and collect their fee. Although each courier risks arrest and might receive only a few thousand dollars for his or her trouble, that represents more than ten years' earnings for an average Nigerian worker.

It seems that as long as there is an illicit market and there are poor people anywhere in the world, some of them will be willing to take the risk to earn high profits.

---

heating the heroin and inhaling the vapors from a "crack pipe." The increased purity of available heroin has allowed smoking, as well as snorting, to produce the effects users want, while they avoid the use of needles that might spread AIDs or other diseases. However, a couple of mysterious cases of brain damage appeared in New York in 1996, and these were tentatively attributed to smoking heroin by heating it in aluminum foil.[26]

PHARMACOLOGY OF THE OPIATES

Chemical Characteristics

Raw opium contains about 10 percent morphine by weight and a smaller amount of codeine. The addition of two acetyl groups to the morphine molecule results in diacetylmorphine, or heroin (figure 15.2). The acetyl groups allow heroin to penetrate the blood-brain barrier more readily, and heroin is therefore two to three times more potent than morphine.

Medicinal chemists have worked hard over the decades to produce compounds that would be effective painkillers, trying to separate

the analgesic effect of the opiates from their dependence-producing effects. Although the two effects could not be separated, the research has resulted in a variety of synthetic opiates that are sold as pain relievers (table 15.1). Especially interesting among these is fentanyl, which is approximately a hundred times as potent as morphine. Fentanyl is used primarily in conjunction with surgical anesthesia, although both fentanyl and some of its derivatives have also been manufactured illegally and sold on the streets. In 1994, Abbott Laboratories began to market a prescription fentanyl "lollipop" for children who are facing surgery or other painful procedures. This drug is so potent that if a child sucks on the lozenge, which is supplied on a plastic stick, within 5 to 15 minutes significant sedation and analgesia are obtained. Apparently Abbott is betting that such a device will find use when children are frightened and in pain and the threat of receiving an anesthetic injection would only increase the child's distress.

In addition to the opiate analgesics, this search for new compounds led to the discovery of **narcotic antagonists**, drugs that block the

Morphine   Codeine   Heroin

■ carbon ■ oxygen ■ nitrogen (hydrogen omitted)

Figure 15.2 Narcotic agents isolated or derived from opium

action of morphine, heroin, or other opiates. The administration of a drug such as **naloxone** or *nalorphine* can save a person's life by reversing the depressed respiration resulting from a narcotic overdose. If given to an individual who has been taking narcotics and who has become physically dependent, these antagonists can precipitate an immediate withdrawal syndrome. Both naloxone and the longer-lasting *naltrexone* have been given to addicts to prevent them from experiencing a "high" if they then use heroin.

Mechanism of Action

In the early 1970s, techniques were developed that led to the discovery of selective opiate receptors in rat brain tissue. For decades before this, theories of opiate drug action had relied on the concept of an opiate receptor, but the finding that such structures actually exist in the membranes of neurons led to the next question: What are opiate receptors doing sitting around in the synapses of the brain? Waiting for someone to extract the juice from a poppy? The distribution of these receptors didn't agree with the distribution of any known neurotransmitter substance, so scientists all over the world went to work looking for a substance in the brain that could serve as the natural activator of these opiate receptors. Groups in England and in Sweden succeeded in 1974: a pair of molecules, leu-enkephalin and met-enkephalin, were isolated from brain extracts. These **enkephalins** acted like morphine and were many times more

> **narcotic antagonists:** drugs that can block the actions of narcotics.
>
> **naloxone:** (nal *ox* own) a narcotic antagonist.
>
> **enkephalins:** (en *kef* a lins) morphine-like neurotransmitters found in the brain and adrenals.

TABLE 15.1

Some Prescription Narcotic Analgesics

Generic name	Trade name(s)	Recommended dose (mg)
Natural products		
Morphine		10–30
Codeine		30–60
Semisynthetics		
Heroin, diamorph	(not available in the US)	5–10
Synthetics		
Methadone	Dolophine	2.5–10
Meperidine	Demerol	50–150
Oxycodone	Percodan	2.25–4.5
Oxymorphone	Numorphan	1–1.5
Hydrocodone		5–10
Hydromorphone	Dilaudid	1–4
Dihydrocodeine		32
Propoxyphene	Darvon	32–65
Pentazocine	Talwin	30
Fentanyl	Sublimaze	0.05–0.10

potent. Next came the discovery of a group of **endorphins** (endogenous morphine-like substances) that are also found in brain tissue and also have potent opiate effects.

These discoveries opened a number of doors for scientists, some of which have helped to answer questions and others of which have led only to more questions. It is now clear that endorphins and enkephalins are contained within neurons and released from terminals to act as neurotransmitters or as modulators of neural activity.[27] Beta-endorphin is contained in a relatively small number of long-axon neurons that interconnect the hypothalamus, forebrain limbic structures, the medial thalamus, and the locus ceruleus. Enkephalins are found in a larger number of short-axon neurons within the basal ganglia, hypothalamus, amygdala, substantia nigra, and other areas. In addition to these two major types of endogenous opiates, there are dynorphins and other substances that have some actions similar to morphine. The search for a single endogenous opioid led to the discovery of a wide variety, and another new ag-

onist was reported in 1997.[28] These substances, as well as the natural and synthetic opiate drugs, have actions on at least three different types of opiate receptors, the structures of which were discovered in the early 1990s. One of the most important sites of action may be the midbrain central gray, a region known to be involved in pain perception. However, there are many other sites of interaction between these systems and areas that relate to pain, and pain itself is a complex psychological and neurological phenomenon, so we cannot say that we understand completely how the opiates act to reduce pain.

In addition to the presence of these endogenous opiates in the brain, we know that large amounts of endorphins are released from the pituitary gland in response to stress. Also, enkephalins are released from the adrenal gland. The functions of these peptides circulating through the blood as hormones are not understood at this point. They could perhaps reduce pain by acting in the spinal cord, but they are unlikely to produce direct effects in the brain because they probably do not cross the blood-brain barrier. In the late 1970s, it was speculated that long-distance runners experience a release of endorphins that might be responsible for the so-called runner's high. Unfortunately, the only evidence in support of this notion was measurements of blood levels of endorphins that seemed to be elevated in some, but not all, runners. These endorphins were presumably from the pituitary and might not be capable of producing a high. It is not known whether exercise alters *brain* levels of these substances.

BENEFICIAL USES

Pain Relief

The major therapeutic indication for morphine and the other narcotics is the reduction of pain. After the administration of an analgesic dose of morphine, some patients report that they are still aware of pain but that the pain is no longer aversive. The narcotic agents seem to have their effect in part by diminishing the patient's awareness of and response to the aversive stimulus. Morphine primarily reduces the emotional response to pain (the suffering), and to some extent also the knowledge of the pain stimulus.

The effect of narcotics is relatively specific to pain. Fewer effects on mental and motor ability accompany analgesic doses of these agents than accompany equipotent doses of other analgesic and depressant drugs. Although one of the characteristics of these drugs is their ability to reduce pain without inducing sleep, drowsiness is not uncommon after a therapeutic dose. (In the addicts' vernacular, the patient is "on the nod.") The patient is readily awakened if she sleeps, and dreams during the sleep period are frequent.

Intestinal Disorders

Narcotics have long been valued for their effects on the gastrointestinal system. They quiet colic and save lives by counteracting diarrhea. In years past and today in many underdeveloped countries, contaminated food or water has resulted in severe intestinal infections (dysentery). Particularly in the young and the elderly, the diarrhea and resulting dehydration can be a major cause of death.

Narcotic drugs decrease the number of peristaltic contractions, which is the type of contraction responsible for moving food through the intestines. Considerable water is absorbed from the intestinal material; this fact, plus the decrease in peristaltic contractions, often results in constipation in patients taking the drugs for pain relief. This side effect is what has saved many lives of dysentery victims. Although modern synthetic narcotic derivatives are now sold for this purpose, good old-fashioned paregoric, an opium solution, is still available for the symptomatic relief of diarrhea.

Cough Suppressants

The narcotics also have the effect of decreasing activity in what the advertisers refer to as the cough control center in the medulla. Although coughing is often a useful way of clearing unwanted material from the respiratory passages, at times "nonproductive" coughing can itself become a problem. Since it was first purified from opium, codeine has been widely used for its *antitussive* properties and is still available in a number of prescription cough remedies. Nonprescription cough remedies contain dextromethorphan, a narcotic analogue that is somewhat more selective in its antitussive effects.

---

endorphins: (en *dor* fins) morphine-like neurotransmitters found in the brain and pituitary gland.

CAUSES FOR CONCERN

Dependence Potential

Tolerance

Tolerance develops to most of the effects of the narcotic drugs, although with different effects tolerance can occur at different rates. If the drug is used chronically for pain relief, for example, it will probably be necessary to increase the dose to maintain a constant effect. The same is true for the euphoria sought by recreational users: repeated use results in a decreased effect that can be overcome by increasing the dose. Cross-tolerance exists among all the narcotics: tolerance to one reduces the effectiveness of each of the others. Siegel[29] and others have shown that psychological processes can play an important role in the tolerance to narcotics. When a user repeatedly injects an opiate, various physiological effects occur (changes in body temperature, intestinal motility, respiration rate, and so on). With repeated experience the addict might unconsciously learn to anticipate those effects and to counteract them. Animal experiments have shown that, after repeated morphine injections, a placebo injection produces changes in body temperature opposite to those originally produced by morphine. Thus some of the body's tolerance to narcotics results from conditioned reflex responses to the stimuli associated with taking the drug. To demonstrate how important these conditioned protective reflexes can become, Siegel and his colleagues injected rats with heroin every other day in a particular environment. After fifteen such injections, rats were given a much larger dose of heroin, half in the environment previously associated with heroin and half in a different environment. Of the group given the heroin injection in the different environment, most of the rats died. However, of the group given heroin in the environment that had previously predicted heroin, most of the rats lived.[30] Those rats had presumably learned to associate that environment with heroin injections, and conditioned reflexes occurred that counteracted some of the physiological effects of the drug. This is one example of behavioral tolerance.

Physical dependence

Concomitant with the development of tolerance is the establishment of physical dependence: in a person who has used the drug chronically and at high doses, as each dose begins to wear off, certain withdrawal symptoms begin to appear. These symptoms and their approximate timing after heroin or methadone use are listed in table 15.2. This list of symptoms might have more personal meaning for you if you compare it to a good case of the "24-hour" or "intestinal" flu: combine nausea and vomiting with diarrhea, aches, pains, and a general sense of misery, and you have a pretty good idea of what a moderate case of narcotic withdrawal is like: rarely life-threatening but most unpleasant. If an individual has been taking a large amount of the narcotic, then these symptoms can be much worse than those caused by "24-hour flu" and last at least twice as long. Note that **methadone**, a longer-lasting synthetic narcotic, produces withdrawal symptoms that are usually less severe and always appear later than with heroin. Cross-dependence is seen among the narcotics: no matter which of them was responsible for producing the initial dependence, withdrawal symptoms can be prevented by an appropriate dose of any narcotic. This is the basis for the use of methadone in treating heroin addicts, because substituting legal methadone prevents withdrawal symptoms for as much as a day.

An interesting clue to the biochemical mechanism of withdrawal symptoms has been the finding that *clonidine*, an alpha-adrenergic agonist that is used to treat high blood pressure, can diminish the severity of narcotic withdrawal symptoms. Studies on brain tissue reveal that opiate receptors and alpha-adrenergic receptors are found together in some brain areas, including the norepinephrine-containing cells of the locus

TABLE 15.2

Sequence of Appearance of Some of the Abstinence Syndrome Symptoms

Signs	Approximate hours after last dose	
	Heroin and/or morphine	Methadone
Craving for drugs, anxiety	6	24
Yawning, perspiration, running nose, teary eyes	14	34 to 48
Increase in above signs plus pupil dilation, goose bumps (pilorection), tremors (muscle twitches), hot and cold flashes, aching bones and muscles, loss of appetite	16	48 to 72
Increased intensity of above, plus insomnia; raised blood pressure; increased temperature, pulse rate, respiratory rate and depth; restlessness; nausea	24 to 36	
Increased intensity of above, plus curled-up position, vomiting, diarrhea, weight loss, spontaneous ejaculation or orgasm, hemoconcentration, increased blood sugar	36 to 48	

ceruleus. Clonidine and morphine produce identical effects on the enzyme activity and neurophysiology of these cells. In other brain areas, opiate receptors are found that are not associated with alpha-adrenergic receptors, which is why clonidine does not produce narcotic-like euphoria and is not a good analgesic.[27]

Psychological dependence

That the opiates produce psychological dependence is quite clear; in fact, experiments with the opiates were what led to our current understanding of the importance of the reinforcing properties of drugs (see chapter 3). Animals allowed to self-administer low doses of morphine or heroin intravenously will learn the required behaviors quickly and perform them for prolonged periods, even if they have never experienced withdrawal symptoms. This is an example of what psychologists refer to as *positive reinforcement*: a behavior is reliably followed by the presentation of a stimulus, leading to an increase in the probability of the behavior and its eventual maintenance at a higher rate than before. Remember that the rapidity with which the reinforcing stimulus follows the behavior is an important factor, which is why fewer experiences are needed with a narcotic in-

jected intravenously (fast acting) than with the same drug taken orally (the action is delayed).

Once physical dependence has developed and withdrawal symptoms are experienced, the conditions are set up for another behavioral mechanism, *negative reinforcement*. In this situation an act (drug taking) is followed by the *removal* of withdrawal symptoms, leading to further strengthening of the habit. In heroin addiction the rapid and potent euphoric effect resulting from intravenous injection combined with the appearance of early withdrawal symptoms after only a few hours and their rapid alleviation by another injection leads to the development of strong dependence in many users. Remember, however, that heroin was prescribed in low doses and taken orally by many patients for several years during which it was believed to be nonaddictive. Although heroin is more potent than morphine and can be slightly more addictive because of its more rapid access to the brain, morphine taken intravenously is clearly more addicting than heroin taken orally.

---

methadone: (*meth* a doan) a long-lasting synthetic opiate.

The needle habit

Each heroin administration is followed by a decrease in discomfort, an increase in pleasure, or both. As a result, the behavior itself of preparing and injecting the drug and the setting in which it occurs acquire pleasurable, positive associations through learning mechanisms. Because of this conditioning, the process of using heroin also becomes rewarding. One occasional user commented on the ritual of heroin use:

> Once you decide to get off it's very exciting. It really is. Getting some friends together and some money, copping, deciding where you're going to do it, getting the needles out and sterilizing them, cooking up the stuff, tying off, then the whole thing with the needle, booting, and the rush, that's all part of it. . . . Sometimes I think that if I just shot water I'd enjoy it as much.[31]

Though it might seem strange to the reader, that last statement is true for some individuals who label themselves addicts. These individuals have been called "needle freaks"—at least part of the relief and pleasure they obtain from injecting is a conditioned response to the stimuli (such as needles) associated with heroin use.

A research team headed by a psychiatrist, Charles O'Brien, studied the process of eliminating (extinguishing) the needle habit. A long-acting, experimental narcotic antagonist was administered and the patients were allowed to shoot up using their own equipment and rituals. Most addicts usually shoot up in a bathroom, so the researchers provided a special bathroom where the patients could inject their drugs. Under double-blind conditions the users injected either saline or a high or low dose of a narcotic. No matter which the patient injected, there was no effect because of the administration of the antagonist. Both objective and subjective measures were used, and "all of the self-injections are rated by the patients as pleasurable at first."[32] Only after three to five injections were the subjective reports neutral. Continued self-injections under these conditions

A business woman shooting up heroin in her office. Heroin users come from all walks of life.

resulted in the patients reporting that they hated the whole process. Remember always that there is variability in any biological system: one patient continued to report euphoria after each injection for twenty-six trials, and he regularly showed the pupillary constriction that accompanies the injection of a narcotic! That patient was one of those receiving saline, so it was not a question of the narcotic dose being high or the antagonist dose being low.

Toxicity Potential

Acute toxicity

One specific effect of the narcotics is to depress the respiratory centers in the brain so that respiration slows and becomes shallow. This is perhaps the major side effect of the narcotic agents and one of the most dangerous, because death resulting from respiratory depression can easily follow an excessive dose of these drugs. The basis for this effect is that the respiratory centers become less responsive to carbon dioxide levels in the blood. It is this effect that keeps heroin/morphine and methadone near the top of the list of mentioned drugs in DAWN coroners' reports. Remember that this respiratory depression is additive with the effects of alcohol or other sedative-hypnotics, and there is evidence that a large fraction of those who die from heroin overdose have elevated blood alcohol concentrations and might better be described as dying from a combination of heroin and alcohol. Narcotic overdose can be diagnosed on the basis of the *narcotic triad:* coma, depressed respiration, and pinpoint pupils. Emergency medical treatment calls for the use of naloxone (Narcan), which antagonizes the narcotic effects within a few minutes.

The behavioral consequences of having opiates in the brain are probably less dangerous. Those who inject heroin might "nod off" into a dream-filled sleep for a few minutes, and opium smokers are famous for their "pipe dreams." It is perhaps not surprising that individuals under the influence of narcotics are likely to be less active and less alert than they otherwise would be. There is a clouding of consciousness that makes mental work more difficult. And opiate users are not only less likely to be interested in sex, men can even suffer primary impotence as a direct effect of the drug.

Opiates also stimulate the brain area controlling nausea and vomiting, which are other frequent side effects. Nausea occurs in about half of ambulatory patients given a 15 mg dose of morphine. Also, nausea and vomiting are a common reaction to heroin injection among street users.

Chronic toxicity

Although early in this century many medical authorities believed that chronic narcotic use weakened the user both mentally and physically, there is no scientific evidence that exposure to opiate drugs per se causes long-term damage to any tissue or organ system. Many street users of narcotics do suffer from sores and abscesses at injection sites, but these can be attributed to the lack of sterile technique. Also, the practice of sharing the same needle to inject drugs into the veins can result in the spread of such blood-borne diseases as serum hepatitis and the HIV virus. Again, this is a result not of the drug, but of the technique used to inject it.

Patterns of Abuse

The heroin addict

Only a glimpse of some of the mechanics of a heroin user's life can be presented here. Withdrawal signs might begin about 4 hours after the last use of the drug, but many addicts report that they begin to feel ill only 6 to 8 hours after the last dose. That puts most addicts on a schedule of three to four injections every day. Today's addict is not spending a lot of time nodding off in opium dens as in the good old days. When you have a very important appointment to keep every 6 to 8 hours, every day of the week, every day of the year, you've got to hustle not to miss one of them. Remember, there are no vacations, no weekends off for the regular user, just 1,200 to 1,400 appointments per year to keep.

And each one costs money. Heroin is frequently sold on the street in "dime" bags: $10 for a small plastic bag containing . . . good question—what's in the bag? The material in a $10 bag might have 3 mg or 30 mg. Of course, you might not get *any* heroin, and you can't complain to the Better Business Bureau. At any rate, your addiction can cost you $30 to $100 a day.

The variability in amount of heroin is a problem because of the possibility of an overdose (OD). Addicts should worry about an OD with each new batch of drug used. A sophisticated user buying from a new or questionable source will initially try a much smaller than normal amount of the powder to evaluate its potency.

Once the user has acquired the drug, he prepares it for injection. Usually, the user mixes the powder with unsterile water, heats the mixture briefly in a spoon or bottle cap with a match or lighter, then draws the heroin into a syringe or eyedropper through cotton, thus filtering out the larger impurities. The heroin is then injected intravenously without any attempt at skin cleansing.[33]

Under these conditions it is not surprising that infections do occur. Some users prefer to use an eyedropper with a hypodermic needle attached, because the rubber bulb of the dropper is easier to operate than the plunger of a syringe.

The most common form of heroin use by male addicts is to inject the drug intravenously, that is, to "mainline" the drug. A convenient site is the left forearm (for right-handed users), and the frequent use of dirty needles will leave the arm marked with scar tissue. If the larger veins of the arm collapse, then other body areas will be used. Many beginning addicts start by "skin-popping"—subcutaneous injections. "Skinpopping" increases the danger of tetanus but decreases the risk of hepatitis compared with mainlining. Because of the lack of sterility or even cleanliness, hepatitis, tetanus, and abscesses at the site of injection are not uncommon in street users who inject drugs.

If the addict survives the perils of an overdose, escapes the dangers of contaminated equipment, and avoids being caught, there are still other dangers. Heroin is a potent analgesic, and its regular use can conceal the early symptoms of an illness such as pneumonia. The addict's lack of money for, or interest in, food frequently results in malnutrition. With low resistance from malnutrition and the symptoms of illness going unnoticed as a result of heroin use, the addict becomes quite susceptible to serious disease.

If all these dangers are overcome, the addict might continue to use opiates to an advanced age. Sometimes, however, the addict who avoids illness, death, or arrest and who does not enter and stay in a rehabilitation program or with-

draw himself from the drug might no longer feel the need for the drug and gradually stop using it. The data are still very much debated, but this "maturing out" is probably what happens to a large number of addicts. One authority reports that the addict who survives remains addicted for only about 8 or 9 years. This is an average, however, and according to this report the earlier users start, the longer they remain addicted, with maturing out generally occurring around 35 to 45 years of age.[34] Even if the user lives, the street life of an addict isn't a rose garden.

Misconceptions and preconceptions

Although heroin addicts haven't received as much press in recent years as crack users, most people have some pretty strongly held beliefs about heroin, derived from television, magazines, movies, or conversations. This section deals with some of the major misconceptions that most people, including many professionals, have about nonmedical use and misuse of narcotics. One of the most common misconceptions is that mainlining heroin or morphine induces in everyone an intense pleasure unequaled by any other experience. Often it is described as similar to a whole-body orgasm that persists up to five or more minutes. Some addicts report that they try with every injection to reexperience the extreme euphoria of the first injection but they always have a lesser effect. There are studies, however, as well as clinical and street reports, that some people experience only nausea and discomfort after the initial intravenous administration of morphine or heroin. For whatever reasons, some of these users persist and the discomfort decreases, that is, it shows tolerance more rapidly than the euphoric effects. Under these conditions the injections soon result primarily in pleasant effects. To maintain these pleasurable feelings, though, the dose level must gradually be increased. It is true, however, that even with the narcotics some addicts must partially learn which experiences are defined as pleasurable. One author has referred to the two "powerfully pleasurable effects"—the initial brief rush and then the longer tranquility—and then commented:

> This sequence of events occurs with virtually every nontolerant person, although the first few experiences may be accompanied by vomiting. Even so, the sensations are often pleasurable ("You don't mind vomiting behind smack").[35]

Another misconception has to do with the development of withdrawal symptoms. The addict undergoing withdrawal without medication is always portrayed as being in excruciating pain, truly suffering. It depends. With a large habit, withdrawal without medication is truly hell. The opiate addiction scene is changing too rapidly to be definite about today's user, but many street addicts are described as having "ice cream habits"—they use a low daily drug dose. In one study of individuals who applied for treatment, after being given an injection of the narcotic antagonist naloxone, about one-fifth of the clients showed no withdrawal at all, and about another fifth showed only very mild reactions.[31]

Perhaps the most common misconception about heroin is that after one shot, you are hooked for life. None of the narcotics, or any other drug, fits into that fantasized category. Becoming addicted takes some time, perhaps a week or more, and persistence on the part of the beginner. Regular use of the drug seems to be more important in establishing physical dependence than the size of the dose used. Becoming physically dependent is possible on a weekend, but it frequently requires a longer period with three or four injections a day.

There are probably about 500,000 narcotic addicts in the United States. There may be two to three times as many heroin *chippers*—occasional users. Several reports and studies have appeared on the characteristics of these occasional users, but no consistent differences, compared with addicts, have yet been found other than the pattern of use.

New users, new drugs

Heroin addiction will continue to appear in various groups in each new generation. In each generation low-class junkies are joined by a small group of young, wealthy, "respectable" heroin users, both in the United States and Europe. A new, very pure form of heroin called black tar appeared on the streets in 1986. As if the variable nature of street heroin coming from different sources around the world weren't confusing enough, the street scene became further complicated by the presence of various synthetic drugs. Street users learned about fentanyl, a potent prescription narcotic available in sterile solution for injection. Illicit chemists developed derivatives of fentanyl and sold them on the streets as "China White" or "synthetic heroin." The interesting thing about these "designer drugs" is that the chemists were able to vary the molecule to produce drugs that had not yet been listed as controlled substances. Since 1988, it has been illegal to make or sell such designer drugs, if they have a chemical structure or a pharmacological effect similar to an already controlled substance.

Another synthetic heroin, MPPP, which is a derivative of meperidine (Demerol), was produced by a few illicit laboratories. However, there is substantial danger of trace amounts of the impurity MPTP being included, and this incredibly toxic substance was responsible for the occurrence of permanent brain damage in several users in the 1980s. MPTP results in destruction of dopamine neurons, leading to a form of Parkinson's disease.

By the 1990s heroin was being brought into the United States in larger quantities through a variety of routes. The increased purity of most of the samples increased the danger of overdoses, and the DAWN emergency room and coroners' reports reflected that increased danger. Anyone buying heroin on the street these days faces multiple risks, and the only regulation seems to be that famous old free-market concept, *caveat emptor* ("let the buyer beware").

TREATMENT OF NARCOTIC ADDICTS

History

Dependence on opium, and later on morphine and heroin, is also a very old problem with a long history of varied treatments. A 1902 medical book on the subject of morphinism described a variety of approaches to treatment, mainly concerned with reducing the morphine intake either slowly or more rapidly (over a few days' time) and dealing with the withdrawal symptoms.[36] The danger of relapse was recognized, with the author recommending cold showers, travel abroad, or a temporary change of lifestyle, such as going west to work on a cattle ranch or in a mine. A few years later, the accepted medical "cure" involved the use of high doses of belladonna or some other anticholinergic to maintain a state of delirium for several days, after which the patient was felt to be cured of the addiction![37]

After the Harrison Act was passed in 1914, narcotics became less freely available and somewhat more expensive, even through legal sources. This had the purpose of preventing further addictions, but not all those already addicted could afford frequent visits to a private physician. Cities around the country established public narcotic clinics to help these people. Most of the clinics gradually "detoxified" their clients, but some clients (such as those with chronic pain conditions) were considered incurable and were offered "social adjustment" treatment, which meant continued maintenance on a narcotic. After the passage of alcohol prohibition and the establishment of a Bureau of Narcotics, these clinics were all closed down under pressure from federal agents, and by 1925 there was no longer a legal source of

treatment that included providing narcotics for maintenance.

Federal prisons became choked with narcotic addicts by 1930. That and the repeal of Prohibition led to the reorganization of the Bureau of Narcotics under Harry Anslinger and the establishment of two federal treatment facilities, one in Lexington, Kentucky, and the other in Fort Worth, Texas. The center at Lexington was the first and the more important and served as a combination prison farm, treatment center, and research center where the medical and psychological staff searched for a cure for narcotic addiction. The treatment consisted of gradual withdrawal using morphine, followed by a stay of up to a year, during which the clients would work on the farm and take advantage of the recreational facilities, all the while undergoing psychotherapy and participating in various tests and experiments. The relapse rate after this type of treatment appeared to be above 80 percent and never got much better than that.[37] This was the major approach to treating narcotic addicts into the 1960s, at least partly because Anslinger remained adamantly opposed throughout his career, which ended in 1962, to any outpatient treatment program that included giving narcotics to clients.

Current Medical Approaches

Narcotic antagonists

Research at Lexington revealed some interesting properties of drugs such as nalorphine, naloxone, and cyclazocine. When given to addicts who had been taking morphine, these drugs precipitated a withdrawal syndrome immediately. And these drugs blocked the effects of morphine, heroin, and other narcotics. Could these narcotic antagonists be a cure for addiction? If an addict were first withdrawn from the narcotic and then given the antagonist on a chronic basis, relapse should not be a problem. If a person did try taking heroin, it would have no effect. Although there would be no negative consequence, other than the waste of money, eventually the addict would learn to stop taking heroin, thus curing the addiction. The problem is, of course, that the addict must be highly motivated to take the antagonist. Some of the antagonists, particularly cyclazocine, produce unpleasant side effects. Naloxone, which produces fairly pure antagonism with few side effects, is a short-acting drug that must be taken several times a day to maintain constant antagonism.

With all these difficulties, reports on the effectiveness of narcotic antagonist treatment have not been very promising. More recent experiments have used naltrexone, a long-acting antagonist that was released for marketing as a prescription drug under the brand name Trexan in 1985. A 50 mg tablet can antagonize the effects of a large dose of heroin for twenty-four hours and a smaller dose for two days or more, and it can therefore be given as infrequently as three times a week. Although it is clear that naltrexone therapy is not for everyone, some highly motivated clients who tend to relapse impulsively might buy themselves some time with it. Also, a court-ordered client could be mandated to come to a clinic three or four times a week and take naltrexone. At least for the duration of the treatment, the client would not be able to become readdicted to heroin or other narcotics. We can expect to see this antagonist receive continued but fairly restricted use. An interesting problem arises if a patient on naltrexone is involved in an accident and requires some pain relief. Current practice would be to give high doses of hydromorphone (Dilaudid) to overcome the antagonism. This should, of course, be done only in a hospital and with extreme caution.

Methadone maintenance

Methadone (Dolophine) is a synthetic narcotic analgesic developed in Germany during World War II and found to be a substitute for the then-unavailable opium-based agents. It is quite effective when taken orally, and it has

a long duration of action. The long duration means not only that it needs to be taken less frequently to prevent withdrawal symptoms, but because the drug leaves the body slowly the withdrawal symptoms are less severe. Although long approved as a narcotic analgesic, methadone gained fame as a drug useful in treatment programs for heroin addicts.

The initial study in this area was started in 1964 by Dole and Nyswander, a husband-wife team in New York City. In their initial work, heroin addicts were given 20 to 30 mg of methadone orally every day; this was gradually increased over four to six weeks to 80 to 120 mg given orally once a day. The theory behind the use of methadone to help rehabilitate addicts is that the long-lasting effects of methadone prevent withdrawal symptoms and block the pleasurable effects of opiates. It disrupts the

> pattern of swinging between the states of heroin intoxication and the withdrawal syndrome. "There are three states in the heroin addict's life," says Dr. Dole. "He's either 'straight' (feeling normal), 'high,' or 'sick.' He wakes up sick, takes a shot, and gets high. That lasts a couple of hours, maybe, until he begins coming off the high, and then he'll take another shot if he can get it. He spends very little time being straight, so he usually is not able to hold a job or live normally; he's pretty much a lost soul."[38]

The initial report of the effectiveness of this treatment program on 750 criminal addicts was spectacular.

> A four year trial of methadone blockade treatment has shown 94% success in ending the criminal activity of former heroin addicts. The majority of these patients are now productively employed, living as responsible citizens, and supporting families. The results show unequivocally that criminal addicts can be rehabilitated by a well-supervised maintenance program.[39]

Methadone programs expanded rapidly after these reports. Why did we so readily accept the switching of addicts from one narcotic to another? Could we really condone having government-supported narcotic addicts walking around the streets? Perhaps programs of this type would not have been possible if Harry Anslinger had not retired in 1962, but one of his major concerns could be avoided. Because methadone can be effective if taken only once or twice a day, the addicts could be required to come to the clinic and take the drug under supervision. Thus addicts were not being supplied with drugs that they could take out on the streets and sell or give to others. Also, there was some confusion over whether methadone was acting purely as a narcotic or whether it had some antagonist properties as well. Note that it was indicated that methadone treatment tended to block the pleasurable effects of heroin and that the program was referred to as methadone "blockade" treatment by its proponents. This apparent blockade was probably a result of the buildup to high doses of methadone used in the initial studies. The addicts became tolerant to greater levels of narcotic, and the rather small amount of heroin available in most street "bags" at that time had little effect in a person with such a tolerance. It could be seen as ironic that we were treating narcotic addiction by creating an even greater level of tolerance. Current programs use lower doses, usually under 100 mg per day.

The ethics and morality of the methadone approach were raised early:

> although there is no question that methadone maintenance treatment is an effective way of reducing the criminalistic activities of drug addicts, it is a question who is being treated: society or the drug takers . . . each physician who prescribes methadone to a narcotic addict has this moral question to answer: Is he maintaining the patient on drugs for the good of society or for the good of his individual patient? Is he encouraging a kind of "cop out" by reinforcing the hopeless feeling of drug addicts when he wonders whether he can renounce drug use?[40]

Remember too that the 1960s were a time when the majority of addicts were black and there was simultaneously a focus on racial awareness. The idea that large numbers of people might be expected to spend the rest of their lives dependent on a substance, becoming passive supplicants who report to a clinic twice daily for counseling, appeared to some minority leaders to be a frightening experiment in social control.

Despite these concerns, methadone maintenance continues to be accepted as the most effective approach to heroin addiction. Available methadone programs take on a wide variety of forms, ranging from simple storefront drug handouts to more elaborate evaluation, treatment, and job counseling programs.[41] The effectiveness of methadone treatment can be measured in several ways: heroin use declines dramatically, drug-related problems drop, measures of psychological depression decline, commission of nondrug-defined crimes is reduced significantly, and permanent employment is increased. There is some division over the primary reason for the effectiveness of methadone. Early workers emphasized the chemical aspects of the program: preventing withdrawal symptoms and craving and blocking the pleasurable effects of heroin. Others see the need for daily appearances at the clinic and the opportunities for frequent counseling as the major reasons for success, with the methadone merely providing a reason for such tight control. A recent report indicated that some supplementary counseling is beneficial but that high levels of additional support are not cost-effective.[42]

LAAM

In 1993 the FDA approved another synthetic opiate, L-alpha-acetyl-methadol (**LAAM**), for use in treating narcotic addicts. Because LAAM is metabolized in the liver to an active metabolite, it has much longer-lasting effects than methadone. Instead of daily visits, treatment clients are able to take the drug only three times a week, which is the major advantage of LAAM. In addition, however, clients report feeling less of a narcotic effect from LAAM, which, it is hoped, will ease the transition to a drug-free state.[43]

Both methadone and LAAM maintenance are tightly controlled by the DEA and FDA. Methadone is a regular prescription drug available in both injectable and oral forms for pain relief. But maintenance of addicts has now been formally defined in federal law, and only oral methadone and now LAAM are considered "safe and effective" for this use by the FDA. And this use is not available to every physician, because the FDA still classifies even methadone maintenance as investigational, allowing its use only under approved protocols and by approved clinics. The average American physician is still prohibited from providing any narcotic to an addict for the purpose of maintaining the addiction.

Why don't all heroin addicts simply come in and sign up for free methadone instead of taking heroin? If their drug-taking behavior were motivated only by the "need" for a narcotic, this would make sense. But let's not forget why most of these people use heroin in the first place: to be part of a subculture, to make a statement about their relationship to the dominant society, or for the experience. And let's not forget that the major reason for continuing to use heroin is probably the positive reinforcement produced by the rapid rise in blood levels of heroin immediately after an intravenous injection (the "rush"). Slow-acting oral methadone or LAAM won't produce any of these effects.

Heroin/morphine maintenance

If we are now willing to supply addicts with narcotics, and if addicts want heroin, why don't we just supply them with heroin and clean syringes and let them inject it intravenously? There are some obvious inconveniences compared with methadone, including the need to administer the drug several times a day, and the use of the needles for intravenous injection. Also, there's the aspect of heroin use mentioned by Dole and Nyswander—the intravenous heroin user spends a lot of time reacting to the last

shot or worrying about the next one, with relatively brief periods (only a few hours at a time) of feeling "straight." Oral methadone produces less "up and down" in the blood level of the narcotic and can be more conducive to participating in work, school, or other productive activities. But the major impediment to such an approach is probably the long history Americans have of viewing heroin as an evil substance rather than seeing it as just another narcotic.

Actually, the public clinics that existed in several cities until around 1920 can give us some idea of the utility of providing the addict's "drug of choice," which was usually morphine but was in some cases heroin or codeine. Although Harry Anslinger said many times in later years that these clinics did not work and were hotbeds of criminal activity, a 1974 in-depth review of the clinic in Shreveport, Louisiana, gave a more positive assessment.[44] Most of the clients of that program were employed, most were middle-aged, and most had become addicted as a result of medical treatment. The clinic apparently provided an important service for those individuals and has been viewed as a model of what "might have been." Of course, that clinic refused admission to people suspected of being criminals and encouraged "bums" or "loafers" to leave town instead of offering them treatment. The addicts it did serve could in no way be seen as representative of today's addict population.

A great deal has been said about the British system, in which addicts may register and receive heroin for purposes of maintenance of their addiction. Actually, over the years there really hasn't been a system at all. Britain simply never took the step of outlawing the medical use

---

LAAM: L-alpha-acetyl methadol; a very long-lasting synthetic opiate recently approved for maintenance treatment of opiate addicts.

Tough Moral Stances versus "Harm Reduction"

Several authors over the years have pointed out that legal restrictions on the availability of a drug often lead to the use of a more potent (more easily smuggled) and therefore likely more dangerous form of drug use. Examples abound in the history of the opiates: the Chinese tobacco smokers who switched to opium smoking and the opiate addicts in this country who switched to intravenous heroin when narcotics became so expensive.

A more contemporary issue has to do with the availability of sterile needles for intravenous drug users. In several cities, needle exchange programs have been developed whereby addicts are able to obtain clean needles. In other cities, these programs have been met with scorn.

The needle-exchange program in Liverpool, England, was one of the first successful demonstrations that the spread of HIV could be slowed if clean needles were readily available, and its designers based their approach on what they call a "harm reduction" model of drug control. At issue is the ultimate goal of our drug control policies. If it is to reduce the amount of danger and harm to the population in general, then perhaps needle exchange programs and other changes in enforcement practices would be in order.

How do you feel? Is it more important to reduce the amount of harm done by drug use, or is it more important for our society to take a firm moral stand in hopes of preventing the further spread of drug use?

of heroin or the prescribing of narcotics to addicts by physicians. Thus until 1968 there was no program: British heroin addicts simply obtained a prescription from their physician just as they would for any other drug. Some Americans, noting that there were few narcotic addicts in Britain before the 1960s, had suggested that the major cause of our much greater narcotic addiction problem lay in our attempts to control it![16] We'll never know the answer to that one: even though America and England seem quite similar in many ways, they are far from the same society, either now or in the 1920s.

The British were not immune to the social change of the 1960s, and one reflection of that change was that some British youth began to experiment with drugs. Individuals who went to their physicians for heroin and who had developed the addiction recreationally were reported to the Home Office as "nontherapeutic" heroin addicts. The number of such addicts increased from 47 in 1959 to 222 in 1963. That might not seem like many compared with half a million in the United States, but the increase gave support to those who wanted tighter controls. Noting that a few physicians were writing prescriptions for large amounts of heroin, it was concluded that not every physician should be trusted completely where narcotics addicts were concerned. By 1968 the new system was in place: British physicians could still prescribe any medication, including heroin, to nonaddicts. But addicts now had to register as such and could receive heroin or cocaine only from specially licensed physicians in "drug-dependence clinics," which were established in several areas.

During the 1970s these clinics dispensed less and less heroin and more and more counseling and oral methadone. By 1978 only 9 percent of the clinic clients were receiving heroin, either alone or in combination with other drugs.[45]

In Britain, narcotic addiction has continued to increase, an illicit market for heroin has developed, and crime rates have increased. However, the British still have a much smaller heroin problem than the United States: with a total population about one-fourth that of the United States, Britain probably has less than one-thirtieth the number of heroin addicts.[23] It is certainly ironic that the United States, viewed as the world leader in the control of opiates and in narcotic treatment, continues to be the leader in numbers of heroin addicts.

Recently several other countries have explored the idea of providing heroin to addicts. Switzerland began a program of heroin prescription in 1993, and by 1995 reported a drop in the proportion of burglaries, robberies, and auto thefts committed by drug users.[46] The Australian parliament voted in 1997 to try such an experiment, but it was vetoed by the prime minister.

RAPID OPIATE DETOXIFICATION

The old idea from the early 1900s of using some other drug to help the addict through withdrawal has come back in a big way in the 1990s with a new twist. Heroin (or methadone) addicts are anesthetized and, while unconscious, are given naltrexone so that they will experience immediate withdrawal. After twenty-four hours the patients are released and enter a period of counseling combined with continued naltrexone treatment. The treatment costs about $7,500 in New York, and could obviously generate quite a profit for the providers, who are typically organized as businesses. Although the proponents have made claims of very high success rates with this treatment, traditional treatment specialists are skeptical that this rapid technique will produce long-term abstinence.[47]

SUMMARY

- Opium was used in its raw form for centuries, both medicinally and for pleasure.
- Opium had significant influences on medicine, literature, and world politics through the 1800s.
- Addiction to opiates has been recognized for a long time, but no concerted effort to control addiction was tried until the patent medicine era of the late 1800s, combined with opium smoking by Chinese Americans, led to federal regulations in the early 1900s.
- The typical opiate addict changed from being a middle-aged, middle-class woman using narcotics by mouth to being a young, lower-class man using heroin by intravenous injection.
- Various synthetic narcotics are now available along with the natural products of the opium poppy. These drugs all act at opiate receptors in the brain.
- Opiate receptors are normally acted on by the naturally occurring opiate-like products of the nervous system and endocrine glands, endorphins and enkephalins.
- The narcotic overdose triad consists of coma, depressed respiration, and pinpoint pupils. Death occurs because breathing ceases.
- Illicit heroin comes primarily from Southeast Asia, Southwest Asia, and Mexico.
- Opiate addicts have been offered a wide variety of treatments, but the most effective in reducing crime and relapse has been methadone maintenance.
- A longer-acting synthetic opiate, LAAM, is now available for maintenance treatment.
- Although the British continue to make heroin available for pain relief and to maintain addicts, most British addicts in treatment are now maintained on methadone.

REVIEW QUESTIONS

1. What two chemicals are extracted from the opium poppy?

2. What was the significance of De Quincey's writing about "opium eating"?
3. What were the approximate dates and who were the combatants in the Opium Wars?
4. How is it possible that heroin was at first sold as a nonaddicting pain reliever?
5. How did the "typical" opiate addict change from the early 1900s to the 1920s?
6. Why and when did private physicians and public clinics stop "maintaining" addicts with morphine and other opiates?
7. What were some of the lessons learned about heroin addiction as a result of the Vietnam experience?
8. What two factors were probably responsible for the increase in the smoking of heroin in 1989 and 1990?
9. What is the effect of a narcotic antagonist on someone who has developed a physical dependence on opiates?
10. What are the enkephalins and endorphins, and how do they relate to plant-derived opiates such as morphine?
11. What are the relative advantages and disadvantages of methadone, LAAM, and heroin maintenance?

Related Internet Sites on Opiates

Office of National Drug Control Policy: http://www.whitehousedrugpolicy.gov/

National Institute on Drug Abuse: http://www.nida.nih.gov/

Pain and its treatment: We are not addicts! http://home.ptd.net/~paulbarb/narc.htm

And our own "painless" *Drugs, Society, and Human Behaviour* site: http://www.uwyo.edu/A&S/psyc/dshb.htm

---

REFERENCES

1. Baum LF: *The new wizard of Oz*, New York, 1944, Grosset & Dunlap.
2. Scott JM: *The white poppy: a history of opium*, New York, 1969, Funk & Wagnalls.
3. Hamarneh S: Sources and development of Arabic medical therapy and pharmacology, *Sudhoffs Archiv fur Geschichte der Medizin und der Naturwissenschaften* 54:34, 1970.
4. De Quincey T: *Confessions of an English opium-eater*, New York, 1907, EP Dutton.
5. Turk MH: *Selections from De Quincey*, Boston, 1902, Ginn & Co.
6. De Quincey works, vol 206. Quoted in Lowes JL: *The road to Xanadu*, Boston, 1927, Houghton Mifflin.
7. Blair W: An opium-eater in America, *The Knickerbocker* 20:47-57, 1842.
8. Kramer JC: Opium rampant: medical use, misuse and abuse in Britain and the West in the 17th and 18th centuries, *Br J Addiction*, p 377, 1979.
9. Kramer JC: Heroin in the treatment of morphine addiction, *J Psychedelic Drugs* 9(3):193-197, 1977.
10. Dott DB, Stockman R: *Proceedings of the Royal Society of Edinburgh*, p 321, 1890.
11. Manges M: A second report on the therapeutics of heroine, *New York Medical Journal* 71:51, 82-83, 1900.
12. Wilcox RW: *Pharmacology and therapeutics*, ed 6, Philadelphia, 1905, P. Blakiston's Son.
13. Lindesmith AR: *Addiction and opiates*, Chicago, 1968, Aldine.
14. Kebler LF: The present status of drug addiction in the United States. In *Transactions of the American Therapeutic Society*, Philadelphia, 1910, FA Davis.
15. Black JR: Advantages of substituting the morphia habit for the incurably alcoholic, *The Cincinnati Lancet—Clinic* 22:538-541, 1889.
16. Lindesmith AR: *The addict and the law*, Bloomington, Ind, 1965, Indiana University Press.
17. Smith R: Status politics and the image of the addict, *Iss Crimin* 2(2):157-175, 1966.
18. Preble E, Casey JJ Jr: Taking care of business—the heroin user's life on the street, *Int J Addict* 4(1):1-24, 1969.
19. Isbell H: Discussion, Symposium on Problems of Drug Dependence, Fourteenth Annual Conference Veterans Administration Cooperative Studies in Psychiatry, Houston, Texas, April 1, 1969, Highlights of the Conference, Veterans Administration, Washington, DC, 1969, US Government Printing Office.
20. *Inquiry into alleged drug abuse in the armed services*, Report of a special subcommittee of the Committee on Armed Services, House of Representatives, Ninety-

second Congress, First Session, Apr 23, 1971, Washington, DC, 1971, US Government Printing Office.

21. *The world heroin problem.* Committee Print, House of Representatives, Committee on Foreign Affairs, Ninety-second Congress, First Session, May 27, 1971, Washington, DC, 1971, US Government Printing Office.

22. Robins LN: *The Vietnam drug user returns*, Special Action Office for Drug Abuse Prevention Monograph, Series A, No 2, May 1974, Contract No HSM-42-72-75.

23. Brodsky MD: History of heroin prevalence estimation techniques. *In Self-report methods of estimating drug use*, NIDA Research Monograph No 57, Washington, DC, 1985, US Government Printing Office.

24. National Narcotics Intelligence Consumers Committee: *The supply of illicit drugs to the United States*, Washington, DC, 1996.

25. Schoemer, K: Rockers, models, and the new allure of heroin, *Newsweek*, Aug 26, 1996.

26. Wren CS: View that smoking heroin is safer than injecting is questioned, *New York Times*, Dec 1, 1996.

27. Feldman RS, Meyer JS, Quenzer LF: *Principles of neuropsychopharmacology*, Sunderland, Mass, 1997, Sinauer.

28. Zadina JE and others: A potent and selective endogenous agonist for the μ-opiate receptor. *Nature* 386:499, 1997.

29. Siegel S: Morphine analgesic tolerance: its situation specificity supports a pavlovian conditioning model, *Science* 193:323–325, 1976.

30. Siegel S and others: Heroin "overdose" death: contribution of drug-associated environmental cues, *Science* 216:436–437, 1982.

31. Powell DH: A pilot study of occasional heroin users, *Arch Gen Psychiatry* 28:586–594, 1973.

32. O'Brien CP: "Needle freaks": psychological dependence on shooting up. In *Medical World News*, Psychiatry Annual, New York, 1974, McGraw-Hill.

33. Louria DB, Hensle T, Rose J: The major medical complications of heroin addiction, *Ann Intern Med* 67:1–22, 1967.

34. Winick C: Maturing out of narcotic addiction, *Bull Narc* 14(1):1–8, 1962.

35. Goldstein A: Heroin addiction and the role of methadone in its treatment, *Arch Gen Psychiatry* 26:291–297, 1972.

36. Crothers TD: *Morphinism and narcomanias from other drugs*, reprint edition, New York, 1981, Arno Press.

37. Latimer D, Goldberg J: *Flowers in the blood: the story of opium*, New York, 1981, Arno Press.

38. Methadone maintenance: how much, for whom, for how long? *Medical World News*, pp 53–63, March 17, 1972.

39. Dole VP, Nyswander ME, Warner A: Successful treatment of 750 criminal addicts, *JAMA* 206:2708–2714, 1968.

40. Myerson DJ: Methadone treatment of addicts, *N Eng J Med* 281:390–391, 1969.

41. Joe GW and others: Treatment process and relapse to opioid use during methadone maintenance, *Am J Drug Alcohol Abuse* 20:173, 1994.

42. Kraft MK and others: Are supplementary services provided during methadone maintenance really cost-effective? *Am J Psychiatry* 154:1214–1219, 1997.

43. Swan N: Treatment practitioners learn about LAAM, *NIDA Notes* 9(1):5, 1994.

44. Waldorf D, Orlich M, Reinerman C: *Morphine maintenance: the Shreveport clinic 1919–1923*, Washington, DC, 1974, The Drug Abuse Council.

45. Trebach AS: *The heroin solution*, New Haven, 1982, Yale University Press.

46. Killias M, Uchtenhagen A: On the evaluation of the Swiss heroin prescription projects and its methodology. In *Studies on crime and crime prevention*, Vol. 5. National Council for Crime Prevention, 1996.

47. Mathews J: A solution of substance for substance abuse? *The Washington Post*, Dec 3, 1996.

Hallucinogens

KEY TERMS

- animism
- phantastica
- psychedelic
- psychotomimetic
- indole
- synesthesia
- psilocybin
- peyote
- mescaline
- PCP
- angel dust

OBJECTIVES

After reading this chapter, you should be able to:

- Explain why psychoactive drugs have played an important role in many of the world's religions.
- Describe the history of the discovery and use of LSD.
- Identify the psychological similarities between the indole and catechol hallucinogens, and explain the current scientific view of how they work in the brain.

- Describe several psychoactive plants, the chemicals contained in them, the class of hallucinogen to which they belong, and their psychological effects.

From the soft, quiet beauty of the sacred *Psilocybe* mushroom to the angry, mottled appearance of the toxic *Amanita,* from the mountains of Mexico to the streets of Anytown, USA, from before history to the end of the twentieth century, humans have searched for the perfect aphrodisiac, spiritual experiences, other worlds. The plants have been there to help; it's worth repeating that plants have evolved to produce chemicals that alter the biochemistry of animals. If they make us feel sick, we are unlikely to eat them again, and if they kill us, we are certain not to eat them again. But humans long ago learned to "tame" some of these plants, to use them in just the right ways and in just the right amounts to alter perceptions and emotions without too many unpleasant consequences.

ANIMISM AND RELIGION

Animism, the belief that animals, plants, rocks, streams, and so on derive their special characteristics from some spirit contained within the object, is a common theme in most of the world's religions. Plants that are able to alter our perception of the world and of ourselves fit right into such a view. If the plant contains a spirit, then eating the plant transfers that spirit to the person who ate it, and the spirit of the plant can speak to the consumer, make her feel the plant's joy or provide her with special powers or insights.

In primitive societies, certain individuals became specialists in the ways of these plants, learning when to harvest them and how much to use under what circumstances. These traditions were passed down from one generation to another, and colorful stories were used to teach the principles to apprentices. Our modern term for these individuals is *shaman* or *medicine man/woman* because of their knowledge of drug-containing plants. But because they also were the experts on obtaining power from the spirit world, their function in primitive societies had as much to do with the origins of religion as with the origins of modern medicine. These plants and their psychoactive effects were probably important reasons for the development of spiritual and religious traditions and folklore in many different societies all over the world.[1]

TERMINOLOGY AND TYPES

The issue of what to call this group of drugs is an old one. In 1931, Lewin referred to a class of **phantastica,** drugs that can create in our minds a world of fantasy. Peyote, psilocybin, and LSD all produce this type of effect. In the 1960s, these drugs were described by enthusiastic users as allowing them to see into their own minds, and the term **psychedelic** ("mind-

viewing") was widely used. The term itself implies a beneficial, visionary type of effect, and there is considerable disagreement over whether such effects are really beneficial. Because the drugs are capable of producing hallucinations and some altered sense of reality, a state that could be called psychotic, they have also been referred to as **psychotomimetic** drugs. This term implies that the drugs produce dangerous effects and produce a form of mental disorder, which is also a controversial conclusion. In the 1990s, proponents have made popular a new term, *entheogen,* implying that the substances create spiritual or religious experiences. Is there a descriptive and unbiased term that will allow us to categorize the drugs and then to examine their effects without prejudice? One thing common to these drugs is some tendency to produce hallucinations, so we will refer to them by the name *hallucinogens.*

PHANTASTICA

Although we will call all of these drugs hallucinogens, there are important differences among them. They can be classified according to their chemical structures, known pharmacological properties, how much loss of awareness occurs under their influence, and how dangerous they are. The first types we will review are the classical phantastica: they are capable of altering perceptions while allowing the person to remain

Various psychedelic pills and capsules

animism: the belief that objects attain certain characteristics because of spirits.

phantastica: (fan *tass* tick a) drugs that create a world of fantasy.

psychedelic: (sy ka *dell* ick) "mind-viewing."

psychotomimetic: (sy cot o mim *et* ick) mimicking psychosis.

in communication with the present world. The individual under the influence of these drugs will often be aware of both the "fantasy" world and the "real" world at the same time, might talk avidly about what is being experienced, and will be able to remember much of it later. These drugs can be seen as having more purely hallucinogenic effects in that they do not produce much acute physiological toxicity, that is, there is relatively little danger of dying from an overdose of LSD, psilocybin, or mescaline. The two major classes of phantastica, the indole and catechol hallucinogens, are grouped according to their chemical structures.

INDOLE HALLUCINOGENS

The basic structure of the neurotransmitter serotonin is referred to as an **indole** nucleus. Figure 16.1 illustrates that the hallucinogens LSD and psilocybin also contain this structure. For that reason and the fact that some other

The indole nucleus

Psilocyblin (3-[2-{dimethylamino} ethyl] - indol - 4 - ol dihydrogen phosphate ester)

d-lysergic acid diethylamide (LSD) (9, 10 - didehydro - N, N - diethyl - 6 - methyl - ergoline - 8b - carboxamide)

■ carbon
■ oxygen
■ hydrogen
■ nitrogen
□ phosphorus

Figure 16.1 Indole hallucinogens

chemicals with this structure have similar hallucinogenic effects, we refer to one group of the phantastica as the indoles.

d-Lysergic Acid Diethylamide (LSD)

The most potent and notorious of the hallucinogens, and the one that brought these drugs into the public eye in the 1960s, is not found in nature at all. Although there are naturally occurring compounds that resemble the indole *d*-lysergic acid diethylamide (LSD), their identity as hallucinogens was not known until after the discovery of LSD. LSD was originally synthesized from ergot alkaloids extracted from the ergot fungus *Claviceps purpurea*. This mold occasionally grows on grain, especially rye, and eating infected grain results in an illness called *ergotism*.

Saint Anthony's fire

Grain that has been infected with the ergot fungus is readily identified and is usually destroyed. During periods of famine, however, the grain might be used in making bread. In France between A.D. 945 and 1600 there were at least twenty outbreaks of ergotism, the illness that results from eating infected bread. Although the cause of the illness was established before 1700, only symptomatic treatment exists even today. There are two forms of the disease. In one, there are tingling sensations in the skin and muscle spasms that develop into convulsions, insomnia, and various disturbances of consciousness and thinking. In the other form, gangrenous ergotism, the limbs become swollen and inflamed, with the individual experiencing "violent burning pains" before the affected part becomes numb. Sometimes the disease moves rapidly, with less than twenty-four hours between the first sign and the development of gangrene. Gangrene develops because the ergot causes a contraction of the blood vessels, cutting off blood flow to the extremities.

During the twelfth century, ergotism became associated with Saint Anthony, although the reason for this is not completely clear. It might be that the hospital for the treatment of ergotism was built near the shrine of Saint Anthony because he had suffered from a minor attack of ergotism. Some suggest that the demons he reported battling were the result of the disease.[2] Others believe the illness was called Saint Anthony's fire because those who made the pilgrimage to Egypt, where Saint Anthony had lived, were cured. No matter, those who journeyed to Egypt and those who entered the hospital did lose their symptoms, probably as a result of a diet that did not include ergot-infected rye.

Two interesting articles discussed a possible link between convulsive ergotism and the Salem witch trials of 1692 in which twenty people were executed. The first article[3] built a very strong case that (1) the original symptoms exhibited by the "possessed" eight girls were similar to those seen in convulsive ergotism and (2) the conditions were right for the growth of the ergot fungus on the rye that was the staple cereal. The second article[4] constructed an equally convincing case that ergotism could not have been involved and that the "possession" was psychological in origin. In fact, we will never know for sure; there are, however, enough similarities and lingering doubts that ergotism seems to remain a possible basis for the Salem incident.

LSD discovery and early research

In the Sandoz Laboratories in Basel, Switzerland, in 1938, Dr. Albert Hofmann synthesized *lysergsaurediethylamid*, the German word

---

indole: (*in* dole) a particular chemical structure found in serotonin and LSD.

from which *LSD* comes and that names the substance known in English as *d*-lysergic acid diethylamide. Hofmann was working on a series of compounds derived from ergot alkaloids that had as their basic structure lysergic acid. LSD was synthesized because of its chemical similarity to a known stimulant, nikethamide. It was not until 1943, however, that LSD entered the world of biochemical psychiatry, when Hofmann recorded this in his laboratory notebook:

> Last Friday, April 16, 1943, I was forced to stop my work in the laboratory in the middle of the afternoon and to go home, as I was seized by a peculiar restlessness associated with a sensation of mild dizziness. Having reached home, I lay down and sank in a kind of drunkenness which was not unpleasant and which was characterized by extreme activity of imagination. As I lay in a dazed condition with my eyes closed (I experienced daylight as disagreeably bright) there surged upon me an uninterrupted stream of fantastic images of extraordinary plasticity and vividness and accompanied by an intense, kaleidoscope-like play of colors. This condition gradually passed off after about two hours.[5]

Hofmann later said, "The first experience was a very weak one, consisting of rather small changes. It had a pleasant, fairy tale–magic theater quality."[6] He was sure that the experience resulted from the accidental absorption, through the skin of his fingers, of the compound with which he was working. The next Monday morning Hofmann prepared what he thought was a very small amount of LSD, 0.25 mg, and made the following record in his notebook:

> April 19, 1943: Preparation of an 0.5% aqueous solution of *d*-lysergic acid diethylamide tartrate.
>
> 4:20 P.M.: 0.5 cc (0.25 mg LSD) ingested orally. The solution is tasteless.
>
> 4:50 P.M.: no trace of any effect.
>
> 5:00 P.M.: slight dizziness, unrest, difficulty in concentration, visual disturbances, marked desire to laugh.

At this point the laboratory notes are discontinued:

> The last words could only be written with great difficulty. I asked my laboratory assistant to accompany me home as I believed that my condition would be a repetition of the disturbance of the previous Friday. While we were still cycling home, however, it became clear that the symptoms were much stronger than the first time. I had great difficulty in speaking coherently, my field of vision swayed before me, and objects appeared distorted like images in curved mirrors. I had the impression of being unable to move from the spot, although my assistant told me afterwards that we had cycled at a good pace.
>
> Six hours after ingestion of the LSD-25 my condition had already improved considerably. Only the visual disturbances were still pronounced. Everything seemed to sway and the proportions were distorted like the reflections in the surface of moving water. Moreover, all objects appeared in unpleasant, constantly changing colors, the predominant shades being sickly green and blue. When I closed my eyes, an unending series of colorful, very realistic and fantastic images surged in upon me. A remarkable feature was the manner in which all acoustic perceptions (e.g., the noise of a passing car) were transformed into optical effects, every sound causing a corresponding colored hallucination constantly changing in shape and color like pictures in a kaleidoscope. At about 1 o'clock I fell asleep and awakened the next morning somewhat tired but otherwise feeling perfectly well.[5]

The amount Albert Hofmann took orally is 5 to 8 times the normal effective dose, and it was the potency of the drug that attracted attention to it. Mescaline had long been known to cause strange experiences, alter consciousness, and lead to a particularly vivid kaleidoscope of colors, but it takes 4,000 times as much mescaline as LSD. LSD is usually active when only 0.05 mg (50 µg) is taken, and in some people a dose of 0.03 mg is effective.

The first report on LSD in the scientific literature came from Zurich in 1947, but it was 1949 before the first North American study on its use in humans appeared. In 1953, Sandoz applied to the Food and Drug Administration to study LSD as an investigational new drug. Between 1953 and 1966 Sandoz distributed large quantities of LSD to qualified scientists throughout the world. Most of this legal LSD was used in biochemical and animal behavior research.

Besides an interest in trying to develop "model psychoses" in animals and humans so that treatments could be developed, the major thrust of LSD research had to do with its alleged ability to access the "subconscious mind." This notion probably derived from the dreamlike quality of the reports of LSD experiences and the long-held psychoanalytic view that dreams represent subconscious thoughts trying to express themselves. Thus LSD was widely used as an adjunct to psychotherapy. When a psychiatrist felt that a patient had reached a roadblock and was unable to dredge up repressed memories and motives, LSD might be used for its psychedelic (mind-viewing) properties. Thus LSD took over as a modern truth serum, replacing sodium pentothal and scopolamine. Whether LSD actually helped these patients in the long run or only seemed helpful to the psychiatrists who believed in it is still being debated in the 1990s.

Two other potentially therapeutic uses were studied: for various theoretical reasons it was believed that LSD might be a good treatment for alcoholics, and initial reports of its effectiveness were quite positive. Later, it was hoped that LSD would allow terminal cancer patients to achieve a greater understanding of their own mortality. Thus many such patients were allowed to explore their feelings while under the influence of this fantasy-producing agent.

In April 1966 the Sandoz Pharmaceutical Company recalled the LSD it had distributed and withdrew its sponsorship for work with LSD. Large quantities of illegally manufactured LSD of uncertain purity were being used in the street, and Sandoz decided to give the responsibility for the legal distribution of LSD to the federal government.

Scientific study of the hallucinogens declined in the 1970s. The Reverend Walter Clark, a theologian and well-known advocate of controlled research on psychedelic drugs, provided data to support what he wrote in 1975:

> Because of bureaucratic restrictions and public fear of the highly publicized dangers of the drugs both real and supposed, responsible investigators have too often retired from the field, despite their interest in the drugs and the conviction of many that these drugs are exceedingly promising tools in mental health and for the study of the human mind and development.[7]

Dr. Clark was partially whistling in the dark, because marijuana and its active ingredients had the same bureaucratic restrictions and they had been legally studied by thousands of scientists. More probably, hallucinogenic research had reached a dead end where new ideas were needed and not forthcoming. A 1974 report by a National Institute of Mental Health (NIMH) research task force on hallucinogenic research stated:

> Virtually every psychological test has been used to study persons under the influence of LSD or other such hallucinogens, but the research has contributed little to our understanding of the bizarre and potent effects of this drug.[8]

Partly as a reality-oriented response to this type of evaluation and partly because of the dead ends, the NIMH stopped its in-house LSD research on humans in 1968 and stopped funding university human research on LSD in 1974. The National Cancer Institute and the National Institute on Alcohol Abuse and Alcoholism stopped supporting psychedelic research in 1975 because it was nonproductive. Most of the research since that time has been conducted on animals in an effort to better understand the mechanism of action at a neural level.

Secret army/CIA research with LSD

The unveiling of CIA/army human research programs using hallucinogens began with a June 1975 report by the Rockefeller Commission on the CIA. A forty-three-year-old biochemist, Frank Olson, had committed suicide on November 28, 1953, less than two weeks after CIA agents had secretly slipped LSD into his after-dinner drink. This drug caused a panic reaction in Dr. Olson, and he was taken to New York City for psychiatric treatment. After his suicide, his family had been told only that he had jumped or fallen from his tenth-story hotel room in Manhattan. In 1975 when this was uncovered, President Ford quickly apologized to the Olson family at the White House and said the incident was "inexcusable and unforgivable. . . . a horrible episode in American history."[9] It was not until October 1976 that enough government red tape was cut through to make it possible to award $750,000 to the Olson family.

Awareness of the Olson death started Congress and journalists digging for more, this time into the military as well. The army's interest in, and human experiments on, the use of psychedelics for warfare and for interrogation of prisoners and spies was not hidden. It was open knowledge in the scientific and military communities that such research was conducted at Edgewood Arsenal in Maryland, where Dr. Olson was poisoned, and at several major universities in the United States.

It was easy to see how the military and intelligence agencies got involved in this work. "American military and intelligence officials watched men with glazed eyes pouring out rambling confessions at the Communist purge trials in Eastern Europe after World War II, and for the first time they began to worry about the threat of mind-bending drugs as weapons."[10] They worried enough to repeatedly contact Dr. Hofmann about the feasibility of large-scale production of LSD,[11] and the CIA considered buying 10 kg in 1953 for $240,000. We can all be pleased that they decided against the purchase, which would have provided 100 million doses!

As the information kept pouring out of government files in the 1975 to 1976 period, it became clear that the army-sponsored research on 585 soldiers and 900 civilians between 1956 and 1967 had been very poorly done. The army and some of the university scientists had violated many of the ethical codes established as a result of the Nuremberg war crimes trials after World War II. Three failures were especially blatant: many of the volunteers were not really volunteers, many of the participants could not quit an experiment if they wanted to, and the participants were not told the nature of the experiment.

This horror story could go on almost without end; mention could be made of CIA agents picking up patrons in bars and secretly putting LSD in their drinks or of the administration of LSD to unsuspecting civilians around the world. The inspector general of the army issued a long report that criticized almost every aspect of the army's involvement with human LSD research: its conception, its execution, and its productivity.[12] This story should all too strikingly bring home the dangers of giving drugs to persons without their knowledge. These drugs can literally be mind-breaking when used incautiously.

Recreational use

The illegal LSD story starts with legal psilocybin, or perhaps at West Point, where Timothy Leary discovered Asian mysticism.

The story proper starts in the summer of 1960 in Mexico, where for the first time Leary used the magic mushrooms containing psilocybin. As he later said, he realized then that the old Timothy Leary was dead; the "Timothy Leary game" was over. Working at Harvard University, Leary collaborated with Dr. Richard Alpert and discussed the meaning and implication of this new world with Aldous Huxley.

During the 1960–1961 school year Leary and Alpert began a series of experiments on Harvard graduate students using pure psilocybin, which they had obtained through a physician. Leary's original work was apparently done under proper

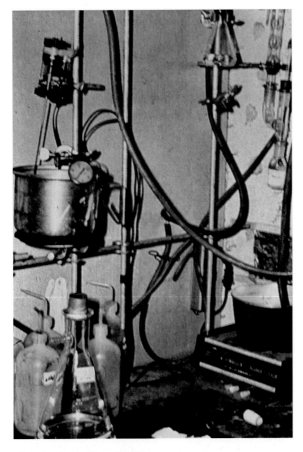

Illegal production of LSD.

scientific controls and with a physician in attendance because drugs were used. The use of a physician was later eliminated, and then other controls were dropped. In fact, Leary believed strongly that the experimenter should use the drug along with the subject, in order to be able to communicate with the subject. This practice removes the experimenter from the role of objective observer and can hardly be classified as seriously scientific.

Leary's drug-taking in the role of experimenter and the apparent abandonment of any

semblance of a scientific approach were questioned by Harvard authorities and other scientists. Some of the major issues were that no physician was present when drugs were administered, undergraduates were used in drug experiments, and drug sessions were conducted outside the laboratory in Leary's home and at other places off campus. As a result of many factors, Alpert and Leary were dismissed from their academic positions in the spring of 1963.[13]

All was reasonably quiet in 1964 and 1965. Alpert, now known as Baba Ram Dass, separated from Leary and lectured on the West Coast, while Leary settled at an estate in Millbrook, New York, that was owned by a wealthy supporter of Leary's beliefs. In 1964, Leary announced that drugs were not necessary to rise above and go beyond one's ego. He reiterated this again in 1966 after he was arrested for possession of marijuana at the Millbrook estate.

Also in 1966 Leary started his religion, the League of Spiritual Discovery, with LSD as the sacrament. The League got off to a slow start, and Leary's home base at Millbrook was under attack around the same time. The concern was that Leary would attract "drug addicts to Millbrook. When their money runs out, they will murder, rob and steal, to secure funds with which to satisfy their craving."[14]

Leary was the guru of the age, but his sacrament was already being secularized. Increasing numbers of young people were responding to the motto of the League for Spiritual Discovery: Turn On, Tune In, and Drop Out. Leary phrased it meaningfully:

> Turning on correctly means to understand the many levels that are brought into focus; it takes years of discipline, training, and discipleship. To turn on a street corner is a waste. To tune in means you must harness rigorously what you are learning. . . .
> To drop out is the oldest message that spiritual teachers have passed on. You can get only by giving up.[15]

Noble words, perhaps, but street corner turnons were becoming more frequent. A combination of many things increased the use of hallucinogens, and especially LSD, during the early and mid 1960s. LSD's promise of new sensations (which were delivered), of potent aphrodisiac effects (which were not forthcoming),[16] of feelings of kinship with a friendly peer group (which occurred) spread the drug rapidly.

In the summer of 1966, delegates to the annual convention of the American Medical Association passed a resolution urging greater controls on hallucinogens. They were a little uptight, as was the nation; in part, the resolution stated:

> these drugs can produce uncontrollable violence, overwhelming panic . . . or attempted suicide or homicide, and can result, among the unstable or those with preexisting neurosis or psychosis, in severe illness demanding protracted stays in mental hospitals.[17]

LSD use appears to have peaked in 1967 and 1968, after which it tapered off. Several factors probably contributed to this decline, including widely publicized "bad trips," prolonged psychotic reactions, chromosome damage, self-injurious behavior, and "flashbacks." Concerned, many people began to avoid hallucinogens, whereas others shunned the synthetic LSD for the natural experiences produced by psilocybin or mescaline (actually, into the mid 1970s these natural substances, although in demand, were in short supply, and most street samples of either psilocybin or mescaline contained primarily LSD or PCP).

After a series of arrests on drug charges, Timothy Leary was sent to a minimum security prison in 1969, from which he escaped in 1970. After wandering around the world for a couple of years, he surrendered and was sent back to prison. Before his release in 1976, he stated that he was "totally rehabilitated" and would "never, under any circumstances, advocate the use of LSD or any drug."[18] Touring college campuses on the lecture circuit in the early 1980s, Leary talked about "how to use drugs without abusing them."[19]

LSD pharmacology

LSD is odorless, colorless, tasteless, and one of the most potent psychochemicals known. Let's remind ourselves about the pharmacological meaning of *potent:* it takes little LSD to produce effects. A drug could be highly potent and yet not produce much in the way of effects. For example, LSD has never been definitely linked to even one human overdose death. In rats, reliable behavioral effects can be produced by 0.04 mg/kg, whereas the LD_{50} is about 16 mg/kg, 400 times the behaviorally effective dose.

Absorption from the gastrointestinal tract is rapid, and most humans take LSD through the mouth. At all postingestion times, the brain contains less LSD than any of the other organs in the body, so it is not selectively taken up by the brain. Half of the LSD in the blood is metabolized every three hours, so blood levels decrease fairly rapidly. LSD is metabolized in the liver and excreted as 2-oxy-lysergic acid diethylamide, which is inactive.

Tolerance develops rapidly, repeated daily doses becoming completely ineffective in three to four days. Recovery is equally rapid, so weekly use of the same dose of LSD is possible. Cross-tolerance has been shown between LSD, mescaline, and psilocybin, and the effects of each can be blocked or reversed with chlorpromazine. Physical dependence or addiction to LSD or to any of the hallucinogens has not been shown.

LSD is a sympathomimetic agent, and the autonomic signs are some of the first to appear after LSD is taken. Typical symptoms are dilated pupils, elevated temperature and blood pressure, and an increase in salivation.

The fact that the indole structure of LSD resembles that of serotonin led first to the idea that LSD works by acting at serotonin receptors. Injections of radioactive LSD into animals demonstrate that serotonin receptors are the primary, but not the only, binding sites for LSD.[20] Electrophysiological recordings from serotonin-containing neurons in the raphe nuclei of rats reveal that LSD injections cause a complete cessation of spontaneous electrical activity at doses comparable to those producing behavioral effects.[21] Thus there is fairly general agreement that many of the primary CNS effects of LSD are by actions on the serotonin systems.

However, there are several problems with this explanation of LSD effects. A basic problem relates to the fact that mescaline and other catechol hallucinogens have chemical structures more similar to the neurotransmitters dopamine and norepinephrine than to serotonin. However, they have psychological effects that are very similar to those of LSD. Rats trained to press one lever after an injection of LSD and another lever after a saline (placebo) injection will respond on the LSD lever if given other indole or catechol hallucinogens, but not if given PCP, anticholinergics, stimulants, sedatives, or opiates.[22] Thus the highly specific "LSD stimulus" in a rat appears to be similar to the stimuli produced by other indole and catechol hallucinogens. It has been suggested that the catechol hallucinogens are flexible enough to assume a shape that would allow them to fit the "LSD receptor," which could be a serotonin receptor.[23]

Whereas most of the behavioral effects of LSD and the catechol hallucinogens can be blocked by drugs that act as serotonin-receptor antagonists, others cannot. Add to this that there are several subtypes of serotonin receptors, some of which are excitatory and others inhibitory, and that LSD can act as either an agonist or an antagonist at different serotonin receptors, and you can begin to see how complicated this issue becomes. At the present time, the best evidence seems to indicate that LSD and other hallucinogens, including mescaline and psilocybin, act by stimulating the "serotonin-2" subtype of receptors.[24] Among a large group of hallucinogenic chemicals, there is a high correlation between their potency in binding to this type of receptor from rat brains and their potency in producing hallucinogenic effects in humans.

The LSD experience

Regardless of the chemical mechanism, most scientists feel that the most important effect is the modification of perception, particularly of visual images. Some of the experiences reported, especially after low doses, might best be described as illusions, or perceptual distortions, in which an object that is in fact present is seen in a distorted form (brighter than normal, moving, multiple images of the same object). Siegel,[25] who conducted laboratory research on the visual images reported after the ingestion of various drugs, reported that some images can be seen with eyes open or closed and thus are hallucinations rather than illusions. One stage of such hallucinogen-induced imagery consists of form-constants: lattices, honeycomb or chessboard designs, cobwebs, tunnel, alley or cone shapes, and spiral figures. These shapes were generally combined with intense colors and brightness. At another stage, complex images, such as landscapes, remembered faces, or objects, might be combined with the form-constants (e.g., a face might be seen "through" a honeycomb lattice, or multiple images of the face might appear in a honeycomb configuration). Siegel suggested that the perceptual processing mechanisms might be activated at the same time as the sensory inputs are either reduced or impaired, thus allowing vivid perception of images that come from inside, rather than outside, the brain.

Besides changes in visual perception, users also report an altered sense of time, changes in the perception of one's own body (perhaps indicating a reduction in somatic sensory input), and some alterations of auditory input. A particularly interesting phenomenon is that of **synesthesia**, a "mixing of senses," in which sounds might appear as visual images (as reported by Dr. Hofmann on the first-ever LSD "trip"), or the visual picture might alter in rhythm with music.

Altered perception is combined with enhanced emotionality, perhaps related to the arousal of the sympathetic branch of the autonomic nervous system. Thus one might interpret the images as exceptionally beautiful or awe inspiring because of an enhanced tendency to react with intense emotion. Alternatively, an object appearing to break apart or move away from or toward the perceiver might be reacted to with intense sadness or with fear. This fear can result in a pounding heart and rapid, shallow breathing, which further frightens the tripper and can lead to a full-blown panic reaction.

Part of the wonder of these agents is that they do not give repeat performances. However, even though each trip differs, the general type of experience and the sequence of experiences are reasonably well delineated. When an effective dose (30 to 100 μg) is taken orally, the trip will last six to nine hours. It can be greatly attenuated at any time through the administration of chlorpromazine intramuscularly.

The initial effects noticed are autonomic responses that develop gradually over the first 20 minutes. The individual might feel dizzy or hot and cold; his mouth might be dry. These effects diminish and, in addition, are less and less the focus of attention as alteration in sensations, perceptions, and mood begin to develop over the following 30 to 40 minutes. In one study, after the initial autonomic effects, the sequence of events over the next 20 to 50 minutes consisted of mood changes, abnormal body sensation, decrease in sensory impression, abnormal color perception, space and time disorders, and visual hallucinations. One visual effect was described beautifully:

> The guide asked me how I felt, and I responded, "Good." As I muttered the word "Good," I could see it form visually in the air. It was pink and fluffy like a cloud. The word looked "Good" in its appearance and so it had to be "Good." The word and the thing I was trying to express were one, and "Good" was floating around in the air.[26]

About one hour after taking LSD, the intoxication is in full bloom, but it is not until near the end of the second hour that changes occur in the perception of the self. Usually these changes center around a depersonalization. The individual might feel that the sensations she experiences are not from her body or that she has no body. Body distortions are common, the sort of thing suggested by the comment of one user: "I felt as if my left big toe were going to vomit!" Not unusual is a loss of self-awareness and loss of control of behavior.

Two frequent types of overall reactions in this stage have been characterized as "expansive" and "constricted." In the expansive reaction (a good trip) the individual can become excited and grandiose and feel that he is uncovering secrets of the universe or profundities previously locked within himself. Feelings of creativity are not uncommon: "If I only had the time, I could write the truly great American novel." The other end of the continuum is the constricted reaction in which the user shows little movement and frequently becomes paranoid and exhibits feelings of persecution. The prototype individual in this situation is huddled in a corner fearful that some harm will come to him or that he is being threatened by some aspect of the hallucinations. As the drug effect diminishes, normal psychological controls of sensations, perceptions, and mood return.

Adverse reactions

The adverse reactions to LSD ingestion have been repeatedly emphasized in the popular and scientific literature. Because there is no way of knowing how much illegal LSD is being used or how pure the LSD is that people are taking, there is no possibility of determining the true incidence of adverse reactions to LSD. Adverse reactions to the street use of what is thought to be LSD can result from many factors. It is important to always remember that drugs obtained on the street frequently are not what they are claimed to be—in purity, chemical composition, or quantity.

A 1960 study surveyed most of the legal U.S. investigators studying LSD and mescaline effects in humans. Data were collected on 25,000 administrations of the drug to about 5,000 individuals. Doses ranged from 25 to 1,500 µg of LSD and 200 to 1,200 mg of mescaline. In some cases the drug was used in patients undergoing therapy; in other cases the drug was taken in an experimental situation to study the effects of the drug. Only LSD and mescaline used under professional supervision were surveyed. Some results are noted in table 16.1.

A 1964 article, "The LSD Controversy,"[27] stated:

> It would seem that the incidence statistics better support a statement that the drug is exceptionally safe rather than dangerous. Although no statistics have been compiled for the dangers of psychological therapies, we would not be surprised if the incidence of adverse reactions, such

as psychotic or depressive episodes and suicide attempts, were at least as high or higher in any comparable group of psychiatric patients exposed to any active form of therapy.

but then went on to say:

> It is also important to distinguish between the proper use of this drug in therapeutic or experimental settings and its indiscriminate use and abuse by thrill seekers, "lunatic fringe," and drug addicts. More dangers seem likely for the unstable character who takes the drug for "kicks," curiosity, or to escape reality and responsibility than someone taking the drug for therapeutic reasons under strict medical aegis and supervision.

- **Panic reactions.** One type of adverse reaction that can develop during the drug-induced experience is the panic reaction, which is typified in the following case history:

> A 21-year-old woman was admitted to the hospital along with her lover. He had had a number of LSD experiences and had convinced her to take it to make her less constrained sexually. About half an hour after ingestion of approximately 200 microgm., she noticed that the bricks in the wall began to go in and out and that light affected her strangely. She became frightened when she realized that she was unable to distinguish her body from the chair she was sitting on or from her lover's body. Her fear became more marked after she thought that she would not get back into herself. At the time of admission she was hyperactive and laughed inappropriately. Stream of talk was illogical and affect labile. Two days later, this reaction had ceased. However, she was still afraid of the drug and convinced that she would not take it again because of her frightening experience.[28]

- **Prolonged psychotic reaction.** When an overt psychosis develops, remedial treatment

TABLE 16.1

Estimated Rates of Major Complications Associated with LSD

Groups studied	Number per 1,000 persons		
	Attempted suicide	Completed suicide	Psychotic reaction over 48 hours
Subjects in experiments	0	0	0.8
Patients undergoing psychotherapy	1.2	0.4	1.8

synesthesia: (sin ess *thees* ya) the blending of different senses, such as "seeing" sounds.

is not usually so rapid, and the next individual to be described was hospitalized for prolonged treatment. Usually such psychosis occurs in individuals with a precarious hold on reality in the nondrug condition. The flood of new experiences and feelings is too much for this type of person to integrate.

A 23-year-old man was admitted to the hospital after he stood uncertain whether to plunge an upraised knife into his friend's back. His wife . . . reported that he had been acting strangely since taking LSD approximately 3 weeks before admission. He was indecisive and often mute and shunned physical contact with her. On admission he was catatonic, mute and echopractic. He appeared to be preoccupied with auditory hallucinations of God's voice and thought he had achieved a condition of "all mind." On transfer to another hospital 1 month after admission, there was minimal improvement.

During his adolescence the patient had alternated between acceptance of and rebellion against his mother's religiosity and warnings of the perils of sex and immorality. He had left college during his 1st year after excessive use of amphetamines. He attended, but did not complete, art school. His marriage of 3 years had been marked by conflict and concern about his masculinity. Increasing puzzlement about the meaning of life, his role in the universe and other cosmic problems led to his ingestion of LSD. Shortly after ingestion he was ecstatic and wrote to a friend, "We have found the peace, which is life's river which flows into the sea of Eternity." Soon afterward, in a brief essay, he showed some awareness of his developing psychosis, writing, "I am misunderstood, I cried, and was handed a complete list of my personality traits, habits, goals, and ideals, etc. I know myself now, I said in relief, and spent the rest of my life in happy cares asylum. AMEN."[28]

It would be easy to blame this young man's psychosis on LSD, but it is also easy to find evidence in his case history of a possible developing schizophrenia that might have been partly responsible for his wanting to try LSD. Statistically, there is no evidence that LSD use results in increased likelihood of prolonged psychosis (see table 16.1).

- **Flashbacks.** One of the frightening and interesting adverse reactions to LSD is the flashback. More than any other reaction, the recurrence of symptoms weeks or months after an individual has taken LSD brings up thoughts of brain damage and permanent biochemical changes. Flashbacks consist of the recurrence of certain aspects of the drug experience after a period of normalcy and in the absence of any drug use. The frequency and duration of these flashbacks are quite variable and seem to be unpredictable. They are most frequent just before going to sleep, while driving, and in periods of psychological stress. They seem to diminish in frequency and intensity with time if the individual stops using psychoactive drugs.

Although some of the reactions reported as "flashbacks" might be nothing more than intense memories or experiences that non-LSD users can also have, such as déjà vu, there remain many reports of "reexperiencing" LSD-like reactions in a frightening way. One group continued to study this phenomenon and reported that psychophysical tests of visual function showed measurable impairments several years after the last use of LSD.[29] A group of 24 ex-LSD users was compared with 20 control subjects. Although there were no differences between the groups in visual acuity, color vision, or several other measures, a significant difference was found in the rate at which a flickering light appeared to "fuse" into a continuous light, especially when the light was presented to the peripheral parts of the visual field. The LSD group also did not adapt to darkness as well as the control group. The authors concluded that their results are consistent with long-term changes in the central nervous system of LSD users.

Beliefs about LSD

LSD is truly a legend in its own time—actually, there are many legends. People probably have more ideas about what LSD does and does not do than they have about any other drug. Only a few of these beliefs can be mentioned.

- **Creativity.** One of the most widely occurring beliefs is that these hallucinogenic agents increase creativity or release creativity that our inhibitions keep bottled inside us. There have been several experiments that have attempted to study the effects of LSD on creativity, but there is no good evidence that the drug increases it. In one laboratory study using LSD at doses of 0.0025 or 0.01 mg/kg body weight, "the authors concluded that the administration of LSD-25 to a relatively unselected group of people for the purpose of enhancing their creative ability is *not* likely to be successful."[30] An experiment with professional artists under the influence of LSD concluded: "for the creative artist, drugs are likely to produce more negative than positive results."[31]

- **Therapy.** Another common belief is that LSD has therapeutic usefulness, particularly in the treatment of alcoholics, even though reports of results with LSD in alcoholism gradually changed from glowing and enthusiastic to cautious and disappointing. One well-controlled study compared the effectiveness of one dose of either 0.6 mg of LSD or 60 mg of dextroamphetamine in reducing drinking by alcoholics. No additional therapy, physical or psychological, was used. The authors found that "LSD produced slightly better results early, but after six months the results were alike for both treatment groups."[32]

Some investigators reported considerable success with LSD in reducing the pain and depression of patients with terminal cancer. The LSD experiences were part of a several-day program involving extensive verbal interaction between the therapist and patient. Although not successful in every case, the LSD therapy was followed by a reduction in the use of narcotics, "less worry about the future," and "the appearance of a positive mood state." The authors

Attitudes toward LSD

In light of what you have learned about LSD, it will be interesting for you to see how other people view it, preferably people who have not recently studied the topic. Make up a list of questions covering both knowledge about and attitudes toward LSD. Be sure to include questions about why people took LSD in the 1960s, benefits, risks, and whether its use is still prevalent. Then find time to conduct interviews with several people, asking the questions you have developed. See if you can summarize consistencies in the knowledge and beliefs of these people, comparing the summary with the facts as presented in the text.

concluded that they have a treatment "which may be highly promising for patients facing fatal illness if implemented in the context of brief, intensive, and highly specialized psychotherapy catalyzed by a psychedelic drug such as LSD." A scientific peer review by NIMH[33] concluded: "Research on the therapeutic use of LSD has shown that it is not a generally useful therapeutic drug as an adjunct to a routine psychotherapeutic approach or as a treatment in and of itself."

- **Chromosome damage.** A credibility gap in the world of drugs developed in 1967 between the press and the public with the publication of a scientific report that LSD caused damage to chromosomes of white blood cells (leukocytes) in vitro. This report was quickly followed by a study showing a higher than normal incidence of chromosomal damage in the white blood cells of LSD users. These data received much attention in the mass media and are thought to be one of the reasons for the decrease in LSD use that has occurred since 1967. Not so widely publicized were the many follow-up reports that did *not* show any relationship in vitro or in vivo between white blood cell chromosome damage and LSD use.

The popular reports also had a way of neglecting to emphasize (or mention) that the effects were on white blood cells and not on the germ cells, which are the important cells for reproduction. The weight of evidence gathered over the years does *not* support the claim that LSD can cause birth defects or cancer in its human users.

Psilocybin

The magic mushrooms of Mexico have a long history of religious and ceremonial use. These plants, as well as peyote, dropped from Western sight (but not from native use) for three hundred years after the Spanish conquered the Aztecs and systematically destroyed their writings and teachings. The mushrooms were to be particularly suppressed. The name *teonanacatl* can be translated as "God's flesh" or as "sacred mushroom," and either name was very offensive to the Spanish priests.

It was not until the late 1930s that it was clearly shown that these mushrooms were still being used by natives in southern Mexico and the first of many species was identified. The real breakthrough came in 1955. During that year a New York banker turned ethnobotanist and his wife established rapport with a native group still using mushrooms in religious ceremonies. Gordon Wasson became the first outsider to participate in the ceremony and to eat of the magic mushroom. In language quite unlike that of a banker you can almost hear Wasson's soul cry out as he tries to describe the experience:

It permits you to travel backwards and forward in time, to enter other planes of existence, even (as the Indians say), to know God.[34]

Psilocybe mushroom containing psilocybin, which is chemically related to lysergide (LSD).

The mushroom that seems to have the greatest psychoactive effect is *Psilocybe mexicana*. The primary active agent in this mushroom is **psilocybin,** an indole that the discoverer of LSD, Albert Hofmann, isolated in 1958 and later synthesized.

The dried mushrooms are 0.2 to 0.5 percent psilocybin. The hallucinogenic effects of psilocybin are quite similar to those of LSD and the catechol hallucinogen mescaline, and cross-tolerance exists among these three agents.[35]

The psychoactive effects are clearly related to the amount used, with up to 4 mg yielding a pleasant experience, relaxation, and some body sensations. Higher doses cause considerable perceptual and body-image changes with hallucinations in some individuals. Accompanying these psychic changes are dose-related sympathetic arousal symptoms. There is some evidence that psilocybin has its central nervous system effects only after it has been changed in the body to psilocin. Psilocin is present in the mushroom only in trace amounts but is about 1.5 times as potent as psilocybin. Perhaps the greater CNS effect of psilocin is the result of its higher lipid solubility.

One of Leary's followers used psilocybin in the now-classic Good Friday study. The Good Friday study was designed to investigate the ability of psilocybin to induce meaningful religious experiences in individuals when the drug is used in a religious setting. Twenty seminarians participated in a double-blind study, with half receiving 30 mg of psilocybin and half placebos, ninety minutes before attending a religious service. Tape recordings of the subjects' experiences were made immediately after the 2½-hour service, which was held in a chapel. Within a week a questionnaire was completed, followed by a similar one six months later. The first was directed at determining the magnitude and type of change that occurred during the experiment, and the later one at assessing the durability of the change. Leary later summarized the outcome of the Good Friday study by saying:

> the results clearly support the hypothesis that, with adequate preparation and in an environment which is supportive and religiously meaningful, subjects report mystical experiences significantly more than placebo controls.[36]

Given access to some spores of the mushroom and proper growing conditions, it is possible to cultivate *psilocybe M.* in a closet. As a consequence of illegal production in the United States, the use of this mushroom has continued into the 1990s, with sporadic outbursts of availability. Although occasionally a major mushroom producer will be discovered, most of the production seems to be on a local, amateur basis. Young people might obtain a few "shrooms" to consume at a party, usually in small quantities and in combination with alcoholic beverages. Under such circumstances it is difficult to tell how much of an effect is produced by the mushrooms and how much by the social situation and the alcohol.

Morning Glory

Of the psychoactive agents used freely in Mexico in the sixteenth century, *ololiuqui,* seeds of the morning glory plant *Rivea corymbosa,* perhaps had the greatest religious significance. These seeds tie America to Europe even today. When Albert Hofmann analyzed the seeds of the morning glory, he found several active alkaloids as well as *d*-lysergic acid amide, which is about one-tenth as active as LSD. The presence of *d*-lysergic acid amide is really quite amazing (to botany majors), because before this discovery in 1960, lysergic acid had been found only in much more primitive groups of plants such as the ergot fungus.[37]

A different species of morning glory, *Ipomoea violacea,* seems to be the primary source in the United States of most commercial morning glory seeds containing effective amounts of these alkaloids. Considering the psychoactivity of these seeds, the commercial names seem quite appropriate: Pearly Gates, Flying Saucers, Heavenly Blue!

DMT

Dimethyltryptamine (DMT) has never been widely used in the United States, although it has a long, if not noble, history. In fact, on a worldwide basis, DMT is one of the most important naturally occurring hallucinogenic compounds, and it occurs in many plants. DMT is the active agent in Cohoba snuff, which is used by some South American and Caribbean Indians in hunting rituals. Although DMT was synthesized in the 1930s, its discovery as the active ingredient in cohoba first led to human examination of its psychoactive properties in 1956.

DMT is ineffective when taken orally and must be snuffed, smoked, or taken by injection. The effective intramuscular dose is about 1 mg/kg body weight. Intravenously, hallucinogenic effects are seen within 2 minutes after

---

psilocybin: (sill o *sy* bin) active chemical in psilocybe mushrooms from Mexico.

Although morning glory seeds were used as religious plants in Mexico before Columbus, the seeds of most types of morning glories available in the United States have little or no hallucinogenic action.

doses of 0.2 mg/kg or more, and last for less than 30 minutes.[38] The freebase form of DMT can be "smoked" by adding the crystals to some type of plant, and 20 to 40 mg is the usual dose. The effect is brief no matter how it is used, and rapid tolerance limits one's ability to prolong the experience with repeated doses.

Interest in DMT has recently been rekindled by the discovery that it is a common ingredient in psychoactive mixtures known as ayahuasca based principally on a plant containing the MAO inhibitor harmaline. The combination of DMT with the MAO inhibitor (see chapter 9 for a description of MAO inhibitors as antidepressants) apparently intensifies and prolongs the DMT effect. Modern-day pilgrims are traveling to the Amazon to experience this apparently rather dramatic combination of plant substances.[39]

CATECHOL HALLUCINOGENS

This second group of phantastica, although having psychological effects quite similar to those of the indole types, is based on a different structure, that of the catechol nucleus. That nucleus forms the basic structure of the catecholamine neurotransmitters, norepinephrine and dopamine. Figure 16.2 shows the catechol structure and the structures of some catechol hallucinogens. Look for the catechol nucleus in each of the hallucinogens, and then compare these structures with the structure of amphetamine and other stimulants shown in chapter 7.

Mescaline

Peyote (from the Aztec *peyotl*) is a small, spineless, carrot-shaped cactus, *Lophophora williamsii* Lemaire, that grows wild in the Rio Grande Valley and southward. It is mostly subterranean, and only the grayish-green pincushion-like top appears above ground.[40]

In pre-Columbian times the Aztec, Huichol, and other Mexican Indians ate the plant ceremonially either in the dried or green state. This produces profound sensory and psychic derangements lasting twenty-four hours, a property which led the natives to value and use it religiously.[41]

The basic catecholamine structure (dopamine)

3,4,5 trimethoxyphenylethylamine (mescaline)

■ carbon
■ oxygen
■ hydrogen
■ nitrogen

2', 5' dimethoxy -4'- methylamphetamine (DOM)

3, 4 methylenedioxy ampetamine (MDA)

3,4 methylenedioxy methampetamine (MDMA)

Figure 16.2 Cathechol hallucinogens

Only the part of the cactus that is above ground is easily edible, but the entire plant is psychoactive. This upper portion, or crown, is sliced into disks that dry and are known as "mescal buttons." These slices of the peyote cactus remain psychoactive indefinitely and are the source of the drug between the yearly harvests. The journey by Indians in November and December to harvest the peyote is an elaborate ceremony, sometimes taking almost a month and a half. When the mescal buttons are to be used, they are soaked in the mouth until soft, then formed by hand into a bolus and swallowed.

peyote: (pay *oh* tee) a type of hallucinogenic cactus.

Peyote cactus.

Mescal buttons should not be confused with mescal beans—or with mescal liquor, which is distilled from the fermentation of the agave cactus. Mescal buttons are slices of the peyote cactus and contain **mescaline** as the primary active agent. Mescal beans, however, are dark red seeds from the shrub *Sophora secundiflora*. These seeds, formerly the basis of a vision-seeking cult, contain a highly toxic alkaloid, cytisine, the effects of which resemble those of nicotine, causing nausea, convulsions, hallucinations, and occasionally death from respiratory failure. The mescal bean has a long history, and there is some evidence that use of the bean diminished and ceased when the safer peyote became available in the southwestern United States. In the transition from a mescal bean to a mescal button cult there appeared, in some tribes, a period in which a mixture of peyote and mescal seeds was concocted and drunk. These factors contributed to considerable confusion in the early (and some recent) literature.[37]

Although there was evidence that the use of peyote had moved north into the United States as early as 1760, it was not until the late nineteenth century that a peyote cult was widely es-tablished among the Indians of the plains. From that time to the present, Indian missionaries have spread the peyote religion to almost a quarter of a million Indians, some as far north as Canada. The development of the present form of this sect has been summarized:

> The independent groups of the Peyote Religion have federated into the Native American Church during the 20th century, like the independent congregations of the Jesus Cult federated into the Catholic Church during the 4th century. However, just as not all congregations accepting the basic doctrines of Christianity belonged to the Catholic Church, so not all groups accepting the basic doctrines of Peyotism belong to the Native American Church.[42]

The *Native American Church* of the United States was first chartered in Oklahoma in 1918 and is an amalgamation of Christianity and traditional beliefs and practices of the Indians. Its basic beliefs are simply stated in the articles of incorporation:

> The purpose for which this corporation is formed is to foster and promote religious believers in Almighty God and the customs of the several Tribes of Indians throughout the United States in the worship of a Heavenly Father and to promote morality, sobriety, industry, charity, and right living and cultivate a spirit of self-respect and brotherly love and union among the members of the several Tribes of Indians throughout the United States . . . with and through the sacramental use of peyote.[43]

In 1960, peyotism was "the major religious cult of most Indians of the United States between the Rocky Mountains and the Mississippi."[40] As in all religions a variety of rituals has developed surrounding the use of peyote in religious ceremonies. Peyote is also used in other ways because the Indians attribute spiritual power to the peyote plant. As such, peyote is believed to be helpful, along with prayers and modern medicines, in curing illnesses. It is also worn as an amulet, much as some Christians

Kickapoo peyote ceremony.

wear a Saint Christopher's medal, to protect the wearer from harm.

For many years the use of peyote as a sacrament by the Native American Church was protected by the constitutional guarantee of freedom of religion. In fact, it was that protection that had inspired Timothy Leary to attempt a similar exclusion for LSD in his newly founded 1960s League of Spiritual Discovery. However, in 1990 the Supreme Court ruled that the State of Oregon could prosecute its citizens for using peyote, and the freedom of religion argument was not allowed.[44] A large group of religious and civil liberties organizations asked the Court to reconsider its decision, but they declined to do so. The two defendants in the case were American Indians and members of the Native American Church. Federal law and many state laws specifically exclude sacramental peyote use, and the Court pointed out that Oregon could exclude such use, too. It is not clear what the long-term implications of this ruling might be. That will depend to some extent on whether other states decide to outlaw all use of peyote.

Nonreligious use of mescaline

Near the end of the nineteenth century, Arthur Heffter isolated several alkaloids from peyote and showed that mescaline was the primary agent for the visual effect induced by peyote. Mescaline was synthesized in 1918, and most experiments on the psychoactive and/or behavioral effects since then have used synthesized mescaline. More than thirty psychoactive alkaloids have now been identified in peyote, but mescaline does seem to be the agent responsible for the vivid colors and other visual effects. The fact that mescaline is not equivalent to peyote is not always made clear in the literature.[45]

> **mescaline:** (*mess* **ka lin**) active chemical in the peyote cactus.

One of the early investigators of the effects of peyote was Dr. Weir Mitchell, who used an extract of peyote and who reported, in part:

> The display which for an enchanted two hours followed was such as I find it hopeless to describe in language which shall convey to others the beauty and splendor of what I saw. Stars, delicate floating films of color, then an abrupt rush of countless points of white light swept across the field of view, as if the unseen millions of the Milky Way were to flow in a sparkling river before my eyes . . . zigzag lines of very bright colors . . . the wonderful loveliness of swelling clouds of more vivid colors gone before I could name them.[46]

Another early experimenter was Havelock Ellis. Interestingly, he took his peyote on Good Friday in 1897, sixty-five years before the much-noted Good Friday experiment with psilocybin. His experience is described in detail in a 1902 article titled "Mescal: A Study of a Divine Plant"[47] in *Popular Science Monthly*, but a brief quotation gives the essence of the experience:

> On the whole, if I had to describe the visions in one word, I should say that they were living arabesques. There was generally a certain incomplete tendency to symmetry, the effect being somewhat as if the underlying mechanism consisted of a large number of polished facets acting as mirrors. It constantly happened that the same image was repeated over a large part of the field, though this holds good mainly of the forms, for in the colors there would still remain all sorts of delicious varieties. Thus at a moment when uniformly jewelled flowers seemed to be springing up and extending all over the field of vision, the flowers still showed every variety of delicate tone and tint.

Not every individual wants every educational opportunity. William James, surprisingly, was one who did not. He wrote to his brother Henry: "I ate one but three days ago, was violently sick for twenty-four hours, and had no other symptoms whatever except that and the Katzenjammer the following day. I will take the visions on trust." Even Dr. Weir Mitchell, who had the effect previously recorded, said: "These shows are expensive. . . . The experience, however, was worth one such headache and indigestion but was not worth a second."

Even if you get by without too much nausea and physical discomfort, which the Indians also report, all might not go well. Huxley, whose 1954 *The Doors of Perception*[48] made him a guru in this area, admitted: "Along with the happily transfigured majority of mescaline takers there is a minority that finds in the drug only hell and purgatory." It is reported that natives sometimes wished for "bad trips" when taking this or other plants. By meeting their personal demons, they hoped to conquer them and remove problems from their lives.

Pharmacology of mescaline

Mescaline is readily absorbed if taken orally, but it only very poorly passes the blood-brain barrier (which explains the high doses required). There is a maximal concentration of the drug in the brain after 30 to 120 minutes. About half of it is removed from the body in 6 hours, and there is evidence that some mescaline persists in the brain for up to 9 to 10 hours. Similar to the indole hallucinogens, the effects obtained with low doses, about 3 mg/kg body weight, are primarily euphoric, whereas doses in the range of 5 mg/kg give rise to a full set of hallucinations. Most of the mescaline is excreted unchanged in the urine, and the metabolites identified thus far are not psychoactive.

A dose that is psychoeffective in humans causes pupil dilation, pulse rate and blood pressure increases, and an elevation in body temperature. All of these effects are similar to those induced by LSD, psilocybin, and most other alkaloid hallucinogens. There are other signs of central stimulation, such as EEG arousal, after mescaline intake. In rats the LD_{50} is about 370 mg/kg body weight, ten to thirty times the dose that causes behavioral effects. Death results from convulsions and respiratory arrest. Tolerance develops more slowly to mescaline than to LSD, and there is cross-tolerance between them. As with LSD, mescaline intoxication can be blocked with chlorpromazine.

Although mescaline and the other catechol hallucinogens have a structure that resembles the catecholamine neurotransmitters, it has been proposed that they might in fact operate via the same mechanism as LSD, perhaps mainly via serotonin actions. The fact that the psychological effects of these two chemical classes of phantastica are so similar in humans, and also that the behavioral effects of either drug in rats are blocked by serotonin antagonists, suggest a common mechanism, and studies of the structures of catechol hallucinogens indicate certain similarities to the overall LSD structure.[23]

Amphetamine Derivatives

There is a large group of synthetic hallucinogens that are chemically related to amphetamine. However, most of these drugs have little amphetamine-like stimulant activity. Thanks to certain chemical substitutions on the ring part of the catechol nucleus, these drugs are more mescaline-like (figure 16.2).

DOM (STP)

DOM is 2,5-dimethoxy-4-methylamphetamine. In the 1960s and 70s, DOM was called STP, and street talk was that the initials stood for serenity, tranquility, and peace. Its actions and effects are highly similar to those of mescaline and LSD, with a total dose of 1 to 3 mg yielding euphoria and 3 to 5 mg a six- to eight-hour hallucinogenic period. This makes DOM about a hundred times as potent as mescaline but only one thirtieth as potent as LSD.

DOM has a reputation for inducing an extraordinarily long experience, but this seems to be caused by the very large amounts being used. Some pills of DOM bought on the street contained about 10 mg—a very big dose. Reports by users had suggested that DOM was unlike other hallucinogens and that its effects were enhanced

rather than blocked by chlorpromazine. Controlled laboratory work with normal volunteers, however, has clearly shown that the effects of DOM are similar to those of other hallucinogens and that chlorpromazine does attenuate the DOM experience.[49]

An excellent review from the Haight-Ashbury Clinic contains most of the essential information about the rise and fall of DOM use:

> It appears then that DOM produces a higher incidence of acute and chronic toxic reactions than any of the other commonly used hallucinogens. . . . It appears that the effects of DOM are like a combination of amphetamine and LSD with the hallucinogenic effects of the drug very often putting the peripheral amphetamine-like physiological effects out of perspective.[50]

MDA and others

In addition to DOM, many other amphetamine derivatives have been synthesized and shown to have hallucinogenic properties. Most of these, such as DOET, TMA-2, and the various MDAs, have effects very similar to those of DOM and mescaline, as well as LSD and the indole types. There is some indication that one type of derivative, MDA (see figure 16.2), has effects that are subjectively somewhat different.[23] MDA, which is somewhat more potent than mescaline, has seen some recreational use through illicit manufacture. Because of the variety of possible hallucinogenic amphetamine derivatives and because most of these chemicals are not specifically listed as controlled substances, illicit drug makers were drawn to this group of chemicals in the production of various "designer drugs" to be sold on the street as hallucinogens.

MDMA

One of the amphetamine derivatives received special attention in July 1984 when the DEA proposed scheduling it. MDMA is similar in structure to MDA but is apparently quite different from the other hallucinogens. Rats trained to discriminate DOM from saline did show some generalization from the DOM stimulus to MDA but not to MDMA. Furthermore, there is no cross-tolerance between MDA and MDMA.[23] Although there was some use of MDMA on the streets (it was called "Ecstasy" or "XTC"), what was surprising was that a number of psychiatrists came forth who had been quietly using MDMA, a drug that, although not approved by the FDA, was not illegal. These psychiatrists testified against the scheduling of MDMA, insisting that it was not a true hallucinogen and that it had a special ability to promote empathy, thus aiding the psychoanalytic process.[51]

There is some evidence supporting this claim of increased empathy: in a 1987 study, a hundred people completed detailed questionnaires describing the effects of their previous use of MDMA.[52] Although such retrospective reports are less reliable than reports obtained during or immediately after the experience, a remarkably common report (90 percent of the individuals) was that they experienced a heightened sense of "closeness" with other people. Other common effects were an increased heart rate, dry mouth, grinding of the teeth, profuse sweating, and other autonomic effects. Although several people reported that objects seemed more "luminescent," very few reported actual visual hallucinations.

The bad news is that this otherwise fairly benign drug might cause permanent brain damage. Several laboratories have reported that rats given MDMA injections show a selective destruction of serotonin neurons in their brains. Then a similar effect was reported in monkeys at only two to three times the normal human dose, and this led many observers to conclude that similar brain damage could occur in human MDMA users.[53] It should be stressed that this effect is *not* caused by LSD, mescaline, psilocybin, or most other drugs, and that the evidence that MDMA causes damage is strong enough to be taken seriously. The serotonin re-uptake inhibitor fluoxetine (Prozac; see chapter 9) blocks the neurotoxicity in rats but does not appear to block the psychoactive effect in humans, and some human users have begun using fluoxetine with MDMA to reduce the chances of brain damage.[54] MDMA has been listed as a Schedule I controlled substance since 1988.

PCP

In the 1950s, Parke, Davis & Company investigated a series of drugs in the search for an efficient intravenous anesthetic. On the basis of animal studies, they selected 1-(1-phenylcyclohexyl) piperidine hydrochloride (PCP, generic name *phencyclidine*) for testing in humans. The studies on monkeys had indicated that **PCP** was a good analgesic but did not produce good muscle relaxation nor did it produce sleep. Instead, the animals showed a sort of "dissociation" from what was happening: "During the operation the animal had its eyes open and looked about unconcernedly." In 1958 the first report was published on the use of PCP (brand name Sernyl) for surgical anesthesia in sixty-four humans.[55] Sernyl produced good analgesia without depressing blood circulation or respiration and did not produce irregularities in heartbeat. Loss of sensation occurred within two or three minutes of beginning the intravenous infusion, after about 10 mg of the drug had been delivered. The patients later had no memory of the procedure, did not remember being spoken to, and remembered no pain. Compared with existing anesthetics, which tend to depress both respiration and circulation through general depression of the CNS, this type of "dissociative" anesthetic seemed to be quite safe. However, the psychological reactions to the drug were unpredictable. During administration of the drug a few patients became very excited, and a different anesthetic had to be used. Several patients were "unmanageable" as they emerged from the anesthetic, exhibiting severely manic behavior. This and later reports indicated that many people given anesthetic doses of Sernyl reported changes in body perception and hallucinations, and in about 15 percent of the patients, experienced a "prolonged confusional psychosis," lasting up to four days after the drug was given. This period of confusion was characterized by feelings of unreality, depersonalization, persecution, depression, and intense anxiety.

News of this new hallucinogen soon reached Dr. Luby, a psychiatrist, who began testing it in both normal and schizophrenic subjects.[56] All the subjects reported changes in perception of their own bodies, with one normal subject saying, "my arm feels like a 20-mile pole with a pin at the end." Another said, "I am a small . . . not human . . . just a block of something in a great big laboratory." There were a number of reports of floating, flying, dizziness, and of alternate contraction and expansion of body size. All subjects also showed some type of thought disorder. Some made up new words, uttered strings of unrelated words, or repeated words or simple phrases over and over. Also, all became increasingly drowsy and apathetic. At times a subject would appear to be asleep but when asked a direct question would respond. When asked, "Can you hear me?" subjects often responded, "No." The majority became either angry or uncooperative. Many of the normal subjects said they felt as if they were drunk from alcohol. All subjects displayed diminished pain, touch, and position sense, and all showed nystagmus (rapid oscillations of the eyes) and a slapping, ataxic walk. Luby and his colleagues felt that PCP was different from LSD or mescaline in that there were few reports of intense visual experiences and many more reports of body image changes. The disorganized thinking, suspiciousness, and lack of cooperation made the PCP state resemble schizophrenia much more than the LSD state.

Thus by 1960 PCP was well characterized as an excellent anesthetic for monkeys, a medically safe but psychologically troublesome anesthetic for humans, and a hallucinogen different from LSD and mescaline, with profound effects on body perception. Parke, Davis withdrew Sernyl as an investigational drug for humans in 1965 and in 1967 licensed another company to sell Sernylan as an animal anesthetic. It was particularly used with primates, in both research laboratories and zoos. Also, because of its rapid action and wide safety margin, Sernylan was used in syringe bullets to immobilize stray, wild, or dangerous zoo animals. Because of the popular term *tranquilizer gun* for this use, PCP became popularly, and inaccurately, known as an animal "tranquilizer."

Even though Sernyl was never marketed for human use, a related chemical from the same series was marketed as an anesthetic. Ketamine, which has somewhat more depressant activity than PCP and fewer prolonged reactions, is nevertheless quite similar. The 1994 *Physician's Desk Reference* contained the following special note about ketamine:

> Emergence reactions have occurred in approximately 12 percent of patients. The psychological manifestations vary in severity between pleasant dream-like states, vivid imagery, hallucinations, and emergence delirium. In some cases these states have been accompanied by confusion, excitement, and irrational behavior which a few patients recall as an unpleasant experience. The duration ordinarily is no more than a few hours; in a few cases, however, recurrences have taken place up to 24 hours postoperatively.[57]

In late 1967, workers at the Haight-Ashbury Medical Clinic obtained samples of a substance being distributed as the "Peace Pill." The drug was analyzed, determined to be PCP, and its identity and dangers were publicized in the

---

PCP: phencyclidine; originally developed as an anesthetic; has hallucinogenic properties.

Angel dust: phencyclidine (PCP) on plant material for smoking.

community in December 1967. By the next year it was reported that this drug had enjoyed only brief popularity and then disappeared. It appeared briefly in New York in 1968 as "hog" and at other times as "trank." Into the early 1970s, PCP was apparently regarded as pretty much a "garbage" drug by street people. In the early 1970s, PCP crystals were sometimes sprinkled onto oregano, parsley, or alfalfa and sold to unsuspecting youngsters as marijuana. In this form, it became known as **angel dust.** Because PCP can be made inexpensively and relatively easily by amateur chemists, when it is available it usually doesn't cost much. Eventually, the rapid and potent effects of angel dust made it a desired substance in its own right. Joints made with PCP sometimes contained marijuana, sometimes another plant substance, and were known as "killer joints" or "sherms" (because they hit you like a Sherman tank). By the late 1970s, PCP use was the most common cause of drug-induced visits to hospital emergency rooms in many communities, and in some neighborhoods young users could be seen "moonwalking" down the street (taking very high, careful, and slow steps) on any Saturday night.

Some users develop a profound psychological dependence on PCP, in spite of its unpredictability and the behavioral impairment it produces. One user reported:

Immediately after smoking the Dust I started experiencing the effects. All my troubles seemed to go away. I felt a little drunk and had some trouble walking around the apartment. Objects appeared either very far away or very close and I couldn't really judge distance at all. . . . I liked being apart from things, and felt outside my body for most of the trip. That was fun. Before I smoked I had been troubled about some exams coming up and felt I wasn't really prepared. . . . All that anxiety vanished with the Dust. . . . I felt at peace. It was a good feeling. . . . I want to be there always.[58]

That individual was unusually descriptive about the experience. Most often, a PCP user doesn't say much that makes sense while the drug is having its effects, and later the user doesn't remember much of what happened.

The dependence-producing properties of PCP have also been studied in monkeys, which will learn to respond to produce intravenous injections of the drug.[59] This is in contrast to LSD and other hallucinogens, which will not support animal self-administration and do not produce psychological dependence in most users.

Because some PCP users have been reported to behave violently, there is a question as to whether PCP tends to promote violence directly or whether violence is a side effect of the suspicion and anesthesia produced by the drug. Most users do not report feeling violent and feel so uncoordinated that they can't imagine "picking a fight." However, police who have tried to arrest PCP users have had trouble subduing them because many of the commonly used arrest techniques rely on restraining holds that result in pain if the arrestee resists. Because the PCP user is anesthetized, these restraint techniques are less effective.[60] Manual restraint by more than one officer might be required to arrest some PCP users, although one might question how different this is from the problem of arresting a violent drunk who is "feeling no pain."

That PCP users might not feel pain has resulted in some gruesome legends about users biting or cutting off their own fingers and so forth. Like earlier stories about LSD users blinding themselves by staring at the sun, these legends cannot be substantiated and most likely did not really occur. One oft-repeated story probably falls into the category of "police folklore." Every cop knows for a fact the story about the PCP user who was so violent, had such superhuman strength, and was so insensitive to pain that he was shot twenty-eight times (or some similar large number of times) before he fell. Although everyone knows that this happened, no one can tell you exactly when or where. One might dismiss such folklore as harmless, unless it contributes to events such as the shooting, six times at close range, of an unarmed, naked, thirty-five-year-old biochemist who was trying to climb the street sign outside his laboratory. This story really did happen, on August 4, 1977, during the height of the PCP epidemic. The lethal shots were fired by a Los Angeles police officer. The coroner's office reported that the victim's blood did contain traces of a drug similar to PCP.[61] More recently, Los Angeles police officers involved in the widely publicized videotaped beating of Rodney King said during their trial that they used such force because they believed King might have been "dusted"—under the influence of PCP.

The mechanism of PCP's action on the brain was a mystery for several years, because PCP does alter many neurotransmitter systems but did not appear to act directly on any of them. In 1979, it was reported that a specific receptor for PCP was present in the brain, and in 1981 the identity between the receptor and another that had previously been considered a subtype of opiate receptor was reported.[62] The drug cyclazocine, which has some opiate activity and has also been reported to produce hallucinations, binds well to this PCP receptor, but morphine,

Ibogaine as an Addiction Treatment

Ibogaine is a less well known indole drug that comes from the African shrub *Tabernanthe iboga*. The drug has been used by the local natives as a stimulant at lower doses and a hallucinogen at higher doses.[73] Animal experiments have demonstrated a short-term effect of reducing the self-administration of opioids or of cocaine, although the finding is not consistent. Also, there have been claims that humans who use ibogaine lose their craving for whatever drug they have been addicted to. This has led to proposals to carry out full-scale testing of ibogaine as a possible teatment for addiction. However, these suggestions have been met by a great deal of skepticism from people with long experience in treating addiction, who are used to periodic claims of a "miracle cure." Also, there has been considerable reluctance on the part of the federal drug-abuse research agency, NIDA, to promote a large-scale study of ibogaine. This might be partly due to the drug's reputation as an hallucinogen and partly due to the inconsistent nature of the animal research findings.

naloxone, and other opiates do not. Thus the receptor is probably better characterized as being selective for PCP, ketamine, and other similar drugs rather than as a type of opiate receptor. The presence of such a receptor has led to speculation about a possible endogenous substance,

angel dust: street name for PCP sprinkled on plant material.

facetiously called "angel-dustin," that would normally act on the receptor. It is not far from there to the speculation that excessive amounts of this hypothetical "angel-dustin" in some individuals might be responsible for schizophrenia, but as of yet there is no good clinical evidence in support of such a notion.

The PCP receptor is found in close association with receptors for glutamate, an excitatory neurotransmitter, where PCP antagonizes the excitatory action of the normal transmitter. Thus the mechanism by which PCP produces its effects is becoming clearer even if the proposed endogenous PCP-like substance has not yet been found.

ANTICHOLINERGIC HALLUCINOGENS

The potato family contains all the naturally occurring agents to be discussed here. Three of the genera—*Atropa, Hyoscyamus,* and *Mandragora*—have a single species of importance and were primarily restricted to Europe. The fourth genus, *Datura,* is worldwide and has many species containing the active agents.

The family of plants in which all these genera are found is *Solanaceae,* "herbs of consolation," and three pharmacologically active alkaloids are responsible for the effects of these plants. *Atropine,* which is *dl*-hyoscyamine, scopolamine or *l*-hyoscine, and *l*-hyoscyamine are all potent central and peripheral cholinergic blocking agents. These drugs occupy the acetylcholine receptor site but do not activate it; thus their effect is primarily to block muscarinic cholinergic neurons, including the parasympathetic system.

These agents have potent peripheral and central effects, and some of the psychological responses to these drugs are probably a reaction to peripheral changes. These alkaloids block the production of mucus in the nose and throat. They also prevent salivation, so the mouth becomes uncommonly dry, and perspiration stops.

Temperature can increase to fever levels (109 °F has been reported in infants with atropine poisoning), and heart rate can show a fifty-beat-per-minute increase with atropine. Even at moderate doses these chemicals cause considerable dilation of the pupils of the eyes with a resulting inability to focus on nearby objects. With large enough doses, there develops a behavioral pattern that resembles toxic psychosis; there is delirium, mental confusion, loss of attention, drowsiness, and loss of memory for recent events. These two characteristics—a clouding of consciousness and no memory for the period of intoxication—plus the absence of vivid sensory effects separate these drugs from the indole and catechol hallucinogens. Instead of phantastica, a better term for the anticholinergics might be *deliriants.*

Belladonna

Atropine, which was isolated in 1831, is the active ingredient in deadly nightshade, *Atropa belladonna.* The name of the plant reflects two of its major uses in the Middle Ages and before. The genus name reflects its use as a poison. Deadly nightshade was one of the plants used extensively by both professional and amateur poisoners; fourteen of its berries contain enough of the alkaloid to cause death.

Belladonna, the species name, meaning "beautiful woman," comes from the use of the extract of this plant to dilate the pupils of the eyes. Interestingly, Roman and Egyptian women knew something that science did not learn until quite recently. In the 1950s, it was demonstrated, by using pairs of photographs identical except for the amount of pupil dilation, that most people judge the girl with the more dilated eyes to be prettier.

Of more interest here than pretty girls or poisoned men is the sensation of flying reported by witches. The first step toward completing this experiment is to make an ointment. Although there are many recipes, a good one seems to be infant's fat, juice of water parsnip, aconite, cinquefoile, deadly nightshade, and soot.

When the ointment is made, it is rubbed on the body and especially liberally between the legs and on a stick that is to be straddled. This stick served as a phallic symbol during the ceremony of the Sabbat. The Sabbat, or Black Mass, worshipped Satan, and both men and women engaged in a nightlong orgy. Straddling the stick and hopping and shrieking around a circle they felt able "to be carried in the aire, to feasting, singing, dansing, kissing, culling and other acts of venerie, with such youthes as they love and desire most!"[63] The feeling of levitation perhaps comes from the irregular heartbeat in conjunction with drowsiness. Some have reported that changes in heart rate coupled with falling asleep sometimes results in a sensation of falling (or flying),[64] but a more likely explanation is simply the power of suggestion.

Other actions were important in causing the effects of the Sabbat. The pounding of the heart would certainly convey excitement, and the excitement might cause sexual arousal. One of the reputations of belladonna was as an aphrodisiac, so it might all fit together. Perhaps the physiological effects of the agents coupled with a good placebo effect was enough for the witches who attended the Sabbat.

Mandrake

The famous *mandrake* plant *(Mandragora officinarum)* contains all three alkaloids. Although many drugs could be traced to the Bible, it is particularly important to do so with mandrake because its close association with love and lovemaking has persisted from Genesis to recent times.

> In the time of wheat-harvest Reuben went out and found some mandrakes in the open country and brought them to his mother Leah. Then Rachel asked Leah for some of her son's mandrakes, but Leah said, "Is it so small a thing to have taken away my husband, that you should take my son's mandrakes as well?" But Rachel said, "Very well, let him sleep with you tonight in exchange for your son's mandrakes." So when Jacob came in from the country in the evening, Leah went out to meet him and said, "You are to sleep with me tonight; I have hired you with my son's mandrakes." That night he slept with her.[65]

The mandrake root is forked and, if you have a vivid imagination, resembles a human body. The root contains the psychoactive agents and was endowed with all sorts of magical and medical properties. The association with the human form is alluded to in Juliet's farewell speech: "And shrieks like mandrakes torn out of the earth, That living mortals hearing them run mad."

Henbane

Compared with deadly nightshade and mandrake, *Hyoscyamus niger* has had a most uninteresting life. This is strange, because it is pharmacologically quite active and contains both scopolamine and *l*-hyoscyamine. Other plants of this genus contain effective levels of the alkaloids, but it is *Hyoscyamus niger* that appears throughout history as *henbane,* a highly poisonous substance and truly the bane of hens, as well as other animals.

Pliny in A.D. 60 said: "For this is certainly known, that, if one takes it in drink more than four leaves, it will put him beside himself." Hamlet's father must have had more than four leaves because it was henbane that was used to poison him.

Datura

The distribution of the many *Datura* species is worldwide, but they all contain the three alkaloids under discussion—atropine, scopolamine, and hyoscyamine—in varying amounts. Almost as extensive as the distribution are its uses and its history. Although it is not clear when the Chinese first used *Datura metel* as a medicine to treat colds and nervous disorders, the plant was important enough to become associated with Buddha:[66]

> The Chinese valued this drug far back into ancient times. A comparatively recent Chinese medical text, published in 1590, reported that "when Buddha preaches a sermon, the heavens bedew the petals of this plant with rain drops."

Halfway around the world 2,500 years before the Chinese text, virgins sat in the temple to Apollo in Delphi and, probably under the influence of *Datura*,[66] mumbled sounds that holy men interpreted as predictions that always came true. The procedure was straightforward, and

> preliminary to the divine possession, she appears to have chewed leaves of the sacred laurel . . . prior to speaking . . . she was supposed to be inspired by a mystic vapour that arose from a fissure in the ground.[67]

Probably either the plant material eaten was one of the *Datura* species or the burning seeds and leaves of the *Datura* plant formed the mystic vapor she inhaled. It should not go unnoticed, as we search for the beyond within, that engraved on the temple at Delphi were the words "Know thyself."

Datura is associated with the worship of Shiva in India, where it has long been recognized as an ingredient in love potions and also has been known as "deceiver" and "foolmaker." In Asia the practice of mixing the crushed seeds of *Datura metel* in tobacco, cannabis, and food persists even today.

The ever-busy chronicler Hernandez mentioned the use of *Datura inoxia* (loco weed) by the Aztecs, and the use of various *Datura* species by Indians of the United States Southwest for magical and religious purposes is well substantiated.[36] One of the interesting uses of *Datura stramonium,* which is native and grows wild in the eastern United States, was devised by the Algonquin Indians. They used the plant to solve the problem of the adolescent search for identity.

The youths are confined for long periods, given ". . . no other substance but the infusion or decoction of some poisonous, intoxicating roots . . ." and "they became stark, staring mad, in which raving condition they were kept eighteen or twenty days." These poor creatures drink so much of that water of Lethe that they perfectly lose the remembrance of all former things, even of their parents, their treasure and their language. When the doctors find that they have drunk sufficiently of the wysoccan . . . they gradually restore them to their senses again. . . . Thus they unlive their former lives and commence men by forgetting that they ever have been boys.[66]

This same plant is now called Jamestown weed, or jimsonweed, as a result of an incident in the seventeenth century. This was fortunately recorded for history in the famous book *The History and Present State of Virginia,*[68] published first in 1705 by Robert Beverly.

> The *James-Town* Weed (which resembles the Thorny Apple of *Peru,* and I take to be the Plant so call'd) is supposed to be one of the greatest Coolers in the World. This being an early Plant, was gather'd very young for a boil'd Salad, by some of the Soldiers sent thither, to pacifie the Troubles of *Bacon*; and some of them eat plentifully of it, the Effect of which was a very pleasant Comedy; for they turn'd natural Fools upon it for several Days.

Although there has been some recent abuse of jimsonweed, the unpleasant and dangerous side effects of this plant serve to limit its recreational use.

Synthetic Anticholinergics

Anticholinergic drugs were once used to treat Parkinson's disease (before the introduction of L-dopa) and are still widely used to treat the pseudoparkinsonism produced by antipsychotic drugs (see chapter 9). Particularly in older people there is concern about inadvertently producing an "anticholinergic syndrome," characterized by excessive dry mouth, elevated temperature, delusions, and hallucinations. Anticholinergic drugs such as trihexyphenidyl (Artane) and benztropine (Cogentin) have only rarely been abused for their delirium-producing properties.

AMANITA MUSCARIA

The *Amanita muscaria* mushroom is also called "fly agaric," probably because of what it does to flies. It doesn't kill them, but when they suck its juice, it puts them into a stupor for two to three hours. It is one of the common "poisonous" mushrooms found in forests in many parts of the world. The older literature suggests that eating five to ten *Amanita* mushrooms results in severe effects of intoxication such as muscular twitching leading to twitches of limbs and raving drunkenness with agitation and vivid hallucinations. Later follow many hours of partial paralysis with sleep and dreams.

When the ancient Aryan invaders swept down from the north into India 3,500 years ago, they brought Soma, itself considered a deity. The cult of Soma ruled India's religion and culture for many years—the poems of the Rig Veda celebrate the sacramental use of this substance. It has only been within the past 25 years that scholars have discovered and agreed on the identity of Soma as *Amanita*.[1]

The suggestion has been made that the ambrosia ("food of the gods") mentioned in the secret rites of the god Dionysius in Greece was a solution of the *Amanita* mushroom.[69] And based on paintings representing the "tree of life" found in ancient European cave paintings, it has been suggested that *Amanita muscaria* use formed a basis for the cult that originated about 2,000 years ago and today calls itself Christianity.[70]

Until the Russians introduced them to alcohol, many of the isolated nomadic tribes of Siberia had no intoxicant but *Amanita*:

> Use of the Amanita mushroom by Siberian tribes continues today largely free from social control of any sort. Use of the drug has a Shamanist aspect, and forms the basis for orgiastic

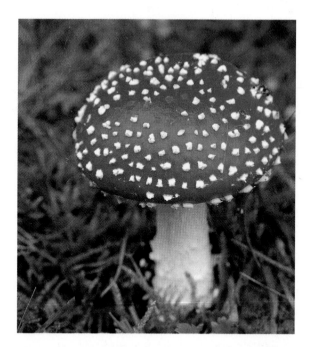

The red- and white-speckled mushroom *Amanita muscaria* played a major role in the early history of Indo-European and Central American religions.

communal indulgences. Since the drug can induce murderous rages in addition to more moderate hallucinogenic experiences, serious injuries frequently result.[71]

In the frozen northland, these mushrooms are expensive; sometimes several reindeer are exchanged for an effective number of the mushrooms. They do have the unique property of being reusable, and during the long winter months they might be worth the price. The mushrooms themselves are not reusable; once eaten, they're gone. But this is a hallucinogen that is excreted unchanged in the urine. When the effect begins to wear off, "midway in the orgy the cry of 'pass the pot' goes out."[72] The active ingredient can be reused four or five times in this way!

There is evidence that *Amanita* was also used as a holy plant by several tribal groups in the

FYI   Toadlicking: An "Urban Legend"

In the late 1980s a story was going around about a substance called *bufotenin,* an indole that looks like it might be hallucinogenic and was originally identified in the skins of toads (genus *Bufo*). In one version of the story, "hippies" living in the hills of Northern California were chasing toads through the woods and licking them to get high: California was said to have listed one species of toad as a controlled substance. In another version, it was the infamous cane toad of Australia, said to be licked or ingested both by aborigines and by Australian hippies.

It's a great story, seemingly plausible enough, and certainly colorful enough to repeat. It found its way into drug abuse lectures and at least one textbook, and the Australian version was passed along as fact by *USA Today* in 1988. The idea even became the plot for one episode of the television program LA Law. The only problem is that the story "ain't necessarily so."

Bufotenin was studied experimentally back in the 1950s, during the heyday of research on hallucinogens as models of schizophrenia. Probably it was studied because it was found in *Amanita* mushrooms and they were known to have been used as hallucinogens. However, when bufotenin was given to "volunteer" prison inmates (by injection, not licking) it was found to be a not very potent hallucinogen. It may have been toxic in other ways because the experimental subjects became quite cyanotic (meaning they turned blue, although the researcher in charge says it was more of a deep purple).[74] That basically ended human research with bufotenin. We can't prove that nobody ever licked a toad in California, but there is no documented evidence for this as a regular practice of any group at any time, nor is there any documented evidence that hallucinatory effects can be gotten in this way.

This legend could have tragic consequences, in that toads do have a variety of toxins in their skins that protect them from being eaten by predators. If a person actually ate toad skins or somehow obtained and used pure bufotenin, they could become quite ill or even die. One Australian youth is reported to have died after eating cane toad eggs.

This story is such a graphically gross one that it doesn't want to go away, in spite of a small story debunking the myth published in *Scientific American* in 1990. Even after that came out, a Georgia legislator referred to "the extreme danger of cane-toad licking becoming the designer drug of choice." A warning was published in the *British Journal of Psychiatry* (November 1990) that "the Australian cane toad is popularly kept as a pet in the US, and licked by its owners for the resulting hallucinatory effects," with the note that two English toads also have the potential to be used in this way.

Two pieces of advice: don't lick strange toads, and be especially cautious about believing any weird story you hear that involves hallucinogenic drugs, unless there is documented evidence (who, what, when, where, why, how, and how much?). The "mystical" nature of these substances has no doubt inspired more untrue legends than any other type of drug.

Americas, ranging from Alaska and the Great Lakes to Mexico and Central America. In several of the legends, its origin is associated with thunder and lightning.[1]

For many years the active agent in this mushroom was thought to be *muscarine* (for which the muscarinic cholinergic receptors were named). This substance activates the same type of acetylcholine receptor that is blocked by the anticholinergics. However, pharmacological studies with other cholinergic agonists did not produce similar psychoactive effects. Next, attention focused on *bufotenin,* an indole that is found in high concentrations in the skins of toads (see the FYI box). However, the hallucinogenic properties of bufotenin have been in doubt, and *Amanita* species contain only small amounts of it. In the mid 1960s, meaningful amounts of two chemicals were found: ibotenic acid and muscimol.

The effects of *Amanita* ingestion are not similar to those of other hallucinogens, and that helped confuse the picture with regard to the mechanism. Muscimol can act as an agonist at GABA receptors, which are inhibitory and also found throughout the CNS. Muscimol is more potent than ibotenic acid, and drying of the mushroom, which is usually done by those who use it, promotes the transformation of ibotenic acid to muscimol. Muscimol has been given to humans, resulting in confusion, disorientation in time and place, sensory disturbances, muscle twitching, weariness, fatigue, and sleep.[37]

It should be stressed that, whereas *Amanita muscaria* and other related poisonous mushrooms are to be found in North America, they are a particularly dangerous type of plant with which to experiment.

SUMMARY

- Hallucinogenic plants have been used for many centuries, not only as medicines, but for spiritual and recreational purposes as well.

- LSD, a synthetic hallucinogen, alters perceptual processes and enhances emotionality so that the real world is seen differently and responded to with great emotion.
- Other chemicals that contain the indole nucleus, such as psilocybin (from the Mexican mushroom), have effects similar to those of LSD.
- Mescaline, from the peyote cactus, and synthetic derivatives of amphetamine represent the catechol hallucinogens. They also have psychological effects quite similar to those of the indole types.
- MDMA is also the only drug in this group that appears likely to be capable of producing permanent brain damage in its users.
- Angel dust, or PCP, produces more changes in body perception and fewer visual effects than LSD.
- Anticholinergics are found in many plants throughout the world and have been used not only recreationally, medically, and spiritually, but also as poisons.

REVIEW QUESTIONS

1. What are the distinctions among phantastica, psychedelics, psychotomimetics, entheogens, and hallucinogens?
2. What is the precise relationship between ergotism and LSD?
3. Why was LSD used in psychoanalysis in the 1950s and 1960s? How does this relate to its proposed use by the army and the CIA?
4. Describe the addictive potential of LSD in terms of tolerance, physical dependence, and psychological dependence.
5. What are three adverse psychological reactions that have been associated with LSD use?
6. What is the active agent in the "magic mushrooms" of Mexico, and is it an indole or catechol?
7. Besides the psychological effects, what other effects are reliably produced by peyote?

8. Contrast MDMA and PCP in terms of how they appear to make people feel about being close to others.
9. Which of the hallucinogenic plants was most associated with witchcraft?
10. Describe what is actually known about bufotenin and the "toad-licking" phenomenon.

WEB WATCH

Related Internet Sites on Hallucinogens

The Ibogaine Dossier: http://www.ibogaine.org/

The Lycaeum: http://www.lycaeum.org/

And the excedingly psychedelic *Drugs, Society, and Human Behavior* site: http://www.uwyo.edu/A&S/psyc/dshb.htm

---

REFERENCES

1. Schultes RE, Hofmann A: *Plants of the gods,* New York, 1979, McGraw-Hill.
2. Hordern A: Psychopharmacology: some historical considerations. In Joyce CRB, editor: *Psychopharmacology: dimensions and perspectives,* Philadelphia, 1968, JB Lippincott.
3. Caporael LR: Ergotism: the Satan loosed in Salem, *Science* 192:21–26, 1976.
4. Gottlieb J, Spanos NP: Ergotism and the Salem village witch trials, *Science* 194:1390–1394, 1976.
5. Hofmann A: Psychotomimetic agents. In Burger A, editor: *Drugs affecting the central nervous system,* vol 2, New York, 1968, Marcel Dekker.
6. Horowitz M: Interview with Albert Hofmann, *High Times,* pp 24–81, July 1976.
7. Clark W: Psychedelic research: obstacles and values, *J Humanistic Psych* 15(3):5–17, 1975.
8. Segal J, editor: *Research in the service of mental health, research on drug abuse,* National Institute on Mental Health, Pub No (ADM) 75-236, US Department of Health, Education, and Welfare, Washington, DC, 1975, US Government Printing Office.
9. Johnston L: Ford signs grant of $750,000 in LSD death in CIA test, *New York Times,* p C43 Oct 14, 1976.
10. Treaster JB: Mind-drug test a federal project for almost 25 years, *New York Times,* p M42, Aug 11, 1975.
11. CIA considered big LSD purchase, *Washington Star,* Aug 4, 1975. See also Knight M: LSD creator says army sought drug, *New York Times,* August 1, 1975.
12. Taylor JR, Johnson WN: *Use of volunteers in chemical agent research,* Inspector General Report No DAIGIN 21-75, Washington, DC, Mar 10, 1976, US Department of Army.
13. Weil AT: The strange case of the Harvard drug scandal, *Look,* pp 38–48, Nov 5, 1963.
14. Blumenthal R: Leary drug cult stirs Millbrook, *New York Times,* p 49, June 14, 1967.
15. Celebration #1, *New Yorker* 42:43, 1966.
16. Masters REL: Sex, ecstasy, and the psychedelic drugs, *Playboy* 14(11):94–226, 1967.
17. Council on Mental Health and Committee on Alcoholism and Drug Dependence: Dependence on LSD and other hallucinogenic drugs, *JAMA* 202:141–144, 1967.
18. Leary, once an LSD advocate, paroled, *New York Times,* p 25, Apr 21, 1976.
19. Leary and Liddy, debating specialists, *New York Times,* p B26, Sept 3, 1981.
20. Hamon M: Common neurochemical correlates to the action of hallucinogens. In Jacobs BL, editor: *Hallucinogens: neurochemical, behavioral and clinical perspectives,* New York, 1984, Raven Press.
21. Aghajanian GK: LSD and serotonergic dorsal raphe neurons: intracellular studies in vivo and in vitro. In Jacobs BL, editor: *Hallucinogens: neurochemical, behavioral and clinical perspectives,* New York, 1984, Raven Press.
22. Appel JB, Rosecrans JA: Behavioral pharmacology of hallucinogens in animals: conditioning studies. In Jacobs BL, editor: *Hallucinogens: neurochemical, behavioral and clinical perspectives,* New York, 1984, Raven Press.
23. Nichols DE, Glennon RA: Medicinal chemistry and structure-activity relationships of hallucinogens. In Jacobs BL, editor: *Hallucinogens: neurochemical, behavioral and clinical perspectives,* New York, 1984, Raven Press.
24. Jacobs BL: How hallucinogenic drugs work, *American Scientist* 75:386–392, 1987.
25. Siegel RK: The natural history of hallucinogens. In Jacobs BL, editor: *Hallucinogens: neurochemical, behavioral and clinical perspectives,* New York, 1984, Raven Press.
26. Krippner S: Psychedelic experience and the language process, *J Psychedelic Drugs* 3(1):41–51, 1970.
27. Levine J, Ludwig AM: The LSD controversy, *Compr Psychiatry* 5(5):318–319, 1964.

28. Forsch WA, Robbins ES, Stern M: Untoward reactions to lysergic acid diethylamide (LSD) resulting in hospitalization, *N Eng J Med* 273:1235–1239, 1965.

29. Abraham HD, Wolf E: Visual function in past users of LSD: psychophysical findings, *J Abnorm Psychol* 97:443–447, 1988.

30. Zegans LS, Pollard JC, Brown D: The effects of LSD-25 on creativity and tolerance to regression, *Arch Gen Psychiatry* 16:740–749, 1967.

31. Painting under LSD, *Time* p 88, Dec 5, 1969.

32. Hollister LE, Shelton J, Krieger G: A controlled comparison of lysergic acid diethylamide (LSD) and dextroamphetamine in alcoholics, *Am J Psychiatry* 125:1352–1357, 1969.

33. NIMH research on LSD, Extramural programs fiscal year 1948 to present, prepared Sept 1, 1975.

34. Crahan ME: God's flesh and other preColumbian phantastica, *Bulletin of the Los Angeles County Medical Association* 99:17, 1969.

35. Wolbach AB Jr, Isbell H, Miner EJ: Cross tolerance between mescaline and LSD-25, with a comparison of the mescaline and LSD reactions, *Psychopharmacologia* 3:1–14, 1962.

36. Leary T: The religious experience: its production and interpretation, *J Psychedelic Drugs* 1(2):3–23, 1967–1968.

37. Schultes RE, Hofmann A: *The botany and chemistry of hallucinogens,* Springfield, Ill, 1980, Charles C Thomas.

38. Strassman RJ, Qualls CR: Dose-response study of N,N-Dimethyltryptamine in humans, *Arch Gen Psychiatry* 51:85, 1994.

39. Ott, J: *Pharmacotheon.* Kennewick, Wash, Natural Products Company, 1993.

40. LaBarre W: Twenty years of peyote studies, *Current Anthropology* 1(1):45, 1960.

41. LaBarre W: *The peyote cult,* Hamden, Conn, 1964, Shoe String Press.

42. Slotkin JS: Religious defenses (the Native American Church), *J Psychedelic Drugs* 1(2):77–95, 1967–1968.

43. LaBarre W and others: Statement on peyote, *Science* 114:524, 582–583, 1951.

44. Greenhouse L: Court is urged to rehear case on ritual drugs, *New York Times,* May 11, 1990.

45. Kapadia GJ, Goyez MBE: Peyote constituents: chemistry, biogenese, and biological effects, *J Pharm Sciences* 59:1699–1727, 1970.

46. De Ropp RS: *Drugs and the mind,* New York, 1957, Grove Press.

47. Ellis H: Mescal: a study of a divine plant, *Popular Science Monthly* 61:59, 65, 1902.

48. Huxley A: *The doors of perception,* New York, 1954, Harper & Row.

49. Snyder SH, Faillace L, Hollister L: 2,5-Dimethoxy-4-methyl-amphetamine (STP): a new hallucinogenic drug, *Science* 158:669–670, 1967.

50. Smith D, Meyers F: The psychotomimetic amphetamine with special reference to STP (DOM) toxicity. In Smith D, editor: *Drug abuse papers,* 1969, Section 4, Berkeley, Calif, 1969, University of California.

51. MDMA: compound raises medical, legal issues, *Brain/Mind Bulletin,* Apr 15, 1985.

52. Peroutka SJ and others: Subjective effects of 3,4-methylenedioxymethamphetamine in recreational users, *Neuropsychopharmacology* 1:273–277, 1988.

53. Mathias R: Like methamphetamine, "ecstasy" may cause long-term brain damage. *NIDA Notes,* Nov/Dec 1996.

54. McGann UD, Ricuarte GA: Reinforcing subjective effects of 3,4-methylenedioxymethamphetamine ("Ecstasy") may be separable from its neurotoxic actions: Clinical evidence, *J Clin Psychopharmacol* 13:214, 1993.

55. Greifenstein FE and others: A study of a l-dryl cycle hexyl amine for anesthesia, *Anesth Analg* 37(5):283–294, 1958.

56. Luby E and others: Study of a new schizophrenomimetic drug—Sernyl, *AMA Arch Neur Psychiatry* 81:113–119, March 1959.

57. *Physician's Desk Reference,* ed 48, Oradell, NJ, 1994, Medical Economics.

58. Siegel RK: Phencyclidine and ketamine intoxication: A study of four populations of recreational users. In Petersen RC, Stillman RC, editors: *Phencyclidine (PCP) abuse: an appraisal,* NIDA Research Monograph No 21, Washington, DC, 1978, US Department of Health and Human Services.

59. Balster RL, Chait LD: The behavioral effects of phencyclidine in animals. In Petersen RC, Stillman RC, editors: *Phencyclidine (PCP) abuse: an appraisal,* NIDA Research Monograph No 21, Washington, DC, 1978, US Department of Health and Human Services.

60. Siegel RK: PCP and violent crime: the people vs peace, *J Psychedelic Drugs* 12(3–4):317, 1980.

61. Overend W: PCP: death in the "dust," *Los Angeles Times,* Sept 26, 1977.

62. Quirion R and others: Phencyclidine (angel dust)/sigma "opiate" receptor: visualization by tritium-sensitive film, *Proc Nat Acad Sci USA* 78:5881–5885, 1981.

63. Briggs KM: *Pale Hecate's team,* New York, 1962, Humanities Press.

64. Langdon-Brown W: *From witchcraft to chemotherapy,* Cambridge, 1941, Cambridge University Press.

65. Genesis 30:14–16, *The New English Bible,* Oxford University Press and Cambridge University Press, 1970.

66. Schultes RE: The plant kingdom and hallucinogens (Part III), *Bull Narc* 22(1):43–46, 1970.

67. *Encyclopedia Brittanica,* vol 16, 1929.

68. Beverly R: *The history and present state of Virginia, 1705,* Chapel Hill, NC, 1947, University of North Carolina Press.

69. Graves R: *Steps,* London, 1958, Cassell.
70. Allegro JM: *The sacred mushroom and the cross,* New York, 1970, Doubleday.
71. Wasson RG: Fly agaric and man. In Efron DH, editor: *Ethnopharmacologic search for psychoactive drugs,* Washington, DC, 1967, National Institute of Mental Health. See also Wasson RG: *Soma, divine mushroom of immortality,* New York, 1971, Harcourt Brace Jovanovich.
72. Hallucinogens, *Columbia Law Review* 68(3):521–560, 1968.
73. Feldman RS, Meyer JS, Quenzer LF: *Principles of Neuropsychopharmacology,* Sunderland, Mass, 1997, Sinauer.
74. Horgan J: Bufo abuse, *Scientific American,* pp 26–27, Aug 1990.

Marijuana and Hashish

KEY TERMS	OBJECTIVES

After reading this chapter, you should be able to:

Cannabis
hashish
sinsemilla
THC
anandamide
dronabinol
Marinol

- List the various cannabis species and some of the ways the plant is prepared for use.
- Describe the history of cannabis use.
- Name the chemical that is the most active ingredient in marijuana.
- Describe the absorption, distribution, and metabolism of THC.

- Discuss the THC receptor and endogenous compounds with marijuana-like actions.
- Explain the basic physiological and behavioral effects of marijuana.
- Discuss the current status of medical uses for marijuana.

Marijuana has meant so many things to so many people over the years that it is hard to describe it from a single perspective. We wind up behaving like that famous committee of blind men examining an elephant: the way you describe it depends on where you're standing. The matter of classifying marijuana among the other psychoactive drugs is so complex that we, like most authors, avoid the issue by setting it off by itself. Marijuana can produce some sedative-like effects, some pain relief, and, in large doses, hallucinogenic effects. Thus many of its users treat it as a depressant; it has been called a narcotic (for both pharmacological, as well as political, reasons); and it is often included among descriptions of hallucinogenic plants. The effects it produces when used as most people use it are, however, sufficiently different from those of other psychoactive drugs to justify its consideration as a unique substance.

CANNABIS

The Plant

Marijuana (or *marihuana;* either spelling is correct) is a preparation of leafy material from the *Cannabis* plant that is used by smoking. The question is, which *Cannabis* plant, because there is still botanical debate over whether there is one, three, or more species of *Cannabis.* In

---

Cannabis: (*can* **a biss**) genus of plant known as marijuana.

Leaves of the *Cannabis* (marijuana) plant.

previous years, there were legal arguments over this issue because the laws mentioned only *Cannabis sativa.* Does that include all marijuana or not? The evidence is strong that there are three separate species. *Cannabis sativa* originated in Asia but now grows worldwide and primarily has been used for its fibers, from which hemp rope is made. This is the species that grows as a weed in the United States and Canada. *Cannabis indica* is grown for its psychoactive resins and is cultivated in many areas of the world, including selected planters and backyards of the United States. The third species, *Cannabis ruderalis,* grows primarily in Russia and not at all in America. The plant Linnaeus named *C. sativa* in 1753 is what is still known as *C. sativa.*[1]

It was *C. sativa* that George Washington grew at Mount Vernon, most likely not to get high but to make rope and possibly for medicinal uses. From his fields and many others like it, *C. sativa* spread across the nation, growing spontaneously.

C. sativa that is cultivated for use as hemp grows as a lanky plant up to eighteen feet high. *C. indica* plants cultivated for their psychoactive effects are more compact and usually only two or three feet tall. The psychoactive potency results from an interaction between genetics and environmental conditions. Plants of different species grown under identical conditions produce different amounts of psychoactive material, and the same plants will vary in potency from year to year, depending on the amount of sunshine, warm weather, and moisture.

Preparations from Cannabis

The primary psychoactive agent, delta-9-tetrahydrocannabinol (THC), is concentrated in the resin of the plant; most of the resin is in the flowering tops, less is in the leaves, and there is little in the fibrous stalks. The psychoactive potency of a cannabis preparation depends on the amount of resin present and therefore varies, depending on the part of the plant used. We describe three traditional cannabis preparations from India, each of which corresponds roughly to preparations available in the United States. The most potent of these is called *charas* in India, and it consists of pure resin that has been carefully removed from the surface of leaves and stems. **Hashish,** or hasheesh, is a substance widely known around the world and in its purest form is pure resin, like charas. It may be less pure, depending on how carefully the resin has been separated from the plant material. Samples of hashish available in the United States vary widely in their THC content, averaging about 7 or 8 percent, and ranging up to about 14 percent THC.

The second most potent preparation is traditionally called *ganja* in India, and it consists of the dried flowering tops of plants with pistillate flowers (female plants). The male plants are removed from the fields before the female plants can become pollinated and put their energy into seed production; this increases the potency of the female plants. This method of production has become increasingly popular in recent years in the United States for producing high-grade marijuana known as **sinsemilla** (Spanish *sin semilla,* "without seeds"). The flowering top portion of the plant is referred to as the "bud" by

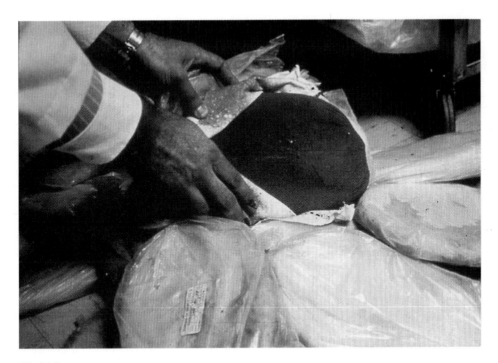

Hashish

American growers. Sinsemilla samples from the United States also vary widely in THC content, averaging around 4 or 5 percent, usually not over 7 or 8 percent maximum, although occasional samples have been reported as high as 10 or 11 percent.

The weakest form in India is *bhang,* which is made by using the entire remainder of the plant after the top has been picked, drying it, and grinding it into a powder. The powder might then be mixed into drinks or candies.[1] Americans don't usually see this type of preparation, but we might consider it somewhat analogous to low-grade marijuana, which consists of the leaves of a plant, perhaps even a *sativa* plant found growing as a weed. Some of this low-grade marijuana contains less than 1 percent THC.

Manually scraping exuded resin off the plant to make hashish is a tedious process, and a more efficient method of separating the resin from plants has been known for many years. The plants are boiled in alcohol, then the solids filtered out and the liquid evaporated down to a thick, dark substance once known medically as "red oil of cannabis" and now referred to as *hash oil.* Again, this product varies widely in its potency but can contain more than 50 percent THC. Until fairly recently, both the medical and the psychological effects of cannabis preparations were variable. All the traditional methods could do was produce relatively pure plant

---

hashish: (hash *eesh* or *hash* eesh) concentrated resin from the *Cannabis* plant.

sinsemilla: (sin se *mee* ya) "without seeds"; a method of growing more potent marijuana.

Hashish oil

resin, but that resin could vary considerably in its THC content.

If we consider only the marijuana available for smoking in the United States, we can see that it can vary widely in potency from a low-grade product containing less than 1 percent THC to a high-grade sinsemilla containing 8 percent or more THC. The usual range of potency for marijuana seems to be 2 to 5 percent, however. Since the mid 1980s there have been repeated statements to the effect that the marijuana available on the streets today is "ten times" more potent than the marijuana of the 1960s. The political message behind this is that the marijuana of the 1960s may have been relatively harmless, but the current marijuana is more dangerous. In fact, the entire range of these traditional preparations has been known, and scientific, literary, and medical descriptions of the wide range of effects have been based on this entire range of potencies, for 150 years. It is

true that U.S. marijuana growers are becoming more sophisticated and producing more sinsemilla, but the overall range of potencies of marijuana available on the streets is still from under 1 percent to about 8 percent, just as in the early 1970s.[2]

A strange kind of "success story" surrounds modern-day American growers of marijuana. In the 1970s, domestic marijuana was typically inexpensive, low-grade sativa leaves, and higher-grade marijuana was usually imported from Mexico, Colombia, or other warm growing regions. As U.S. efforts to arrest drug smugglers intensified, smugglers turned to cocaine, which was easier to conceal and more profitable. U.S. growers attempting to produce sinsemilla figured out that *C. sativa* doesn't flower well in northern climates, and focused on *C. indica*, planting crops in gardens and in small, isolated fields. The Drug Enforcement Administration (DEA) and local law enforcement agencies countered with large-scale efforts to eradicate these plants, driving many growers indoors to use hydroponics, "grow lights", and other technological advances. Experimentation and cross-breeding of indica and sativa plants has resulted in the most sophisticated growers being able to produce very small plants that take up little room but produce large "buds" within two months or so. These days, the most potent, and most expensive, marijuana comes from American growers. Marijuana is now considered to be by far America's number one cash crop, earning something like $30 billion per year.[3]

HISTORY

Early History

The earliest reference to cannabis is in a pharmacy book written in 2737 B.C. by the Chinese emperor Shen Nung. Referring to the euphoriant effects of cannabis, he called it the "Liberator of Sin." There were some medical uses, however, and he recommended it for "female weakness, gout, rheumatism, malaria, beriberi, constipation and absent-mindedness."[4] Social use of the plant spread to the Moslem world and North Africa by A.D. 1000. In this period in the eastern Mediterranean area a legend developed around a religious cult that committed murder for political reasons. The cult was called "hashishiyya," from which our word *assassin* developed. In 1299, Marco Polo told the story he had heard of this group and their leader. It was a marvelous tale and had all the ingredients necessary for a tale to survive through the ages: intrigue, murder, sex, the use of drugs, mysterious lands. The story of this group and their activities was told in many ways over the years, and Boccaccio's *Decameron* contained one story based on it. Stories of this cult, combined with the frequent reference to the power and wonderment of hashish in *The Arabian Nights,* were widely circulated in Europe over the years.

The Nineteenth Century: Romantic Literature and the New Science of Psychology

At the turn of the nineteenth century, world commerce was expanding. New and exciting reports from the world travelers of the seventeenth and eighteenth centuries introduced new cultures and new ideas to Europe. Asia and the Middle East had yielded exotic spices, as well as the stimulants coffee and tea. Europe was ready for another new sensation, and got it. The returning veteran, as usual, gets part of the blame for introducing what Europe was ready to receive.

Napoleon's campaign to Egypt at the beginning of the nineteenth century increased the Romantic's acquaintance with hashish and caused them to associate it with the Near East. . . . Napoleon was forced to give an order forbidding all French soldiers to indulge in hashish. Some of the soldiers brought the habit to France, however, as did many other Frenchmen who worked for the government or traveled in the Near East.[5]

By the 1830s and 1840s, everyone who was anyone was using, thinking about using, or decrying the use of mind-tickling agents such as opium and hashish. One of the earliest (1844) popular accounts of the use of hashish is in *The Count of Monte Cristo* by Alexander Dumas. The story includes a reference to the Assassins story and contains statements about the characteristics of the drug that still sound contemporary. During the 1840s a group of artists and writers gathered monthly at the Hotel Pimodan in Paris's Latin Quarter to use drugs. This group became famous because one of the participants, Gautier, wrote a book, *Le Club de Hachischins,* that described their activities. From this group have come some of the best literary descriptions of hashish intoxication. These French Romantics, like the impressionistic painters of a later period, were searching for new experiences, new sources of creativity from within, new ways of seeing the world outside. A few of the regulars were well-known writers, including Baudelaire, Gautier, and Dumas.

Baudelaire used hashish and was an astute observer of its effects in himself and in others. In his book *Artificial Paradises,* he echoed what Dumas had written about the kind of effect to expect from hashish:

The intoxication will be nothing but one immense dream, thanks to intensity of color and the rapidity of conceptions; but it will always preserve the particular tonality of the individual. . . . The dream will certainly reflect its dreamer. He is only the same man grown larger . . . sophisticate and ingénu . . . will find nothing miraculous, absolutely nothing but the natural to an extreme.[6]

The extent of Baudelaire's actual experience with hashish is debatable, but he did identify (and exaggerate) three stages of intoxication after oral intake. These are still being rediscovered.

At first, a certain absurd, irresistible hilarity overcomes you. The most ordinary words, the simplest ideas assume a new and bizarre aspect. This mirth is intolerable to you; but it is useless to resist. The demon has invaded you. . . .

It sometimes happens that people completely unsuited for word-play will improvise an endless string of puns and wholly improbable idea relationships fit to outdo the ablest masters of this preposterous craft. But after a few minutes, the relation between ideas becomes so vague, and the thread of your thoughts grows so tenuous, that only your cohorts . . . can understand you.

Next your senses become extraordinarily keen and acute. Your sight is infinite. Your ear can discern the slightest perceptible sound, even through the shrillest of noises.

The strangest ambiguities, the most inexplicable transpositions of ideas take place. In sounds there is color; in colors there is a music. . . . You are sitting and smoking; you believe that you are sitting in your pipe, and that *your pipe* is smoking *you;* you are exhaling *yourself* in bluish clouds.

This fantasy goes on for an eternity. A lucid interval, and a great expenditure of effort, permit you to look at the clock. The eternity turns out to have been only a minute.

The third phase . . . is something beyond description. It is what the Orientals call *kef;* it is complete happiness. There is nothing whirling and tumultuous about it. It is a calm and placid beatitude. Every philosophical problem is resolved. Every difficult question that presents a point of contention for theologians, and brings despair to thoughtful men, becomes clear and transparent. Every contradiction is reconciled. Man has surpassed the gods.[6]

As the end of the nineteenth century approached, the use of the anxiety-relieving drugs increased, but the hashish experience held little interest for the dweller in middle America. Just beginning, however, was the new science of psychology, whose interest was in the workings of the mind. The writings of William James and others introduced the possibility of using psychoactive agents in studying psychological processes. In 1899, one of the psychologists who had been using cannabis in experiments said, "To the psychologist it (cannabis) was as useful as the microscope to the naturalist; it magnifies psychological states and in this way is an aid to its study."[7]

"Marijuana, Assassin of Youth"

At the beginning of the twentieth century, public interest in cannabis and its use was not very widespread. In the early 1920s, there were a few references in the mass media to the use by Mexican Americans of something the newspapers called marijuana, but public concern was not aroused. In 1926, however, a series of articles associating marijuana and crime appeared in a New Orleans newspaper. As a result, the public began to take an interest in this "new" drug.

The commissioner of narcotics, Harry Anslinger, said that in 1931 the Bureau of Narcotics' file on marijuana was less than two inches thick. The same year, the Treasury Department stated:

> A great deal of public interest has been aroused by the newspaper articles appearing from time to time on the evils of the abuse of marijuana, or Indian hemp. This publicity tends to magnify the extent of the evil and lends color to an inference that there is an alarming spread of the improper use of the drug, whereas the actual increase in such use may not have been inordinately large.[4]

Even so, by 1935 there were 36 states with laws regulating the use, sale, and/or possession of marijuana. By the end of 1936 all 48 states had similar laws. The federal worm had also turned. In 1937, at congressional hearings, Anslinger stated that "traffic in marihuana is increasing to such an extent that it has come to be the cause for the greatest national concern."[8] In the 1931 to 1937 period, it is true, the use of marijuana had spread throughout the country, but there is no evidence that there was extensive use in most communities. The primary motivation for the congressional hearings on marijuana came not because of the use of marijuana as an inebriant or a euphoriant but because of reports by police and in the popular literature stating: "Most crimes of violence are laid to users of marihuana."[9]

Scientific American[10] reported in March 1936:

> Marijuana produces a wide variety of symptoms in the user, including hilarity, swooning, and sexual excitement. Combined with intoxicants, it often makes the smoker vicious, with a desire to fight and kill.

And *Popular Science Monthly*[11] in May 1936 contained a lengthy article with such statements as this:

> The Chief of Philadelphia County detectives declared that whenever any particularly horrible crime was committed—and especially one pointing to perversion—his officers searched first in marijuana dens and questioned marijuana smokers for suspects.

It hardly seemed necessary for readers to be told that marijuana had arrived as "the foremost menace to life, health, and morals in the list of drugs used in America."[11]

In this period the association was repeatedly made between crime, particularly violent and/or perverted crime, and marijuana use. A typical report,[12] cautiously phrased as were all of them, follows:

> In Los Angeles, Calif., a youth was walking along a downtown street after inhaling a marijuana cigarette. For many addicts, merely a portion of a "reefer" is enough to induce intoxication. Suddenly, for no reason, he decided that someone had threatened to kill him and that his life at that very moment was in danger. Wildly he looked about him. The only person in sight was an aged bootblack. Drug-crazed nerve centers conjured the innocent old shoe-shiner into a destroying monster. Mad with fright, the addict hurried to his room and got a gun. He killed the old man, and then, later, babbled his grief over what had been wanton, uncontrolled murder.
>
> "I thought someone was after me," he said. "That's the only reason I did it. I had never seen the old fellow before. Something just told me to kill him!"

That's marijuana!

However, not all articles condemned marijuana as the precipitator of violent crimes. An article in *The Literary Digest* reported that the chief psychiatrist at Bellevue Hospital in New York City had reviewed the cases of over 2,200 criminals convicted of felonies. Referring to marijuana he said, "None of the assault cases could be said to have been committed under the drug's influence. Of the sexual crimes, there was none due to marihuana intoxication. It is quite probable that alcohol is more responsible as an agent for crime than is marihuana."[13]

There was very poor documentation of the relationship between marijuana and crime, which in the 1930s was stated as if it had been proved. A thorough review[14] of Commissioner Anslinger's writings on marijuana concluded:

> In the works of Mr. Anslinger, there are either no references or references to volumes which my assistants and I have checked and which, in our checking, we find to be based upon much hearsay and little or no experimentation. We found a mythology in which later writers cite the authority of earlier writers, who also had little evidence. We have found, by and large, what can most charitably be described as a pyramid of prejudice, with each level of the structure built upon the shaky foundations of earlier distortions.

Examples of this "pyramid of prejudice" abound, but here's one way it worked: One of Mr. Anslinger's Treasury agents would testify before Congress and relate one of these outrageous stories of marijuana-induced violence. Next, the testimony would be referred to in an editorial in a medical journal, such as the *Journal of the American Medical Association* (*JAMA*). Then Anslinger or one of his people would write a magazine article, citing the prestigious *JAMA* as the source of the information!

With such poor evidence supporting the relationship between marijuana use and crime, it seems strange that the true story was never told. There are probably several reasons. One was the Great Depression, which made everyone acutely sensitive to, and wary of, any new and particularly foreign influences. The fact that it was lower-class Mexican Americans and blacks who had initiated use of the drug made the drug doubly dangerous to the white middle class.

Another contributing factor probably was the regular reference in associating marijuana and crime to the murdering cult of Assassins as suggestive of the characteristics of the drug. The 1936 *Popular Science Monthly*[11] reference to the Assassins is the most concise:

> The origin of the word "assassin" has two explanations, but either demonstrates the menace of Indian hemp. According to one version, members of a band of Persian terrorists committed their worst atrocities while under the influence of hashish. In the other version, Saracens who opposed the Crusaders were said to employ the services of hashish addicts to secure secret murderers of the leaders of the Crusades. In both versions, the murderers were known as "haschischin," "hashshash" or "hashishi" and from those terms comes the modern and ominous "assassin."

In none of the original stories and legends were the murders committed by individuals under the influence of hashish; rather, hashish was part of the reward for carrying out the murders. No matter. As the thirties rolled on, fear of marijuana users and of marijuana itself increased, as did state marijuana-control laws. In the mid 1930s the Narcotics Bureau acted to support federal legislation, and in the spring of 1937 congressional hearings were held.

The Marijuana Tax Act of 1937

Passage of the Marijuana Tax Act was a foregone conclusion. There were few witnesses to testify other than law enforcement officers. People dealing in birdseed had the act modified so they could import sterilized cannabis seed for use in their product. An official of the American Medical Association (AMA) testified on his own behalf, not representing the AMA, against the bill. His reasons for opposing the bill were multiple. Primarily, he thought the state antimarijuana laws were adequate and, also, that the social-menace case against cannabis had not been proved at all. It might be that most other medical doctors didn't associate the old remedies based on cannabis with this new foreign-sounding drug marijuana. The bill was passed in August and became effective on October 1, 1937.

The general characteristics of the law followed the regulation-by-taxation theme of the Harrison Act of 1914. The federal law did not outlaw cannabis or its preparations; it just taxed the grower, distributor, seller, and buyer and made it, administratively, almost impossible to have anything to do with cannabis. In addition, the Bureau of Narcotics prepared a uniform law that many states adopted. The uniform law on marijuana specifically named *C. sativa* as the species of plant whose leafy material is illegal. In later years, there were some court cases in which the defense argued that the material confiscated by the police came from *C. indica* and thus was not illegal. In the usual specimens obtained by police or presented in court, all distinguishing characters between species are either not present or are obliterated by drying and crushing. Because the cannabinoids are present in all species, there is no way of telling what species one has at hand with most confiscated marijuana. The current federal and uniform laws refer only to *Cannabis*.

The state laws made possession and use of cannabis illegal per se. In May 1969, thirty-two years later, the U.S. Supreme Court declared the Marijuana Tax Act unconstitutional and overturned the conviction of Timothy Leary because there was

> in the Federal anti-marijuana law—a section that requires the suspect to pay a tax on the drug, thus incriminating himself, in violation of the Fifth Amendment: and a section that assumes (rather than requiring proof) that a person with foreign-grown marijuana in his possession knows it is smuggled.[15]

After the Marijuana Tax Act

Passage of the Marijuana Tax Act had an amazing effect. Almost immediately there was a sharp reduction in the reports of heinous crimes committed under the influence of marijuana! The price of the merchandise increased rapidly (the war came along, too), so that five years after passage of the act the cost of a marijuana cigarette—a reefer—had increased six to twelve times and cost about a dollar.

The year after the law was enacted, 1938, Mayor Fiorello LaGuardia of New York City remembered what no one else wanted to recall. What he recalled were two army studies on marijuana use by soldiers in the Panama Canal Zone around 1930. Both reports found marijuana to be innocuous and said that its reputation as a troublemaker "was due to its association with alcohol which was always found the prime agent."[16]

Mayor LaGuardia asked the New York Academy of Medicine to study marijuana, its use, its effects, and the necessity for control. The report, issued in 1944, was intensive and extensive and a very good study for its time. The complete report is available,[17] so only a part of the summary is quoted:

> It was found that marihuana in an effective dose impairs intellectual functioning in general. . . .
>
> Marihuana does not change the basic personality structure of the individual. It induces a feeling of self-confidence, but this expressed in thought rather than in performance. There is, in fact, evidence of a diminution in physical activity. . . .
>
> Those who have been smoking marihuana for a period of years showed no mental or physical deterioration which may be attributed to the drug.[17]

This 1944 report, which was completed by a very reputable committee of the New York Academy of Medicine, brought a violent reaction. The AMA stated in a 1945 editorial:[18]

> For many years medical scientists have considered cannabis a dangerous drug. Nevertheless, a book called "Marihuana Problems" by New York City Mayor's Committee on Marihuana submits an analysis of seventeen doctors of tests on 77 prisoners and, on this narrow and thoroughly unscientific foundation, draws sweeping and inadequate conclusions which minimize the harmfulness of marijuana. Already the book has done harm. One investigator has described some tearful parents who brought their 16 year old son to a physician after he had been detected in the act of smoking marihuana. A noticeable mental deterioration had been evident for some time even to their lay minds. The boy said he had read an account of the LaGuardia Committee report and that this was his justification for using marihuana.

As in all such reports and reactions to reports, there is little dispute over the facts, only over the interpretation. The LaGuardia Report is in substantial agreement with the Indian Hemp Commission Report of the 1890s, the Panama Canal Zone reports of the 1930s, and the comprehensive reports in the 1970s by the governments of New Zealand, Canada, Great Britain, and the United States, in addition to the 1981 report to the World Health Organization and the 1982 report by the National Academy of Science to the Congress of the United States, so it is likely that the conclusions of the LaGuardia Report were and are for the most part valid.

The 1950s and 1960s are a unique period in the history of marijuana. There was a hiatus in scientific research on cannabis, but experimentation in the streets increased. With the arrival of the "psychedelic sixties," the popular press emphasized the more sensational hallucinogens. Marijuana, however, became the most common symbol of youthful rejection of authority and identification with a new era of personal freedom. According to the annual high school senior survey and the NIDA household survey (see chapter 1), marijuana apparently peaked in popularity in the United States around 1980.

During the 1980s and early 1990s, marijuana use became much less popular than it had been in the 1970s, but the mid 1990s saw the beginning of a significant rise in the number of young people using marijuana or hashish.

PHARMACOLOGY

Cannabinoid Chemicals

The chemistry of cannabis is quite complex, and isolation and extraction of the active ingredient are difficult even today. The active agent in cannabis is unique among psychoactive plant materials in that it contains no nitrogen and thus is not an alkaloid. Because it lacks nitrogen, the nineteenth-century chemists who had been so successful in isolating the active agents from other plants were unable to identify the active component of cannabis.

There are over 400 different chemicals in marijuana, but only 61 of them are unique to the *Cannabis* plant—these are called cannabinoids. One of them, delta-9-tetrahydrocannabinol **(THC)**, was isolated and synthesized in 1964 and is clearly the most pharmacologically active. Structures of some of these chemicals are shown in figure 17.1. The major active metabolite in the body of THC is 11-hydroxy-delta-9-THC.

Take special note that the relationship of THC to cannabis is probably more similar to the relationship of mescaline to peyote than of alcohol to beer, wine, or distilled spirits. Alcohol is the only behaviorally active agent in alcoholic beverages, but there might be several active agents in cannabis.

Absorption, Distribution, and Elimination

When smoked, THC is rapidly absorbed into the blood and distributed first to the brain, then redistributed to the rest of the body, so that within 30 minutes much is gone from the brain. The psychological and cardiovascular effects occur together, usually within 5 to 10 minutes. The THC remaining in the blood has a half-life of about 19 hours, but metabolites (of which there are at least forty-five), primarily 11-hydroxy-delta-9-THC, are formed in the liver and have a half-life of 50 hours. After one week 25 to 30 percent of the THC and its metabolites might still remain in the body. Complete elimination of a large dose of THC and its metabolites might take two or three weeks. THC taken orally is slowly absorbed, and the liver transforms it to 11-hydroxy-delta-9-THC; therefore much less THC reaches the brain after oral ingestion, and it takes much longer for it to have psychological effects.

The high lipid solubility of THC means that it (like its metabolites) is selectively taken up and stored in fatty tissue to be released slowly. Excretion is primarily through the feces. All of this has two important implications: (1) There is no easy way to monitor (in urine or blood) THC/metabolite levels and relate them to behav-

Δ-9 THC   Anandamide

■ carbon   ■ oxygen   ■ hydrogen   ■ nitrogen

Figure 17.1 Δ-9 THC, the most active substance found in *Cannabis,* and anandamide, isolated from brain tissue ioral and/or physiological effects, as can be done with alcohol, and (2) the long-lasting, steady, low concentration of THC and its metabolites on the brain and other organs might have effects not yet determined.

With the advent of isolated THC, dose-response relationships could be determined and the differential response to oral and inhalation modes of intake evaluated.

> Threshold doses of 2 mg. smoked and 5 mg. orally produced mild euphoria; 7 mg. smoked and 17 mg. orally, some perceptual and time sense changes occurred; and at 15 mg. smoked and 25 mg. orally, subjects reported marked changes in body image, perceptual distortions, delusions and hallucinations.[19]

Oral intake is more frequently followed by nausea, physical discomfort, and hangover, and the dose level cannot be titrated as accurately as is possible when smoking. There might be other differences in effects between comparable oral and smoking intake, although this has not been studied extensively.

A reminder: Cannabis is a drug that has primarily been used in two dosage forms of very different potency. Hashish and cannabis extracts that give rise to the experiences reported by Baudelaire and others are potent hallucinogenic agents. The drug delivery system that spread through the United States in the 1920s and 1930s was a much less potent form, marijuana. The active ingredient is the same; the amount differs. Both marijuana and hashish are available and used in the United States today, although the great majority of users restrict themselves to marijuana.

Mechanism of Action

Scientists searched for years for a key to help them unlock the mystery of marijuana's action on the nervous system. Of course, the identification and purification of delta-9-THC was a necessary step. A significant breakthrough was made by researchers at the NIMH laboratories in 1988. They developed a technique to identify and measure highly specific and selective binding sites for THC and related compounds in rat brains. One result was the development and testing of more potent marijuana analogues.[20] Another result was the 1992 discovery of a natural substance produced in the body that has marijuana-like effects when administered to animals. This substance, called **anandamide,** started the search for other related chemicals. [21] In 1996 it was reported that chocolate contains chemicals that are structurally and biochemically related to anadamide, but whether these chemicals have similar effects or are present in sufficient amounts remains unclear.[22] Eventually these discoveries will lead to greater understanding of how we naturally cope with stress, pain, and nausea, and might well lead to the development of selective drugs that will be more practical than THC.

Physiological Effects

Thus far the study of the effects of THC on the physiology of the body has done little more than quantify earlier reports in which resin extracts were used. The established physiological effects of cannabis are dose related, for the most part minor, of indeterminate importance for the psychological effects, and of unknown toxicological significance. For many years there has been substantial agreement on the short-term physiological effects of cannabis.

> Physiological changes accompanying marijuana use at typical levels of American social usage are relatively few. One of the most consistent is an

---

THC: delta-9-tetrahydrocannabinol, the most active chemical in marijuana.

anandamide: (an *and* a mide) a chemical isolated from brain tissue that has marijuana-like properties.

increase in pulse rate. Another is reddening of the eyes at the time of use. Dryness of the mouth and throat are uniformly reported. Although enlargement of the pupils was an earlier impression, more careful study had indicated that this does not occur. Blood pressure effects have been inconsistent.[23]

Except for bronchodilation, acute exposure to marijuana has little effect on breathing as measured by conventional pulmonary tests. Heavy marijuana smoking over a much longer period could lead to clinically significant and less readily reversible impairment of pulmonary function. The smoking of marijuana causes changes in the heart and circulation that are characteristic of stress. But there is no evidence to indicate that it exerts a permanently deleterious effect on the normal cardiovascular system. Marijuana increases the work of the heart, usually by increasing heart rate, and in some persons by increasing blood pressure. This increase in workload poses a threat to patients with hypertension, cerebrovascular disease, and coronary atherosclerosis.[23]

Behavioral Effects

Almost all writers emphasize that a new user has to learn how to smoke marijuana. The first step involves deeply inhaling the smoke and holding it in the lungs for twenty to forty seconds. Then the user has to learn to identify and control the effects and, finally, to label the effects as pleasant. Because of this learning process, most first-time users do not achieve the euphoric "stoned" or "high" condition of the repeater.

The effects accompanying marijuana smoking by the experienced user are relatively well established.

A cannabis "high" typically involves several phases. The initial effects are often somewhat stimulating and, in some individuals, may elicit mild tension or anxiety which usually is replaced by a pleasant feeling of well-being. The later effects usually tend to make the user introspective

and tranquil. Rapid mood changes often occur. A period of enormous hilarity may be followed by a contemplative silence.[18]

One investigator had experienced marijuana smokers indicate how frequently their marijuana intoxication included each of 206 effects listed on a sheet. Although there are great difficulties in looking for generalizations among idiosyncratic responses, the investigator was able to summarize 124 common subjective effects.

Sense perception is often improved, both in intensity and in scope. Imagery is usually stronger but well controlled, although people often care less about controlling their actions. Great changes in perception of space and time are common, as are changes in psychological processes such as understanding, memory, emotion, and sense of identity. . . .

To the extent that the described effects are delusory or inaccurate, the delusions and inaccuracy are widely shared. It is interesting, too, that nearly all the common effects seem either emotionally pleasing or cognitively interesting, and it is easy to see why marijuana users find the effects desirable regardless of what happens to their external behavior.[24]

The subjective effects of smoking marijuana—the high—are quite difficult to study. First, because tolerance does develop, experienced smokers should show *less* effect than beginning smokers. But almost everyone suggests that you have to learn to use marijuana, and you have to learn to appreciate the psychological effects that occur. This would mean that experienced smokers should show *more* effect than beginning smokers. In addition to these factors, or maybe as part of them, there is much learning and association of the high with the smell, feel, taste, and rituals of using marijuana. This would suggest that an experienced user would report *more* effect from a placebo cigarette than would a beginning user. The placebo cigarette would elicit the feelings associated with (conditioned to) the use of marijuana, and there should be more of these associations in the experienced user. It might also be expected that frequent marijuana

TABLE 17.1

Reports of Intoxication and Measured Physiological Changes from Experienced Users Smoking Marijuana and Placebo Cigarettes (n = 100)

	Number of subjects reporting	
Intoxication level (0 sober, 100 maximum)	Marijuana	Placebo
0–19	15	35
20–39	11	28
40–59	20	21
60–79	32	12
80–100	22	4
Average	61	34
Average physiological change (pre- to post-smoking)	Marijuana*	Placebo[†]
Pulse rate (beats/min)	+24.00	−4.00
Salivary flow (ml/5 min)	−1.60	+0.80
Redness of eye (0–4 scale)	+1.92	+0.04

*All significant, $p < 0.05$.

[†]None significant.

users would be *less* sensitive than infrequent users to THC itself, because more of their expectations are involved in the factors related to smoking marijuana. Tables 17.1 and 17.2 speak to these issues. Placebo cigarettes were made for these studies by extracting the THC and other cannabinols from marijuana with alcohol. The marijuana contained 0.9 percent THC, and the cigarettes were made so that they contained 9 mg THC, of which about 5 mg would be delivered to the user. This was midrange potency compared with what was being sold on the streets of San Francisco where these double-blind studies were done.[25]

Table 17.1 shows very nicely that, although experienced users report more intoxication from using a THC-containing marijuana cigarette, there is a moderate level of intoxication reported after the use of a similar smelling, tasting, and feeling cigarette without THC. This should not be too surprising, because some experienced

users report that they can turn themselves on just by thinking about it. It might be possible to fool the psyche, but not the soma. The physiological changes from use of the active cigarette are what you would expect: increase in heart rate, drying of mouth, reddening of eyes. These changes do not occur with the placebo.

The interaction of learning and of tolerance are clear in table 17.2. When the THC-containing cigarettes were smoked, infrequent users reported a bigger effect than frequent users (tolerance). But when placebo cigarettes were smoked, frequent users got a much larger effect than infrequent users (conditioned effect). The same type of response shows up in part B of table 17.2, but it is also interesting that frequent users respond much less to the oral THC than do the infrequent users. This is probably a combination of tolerance and absence of the usual associations with getting high. ("If I don't see, smell, and feel these things, then I can't be intoxicated.") Even though the subjective effects vary with expectancy and other factors, the physiological effects follow the physiology, and the frequent users show smaller physiological changes to the oral THC than infrequent users do.

One of the most consistent effects is on short-term memory, that is, tasks such as learning and remembering new information or remembering and following a sequence of directions. In everyday use while intoxicated, the marijuana user is unable to easily recall information she learned just seconds or minutes before. This memory lapse affects the general thread of conversation among a group of users, as Baudelaire noted. On this issue one of the truly grand old men of the study of drug effects, A. Wikler, commented:

> The drunkard staggers—
> only when he walks,
> The pothead forgets—
> only when he talks.

This impairment of short-term memory is probably the basis for the changes in time sense frequently reported. The user feels that more

TABLE 17.2

Reports of Intoxication and Measured Physiological Changes in Frequent and Infrequent Marijuana Users

	Infrequent users (less than 2 cigarettes a month)	Frequent users (more than 7 cigarettes a month)
Reported level of intoxication after using (averages, range 0–100)		
A. Marijuana cigarette	67	52
Placebo cigarette	22	48
B. Marijuana cigarette	62	56
Oral extract (25 mg THC)	72	32
Placebo cigarette	26	51
Placebo oral extract	2	5
Physiological changes		
Pulse rate (beats/min)	+31.0*	+17.0
Salivary flow (ml/5 minutes)	−1.8*	−0.9
Redness of eye (0–4 scale)	+2.1	+1.5

*Signicant differences, $p < 0.05$, between infrequent and frequent users.

time has passed than actually has. Such over-estimation of the passage of time is the most commonly reported psychological effect of marijuana smoking and has been validated in many experiments.

One particularly important finding is that although reaction time is not greatly affected, if affected at all, there is a great impairment in the ability to engage in *tracking* behavior, such as keeping a pointer on a spot on a rotating turntable. Tracking behavior requires sustained attention, and this ability is decreased considerably by marijuana. Loss of concentration is perhaps also demonstrated by the finding that the quality of interpersonal communication (the richness of the language and attention to feedback from the other person) diminishes under the influence of marijuana.

MEDICAL USES OF CANNABIS

Cannabis never attained the medical status of opium, so its medical report is spotted, but the first report of medical use was by Shen Nung in 2737 B.C. Some 2,900 years after the Shen Nung

report, another Chinese physician, Hoa-tho (A.D. 200) recommended cannabis resin mixed with wine as a surgical anesthetic. Although cannabis preparations were used extensively in medicine in India and after about A.D. 900 in the Near East, there was almost nothing about it in European medicine until the 1800s.

Early reports in European medical journals, such as de Sacy's 1809 article titled "Intoxicating Preparations Made with Cannabis," awakened more interest in the writers and artists of the period than in medical men. In 1839, however, a lengthy article, "On the Preparations of the Indian Hemp, or Gunjah," was published by a British physician working in India.[26] He reviewed the use of cannabis in Indian medicine and reported on his own work with animals, which suggested that cannabis preparations were quite safe. Having shown cannabis to be nontoxic, he used it clinically and found it to be an effective anticonvulsant and muscle relaxant, as well as a valuable drug for the relief of the pain of rheumatism.

In 1860 the Ohio State Medical Society's Committee on *C. indica* reported its successful use in the treatment of stomach pain, chronic cough, and gonorrhea. One physician felt he had to "assign to the Indian hemp a place among the so-called hypnotic medicines next to opium."[27] By the 1890s a medical text included this statement: "Cannabis is very valuable for the relief of pain, particularly that depending on nerve disturbances."[4]

One of the difficulties that has always plagued the scientific, medical, and social use of cannabis is the variability of the product. An 1898 brochure reviewed the assay and standardization techniques used with many of the common plant drugs and stated: "In Cannabis Indica we have a drug of great importance and one which all of materia medica is undoubtedly the most variable."[28] Four years later, Parke, Davis,[29] using new standardization procedures, claimed that "each lot sent out upon the market by us is of full potency and to be relied upon." They listed a variety of cannabis products available for medical use, including "a Chocolate Coated Tablet Extract Indian Cannabis 1/4 grain"!

Passage of the 1937 law resulted in all twenty-eight of the legal cannabis preparations being withdrawn from the market, and in 1941 cannabis was dropped from *The National Formulary* and *The U.S. Pharmacopeia*. Note well that the decline in the medical use of cannabis occurred long before 1937 and that the law did not eliminate an actively used therapeutic agent. Four factors, however, certainly contributed to the declining prescription rate of this plant. One was the development of new and better drugs for most illnesses. Second was the variability of the available medicinal preparations of cannabis, which was repeatedly mentioned in the 1937 hearings.[7] Third, cannabis is very insoluble in water and thus not amenable to injectable preparations. Last, taken orally it has an unusually long (1- to 2-hour) latency to onset of action.

With the recent renewed interest in marijuana as a social drug came some reevaluation and rethinking of the implications of some of the older therapeutic reports. Scientists looked again at some of the most interesting reported therapeutic effects of cannabis. One is its anticonvulsant activity. A 1949 report[30] found it effective in some cases where phenytoin (Dilantin), the anticonvulsant of choice both then and now, was ineffective. The fact that both Queen Victoria's physician and Sir William Osler, as well as others, found cannabis to be very effective against tension headaches or migraine has caused some interest.[31]

A 1972 report showed that marijuana smoking was effective in reducing the fluid pressure of the eye in a glaucoma patient.[32] That report became a cause célèbre in 1975 when a glaucoma patient was arrested for growing marijuana plants on his back porch for medical purposes. This man fifteen months later (1) saw the charges against him dropped, (2) had his physician certify that the only way for him to avoid blindness was to smoke five joints a day, and (3) had these marijuana joints legally supplied to him by the United States government.[33] This began a very limited program in which the National Institute on Drug Abuse (NIDA) provided medical-grade marijuana cigarettes to patients with the FDA's approval of a "compassionate use" protocol.

A second possible important medical use was reported in 1975. Medication containing THC, the active ingredient in marijuana, was the only kind that was effective in reducing the severe nausea caused by certain drugs used to treat cancer. A 1982 report from the National Academy of Sciences stated:

> Cannabis and its derivatives have shown promise in the treatment of a variety of disorders. The evidence is most impressive in glaucoma . . . ; in asthma. . . ; and in the nausea and vomiting of cancer chemotherapy . . . and might also be useful in seizures, spasticity, and other nervous system disorders.[23]

On the other hand, Dr. Nahas, a medical researcher and prominent foe of marijuana, felt that:

For each of these uses, there are other modern drugs with greater bioavailability, specificity, and effectiveness. . . . Reproducible absorption, consistent and predictable pharmacological effects may not be achieved. . . . It appears that it will not become a useful therapeutic agent.[34]

In 1985 the FDA licensed a small drug company, Unimed, Inc., to begin producing a capsule containing THC for sale to cancer chemotherapy patients who are experiencing nausea. The drug is referred to by the generic name **dronabinol** and the brand name **Marinol**. Dronabinol has helped cancer chemotherapy patients to gain weight, and in 1993 the FDA also approved its use for stimulating appetite in AIDS patients.[35] The National Organization for the Reform of Marijuana Laws (NORML) wants marijuana cigarettes themselves approved, under the theory that the dose can be better controlled and smoking is there-

fore safer. Their position received some support from the DEA's chief administrative law judge in 1988, who recommended that the DEA move marijuana from Schedule I to Schedule II so physicians could use it to treat the nausea produced by cancer chemotherapy and also to relieve suffering in cases of multiple sclerosis. He called natural marijuana "one of the safest therapeutically active substances known to man."[36] The DEA finally decided in 1992 that there was insufficient evidence to justify rescheduling marijuana to Schedule II, so it will remain officially "without medical usefulness"; part of their justification was that because "pure" THC is now available by prescription, there is no justification for providing the raw plant material to be smoked.

Also in 1992, apparently in response to a number of "compassionate use" requests from AIDS patients seeking improved appetites, the

---

FYI **Should Medical Patients Have Access to Marijuana?**

The 1996 Arizona and California ballot initiatives allowing patients to use marijuana on the advice of their physicians reawakened public interest in this topic. The best-demonstrated effects of marijuana (and of THC) are the reduction of the nausea caused by chemotherapy for cancer, and the stimulation of appetite, which might benefit AIDs patients. With such serious illnesses involved, many feel that the compassionate thing is to allow marijuana to be used if it might help, since the risk of dependence seems to be a rather small issue in such cases. In fact, "cannabis buyers clubs" had sprung up in many large cities, most notably San Francisco, and patients who had notes from their physicians could purchase from them. These clubs were illegal, but local law en-

forcement agencies had for the most part left them alone, not wanting to arrest seriously ill patients. Of course, because the clubs were illegal and informally operated, there was no guarantee that everyone purchasing marijuana was in fact seriously ill.

Following the passage of the ballot initiatives, the U.S. government in December 1996 announced that it would move to revoke the DEA registration of any physician who advised a patient to use illegal drugs. This caused some to wonder about violations of the tradition of privileged communications between doctors and patients, and so far the legality of all of this is open to question. In early 1998 the U.S. Justice Department announced plans to shut down all cannabis buyers clubs in California.

FDA quietly terminated the process of reviewing any new compassionate use protocols for marijuana cigarettes.[37] Although thirty-six states had approved legislation allowing for medical use of marijuana under a physician's prescription, only thirteen patients had received FDA approval in the seventeen years the program was in effect.

1996 Ballot Initiatives on Medical Marijuana

The question of medical usefulness for marijuana seemed to some to have been taken away from federal agencies and put in the hands of the public when in November of 1996, both Arizona and California voters passed ballot initiatives allowing physicians to recommend marijuana for serious illnesses, and allowing patients to possess and use marijuana if their physicians recommend it.[38] There was still no legal way for patients to purchase marijuana, of course, and no legal growers or distributers. As noted above, more than half the states had previously passed laws allowing medicinal use of marijuana, so in some sense this was not new. However, those previous laws were passed in the 1970s, when decriminalization and even legalization of marijuana wcrc bcing debated openly. By the mid 1990s, when record numbers of arrests were being made for marijuana law violations, such action by voters came as a big surprise, and elicited some strong reactions from the federal government (see the FYI Box).

Another Institute of Medicine study

The Institute of Medicine (IOM) of the prestigious National Academy of Sciences last issued a comprehensive report on mariujana in 1982. In 1998 the IOM began developing a new report focusing on scientific evidence for the safety and efficacy of marijuana as a medicine. The report was not completed at the time of this writing. An update on the status of this report will be available on our internet web site (see Web Watch).

CAUSES FOR CONCERN

Dependence Potential

Tolerance

For years there was debate over whether tolerance developed to the effects of THC and/or marijuana. Whereas animal studies repeatedly demonstrated tolerance to the behavioral disruption produced by large doses of marijuana, the experiences of human marijuana smokers seemed to indicate that experienced users could get high more readily than inexperienced users, possibly implying reverse tolerance or sensitization to the drug. We now know that learning plays an important role in the psychological reaction, particularly to low doses of marijuana. That, combined with the fact that THC can build up in the tissues of chronic users, might account for any increased reaction. However, a number of human studies have now demonstrated clear evidence of tolerance to some of the physiological effects of THC (see table 17.2). If high levels of marijuana are used regularly over a sustained period of time, tolerance will be obvious.

Physical dependence

Physical dependence has been demonstrated in laboratory experiments with humans given large doses of THC every four hours for ten to twenty days. Beginning several hours after the last oral dose, subjects showed irritability, restlessness, nausea, and vomiting. These symptoms peaked at eight hours and declined over the next three days. Sleep disturbances and loss of appetite were also reported.[39] Such withdrawal symptoms are virtually never reported

---

dronabinol: (dro *nab* i noll) the generic name for prescription THC in oil in a gelatin capsule.

Marinol: (*mare* i noll) brand name for dronabinol.

outside the research laboratory. One reason for this might be that the drug is so long-lasting. Withdrawal signs are always more dramatic when a drug leaves the body quickly. The development of a specific antagonist for the marijuana (or anandamide) receptor has made it possible to demonstrate clear withdrawal symptoms in laboratory animals, because administration of an antagonist has the effect of removing the drug from its receptors almost instantaneously.[40] In animal studies, the withdrawal symptoms resemble those of opiate withdrawal to some extent and might have some mechanisms in common.

Psychological dependence

The strength of a drug's tendency to produce behavioral dependence can be estimated by looking at how many of its users develop patterns of daily, repeated use. With a highly addicting practice like cigarette smoking, the majority of users are daily users of multiple doses. With alcohol and many other drugs, most users avoid such a pattern, but a few develop strong dependence. The marijuana pattern seems to be more similar to that of alcohol use than of cigarette smoking or heroin injection. As Dr. David E. Smith of the Haight-Ashbury Medical Center said in 1982: "Regular heavy users who smoke more than 10 joints a day may be rare, but they do exist."[41]

The picture that emerges is that addiction, in the sense of a constant craving, high-frequency use, the buildup of tolerance, and possible withdrawal symptoms, is not an issue for the majority of marijuana users who engage in occasional smoking of one or two marijuana cigarettes. However, a small fraction of marijuana users do become dependent on daily use of marijuana. This probably has a lot to do with psychosocial variables and is not seen by most researchers as an inevitable consequence of exposure to marijuana. Whatever the causes, drug treatment programs do have clients whose primary drug of abuse is marijuana, and some

are voluntary clients seeking help for what can reasonably be called marijuana addiction. As Smith said, it doesn't happen to most users, but it does happen.

Toxicity Potential

Acute physiological effects

The acute physiological effects of marijuana, primarily an increase in heart rate, have not been thought to be a threat to health. However, as the marijuana-using population ages, there is concern that individuals with high blood pressure, heart disease, or hardening of the arteries might be harmed by smoking marijuana.[23] The lethal dose of THC has not been extensively studied in animals, and no human deaths have been reported from "overdoses" of cannabis.

Impaired driving ability

Behaviorally, the intoxication produced by marijuana does present some danger, especially if the user is driving. Early experiments using weak marijuana and simple reaction-time driving tests found small effects that experienced users seemed to be able to overcome (behavioral tolerance). However, there have now been a large number of studies using more complex and realistic driving tests that show definite impairments with marijuana. In either computer-controlled driving simulators or in actual driving tests on a closed course, these impairments were found to be dose related. The ability to maintain concentration, correct for wind gusts, and maintain a steady speed were all impaired, as was judgment. A telephone survey of nearly 6,000 teenagers found that those who reported driving six or more times per month after smoking marijuana were 2.4 times more likely to be involved in traffic accidents than those who did not drive after smoking marijuana. Studies based on measurements of drugs in the blood of drivers involved in accidents also indicate a role for marijuana in causing accidents, but most who tested positive for THC also tested positive for alcohol, so the results were inconclusive. Laboratory studies have found that smoking two marijuana cigarettes containing fairly high amounts of THC (3.6 percent) does impair performance on standard roadside "sobriety" tests of balance and coordination.[42]

Panic reactions

The other major behavioral problem associated with acute marijuana intoxication is the panic reaction. Much like many of the bad trips with hallucinogens, the reaction is usually fear of loss of control and fear that things will not return to normal. Even our old friend Baudelaire understood this and advised his readers to surround themselves with friends and a pleasant environment before using hashish. Although many people do seek emergency medical treatment for marijuana-induced panic and are sometimes given sedatives or tranquilizers, the best treatment is probably "talking down," or reminding the person of who and where they are, that their reaction is temporary, and that everything will be all right.

Chronic lung exposure

Since a large number of Americans began using marijuana chronically in the 1960s and 1970s, there has been a great deal of concern about the possible long-term effects of chronic marijuana use. There are a couple of physiological concerns that merit attention. One is the effect on lung function and the concern about lung cancer. Experiments have shown that chronic, daily smoking of marijuana does impair air flow in and out of the lungs.[43] It is hard to tell yet whether years of such an effect would result in permanent, major obstructive lung disease in the same way that smoking tobacco cigarettes does. Also, there is no direct evidence linking marijuana smoking to lung cancer in humans. Remember that it took many years of cigarette smoking by millions of Americans before the links between tobacco and lung cancer and other lung diseases were shown.

Marijuana smoke inhaled

Marijuana smoke has been compared with tobacco smoke.[23] Some of the constituents differ (there is no nicotine in marijuana smoke and no THC in tobacco), but many of the dangerous components are found in both. Total tar levels, carbon monoxide, hydrogen cyanide, and nitrosamines are found in similar amounts (except for tobacco-specific nitrosamines, which are carcinogens). Another potent carcinogen, *benzopyrene,* is found in greater amounts in marijuana than in tobacco. Everyone suspects that marijuana smoking will eventually be shown to cause cancer, but how much of a problem this will be compared with tobacco is hard to say. On the one hand, few marijuana smokers smoke twenty marijuana cigarettes every day, whereas tobacco smokers regularly smoke this much. On the other hand, the marijuana cigarette is not filtered and the user generally gets as much concentrated smoke as possible as far down in the lungs as possible and holds it there. So, while some of us wait and see when the data will come out, others are participating in the experiment.

Reproductive effects

The other area of concern seems to be reproductive effects in both men and women. Heavy marijuana smoking can decrease testosterone levels in men, although the levels are still within the normal range and the significance of those decreases is not known. There have been reports of diminished sperm counts or abnormal sperm structure in heavy marijuana users, but again the clinical significance of these reports is not clear.[44] A number of studies have reported either lower birth weight or shorter length at birth for infants whose mothers smoked marijuana during pregnancy.[45] Although these effects are small and inconsistent from one study to the next, it is of course wise to avoid use of all drugs during pregnancy.

The immune system

There have also been reports that marijuana smoking impairs some measures of the functioning of the immune system.[46] Animal studies have found that THC injections can reduce immunity to infection, but at doses well above those obtainable by smoking marijuana. Some human studies of marijuana smokers have suggested reduced immunity, but most have not. If the effect were real, it could result in marijuana smokers being more susceptible to infections, cancer, and other diseases such as genital herpes. One might suspect that such problems would eventually be reflected in the overall death rate of marijuana users. However, a 1997 report examining ten years of mortality data for over 65,000 people found no relationship between mariujana use and overall death rates.[47]

Amotivational syndrome

Since 1971, when some psychiatric case reports were published identifying an *amotivational* syndrome in marijuana smokers, there has been concern about the effect of regular marijuana use on behavior and motivation. A number of experiments and correlational studies have been aimed at answering this question. One thing to remember is the long half-life of marijuana in the body, so that daily smokers can in fact be chronically intoxicated and exhibit behavioral or motivational impairments even

before their daily dose. There does seem to be evidence for this diminished motivation, impaired ability to learn, and school and family problems in some adolescents who are chronic heavy marijuana smokers. If they stop smoking and remain in counseling, the condition improves.[41] This probably implies a constant state of intoxication rather than some long-lasting change in brain function or personality (see also the FYI box).

Insanity

The connection between marijuana use and insanity was one of the main arguments for outlawing the drug in the 1930s, and the notion still remains that marijuana can cause a type of psychosis. There have been reports of psychotic "breakdowns" occurring with rare frequency after marijuana has been smoked, but the causal relationship is in question. The psychotic episodes are generally self-limiting and seem to occur in individuals with a history of psychiatric problems.[41]

Brain damage

For about twenty-five years it has been speculated that amotivational or prolonged psychotic reactions could reflect an underlying damage to brain tissue produced by marijuana. For example, a 1972 report from England indicated that two individuals who demonstrated cerebral atrophy had a history of smoking marijuana. They also had a history of using many other illicit drugs, plus other medical problems, but it was suggested that the brain damage might have been caused by the marijuana. Several experiments have since been done, and all fail to find a relationship between marijuana smoking and cerebral atrophy.

There have been other incomplete or poorly controlled reports of potential brain damage from animal research, and it has been possible to dismiss most of them as inconclusive. However, two experiments on rats, one appearing in 1987 and the other in 1988, gave stronger

FYI   Long-term Effects of Marijuana Smoke in Monkeys

Although there have been some recent, well-controlled, convincing reports that chronic THC exposure may produce permanent changes in neurons in the hippocampus of rats, there have not yet been comparable studies in any primate species. Earlier reports of synaptic changes in the brains of rhesus monkeys have been widely criticized because proper control and sampling techniques were not used.

Recently some results have been reported from a long-term study[56] in which rhesus monkeys were exposed to marijuana smoke through a mask over their faces. The study was well controlled: some monkeys received the smoke from one cigarette each day for a year, others received smoke only on weekends, and others received daily exposure to the smoke from a marijuana cigarette from which the THC had been extracted.

One of the measures taken was how hard the monkeys would work for banana-flavored food pellets: each day the monkey could get one pellet by pressing a plate on the wall of the test cage. The second pellet required two presses, the third three presses, and so on (a progressive-ratio schedule of reinforcement). At some point each day the ratio would become so large that the monkey would stop pressing. At first the monkeys receiving active marijuana were unaffected; however, after several weeks of daily exposure they began to receive fewer pellets than the control monkeys. This effect persisted for a few weeks after the marijuana smoke was stopped. The authors interpreted these results to be a model of the "amotivational syndrome" reported in human marijuana smokers and indicated that the persistent effect may have been due to residual metabolites slowly clearing out of the brain tissue. When the monkeys' brains were examined, neither permanent neurochemical changes[57] nor structural changes in the neurons[58] could be found.

evidence that THC causes permanent changes in the structure of neurons in the hippocampus. One of the reports related these changes to a persistent deficit in the rats' performance on a radial arm maze. The doses used were in the range of what a very heavy marijuana smoker might obtain, and the treatment was given to the rats every day for ninety days. Although it is not clear what the implications might be for human beings smoking less heavily and only occasionally, these are clear effects that should lead to cautious concern.

One thing should be said about research on the adverse consequences of marijuana. There is probably no area of science in which emotion has played such an obvious and influential role. Scientists on both sides have become "crusaders" for their cause. Some individuals seem to think it is their professional duty to seek out and publicize every potential evil associated with marijuana, even if there is not strong scientific evidence in support of their views. Others seem to automatically question the negative reports and look for ways to discredit them. We can predict that the emotion, the premature announcements of new scary findings, the repeating of long discredited stories, and the conflicting reports will continue.

MARIJUANA AND AMERICAN SOCIETY

Remember that our patterns of drug use are but one facet of our evolving society. Our drug use affects and is affected by other social trends in our life. You should at least make note of a couple of important themes from the 1980s, and we'll see how they related to marijuana use. One trend was the increased emphasis on physical health. Jogging, working out, dieting, drinking less alcohol and caffeine, and smoking less are all reflections of our national concern over shaping up. The health trend obviously worked against marijuana use: how many people who won't smoke tobacco will feel good about inhaling marijuana smoke? Second, the 1980s saw a move toward social and political conservatism that also worked against such counterculture behavior as marijuana smoking. And of course, we remember that drug use tends to be faddish. If marijuana was the fashionable drug of the 1970s, then it couldn't be the fashionable drug of the 1980s. However, in the 1990s the drug came back into fashion, at least somewhat.

Data from the yearly survey of high school seniors shows the trends most clearly. After peaking in 1978–1979, the number of high school seniors who have ever smoked marijuana dropped from just over 60 percent to 32 percent in 1992, then rebounded to almost 50 percent by the class of 1997. Equally dramatic were the trends in daily use, which went from 11 percent in 1978 to 2 percent in 1992, and back to almost 6 percent by 1997.[48] The earlier decreases in marijuana use went along with a steady increase in the belief among these students that "people risk harming themselves if they smoke marijuana regularly." Whereas just over one-third of the high school seniors agreed with that statement in 1978, over three-fourths agreed in 1992. Fads being what they are, this downward trend in marijuana use had to end sometime, and the turnaround was seen in the high school

Use of and Attitudes toward Marijuana

Marijuana is not a topic that is discussed as much as it was a few years ago. Unless you belong to a group of people that regularly smokes marijuana, you may not know how your friends feel about the topic. Get together with a small group of your friends and discuss how many have ever smoked marijuana, how they feel about people using marijuana, and how prevalent they think marijuana smoking is among people of their age and status. You might, as a group, come up with a short questionnaire to administer to a larger group to see if your estimates are correct.

senior class of 1992. Significant increases in marijuana use in the 1992–1997 period were accompanied by decreased estimates of risk (see chapter 1).

Although marijuana is not used by most Americans, it is still remarkable how many people have used and continue to use a substance that shouldn't exist at all in our society, according to the Controlled Substances Act and the DEA. That a large fraction of the society continues to violate the laws regarding marijuana is a matter for concern. It is easy to look back and wish that the 1937 Marijuana Tax Act had never happened. Marijuana use was spreading slowly across the United States and with any luck it might have become acculturated. Society would have adapted to marijuana and adapted marijuana to society. Soon it would have become part of society: perhaps most people would never have used it regularly; of those who did use it, most would have known how to use it; some, of course, would have abused it. It has happened before with coffee, tea, tobacco, and alcohol.

The 1937 law prevented all that. It didn't affect most of us a great deal until the 1960s, when a large number of young people began experimenting with drugs. Marijuana, more than anything else, convinced many young people that the government had been lying to them about drugs. They had been told that marijuana would make them insane, enslave them in drug addiction, and lead to violence and perverted sexual acts. Their experience told them that marijuana was pretty innocuous compared with those stories, and it became an important symbol: smoking marijuana struck a blow for truth and freedom. The problem was that laws existed that allowed young people to be sent to jail for twenty years for striking this blow, and that didn't sit well with some people. Voice was given to the millions of marijuana users in 1970 when a young Washington lawyer established the National Organization for the Reform of Marijuana Laws (NORML) with a grant from the Playboy Foundation. As the founder of NORML put it: "The only people working for reform then were freaks who wanted to turn on the world, an approach that was obviously doomed to failure. I wanted an effective, middle-class approach, not pro-grass but antijail."[49]

Also, in 1970 the Comprehensive Drug Abuse Prevention and Control Act of 1970 established the Commission on Marijuana and Drug Abuse. Its 1972 report recommended some legislative changes:

> The Commission recommended that federal and state laws be changed so that private possession of small amounts of marihuana for personal use, and casual distribution of small amounts without monetary profit, would no longer be offenses, though marihuana possessed in public would remain contraband. Cultivation, distribution for profit, and possession with intent to sell would remain felonies. Criminal penalties would be retained for disorderly conduct associated with

marihuana intoxication and driving under the influence of marihuana, and a plea of marihuana intoxication would not be a defense to any criminal act committed under its influence.[50]

The year 1972 was a turning point in the fight to decriminalize marijuana. In June the American Medical Association came out in favor of dropping penalties for possession of "insignificant amounts" of marijuana and noted that "there is no evidence supporting the idea that marijuana leads to violence, aggressive behavior, or crime."[51] In August the American Bar Association called for the reduction of criminal penalties for possession, and a year later the organization recommended decriminalization. Both traditional liberals and conservatives could support the idea, not to declare marijuana legal, but to make possession of marijuana a civil offense, punishable only by a fine. A week before Christmas in 1972 the best known and most literate of American conservatives, William F. Buckley, proclaimed in favor of the decriminalization of marijuana, saying:

> It isn't silly to say that the user should not be molested, even though the pusher should be put in jail. It was so, mostly, under prohibition, when the speakeasy operators were prosecuted, not so the patrons. Thus it is, by and large, in the case of prostitution; and even with gambling; and most explicitly with pornography, the Supreme Court having ruled that you can't molest the owner, even though you can go after the peddler.[52]

In October 1973, Oregon abolished criminal penalties for marijuana use, substituting civil fines of up to $100. Marijuana offenders are given citations that are processed like traffic tickets. Did marijuana use increase in Oregon as a result of the decriminalization? Yes. By leaps and bounds? No. From the fall of 1974, a year after decriminalization, to the fall of 1977, the percentage of adults over eighteen who had "ever used" marijuana went from 19 percent to 25 percent. "Current users" went from 9 percent to 10 percent over the same period. However, marijuana use was increasing toward its 1978 to 1979 peak all over the country at the same time. Possession of a small amount of marijuana was made only a civil offense by eight other states: Maine, Colorado, California, Ohio, Minnesota, Mississippi, New York, and North Carolina. In Alaska, private possession of up to four ounces of marijuana was not illegal at all. One consequence of changing marijuana possession from a felony to a misdemeanor was that it saved money on court costs, juries, and jails. It has been estimated that the state of California enjoyed an average annual savings of over $95 million between 1976 and 1985 as a result of its citation plan for marijuana possession.[53]

At the federal level, action picked up in 1977. In January, Rosalynn Carter joined her husband, the President, in calling for the decriminalization of marijuana" and revealed that their oldest son had been discharged from the navy for smoking marijuana. Bills to decriminalize marijuana possession were introduced into both houses of Congress, and in August President Carter sent a message to Congress in which he asked them to abolish all federal criminal penalties for the possession of small amounts of marijuana.

If the truth were known, in the late 1970s de facto decriminalization had already occurred in many areas of the country. Law enforcement agencies in many of the larger cities of the United States had stopped arresting marijuana users and did not search out those with small amounts for personal use.

When the Reagan administration came into office in 1980, any hope of federal decriminalization was gone, replaced by a "get tough" attitude toward all illegal drugs. Marijuana was no exception. In addition to increased efforts to intercept marijuana shipments coming from abroad, a nationwide effort was launched in 1985 to combat cultivation of marijuana plants. Over 100 million plants were tugged out of the ground in 1987 by state, local, and federal law-enforcement teams.[54] Add to that the "zero tol-erance" seizures of boats, cars, and planes containing even traces of marijuana and the 1988 legislation putting extra pressure on the user (e.g., $10,000 fines at the federal level; see chapter 4), and we can see that the pendulum had definitely swung back. The states began to follow suit: in 1989 Oregon raised its civil penalty for possession from a $100 maximum to a $500 minimum. In 1990, Alaska voters approved the recriminalization of marijuana possession, making it a misdemeanor punishable by a jail term and up to a $1,000 fine. Increased penalties for distribution of controlled substances has brought us back to a situation where about one-sixth of all federal prisoners were incarcerated for marijuana offenses, and longer sentences are often given for selling marijuana than for murder![55] It was estimated that in 1996 more than 600,000 arrests were made in the United States for violating marijuana laws.

SUMMARY

- ▲ Cannabis has a rich history relating both to its medicinal use and to its recreational uses.
- ▲ Marijuana became famous as the "Assassin of Youth" in the 1930s and was outlawed in 1937.
- ▲ Cannabis contains many active chemicals, but the most active is delta-9-THC.
- ▲ THC is absorbed rapidly by smoking but slowly and incompletely when taken by mouth.
- ▲ THC has a long half-life of elimination, and its metabolites can be found in the body for up to several weeks after THC entered the body.
- ▲ Selective THC receptors exist in brain tissue, leading to the discovery of a naturally occurring brain cannabinoid, anandamide.
- ▲ Marijuana causes an increase in the heart rate and reddening of the eyes as its main physiological effects.

▲ Psychologically, THC has some sedative properties, produces some analgesia, and at high doses can produce hallucinations.

▲ In recreational use, some of marijuana's most important behavioral effects probably relate to its impairment of memory.

▲ Marijuana is useful in the treatment of glaucoma, for reducing nausea in patients undergoing cancer chemotherapy, and for increasing appetite in AIDS patients. A legal form of THC is available by prescription.

▲ Although strong behavioral dependence is not common, it does occur in some individuals.

▲ Marijuana can impair driving, and there is evidence that smoking marijuana leads to an increased frequency of accidents.

▲ Most experts agree that chronic smoking of marijuana impairs lung function somewhat and probably increases the risk of lung cancer.

▲ Long-standing concerns about marijuana-induced brain damage have received some limited support from recent animal studies.

REVIEW QUESTIONS

1. What are the major differences between *C. sativa* and *C. indica*?

2. How are hashish and sinsemilla produced?

3. What were the three stages of hashish intoxication described by Baudelaire?

4. Why were Harry Anslinger's writings on marijuana referred to as a "pyramid of prejudice"?

5. What were the general conclusions of the 1944 LaGuardia Commission?

6. What is meant by "cannabinoid," and about how many are their in cannabis? What is the cannabinoid recently found in brain tissue?

7. How is the action of THC in the brain terminated after about thirty minutes, when the half-life of metabolism is much longer than that?

8. What are the two most consistent physiological effects of smoking marijuana?

9. What two medical uses have been approved by the FDA for dronabinol?

10. What seems to be the best explanation for "amotivational syndrome"?

Related Internet Sites on Marijuana

The Marijuana Policy Project: http://www.mpp.org/

National Organization for the Reform of Marijuana Laws: http://www.norml.org/home.html

Partnership for a Drug-Free America: http://www.drugfreeamerica.org/

And the always-popular *Drugs, Society, and Human Behavior* site: http://www.uwyo.edu/A&S/psyc/dshb.htm

REFERENCES

1. Schultes RE, Hofmann A: *The botany and chemistry of hallucinogens,* Springfield, Ill, 1980, Charles C Thomas.

2. Mikuriya TH, Aldrich MR: Cannabis 1988: old drug, new dangers—the potency question, *J Psychoactive Drugs* 20:47-55, 1988.

3. Pollan M: How pot has grown. *New York Times Magazine,* p 31, Feb 13, 1995.

4. Snyder SH: What we have forgotten about pot, *New York Times Magazine,* p 27, Dec 13, 1970.

5. Mickel EJ: *The artificial paradises in French literature,* Chapel Hill, NC, 1969, University of North Carolina Press.

6. Baudelaire CP: *Artificial paradises; on hashish and wine as means of expanding individuality,* translated by Ellen Fox, New York, 1971, Herder & Herder.

7. Unpublished material in the Archives of the American Psychological Association, Department of Psychology, University of Akron, Akron, Ohio.

8. *Taxation of marihuana, hearings before the Committee on Ways and Means, House of Representatives, Seventy-fifth Congress, First Session, on HR 6385, April 27–30 and May 4, 1937,* Washington, DC, US Government Printing Office.

9. Parry A: The menace of marihuana, *Am Mercury* 36:487–488, 1935.

10. Marihuana menaces youth, *Sci Am* 154:151, 1936.

11. Wolf W: Uncle Sam fights a new drug menace . . . marijuana, *Pop Sci Monthly* 128:14, 1936.

12. Anslinger HJ, Cooper CR: Marijuana: assassin of youth, *Am Magazine* 124:19, 153, 1937.

13. Facts and fancies about marihuana, *Literary Digest* 122:7–8, 1936.

14. Whitlock L: Review: marijuana, *Crime and Delinquency Literature* 2(3):367, 1970.

15. Fort J: Pot: a rational approach, *Playboy,* pp 131, 154, Oct 1969.

16. The marihuana bugaboo, *Military Surgeon* 93:95, 1943.

17. Mayor LaGuardia's Committee on Marijuana. In Solomon D, editor: *The marihuana papers,* New York, 1966, New American Library.

18. Marijuana problems, *JAMA* 127:1129, 1945.

19. *Marihuana and health,* Department of Health, Education, and Welfare, Washington, DC, 1971, US Government Printing Office.

20. Howlett AC and others: The cannabinoid receptor: biochemical, anatomical and behavioral characterization, *Trends Neurosci* 13:420–423, 1990.

21. DiMarzo V and others: Formation and inactivation of endogenous cannabinoid anandamide in central neurons, *Nature* 372:686, 1994.

22. di Tomaso E, Beltramo M, Piomelli D: Brain cannabinoids in chocolate, *Nature* 382:677–678, 1996.

23. *Marijuana and health,* Institute of Medicine, National Academy of Sciences, Washington, DC, 1982, National Academy Press.

24. Tart CT: Marijuana intoxication: common experiences, *Nature* 226:701–704, 1970.

25. Jones RT: Tetrahydrocannabinol and the marijuana-induced social "high," or the effects of the mind on marijuana. In Singer AJ, editor: *Marijuana: chemistry, pharmacology, and patterns of social use, Ann NY Acad Sci* 191:155–165, 1971.

26. O'Shaughnessy WB: On the preparations of the Indian hemp, or gunja, *Trans Med Phys Soc,* Bengal pp 71–102, 1838–1840; pp 421–461, 1842.

27. Mikuriya TH: Marijuana in medicine: past, present and future, *California Medicine* 110:34–40, 1969.

28. *Standardization of drug extracts,* promotional brochure, Detroit, 1898, Parke, Davis & Co.

29. Letter to EP Delabarre, 9 Arlington Ave, Providence, RI, from Parke, Davis & Co, Manufacturing Department, Main Laboratories, Detroit, Superintendent's Office, Control Department, March 10, 1902.

30. Davis JP, Ramsey HH: Antiepileptic action of marihuana-active substances, *Federation Proceedings* 8:284–285, 1949.

31. Lieberman DM, Lieberman BW: *Marihuana–a medical review, New Eng J Med* 284:88–91, 1971.

32. Marijuana smoking said to have power to deter glaucoma, *New York Times,* July 28, 1972.

33. Medical therapy, legalization issues debated at Marijuana Reform Conference, *National Drug Reporter* 7(1):3–5, 1977.

34. Nahas GG: The medical use of cannabis. In Nahas, GG, editor: *Marijuana in science and medicine,* New York, 1984, Raven Press.

35. Levine K: Drug approved for treating appetite loss in AIDS patients, *Drug Topics,* Feb 8, 1993.

36. Conlan MF: Top drug cop weighs use of marijuana as an Rx drug, *Drug Topics,* Dec 12, 1988.

37. Karel R: Hopes of many long-term sufferers dashed as FDA ends medical marijuana program, *Psychiatric News,* May 1, 1992.

38. Trebach AS: Arizona and California voters seize initiatives, *The Drug Policy Letter,* Winter/Spring, 1997.

39. Jones RT, Benowitz N: The 30-day trip-clinical studies of cannabis tolerance and dependence. In Braude MC, Szara S, editors: *Pharmacology of marijuana,* New York, 1976, Raven Press.

40. Swan N: Marijuana antagonist reveals evidence of THC dependence in rats, *NIDA Notes,* Nov/Dec, 1995.

41. Smith DE, Seymour RB: Clinical perspectives on the toxicology of marijuana: 1967–1981. In *Marijuana and youth: clinical observations on motivation and learning,* Washington, DC, 1982, US Department of Health and Human Services, US Government Printing Office.

42. Mathias R: Marijuana impairs driving-related skills and workplace performance, *NIDA Notes,* Jan/Feb, 1996.

43. Tashkin DP and others: Respiratory status of seventy-four habitual marijuana smokers, *Chest* 78:699–706, 1980.

44. Nahas GG: Toxicology and pharmacology. In Nahas GG, editor: *Marijuana in science and medicine,* New York, 1984, Raven Press.

45. Tennes K and others: Marijuana: prenatal and postnatal exposure in the human. In Pinkert TM, editor: *Consequences of maternal drug abuse,* NIDA Research Monograph No 59, Washington, DC, 1985, US Government Printing Office.

46. Hollister LE: Health aspects of cannabis, *Pharmacol Rev* 38:1–20, 1986.

47. Sidney S, Beck JE, Friedman GD: Marijuana use and mortality, *American Journal of Public Health* 87: 585–590, 1997.

48. Johnston LD and others: *University of Michigan press release on National High School Senior Survey,* Dec 18, 1997.
49. Anderson P: The pot lobby, *New York Times Magazine,* pp 8-9, Jan 21, 1973.
50. Farnsworth DL: Summary of the Report of the National Commission on Marijuana and Drug Abuse, *Tracks,* 9:1-2, 1972.
51. The AMA and pot, Stash Capsules 4(4), Aug, 1972.
52. Buckley WF, Jr: Pot, legalization of, conservative division, New York Times, Dec 18, 1972.
53. Aldrich MR, Mikuriya T: Savings in California marijuana law enforcement costs attributable to the Moscone Act of 1976—a summary, *J Psychoactive Drugs* 20:75-81, 1988.
54. *1987 Domestic cannabis eradication/suppression program final report,* Drug Enforcement Administration, US Department of Justice, 1987.
55. Schlosser E: Reefer madness, *Atlantic Monthly,* Aug 1994.
56. Paule MG and others: Chronic marijuana smoke exposure in the rhesus monkey II: Effects on progressive ratio and conditioned position responding, *J Pharmacol Exp Ther* 260:210-222, 1992.
57. Ali SF and others: Chronic marijuana smoke exposure in the rhesus monkey IV: Neurochemical effects and comparison to acute and chronic exposure to D-9-tetrahydrocannabinol (THC) in rats, *Pharmacol Biochem Behav* 40:677-682, 1991.
58. Scallet AC: Neurotoxicology of cannabis and THC: a review of chronic exposure studies in animals, *Pharmacol Biochem Behav* 40:671-676, 1991.

Steroids and Other Drugs in Sport

KEY TERMS	OBJECTIVES

After reading this chapter, you should be able to:

ergogenic
anabolic
androgenic
human growth hormone

- Review the historical development of the use of performance-enhancing drugs by athletes and of attempts to regulate drug use by athletes.
- Be familiar with major concepts and terms such as *ergogenic aids* and *anabolic and androgenic steroids.*
- Understand the importance of psychological factors such as the masking of fatigue in evaluating the performance-enhancing properties of drugs.

- Understand what experimental research and athletes' experiences tell us about the effects of stimulant drugs on performance, as well as the side effects and dangers of stimulant drug use.
- Understand what experimental research and athletes' experiences tell us about the effects of anabolic steroids on muscular development and strength, as well as the side effects and dangers of anabolic steroids.

Why so much concern over drug use by athletes? Why not focus on drug use by clarinet players or muffler repair people? There are several answers to this question, and together they demonstrate that there are special reasons to be concerned about drug use in sport. First, there are those well-known athletes who are seen as role models for young people, portraying youth, strength, and health. When a famous athlete is reported to be using cocaine or some other illicit substance, there is concern that impressionable young people will see drug use in a more positive light. After all, haven't corporate sponsors paid these athletes to endorse their products, from shoes to breakfast cereal, based on this presumed influence over young consumers?

Second, some of the drugs used by athletes are intended to give the user an advantage over the competition, an advantage that is clearly viewed as being unfair. This is inconsistent with our tradition of fair play in sports, and widespread cheating of any kind tends to diminish a sport and to diminish public interest in it. Professional wrestling, which is widely viewed as being "rigged" or "staged," is enjoyed more as a form of comic entertainment than as an athletic contest. Most professional and amateur sportspeople guard their honor carefully, and the use of performance-enhancing drugs is seen as a threat to that honor.

Third, there is a concern that both the famous and the not-so-famous athletes who use drugs are endangering their health and perhaps their lives for the sake of a temporary burst of power or speed. To the extent that there are real risks associated with the use of these drugs, athletes should be aware of those risks. Because these drugs are often obtained illicitly, we can assume that the providers of the drugs do not present a balanced cost/benefit analysis to the potential user but instead probably maximize any possible benefit and minimize the dangers.

HISTORICAL USE OF DRUGS IN ATHLETICS

Ancient Times

Although we tend to think of drug use by athletes as a recent phenomenon, the use of chemicals to enhance performance might be as old as sport itself. As with many early drugs, some of these concoctions seemed to make sense at the time but probably had only placebo value. We no longer think that the powdered hooves of an ass will make our feet fly as fast as that animal's, but perhaps it was a belief in that powder that helped the ancient Egyptian competitor's self-confidence. Also, if the other guys are all using it, why take chances?

The early Greek Olympians did use various herbs and mushrooms that might have had some pharmacological actions as stimulants, and Aztec athletes used a cactus-based stimulant resembling strychnine. Athletic competitions probably developed in tribal societies as a means of training and preparation for war or for hunting, and various psychoactive plants were used by tribal peoples during battles or hunts, so it is not surprising that the drugs were also used in "sports" from the beginning.

Early Use of Stimulants

During the 1800s and early 1900s, three types of stimulants were reported to be in use by athletes. *Strychnine*, which became famous as a rat poison, can at low doses act as a central nervous system stimulant. However, if the dose is too high, seizure activity will be produced in the brain. The resulting convulsions can paralyze respiration, leading to death. At least some boxers were reported to have used strychnine tablets. This might have made them more aggressive and kept them from tiring very quickly, but it was a dangerous way to do it. We'll never know how many of those rugged heroes were killed in this way, but there must have been a few. Thomas Hicks won the marathon in the 1904 St. Louis Olympics, then collapsed and had to be revived. His race was partly fueled by a mixture of brandy and strychnine.[1] Although the availability of amphetamines later made dangerous drugs such as strychnine less attractive, there is some evidence that occasional use of strychnine continued at the level of world competition into the 1960s.

Cocaine was also available in the 1800s, at first in the form of Mariani's Coca Wine (used by the French cycling team), which was referred to in some advertisements as "wine for athletes."[2] When pure cocaine became available, athletes quickly adopted this more potent form. Many athletes used coffee as a mild stimulant, and some added pure *caffeine* to their coffee or took caffeine tablets. There were numerous reports of the suspected "doping" of swimmers, cyclists, boxers, runners, and other athletes during this period. Then, as now, some of the suspicions were raised by the losers, who might or might not have had any evidence of doping. Our use of the word *dope* for illicit drugs is derived from a Dutch word used in South Africa to refer to a cheap brandy, which was sometimes given to racing dogs or horses to slow them down. From this came the idea of "doping" horses and then people, more often in an effort to improve rather than impair performance. Dogs and horses received all the substances used by humans, including coca wine and cocaine, before the days of testing for drugs.

Amphetamine

It isn't clear when athletes first started using amphetamines for their stimulant effects, but it was probably not long after the drugs were introduced in the 1930s. Amphetamines were widely used throughout the world during World War II, and in the 1940s and 1950s there were reports of the use of these "pep pills" by professional soccer players in England and Italy. Boxers and cyclists also relied on this new synthetic energy source. More potent than caffeine, longer-lasting than cocaine, and safer than strychnine, it seemed to be the ideal **ergogenic** (energy-producing) drug for both training and competition.

In 1952 the presence of syringes and broken ampules in the speed-skating locker room at the Oslo Winter Olympics was an indication of amphetamine's presence in international competition. There were other reports from the 1952 summer games in Helsinki and the 1956 Melbourne Olympics. Unfortunately, several deaths during this period were attributed to overdoses of amphetamines or other drugs. By the time of the 1960 Rome games, amphetamine use had spread around the world and to most sports. On opening day a Danish cyclist died during time trials. An autopsy revealed that his death resulting from "sunstroke" was aided by the presence of amphetamine, which reduces blood flow to the skin, making it more difficult for the body to cool itself. Three other cyclists collapsed that day, and two were hospitalized.[1] This and other examples of amphetamine abuse led to investigations and to antidoping laws in France and Belgium. Other nations, including the United States, seemed less concerned.

International Drug Testing

Some sports, especially cycling, began to test competitors for drugs on a sporadic basis. Throughout the 1960s there were instances of athletes refusing to submit to tests or failing tests and being disqualified. These early testing efforts were not enough to prevent the death of cyclist Tommy Simpson, an ex-world champion, who died during the 1967 *Tour de France*. His death was seen on television, and weeks later it was reported that his body contained two different types of amphetamine and that drugs had been found in his luggage. This caused the International Olympic Committee in 1968 to establish rules requiring the disqualification of any competitor who refuses to take a drug test or who is found guilty of using banned drugs. Beginning with fewer than 700 urine tests at the 1968 Mexico City Olympics, each subsequent international competition has had more testing, more disqualifications, and more controversy.

American Football

Most Americans did not seem to be very concerned about drug use by athletes until reports surfaced in the late 1960s and early 1970s that professional football players were using amphetamines during games. Before that time, people might not have been very concerned about it even if they had known. You should remember from chapter 7 that amphetamine underwent a major status change in the United States during the 1960s. For years an increasing number of Americans had used amphetamines to keep them awake, provide extra energy, or lose weight. They were seen by most people as legal, harmless "pep pills." It was in that context that the team physicians for professional football teams ordered large quantities of the drugs as a routine part of their supplies, and trainers dispensed them liberally.

By the end of the 1960s, amphetamine was widely considered to be a drug of abuse and a dangerous drug that could lead to violent behavior. In this context, revelations that many professionals were playing "high" made for sensational headlines. Several National Football League (NFL) players sued their teams for injuries received while playing under the influence of drugs, and the NFL officially banned the distribution of amphetamine by team physicians and trainers in 1971. Although the drugs were no longer condoned by the league, the NFL did little at that time to enforce the ban except to request copies of each team's orders for medical supplies. Athletes who wanted amphetamines still obtained and used them, often through a legal prescription from their own physician. The attitude seemed to be that if the players wanted to use pep pills and obtained them on their own, that was their business, but team physicians and trainers shouldn't be using medications to push the athletes beyond their normal endurance. The current NFL policy, of course, restricts all use of amphetamines, as well as many other drugs, no matter where they are obtained.

Steroids

During and after World War II it was found that malnourished people could gain weight and build themselves up more rapidly if they were given the male hormone testosterone. Although it is easy for an American to be biased about such things, it does appear that the Soviets were the first to put this hormone to use on a wide scale to build up their athletes. An American team physician at the 1956 Olympics reported that the Soviet athletes were using straight

---

ergogenic: (er go *gen* ic) producing work or energy; a general term for performance enhancement.

Winning

Imagine that you have gone out for the track team. You compete in the 3,000-meter races and have been training hard for the past two years. It seems as though you have worked as hard as you could every day, yet it's clear that your times have gotten as fast as they're going to get. The conference championships are tomorrow. Your parents have traveled 300 miles to see you run, and lots of your friends will be there cheering you on. You know your own times, and you know the competition, and, although you expect a close race for the top three spots, you figure to come in fourth. You yourself have never used any type of stimulant drug, but you have heard rumors that several of the fastest runners take amphetamines before the race, and you suspect that it is true. Your conference has not yet adopted a drug-screening program for track, however, so there's no way to know for sure.

Under these circumstances, what would you do if:

1. A guy that you don't know very well but who you heard is a drug dealer offers you some "speed" just for the race?
2. A friend of yours has some prescription diet pills that contain amphetamine, and the friend offers you one?
3. You are offered some cocaine to snort right before the race?
4. You are offered an OTC asthma pill that contains ephedrine?
5. You are offered coffee or tea?

Or would you rather not take artificial stimulants at all, come in fourth, and know you did your best and ran a clean race?

testosterone, sometimes in excessive doses and with unfortunate side effects. Testosterone not only helps both men and women become more muscular, its masculinizing effects on women and enlargement of the prostate gland in men are definite drawbacks. The American physician came back to the United States and helped to develop and test the more selective **anabolic** steroids, which were quickly adopted by American weightlifters and bodybuilders.[3]

American and British athletes in events such as discus and shotput were the first to acknowledge publicly that they had used steroids, and there was evidence that steroid use was widespread during the 1960s in most track and field events. These drugs were not officially banned, nor were they tested for in international competition until the early 1970s, mainly because a sensitive urine test was not available until then. Of the 2,000 urine samples taken during the 1976 Olympics, fewer than 300 were tested for the presence of steroids, and 8 of those were positive.[1] The first international athletes to be found guilty of taking steroids were a Bulgarian discus thrower, a Romanian shot-putter, a Polish female discus thrower, and weightlifters from several countries. By that time, the situation appeared to be that individual Western athletes might have chosen to use steroids, but some of the East European countries seemed to have adopted their use almost as a matter of official policy. When the East German swimming coach was asked during the 1976 Olympics why so many of their women swimmers had deep voices, the answer was, "We have come here to swim, not sing."[4]

Anabolic steroids. Testosterone, the male sex hormone, is sometimes abused by athletes for its protein-building (anabolic) effect.

Cocaine Again

During the 1980s, public revelations of drug use by athletes became commonplace and cocaine was often mentioned. Professional basketball, baseball, and football players in the United States were being sent into treatment centers for cocaine dependence, and several either dropped out or were kicked out of professional sports. Most amateur and professional sports organizations adopted longer and more complicated lists of banned substances and rules providing for more and more participants to be tested. For example, the U.S. National Collegiate Athletic Association (NCAA) adopted in 1986 a list of over three thousand brand-name drugs containing banned substances. All participants are to be tested during the championship contest and after all postseason football games. In many events around the world, all contestants must now be subjected to urine tests as a matter of routine.

By the end of the 1980s, some were beginning to question the wisdom of trying to test every athlete for everything. In spite of the enormous expense to which sport organizations have gone, the use of steroids, stimulants, and other performance-enhancing substances seems to some to be as great as ever. So far, however, both the extent of testing and the ingenuity of athletes trying to beat the tests continue to escalate.

STIMULANTS AS PERFORMANCE ENHANCERS

The first question to be answered about the use of a drug to increase energy or otherwise enhance athletic performance is, Does it work? We might not worry so much about unfair competition if we didn't feel that the use of a drug would really help the person using it. There is another reason why it would be nice if these drugs were ineffective: if we could prove that, then we could presumably convince young people not to take the risk of using drugs because there would be no gain to be had. It is worthwhile pointing out that experiments can never prove that a drug has no effect—you might have done a hundred experiments and not used the right dose or the right test (peak output? endurance? accuracy?). The possibility always exists that someone could come along later with the right combination to demonstrate a beneficial effect. Therefore be wary when someone tries to use scientific evidence to argue that some drug "doesn't work," "has no effect," "is not toxic," or is otherwise inactive.

We've had a pretty good idea of the effectiveness of amphetamine since 1959, when Smith and Beecher published the results of a double-blind study comparing amphetamine and placebo in runners, swimmers, and weight

---

anabolic (**an a** *ball* ick) promoting constructive metabolism; building tissue.

throwers.[5] Their conclusion was that most of the athletes performed better under amphetamine, but the improvement was small (a few percentage points' improvement). There have been several studies that reported no differences or very small differences in performance, and some medical experts in the 1960s wanted to argue that amphetamines were essentially ineffective and there was no reason for people to use them. An excellent 1981 review of the existing literature put it all into perspective.[6] Pointing out that it had been taking athletes an average of about seven years for each 1 percent improvement in the world record speed for the mile run, if amphetamine produces even a 1 percent improvement it could make an important difference at that level of competition. Their conclusion: "There is an amphetamine margin. It is usually small, amounting to a few percent under most circumstances. But even when that tiny, it can surely spell the difference between a gold medal and sixth place."

Whether amphetamine or other stimulants increase physical ability (provide "pep," or energy) or produce their actions only through effects on the brain is an interesting question that might not be answerable. Surely a person who feels more confident might train harder, compete with a winning attitude, try harder, and keep trying longer. With amphetamine, improvements have been seen both in events requiring brief, explosive power (shotput) and in events requiring endurance, such as distance running. In laboratory studies, increases have been found in isometric strength and in work output during endurance testing on a stationary bicycle (the subjects rode longer under amphetamine conditions). This endurance improvement could be due to the masking of fatigue effects, allowing a person to compete to utter exhaustion.

Caffeine has also been shown to improve endurance performance under laboratory conditions. In one experiment, 330 mg of caffeine (approximately equivalent to three cups of brewed coffee) increased the length of a stationary bi-

cycle "ride" by almost 20 percent. In another experiment, when subjects rode for two hours, their total energy output was 7 percent higher after 500 mg caffeine than in the control condition.[7] The effectiveness of caffeine might depend upon other factors: for example, a recent study reported no benefit from caffeine when athletes ran long distances (twelve miles) in hot, humid conditions.[8] Small amounts of caffeine are acceptable in most sports, but a urine level above 12 micrograms/mL will lead to disqualification in many competitions. The doses needed to produce large performance increases will produce much higher levels than that, but there could still be a slight improvement even at "legal" levels.

Apparently there have not been any controlled laboratory or field experiments testing the performance-enhancing capabilities of cocaine, but especially during the 1980s there were many athletes who believed in its power. Cocaine's stimulant properties are generally similar to those of amphetamine, so we can assume that it would be effective under some circumstances. Given cocaine's shorter duration of action, it would not be expected to improve endurance over a several-hour period as well as either amphetamine or caffeine.

With all these and several other CNS stimulants banned by most sport associations, some athletes have continued to use them during training, to allow them to run or ride or swim harder. They then do not use the drug for several days before the competition or during the competition, hoping that traces of the substance will not appear in the urine test. This might make sense, but no one knows whether training under one drug condition has an effect on competition under another condition. Also, overexertion under the influence of a fatigue-masking drug might be most dangerous during training, leading to muscle injury, a fall or other accident, or heat exhaustion.

Athletes and others who use amphetamines or cocaine regularly run the risk of developing a dependence on the drug, developing paranoid or violent behavior patterns, and suffering from the loss of energy and psychological depression that occur as the drugs wear off (see chapter 7).

STEROIDS

The male sex hormone testosterone has two major types of effects on the developing human man. **Androgenic** effects refer to the masculinizing actions: initial growth of the penis and other male sex glands, deepening of the voice, and increased facial hair are examples. This steroid hormone also has *anabolic* effects. These include increased muscle mass, increases in the size of various internal organs, control of the distribution of body fat, increased protein synthesis, and increased calcium in the bones. Beginning in the 1950s, drug companies synthesized various steroids that have fewer of the androgenic effects and more of the anabolic effects than testosterone. These are referred to as *anabolic steroids*, although none of them is entirely free of some masculinizing effect.

Whether or not these drugs are effective in improving athletic performance has been controversial: for many years the medical position was that they are not, whereas the lore around the locker room was that they would make anyone bigger, stronger, and more masculine-looking. A lot of people must have had more faith in the locker-room lore than in the "official" word. The 1989 Physician's Desk Reference contained the following statement in bold-face type: "**Anabolic Steroids Have Not Been Shown To Enhance Athletic Ability**." Try telling that to Ben Johnson, the disqualified winner of the 1988 Olympic gold medal in the 100-meter run, or to the people who ran against him. That disclaimer is no longer required by the FDA.

There is no doubt that testosterone has a tremendous effect on muscle mass and strength during puberty, and experiments on castrated animals clearly show the muscle-developing

ability of the synthetic anabolics.[9] What is not so clear is the effect of adding additional anabolic stimulation to adolescent or adult males who already have high circulating levels of testosterone.

Laboratory research on healthy men who are engaged in weight training and are maintained on a proper diet has often found that anabolic steroids produce small increases in lean muscle mass and sometimes also small increases in muscular strength. There is no evidence for an overall increase in aerobic capacity or endurance in those studies. However, it might never be possible to conduct experiments demonstrating the effectiveness of the high doses used by some athletes. Many athletes report that they take ten or more times the dose of a steroid that has been tested and recommended for treatment of some specific disorder.[10] It is also common practice for athletes to take more than one steroid at a time (both an oral and an injectable form, for example). This practice is known as "stacking." To expose research subjects to such massive doses would clearly be unethical.

Another impediment to doing careful research on this topic is that these steroids do produce detectable psychological effects. When double-blind experiments have been attempted, the subjects almost always know when they are on steroids, thus destroying the blind control.[11] This is important because steroid users report that they feel they can lift more or work harder when they are on the steroids. This may be due to CNS effects of the steroids leading to a stimulant-like feeling of energy and loss of fatigue, or to increased aggressiveness expressed as more aggressive training. There is the further possibility of what is known as an *active placebo effect*, with a belief in the power of steroids, enhanced by the clear sensation that the drug is

---

androgenic (an drow *gen* ick) masculinizing.

FYI   Nutritional Ergogenic Aids

If athletes can't get or refuse to use pharmacological aids in athletic competition, most believe that certain foods or nutritional supplements are a "natural" way to enhance their performance. Following is a very abbreviated description of a more complete review of this topic by Melvin H. Williams, Ph.D. (*Nutrition Today*, Jan/Feb 1989, pp 7–14):

Amino acids are the natural building blocks of muscle, and one certainly requires a basic minimum intake of them in order to maintain normal protein synthesis and other functions (including the synthesis of some neurotransmitters). However, there is no scientific evidence to support the idea that supplementing with amino acids or extra protein above the recommended daily allowance will have any beneficial effect at all on muscle development, strength, speed, or endurance. Marketers of these "muscle-building" dietary supplements walk a fine line by avoiding making specific claims on the product labels, so they do not fall under the FDA's rules for demonstrating effectiveness. Usually nearby posters or pamphlets link amino acids to the idea of muscle growth. These supplements are probably of little or no value to an athlete who is receiving proper nutrition.

Carbohydrates are burned as fuels, especially during prolonged aerobic exercise. Carbohydrates taken immediately before or during an endurance performance lasting for more than an hour may enhance the performance by maintaining blood glucose levels and preventing the depletion of muscle stores of glycogen. Carbohydrate "loading" before marathon runs consists of resting for the last day or two while ingesting extra carbohydrates, increasing both muscle and liver stores of carbohydrates. In either case, there is not much evidence to support the value of carbohydrate supplements for athletic performances lasting less than an hour.

Fats, in experiments with fat supplements, have not been found to be a useful ergogenic aid.

continued

doing something because you can "feel" it. Until recently, many of the scientists studying steroid hormones believed that their main effects are psychological, combined with a "bloating" effect on the muscle, in which the muscle retains more fluids, is larger and weighs more, but has no more physical strength.[1]

Psychological Effects

The reported psychological effects, including a stimulant-like "high" and increased aggressiveness, might be beneficial for increasing the amount of work done during training and for increasing the intensity of effort during competition. However, there are also concerns that these psychological effects might produce great problems, especially at high doses. One concern that has been expressed is that a psychological dependence seems to develop in some users, who feel well when they are on the steroids but become depressed when they are off them. Many users take the drugs in cycles, and their

FYI   Nutritional Ergogenic Aids—continued

Vitamins, especially the water-soluble B vitamins, are necessary for normal utilization of food energy. Deficiencies in these vitamins, such as might result when a wrestler is dieting to meet a weight limit, can clearly impair physical performance. However, once the necessary minimum amount is available for metabolic purposes, further supplements are of no value. Many experiments have been done with supplements of C, E, and B complex vitamins or with multivitamin supplements, the so-called vitamin B_{15}, and with bee pollen, and there is no evidence for enhanced performance or faster recovery after workouts. Again, these supplements are probably of no value to an athlete who is receiving proper nutrition.

Minerals, in the form of various mineral supplements, are widely used by athletes. Once again, most are probably not needed or useful, but there may be some exceptions. Electrolyte drinks are designed to replace both fluids and electrolytes such as sodium and chloride that are lost in sweat. Actually, sweat contains a lower concentration of these

electrolytes than does blood, so it is more important to replace the fluids than the electrolytes under most circumstances. Sodium supplementation may be useful for those engaged in ultraendurance events such as 100-mile runs.

Iron supplements are helpful in athletes who are iron-deficient, as may occur especially in female distance runners. However, if iron status is normal, there is probably no value in iron supplements.

The jury is still out on whether sodium bicarbonate (baking soda) enhances performance in anaerobic events such as 400- to 800-meter runs. Some studies indicate improvements, whereas others do not. The same may be said for phosphate loading, which is currently receiving some research attention.

Water is needed by endurance athletes to keep their body temperatures down, especially in a warm environment. Drinking water both before and during prolonged exercise can deter dehydration and improve performance.

up-and-down mood swings can also interfere with their social relationships and other life functions.

There has been a great deal of discussion about "roid rage," a kind of manic rage that has been reported by some steroid users.[12] We should be careful about attributing instances of violence to a drug on the basis of uncontrolled retrospective reports, especially when the perpetrator of a violent crime might be looking for an excuse.[13] However, there is a sufficient number of reports of violent feelings and actions among

steroid users for us to be concerned and to await further research. Says Dr. William Taylor, a leading authority on anabolic steroids, "I've seen total personality changes. A passive, low-key guy goes on steroids for muscle enhancement, and the next thing you know, he's being arrested for assault or disorderly conduct."[14]

Adverse Effects on the Body

There are also many concerns about the effects of steroid use on the body. In young users who have not attained their full height, these steroids can cause premature closing of the growth plates of the long bones, thus limiting their adult height. For all users the risk of peliosis hepatitis (bloody cysts in the liver) and the changes in blood lipids possibly leading to atherosclerosis, high blood pressure, and heart disease are potentially serious concerns. Acne and baldness are reported, as are atrophy of the testes and the development of feminine breasts in men using anabolic steroids.

There are special considerations when women use these anabolic steroids. Because women usually have only trace amounts of testosterone produced by the adrenals, the addition of even relatively small doses of anabolic steroids can have dramatic effects, in terms of both muscle growth and masculinization. Some of the side effects such as mild acne, decreased breast size, and fluid retention; are reversible. The enlargement of the clitoris might be reversible if steroid use is stopped soon after it is noticed. Other effects, such as increased facial hair and deepening of the voice, could be irreversible.[11]

Regulation of Anabolic Steroids

As we found in chapter 2, when a drug produces dependence, violent crime, and toxic side effects, society may feel justified in trying to place special restrictions on the drug's availability. In 1988, congressional hearings were held on the notion of placing anabolic steroids on the list of controlled substances. Evidence was presented that a large black market has developed for these drugs, amounting to perhaps $100 million per year. In addition, there was concern that adolescent boys, many of whom are not athletic at all, had begun to use steroids in the belief that they would quickly become more muscular and "macho" looking.[15] As part of the Omnibus Crime Control Act of 1990, anabolic steroids became listed as a Schedule III controlled substance, requiring more record-keeping and limited prescription refills.[16]

OTHER HORMONAL MANIPULATIONS

Whereas the anabolic steroids have been in wide use, other treatments have been experimented with on a more limited basis. Female sex hormones have been used to feminize men so that they can compete in women's events. The woman's gold medal sprinter in the 1964 Olympics was shown by chromosome testing to be a man, and she/he had to return the medal. Hormone receptor blocking drugs have probably been used to delay puberty in female gymnasts. In women, puberty shifts the center of gravity lower in the body and changes body proportions in ways that adversely affect performance in some gymnastic events. Smaller women appear to be more graceful, spin faster on the uneven bars, and generally have the advantage, which is why top female gymnasts are usually in their teens. However, the Soviets were suspected of tampering with nature: their top three international gymnasts in 1978 were all seventeen or eighteen years old, but these were their heights and weights: 53 inches, 63 pounds; 60 inches, 90 pounds; and 57 inches, 79 pounds.

We have certainly not seen the end of growth-promoting hormonal treatments. **Human growth hormone**, which is released from the pituitary gland, can potentially increase the height and weight of an individual to gigantic proportions, especially if administered during childhood and adolescence. In fact, in rare instances the excessive production of this hormone creates giants well over seven feet tall. These giants usually die at an early age because their internal organs continue to grow. However, administration of a few doses of this hormone at the right time might produce a more controlled increase in body size. Likewise, the growth-hormone-releasing hormone, and some of the cellular intermediary hormones by which growth hormone exerts its effects, might work to

---

UP FOR DEBATE

Did Creatine Kill Wrestlers?

In 1997, three wrestlers died while in training, and traces of creatine were found in one of the young men. Sensational news articles followed in which the death was linked to creatine use. However, a look at what this athlete had done might indicate a different explanation.[18] Jeff Reese, the twenty-one-year-old wrestler who was found to have elevated levels of creatine in his blood, had worked out for two hours in a 92 °F gym wearing a rubber suit, in an attempt to lose twelve pounds in a single day. The other two wrestlers were undertaking similar extreme measures when they died, and there is no evidence they were using creatine. Clearly, we cannot say that creatine caused Jeff's death. With thousands of users out there, the risk of acute toxicity appears to be small. What we don't yet know is the effect of chronic use for months or years at a time. Although creatine is considered a dietary supplement, it is being used in a druglike manner: a pure chemical taken in doses well above normal physiological ranges. No matter how safe creatine appears to be now, we should be cautious about long-term use until more is known.

---

enhance growth. It is not currently possible to test for the presence of these substances. In spite of the possible dangers, the lure of an otherwise capable basketball player growing a couple of inches taller or of a football player being thirty pounds heavier has no doubt caused many young athletes to experiment with these substances. Experiments in which growth hormone was given to adult men have found no increase in muscle protein synthesis or in strength.[11] The 1990 legislation that placed anabolic steroids on the list of controlled substances also made it a crime to distribute human growth hormone for nonmedical purposes.

BETA-2 AGONISTS

At the beginning of the 1992 Olympics, the leader of the British team was disqualified because of the detection of a new drug most of us had never heard of. Clenbuterol was developed as a treatment for asthma and is a relative of several other bronchodilators that are found in prescription inhalers. These drugs have sympathomimetic effects on the bronchi of the lungs but are designed to be more specific than older sympathomimetics such as ephedrine or amphetamine (see chapter 7). Their specificity comes from a selective stimulation of the beta-2 subtype of adrenergic receptors. Research with cows had revealed an increase in muscle mass, and there was beginning to be speculation that this might represent a new type of nonsteroidal anabolic agent. Apparently someone in Great Britain was keeping an eye on the animal research literature and decided to try out the anabolic actions on at least one Olympic athlete. Presumably it was hoped that such a new drug

---

human growth hormone: a pituitary hormone responsible for some types of giantism.

would not be tested for, but the Olympic officials were also well informed and ready, at least for clenbuterol. More recent human studies have shown some increases in strength of selected muscle types with clenbuterol or a similar drug, but there is no evidence that beta-2 agonists improve athletic performance.[17]

CREATINE

The big news for body builders of late has been creatine, a natural substance found in meat and fish. This is a legal product sold as a food supplement. There is clear evidence that creatine helps to regenerate ATP, which provides the energy for muscle contractions. Users of creatine tend to gain some weight, some of which is water weight. There is considerable evidence now that the use of creatine can improve strength and short-term speed in sprinting. However, studies of longer-distance running, cycling and swimming often find no effect, and in one case a significant slowing was reported, probably due to weight gain.[3]

SUMMARY

- Performance-enhancing drugs have been used by athletes throughout history.
- Athletic use of stimulants appears to have increased and spread to most sports with the use of amphetamines during the 1950s and 1960s.
- Amphetamine and caffeine have both been shown to increase work output and to mask the effects of fatigue.
- Some athletes continue to use stimulants for training, in spite of the dangers of injury and overexertion.
- Anabolic steroids are capable of increasing muscle mass and probably strength, although it has been difficult to separate the psychological stimulant-like effect of these drugs from the physical effects on the muscles themselves.
- Anabolic steroids can also produce a variety of dangerous and sometimes irreversible side effects.
- It is difficult to do ethical and well-controlled research on the effects of steroids.
- Growth hormones and related substances might be the next problem to arise.
- Creatine is a legally available nutritional supplement that can increase strength but might slow distance runners because of resultant weight gain.

REVIEW QUESTIONS

1. What was the first type of stimulant drug reported to be used by boxers and other athletes in the 1800s?
2. What was the first type of drug known to be widely used in international competition and that led to the first Olympic urine-testing programs?
3. When and in what country were the selective anabolic steroids first developed?
4. Do amphetamine and caffeine actually enhance athletic performance? If so, how much?
5. What muscle effect do we know for certain that anabolic steroids can produce in healthy men?
6. What is meant by "roid rage," and what double-blind studies have been done on this phenomenon?
7. What specific effect of anabolic steroids might be of concern to young users? To females?
8. How might the Soviets have kept their female gymnasts under five feet tall?
9. Why do "pituitary giants" often die at an early age?
10. How does creatine work to increase strength?

Related Internet Sites on Drugs in Sport

Steroids and ergogenic aids: http://plainfield.bypass.com/~twilbur/steroids.html

Ergogenic aids: http://www.brianmac.demon.co.uk/drugs.htm

What athletes are using: http://www.physsportsmed.com/issues/1997/04apr/eichner.htm

And don't forget to check our *Drugs, Society, and Human Behavior* site: http://www.uwyo.edu/A&S/psyc/dshb.htm

REFERENCES

1. Donohue T, Johnson N: *Foul play: drug abuse in sports,* Oxford, 1986, Basil Blackwell.
2. Asken MJ: *Dying to win: the athlete's guide to safe and unsafe drugs in sports,* Washington, DC, 1988, Acropolis.
3. Eichner ER: Ergogenic aids: What athletes are using—and why, *Physician and Sportsmedicine* 25:70–83, 1997.
4. Goldman B: *Death in the locker room,* South Bend, Ind, 1984, Icarus Press.
5. Smith GM, Beecher HK: Amphetamine sulfate and athletic performance, *JAMA* 170:542–557, 1959.
6. Laties VG, Weiss B: The amphetamine margin in sports, *Federation Proceedings* 40:2689–2692, 1981.
7. Noble BJ: *Physiology of exercise and sport,* St Louis, 1986, Mosby.
8. Cohen BS and others: Effects of caffeine ingestion on endurance racing in heat and humidity, *European J Appl Physiology* 73:358–363, 1996.
9. Williams MH: *Ergogenic aids in sports,* Champaign, Ill, 1983, Human Kinetics.
10. Marshall E: The drug of champions, *Science* 242:183–184, 1988.
11. Yarasheski KE and others: Short-term growth hormone treatment does not increase muscle protein synthesis in experienced weight lifters, *J Appl Physiology* 74:3073–3076, 1993.
12. Pope HG, Katz DL: Affective and psychotic symptoms associated with anabolic steroid use, *Am J Psychiatry* 145:487–490, 1988.
13. Lubell A: Does steroid abuse cause—or excuse—violence? *Physician and Sportsmedicine* 17:176–185, 1989.
14. Fultz O: 'Roid rage, *Am Health* 10:60, 1991.
15. Toufexis A: Shortcut to the Rambo look, *Time,* p 78, Jan 30, 1989.
16. Nightingale SL: Anabolic steroids as controlled substances, *JAMA* 265:1229, 1991.
17. Spann S: Effect of clenbuterol on athletic performance, *Ann Pharmacother* 29:75, 1995.
18. Tarlach GM: Creatine controversy, *Drug Topics,* Feb 2, 1998.

ASSESS YOURSELF!

Street Names

Draw lines to match these "street names" for drugs and related things (left-hand column) with the appropriate item in the right-hand column:

Mexican brown	red oil of Cannabis
STP	smuggler who carries the drug personally
joint	occasional heroin user
chipper	one type of illicit heroin
sherm	an LSD experience
mule	dimethoxymethamphetamine (DOM)
ganja	heroin
trip	marijuana cigarette
smack	marijuana plus PCP ("angel dust")
acid	marijuana in India (and Jamaica)
hash oil	illicit fentanyl or a derivative
dime bag	MDMA
XTC	LSD
China white	$10 worth of heroin

7

Reducing the Demand

American society has done more than condemn the use of drugs—we have taken steps to reduce the number of young people who begin using illicit drugs, and we have established a variety of public and private treatment methods for helping some users to become ex-users. Section 7 explores some of these methods.

19 Breaking the Cycle

What kinds of prevention programs have been tested in the schools, and which ones seem to be effective? What can parents and communities do?

19

Breaking the Cycle

KEY TERMS	OBJECTIVES

After reading this chapter, you should be able to:

values clarification
alternatives
social influence model
DARE

- Distinguish between the goals of drug education and the goals of drug abuse prevention.
- Describe the evolution of prevention models used in public schools from the 1960s to the 1990s.
- Explain why smoking prevention has become a model for prevention of other drug use.

- Describe the effective components of the social influence model.
- Explain how approaches involving peers, families, and other community agencies can be used to strengthen school-based approaches.
- Discuss a rational approach to prevention programs in your own community.

Why can't we *do* something to keep young people from ruining their lives with drugs? As our society seeks to prevent drug abuse by limiting the availability of such drugs as heroin and cocaine, we are forced to recognize several other facts. First, as long as there is a sizable market for these substances, there will be people to supply them. Thus only if we can teach people not to want the drugs can we attack the source of the problem. Second, these substances will never disappear entirely, so we should try to teach people to live in a world that includes them. Third, our society has accepted the continued existence of tobacco and alcohol, yet some people are harmed by them. Can we teach people to coexist with both legal and illegal substances and to live in such a way that their lives and health are not impaired by them?

DEFINING GOALS AND EVALUATING OUTCOMES

Think about the process you are engaged in while reading and studying from this book. The text is aimed at teaching its readers about drugs: their effects, how they are used, and how they relate to society. The goal of the authors is *education*. A person who understands all this information about all these drugs will perhaps be better prepared to make decisions about personal drug use, more able to understand drug use by others, and better prepared to participate in social decisions about drug use and abuse. We would hope that a person who knew all this would be in a position to act more rationally, neither glorifying a drug and expecting miraculous changes from using it nor condemning it as the essence of evil. But our ultimate goal is not to change the reader's behavior in a particular direction. For example, the chapter on alcohol, although pointing out the dangers of its use and the problems it can cause, did not attempt to influence the readers to avoid all alcohol use. In a purely educational program, the primary goal is not to alter a person's drug-taking behavior. Our success would be measured by how much a person knew about alcohol or tobacco or marijuana, not by whether a reader of this book is convinced never to drink or smoke.

On the other hand, there exists an old tradition, going back to the "demon rum" programs of the late 1800s, of presenting negative information about alcohol or drugs in the public schools with the clear goal of *prevention* of use. Some of these early programs presented information that was so clearly one-sided that they could have been classified as propaganda rather than education. We would not measure the success of such a program by how much objective information the students gained about the pharmacology of the narcotics, for example. A more appropriate index might be how many of the students did subsequently experiment with the drugs against which the program was aimed. Until the early 1970s it was simply assumed that these programs would have the desired effect, and few attempts were made to evaluate them.

STAGES OF PREVENTION

The goals and methods of a prevention program also depend on the drug-using status of those served by the program. The programs designed to prevent young people from starting smoking might be different from those used to try to prevent relapse in smokers who have quit, for example. Borrowing an idea developed in the mental health field, drug-abuse prevention theorists have discussed three levels or stages of prevention (table 19.1).

TABLE 19.1

Stages of Prevention

Stage	Clientele	Example
Primary	Young, little or no experience with psychoactive substances	School-based smoking prevention programs
Secondary	Experienced with some psychoactive substances, not in need of treatment	College-based programs in resposible alcohol use
Tertiary	Postreatment	Relapse prevention

- **Primary** prevention programs are those aimed mainly at young people who have not yet tried the substances in question or who may have tried tobacco or alcohol a few times. As discussed in the previous section, such programs might encourage complete abstinence from specific drugs or might have the broader goal of teaching people how to view drugs and the potential influences of drugs on their lives, emotions, and social relationships. Because those programs are presented to people with little personal experience with drugs, they might be expected to be especially effective. On the other hand, there is the danger of introducing large numbers of children to information about a number of drugs that they might otherwise never have heard of, thus arousing their curiosity about them.
- **Secondary** prevention programs could be thought of as designed for people who have tried the drug in question or a variety of other substances. The goals of such programs are usually the prevention of the use of other, more dangerous substances or preventing the development of more dangerous forms of use of the substances they are already experimenting with. We might describe the clientele here as more "sophisticated" substance users who have not suffered seriously from

their drug experiences and who are not obvious candidates for treatment. Many college students would fall into this category, and programs aimed at encouraging responsible use of alcohol among college students are good examples of this stage of prevention.

• **Tertiary** prevention, in our scheme, is relapse prevention, or follow-up programs. For alcoholics or cocaine or heroin addicts, treatment programs are the first order of priority. However, once a person has been treated or has stopped the substance use without assistance, we enter another stage of prevention. Relapse prevention was discussed under the concept of *aftercare* in chapter 3.

PREVENTION PROGRAMS IN THE SCHOOLS

The Knowledge-Attitudes-Behavior Model

After the increase in the use of illicit drugs by young middle-class people in the 1960s, there was a general sense that we were not doing an adequate job of drug education and most school systems increased their efforts. However, there was confusion over the methods to be used. Traditional antidrug programs had relied heavily on representatives of the local police who came in and told a few horror stories, describing the legal trouble due anyone who got caught with illicit drugs. Sometimes the officers showed what the drugs looked like or demonstrated the smell of burning marijuana so that the kids would know what to avoid. Sometimes, especially in larger cities, a former addict would come in and describe how easy it was to get "hooked," the horrible life of the junkie, and the horror of withdrawal symptoms. The 1960s saw more of that, plus the production of a large number of scary antidrug films.

There was also the awareness that teachers and counselors knew little about these substances, and many of them attended courses taught by experts in the field. Some of the experts were enforcement-oriented and presented the traditional scare-tactics information, whereas others were pharmacologists who presented the "dry facts" about the classification and effects of various drugs. Much of this factual information also found its way into the classrooms of the 1960s. It was later pointed out that the programs of this era were based on an assumed model: that providing information about drugs would increase the students' *knowledge* of drugs and their effects, this increased knowledge would lead to changes in *attitudes* about drug use, and these changed attitudes would be reflected in decreased drug-using *behavior*.[1]

In the early 1970s, this model began to be questioned. A 1971 study indicated that students who had more knowledge about drugs tended to have a more positive attitude toward drug use.[2] Of course, it may have been that pro-drug students were more interested in learning about drugs, so this was not an actual assessment of the value of drug education programs. A 1973 report by the same group indicated that four different types of drug education programs were equally effective in producing increased knowledge about drugs and equally ineffective in altering attitudes or behavior.[3] Nationwide, drug use had increased even with the increased emphasis on drug education. There began to be concern about the possibility that drug education may even have contributed to increased drug use. After all, before the 1960s use of marijuana or LSD was rare among school-age youngsters. Most of them didn't know much about these things, had given them little thought, and had probably never considered using them. Telling them over and over not to use drugs was a bit like telling a young boy not to put beans in his nose.[4] He probably hadn't thought of it before, and your warning gives him the idea. At least one study in 1972 found that junior high school students who were exposed to a "fact-oriented" course actually increased their experimentation with drugs.[5] These concerns led the federal government in 1973 to stop supporting the production of drug-abuse films and educational materials until they could determine what kinds of approaches would be effective.

At this point it seemed clear that the question of effectiveness depended greatly on the goals of the program. Do we want all students *never to experiment* with cigarettes, alcohol, marijuana, or other drugs? Or do we want students to be prepared to *make rational decisions* about drugs? For example, a 1976 report indicated that students in drug education programs did increase their use of drugs over the two years after the program, but they were less likely to show drastic escalation of the amount or type of drug use over that period, when compared with a control group.[6] Perhaps by giving the students information about drugs, we make them more likely to try them, but we also make them more aware of the dangers of excessive use. For a time in the 1970s it seemed as though teaching students to make rational decisions about their own drug use with the goal of reducing the overall harm produced by misuse and abuse could be a possible goal of such programs.

Affective Education

Educators have been talking for several years about education as including both a "cognitive domain" and an "*affective* domain," the domain of emotions and attitudes. One reason that young people might use psychoactive drugs is to produce certain feelings: of excitement, or relaxation, of power, of being in control. Or perhaps an individual child might not really want to take drugs but does so after being influenced by others. Helping children to know their own feelings and to express them, helping them to achieve altered emotional states without drugs, and teaching them to feel valued, accepted, and wanted are all presumed to be ways of reducing drug use.

Values clarification

The values clarification approach made the assumption that what was lacking in drug-using adolescents was not factual information about

drugs, but rather the ability to make appropriate decisions based on that information.[7] It was proposed that drug use should not be "flagged" for the students by having special curricula designed just for drugs, but that instead emphasis should be placed on teaching generic decision-making skills. Teaching students to analyze and clarify their own values in life is accomplished by having them discuss their reactions to various situations that pose moral and ethical dilemmas. It should be pointed out that groups of parents or other citizens who are concerned about drug abuse sometimes have great difficulty understanding and accepting these approaches because they do not take a direct antidrug approach. In the 1970s, when these programs were first developed, it seemed important that the schools not try to impose a particular set of values, but rather to allow for differences in religion, family background, etc. For this reason the programs were often said to be *value-free*. To many parents the purpose of **values clarification** training is not immediately clear, and teaching young children to decide moral issues for themselves may run contrary to the particular set of values the parents want their children to learn. Examples of values clarification strategies are given in the FYI box.

Alternatives to drugs

Along with values clarification, another aspect of affective education involved the teaching of **alternatives** to drug use (table 19.2). Under the assumption that students might take drugs for the experience, for the altered states of consciousness that a drug might produce, students are taught so-called natural highs, or altered states, that can be produced through relaxation

---

values clarification: teaching students to recognize and express their own feelings and beliefs.

alternatives: alternative nondrug activities such as relaxation or dancing.

FYI   Examples of Values Clarification Strategies*

Problem Solving

Kindergarten and first grade: Children are read a short story, "Amy and the Surprise." The children then discuss Amy's choices, learning that for every problem situation there may be many possible solutions.

Senior high: Students perform a play titled Alien Invasion. The students then respond to the proposal that aliens have consumed all drugs on the planet, OTC, prescription, and illegal. We have a chance to start over. Which drugs should we keep?

Coping Skills

Kindergarten and first grade: The puppet "Froggy" helps students explore the concept that there are certain feelings associated with stressful situations. They learn where these feelings come from and how to express them. Senior high: Students listen to songs about friendship, then discuss the qualities they consider important in a friend.

Self-Concept

Kindergarten and first grade: A puzzle, "One of the Bunch," is used to explore the experience of being included and accepted by a group.

Senior high: Students spin a "feel wheel" and disclose how they feel about the situation described on the wheel. A small group discussion focuses on different reactions to the same situation and how feelings can influence behavior.

*A few examples from "Here's Looking At You, Two," Comprehensive Health Education Foundation, Seattle, Wash.

---

exercises, meditation, vigorous exercise, or an exciting sport. Students are encouraged to try these things and to focus on the psychological changes that occur. These alternatives should be discussed with some degree of sensitivity to the audience; for example, it would make little sense to suggest to many inner-city thirteen-year-olds that such activities as scuba diving or snow skiing would be good alternatives to drugs.

Personal and social skills

Several studies have indicated that adolescents who smoke, drink, or use marijuana also get lower grades and are less involved in organized sports or school clubs. One view of this is that students might take up substance use in response to personal or social failure. Therefore teaching students how to communicate with others and giving them success experiences has been another component of affective education approaches. For example, one exercise that has been used is having the students operate a school store. This is done as a group effort with frequent group meetings. The involved students are expected to develop a sense of social and personal competence without using drugs. Another approach has been to have older students tutor younger students, which is again designed to give the older students a sense of competence. An experiment carried out between 1978 and 1983 in Napa, California, combined these approaches with a drug education course, small-group discussions led by teachers, and classroom management techniques designed to teach discipline and communication skills and to enhance the students' self-concepts.[8] Although a small effect on alcohol, marijuana, and cigarette

Adrenaline from exercise: a nondrug high

TABLE 19.2

Some Suggested Alternatives to Drug Use

Level of experience	Motives	Possible alternatives
Physical	Relaxation	Relaxation exercises
	Increased energy	Athletics, dancing
Sensory	Stimulation	Skydiving
	Magnify senses	Sensory awareness training
Interpersonal	Gain acceptance	Instruction in social customs
Spiritual/ mystical	Develop spiritual insight	Study of religions

use was found among the girls, the effects were gone by the one-year follow-up.

"Just Say No!"

A 1984 review[9] of prevention studies concluded that

(1) most substance abuse prevention programs have not contained adequate evaluation components; (2) increased knowledge has virtually no impact on substance abuse or on intentions to smoke, drink, or use drugs; (3) affective education approaches appear to be experiential in their orientation and to place too little emphasis on the acquisition of skills necessary to increase personal and social competence, particularly those skills needed to enable students to resist the various interpersonal pressures to begin using drugs; and (4) few studies have demonstrated any degree of success in terms of actual substance abuse prevention.

This last point is not entirely a criticism of the programs themselves but reflects the difficulty of demonstrating statistically significant changes in behavior over some period of time after the programs.

In response to the third point, that affective education approaches have been too general and experiential, the latest efforts at preventing drug use focus on teaching students to recognize peer pressure to use drugs and also teaching specific ways to respond to such pressures without using drugs. This is sometimes referred to as psychological inoculation. In addition to the focus on substance use, "refusal skills" and "pressure resistance" strategies are taught in a broader context of self-assertion and social skills training. The first successful application of this technique was a film in which young actors act out situations in which one person is being pressured to smoke cigarettes. The film then demonstrated effective ways of responding to the pressure gracefully without smoking. After the film, students discuss alternative strategies and practice the coping techniques presented in the film. This approach has been demonstrated to be successful in reducing cigarette smoking in adolescent populations. It has been adapted for use with groups of various ages and for a wider variety of drugs and other behaviors, and students are taught from kindergarten on to "just say no" when someone is trying to get them to do something they know is wrong.

Drug-Free Schools

In 1986, under the direction of then Secretary of Education William J. Bennett, the federal

Alternatives to Drugs

As one part of many drug education programs, students are taught that they can produce natural highs, that is, altered states of consciousness similar to those produced by drugs, but without using drugs.

One such alternative that has been mentioned in these programs is skydiving. Obviously an activity of that sort has all the glamour, danger, and excitement most of us would want. Maybe if the kids could do this whenever they wanted, they wouldn't want to try cocaine or marijuana. But let's examine this as an alternative for a bunch of junior high school kids. First, there's the matter of cost and availability. How realistic is it to think that most of these kids would have any access at all to skydiving? Second, there's the issue of convenience. Even if you were a little rich kid with your own airplane, parachute, and pilot, it's unlikely that you'd be able to go skydiving every afternoon after school. Drugs or alcohol may not provide the best highs in the world, but often they are easy to get and use compared with some of these other activities.

OK, so maybe skydiving isn't a *practical* alternative to drugs for a lot of people. Still, it seems more wholesome and desirable. Let's become social philosophers and ask ourselves why the image of a person skydiving is more positive than the image of a person snorting cocaine. After all, skydiving doesn't make any obvious contributions to society. Let us play devil's advocate and propose that skydiving is not preferable to taking cocaine. Either way, the person is engaged in dangerous, expensive, self-indulgent activity. Contrast skydiving with cocaine, and see if you can answer for yourself why skydiving has a more positive image than cocaine use. You may have to talk about this with several people before you get a consistent feeling for why our society respects one of these activities so much more than the other. What about skiing? Bungee-cord jumping?

government launched a massive program to support "drug-free schools and communities." Among other things, the government provided millions of dollars' worth of direct aid to local school districts to implement or enhance drug prevention activities. Along with this, the Department of Education produced a small book called *What Works: Schools without Drugs,*[10] which made specific recommendations for schools to follow. This book did not recommend a specific curriculum, and in fact its most significant feature was the emphasis on factors other than curriculum, such as school policies on drug and alcohol use. There are suggestions for policies regarding locker searches, suspension, and expulsion of students. The purpose is not so much to take a punitive approach to alcohol or drug use as to point out through example and through official policy that the school and community are opposed to drug use and to alcohol use by minors. Following this general drug-free lead, schools adopted "tobacco-free" policies stating that not only the students but also teachers and other staff people are not to use tobacco products at school or on school-sponsored trips or activities.

According to this approach, the curriculum should include teaching about the laws against drugs as well as about the school policies. In other words, as opposed to the 1970s values

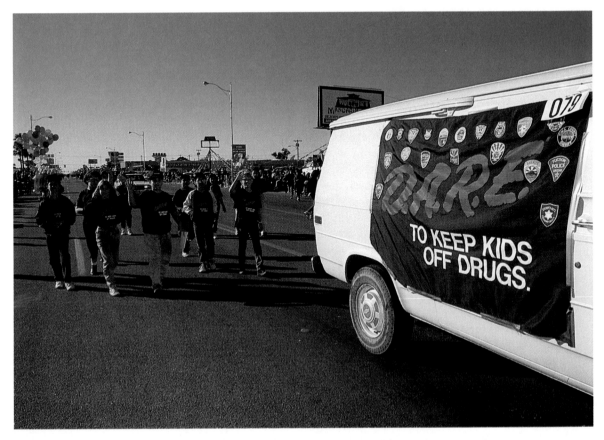

DARE volunteers march in a parade, showing support for the nationwide program.

clarification approach of teaching students how to make responsible decisions for themselves, this approach wants to make it clear to the students that the society at large, the community in which they live, and the school in which they study have already made the decision not to condone drug use or underage alcohol use. This seems to be part of a more general educational trend away from "value-free" schools toward teaching values that are generally accepted in our society. Under the later revisions of this law, for schools to be eligible for funding they must certify that their program teaches that "illicit drug use is wrong and harmful."

Student Assistance Programs

One type of approach that has become popular in high schools and junior high schools is based on the realization that there are many factors that can place a particular child at risk for using illicit drugs (now considered to include alcohol for these young people). These can range from not doing well academically to parental problems (divorce, mental illness, alcoholism) to depression to having friends who drink or use drugs. All students are invited to join or form groups to discuss these issues and to support each other, with the idea that dealing with the

Preventing Inhalant Abuse

The abuse by children of spray paints and other products containing solvents appears to have increased somewhat in recent years (see chapter 8). There are several characteristics of this type of abuse that make it an interesting problem for prevention workers. First, the variety of available products and their ready availability in stores, the home, and even in schools makes preventing access to the inhalants a virtual impossibility. Second, it's probably true that most of the kids who use these substances know it's unhealthy and dangerous to do so, so further information of that sort may not add much in the way of preventing their use. Third, this use is very "faddish"—a group of eighth-graders in one school might start inhaling Scotchguard, a group of sixth-graders in another neighborhood might be into gold paint (in distinct preference to black, yellow, or white).

Given these characteristics, where does a school-based prevention-education program begin to attack the problem? Do you focus on a particular product and try to talk kids out of using gold paint? Do you talk about a whole variety of products and thereby perhaps introduce the kids to new things they hadn't thought of? One very good videotape *(Inhalants: Kids in Danger, Adults in the Dark)* takes the approach of attempting to inform parents and teachers of the varieties of paints, perfumes, solvents, and other spray products used by abusers and also to inform them of some of the subterfuges used by some of the kids (carrying a small cologne vial to school, spraying paint into empty soft drink cans, etc.). However, the video is NOT to be shown to children, because it describes exactly what to do and how to do it. Probably the best idea is to reinforce to children in general terms the dangers of inhalants and not describe any particular substance or method of use in the prevention classes.

risk factor in a direct way should reduce the chances of drug use.

The structures of these groups vary considerably. Some are "facilitated" by professional counselors, others by teachers or parents who have received some specific training in these student support groups.

Peer Counseling

Several formalized programs have been developed for the selection and training of respected student leaders to be made available as "peer counselors" to discuss problems other students may be having. Usually the students are selected for such programs after being nominated by other students or by teachers or counselors. It is best to try to recruit respected students from various social groups in the school (i.e., they shouldn't all be "jocks" or student council leaders). The students are then given training in listening skills, in how to limit the advice or suggestions they provide, and in the resources available for referral of serious problems.

Development of the Social Influence Model

Some of the most sophisticated prevention research in recent years has been focused directly on cigarette smoking in adolescents. This problem has two major advantages over other types of drug use, as far as prevention research is concerned. First, a large enough fraction of adolescents do smoke cigarettes so that measurable behavior change is possible in a group of subjects of reasonable size. In contrast, one would have to perform an intervention with tens of thousands of people before significant alterations in the proportion of heroin users would be statistically evident. Second, the health consequences of smoking are so clear with respect to cancer and heart disease that there is a fairly good consensus over goals: we'd like to prevent adolescents from becoming smokers at all. One research advantage is that there is a relatively simple verification available for self-reported use of tobacco: saliva samples can be measured for cotinine, a nicotine metabolite.

Virtually all the various approaches to drug-abuse prevention have been tried with smoking behavior; in fact, Evans's 1976 smoking prevention paper introduced the use of the psychological inoculation approach based on the **social influence model.**[11] Out of all this research, certain consistencies appear. The most important of these is that it *is* possible to design smoking prevention programs that will be effective in reducing the number of adolescents who begin smoking. Some practical lessons about the components of those programs have also emerged.[12] For example, presenting information about the delayed consequences of smoking (possible lung cancer many years later) is deemed to be relatively ineffective. Information about the immediate physiological effects (increased heart rate, shortness of breath) is included instead. Some of the most important key elements that were shown to be effective were the following.

- **Training refusal skills.** (For example, eight ways to say no.) This was originally based on films demonstrating the kinds of social pressures that peers might use to encourage smoking and modeling a variety of appropriate responses. Then the students engage in role-playing exercises in which they practice these refusal skills. By using such techniques as changing the subject or having a good excuse handy, students learn to refuse to

"cooperate" without being negative. When all else fails, however, they are taught to be assertive and insist on their right to refuse.
- **Public commitment.** Researchers found that having each child stand before his or her peers and promise not to start smoking and signing a pledge not to smoke were effective prevention techniques.
- **Countering advertising.** Students are shown examples of cigarette advertising, and then the "hidden messages" are discussed (young, attractive, healthy, active models are typically used; cigarette smoking might be associated with dating or with sports). Then the logical inconsistencies between these hidden messages and the actual effects of cigarette smoking (e.g., bad breath, yellow teeth, shortness of breath) are pointed out. The purpose of this is to "inoculate" the children against cigarette advertising by teaching them to question its messages.
- **Normative education.** Adolescents tend to overestimate the proportion of their peers who smoke. Presenting factual information about the smoking practices of adolescents provides students with a more realistic picture of the true social norms regarding smoking and reduces the "everybody is doing it" attitude. When possible, statistics on smoking from the specific school or community should be used in presenting this information.
- **Use of teen leaders.** Presenting dry facts about the actual proportion of smokers should ideally be reinforced by example. If you're presenting the program to junior high students, it's one thing to *say* that fewer than one-fifth of the high school students in that community smoke, but it's another to bring a few high school students into the room and

---

social influence model: a prevention model adopted from successful smoking programs.

have them discuss the fact that they don't smoke, their friends don't, their attitude about smokers, and how they have dealt with others' attempts to get them to smoke.

Possible improvements to those approaches are offered by the *cognitive developmental* approach to smoking behavior. McCarthy[13] has criticized the social influence/social skills training model for assuming that all students should be taught social skills or refusal skills without regard to whether they need such training. The model "is that of a defenseless teenager who, for lack of general social skills or refusal skills, passively accedes to social pressures to smoke." An alternative model[14] has been proposed in which the individual makes active, conscious decisions about smoking as part of a process of defining herself or himself as a person experimenting with smoking, becoming a smoker, or as a confirmed smoker. The decision-making processes, and thus the appropriate prevention strategy, might be different at each of these "stages of cognitive development" as a smoker. Furthermore, smokers who begin smoking very young behave differently than smokers who begin as older adolescents (e.g., those who start young show more unanimity in selecting the most popular brand).[13] Given what is known about cognitive and social development, perhaps programs should be tailored for the age group being targeted and for various stages in the development of smoking behavior. This model would not replace the social influence methods, which have been shown to be effective, but would modify them to take into account individual differences in smoking-related attitudes and behavior.

DARE

Perhaps the most amazing educational phenomenon in a long time had fairly modest beginnings in 1983 as a joint project of the Los Angeles police department and school district. Those who are familiar with the Drug Abuse Resistance Education **(DARE)** program will

have recognized its components described under the social influence model of smoking cessation. The difference here was that the educational program was to be delivered by police officers in fifth- and sixth-grade classrooms. By basing the curriculum on sound educational research, by maintaining strict training standards for the officers who were to present the curriculum, and by encouraging the classroom teacher to participate, some of the old barriers to having nonteachers responsible for curriculum were overcome. The officers are in uniform, and they use interactive techniques as described for the social influence model. Most of the components are there: refusal skills, teen leaders, and a public commitment not to use illicit drugs. In addition, some of the "affective education" components are included: self-esteem building, alternatives to drug use, and decision making. The component on consequences of drug abuse is no doubt enhanced by the presence of a uniformed officer who can serve as an information source and symbol for concerns over gang activity and violence and discuss arrest and incarceration. The seventeen-week program is capped by a commencement assembly at which certificates are awarded.

This program happened to be in place at just the right time, both financially and politically. With the assistance of drug-free schools money and with nationwide enthusiasm for new drug prevention activities in the 1980s, the program spread rapidly across the United States. By 1988 there were over 500 programs in 38 states reaching 1.5 million students annually. By the early 1990s DARE programs were found in every state, and the federal Drug-Free Schools and Communities reauthorization bill of 1991 mandated that 10 percent of each state's share of the funds be used to support DARE.

The interesting thing about this program is that it was accepted so quickly by so many schools, and it is endorsed enthusiastically by educators, students, parents, and police participants. All this has occurred in spite of the fact that DARE's effectiveness in preventing drug use was not evaluated extensively until 1994. A review of this phenomenon pointed out that the program's expansion was due to meeting the needs of the communities, agencies, school districts, and officials to conduct prevention activities rather than in demonstrating an impact on drug use.[15] In 1994, two important, large-scale studies of the effects of DARE were reported. One was based on a longitudinal study in rural, suburban, and urban schools in Illinois comparing students exposed to DARE with students who were not.[16] Although the program had some effects on reported self-esteem, there was no evidence for long-term reductions in self-reported use of drugs. The other report was based on a review of eight smaller outcome evaluations of DARE, selected from eighteen evaluations based on whether the reports had a control group, a pretest-posttest design, and reliable outcome measures.[17]

The overall impact of these eight programs was to increase drug knowledge and knowledge about social skills, but the effects on drug use were marginal at best. There was a very small but statistically significant reduction of tobacco use and no reliable effect on alcohol or marijuana use. The repeated failures to demonstrate an impact of the DARE program on drug use remain a dilemma in light of its widespread popularity. Communities have not abandoned the program. Instead, DARE America has encouraged additional programming outside the original fifth- or sixth-grade. "Booster" programs in junior high and high school, and introductions at earlier grades, are becoming more and more common.

Programs that work

Several school-based drug-use-prevention programs have been modeled after the successful social influence model and have components similar to DARE. A few of these programs have now been demonstrated to have beneficial effects on actual drug use.

Project ALERT was first tested in thirty junior high schools in California and Oregon.[18] The program targeted cigarette smoking, alcohol use, and marijuana use. Before the program, each student was surveyed and classified as a nonuser, experimenter, or user for each of the three substances. The curriculum was taught either by health educators or by educators with the assistance of trained teen leaders. Control schools simply continued whatever health or drug curriculum they had been using. The program was delivered in the seventh grade, and follow-up surveys were done 3, 12, and 15 months later. Three "booster" lessons were given in the eighth grade.

The program surprisingly had no measurable effect on initiation of smoking by nonusers. However, those who were cigarette experimenters before the program began were more likely to quit or to maintain low rates of smoking than the control group. The group with teen leader support showed the largest reduction: 50 percent fewer students were weekly smokers at the 15-month follow-up.

The experimental groups drank less alcohol soon after the program was presented, for previous alcohol nonusers, experimenters, and users. However, this effect diminished over time and disappeared by the end of the study.

The most consistent results were in reducing initiation of marijuana smoking and reducing levels of marijuana smoking. For example, among those who were marijuana nonusers at the beginning, about 12 percent of the control group students had begun using marijuana by the 15-month follow-up. In the treatment groups only 8 percent began using during that time period, representing a one-third decrease in initiation to marijuana use.

DARE: Drug Abuse Resistance Education, the most popular prevention program in schools.

Two programs have shown positive effects over longer peiods of time. Project STAR is a middle-school or junior-high-age program that is also based on the social influence model. It is done in classrooms over a two-year period, and includes parents in shared homework and communication training. High school seniors who began this program in junior high used 30 percent less marijuana, 25 percent fewer cigarettes, and 20 percent less alcohol than students in schools that did not use the program.[19]

The Life Skills Training Program has been subjected to several tests and has shown long-term positive results. This three-year program is based on the social influence model and teaches resistance skills, normative education, and media influences. Self-management skills and general social skills are also included. One of the studies found significantly lower use of marijuana, alcohol, and tobacco after six years. A recent application of this program among ethnic minority youth (Latino and African American) in New York City found reduced use on a two-year followup.[20]

PEERS, PARENTS, AND THE COMMUNITY

Our nation's public schools clearly are the most convenient conduit for attempts to achieve widespread social changes among young people, and that is why most efforts at drug-abuse prevention have been carried out there. However, there has also been a recognition that peers, parents, and the community at large also exert powerful social influences on young people. Because these groups are less accessible than the schools, there have been fewer prevention programs based on using their influences. Nevertheless, important efforts have been made in all these areas.

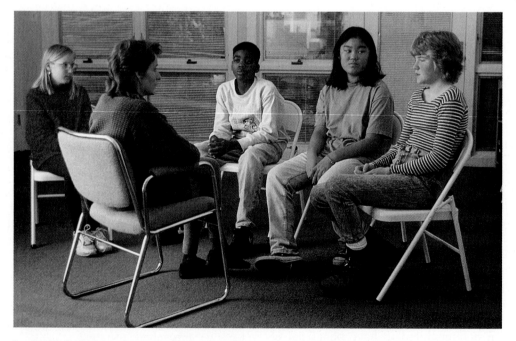

Junior high students in counseling

Peer Programs

Most such programs have taken place in the school setting, but some have used youth-oriented community service programs (such as YMCA, YWCA, and recreation centers) or have focused on "street" youth by using them in group community service projects. The content of peer programs runs the gamut from specific drug information to generic affective training involving social skills and so on.[21]

• **Peer influence** approaches start with the assumption that the opinions of an adolescent's peers are significant influences on the adolescent's behavior. Often using an adult group facilitator/coordinator, the emphasis is on open discussion among a group of children or adolescents. These discussions might focus on drugs, with the peer group discussing dangers and alternatives, or they might simply have the more general goal of building positive group cohesiveness, a sense of belonging, and communication skills.

• **Peer participation** programs often focus on groups of youth in high-risk areas. The idea here is that young people participate in making important decisions and in doing significant work, either as "peers" with cooperating adults or in programs managed almost entirely by the youths themselves. Sometimes participants are paid for community service work, in other cases they engage in money-making businesses, and sometimes they provide youth-oriented information services. These groups almost never focus on drug use in any significant way; rather, the idea is to help people become participating members of society.

The benefits of all these "extracurricular" peer approaches are measurable in terms of acquired skills, improved academic success, higher self-esteem, and a more positive attitude toward peers and school. As to whether they alter drug use significantly, the data either are not available or are inconclusive for the most part.

Parent Programs

The various programs that have worked with parents have been described as taking at least one of four approaches.[22] Most of the programs include more than one of these approaches.

• **Informational** programs provide parents with basic information about alcohol and drugs, as well as information about their use and effects. Although the parents often want to know simply what to look for, how to tell if their child is using drugs, and what the consequences of drug abuse are, the best programs provide additional information. One important piece of information is the actual extent of use of various types of drugs among young people. Another goal might be to make parents aware of their own alcohol and drug use to gain a broader perspective of the issue. A basic rationale is that well-informed parents will be able to teach appropriate attitudes about drugs beginning when their child is young and be better able to recognize potential problems relating to drug or alcohol use.

• **Parenting skills** might be taught through practical training programs. Communicating with children, decision-making skills, how to set goals and limits, and when and how to say "no" to your child can be learned in the abstract and then practiced in role-playing exercises. One risk factor for adolescent drug and alcohol use is poor family relationships, and improving family interaction and strengthening communication can help prevent alcohol and drug abuse.

• **Parent support groups** can be important adjuncts to skills training or in planning community efforts. Groups of parents meet regularly to discuss problem solving, parenting skills, their perceptions of the problem, actions to be taken, and so on.

• **Family interaction** approaches call for families to work as a unit to examine, discuss, and confront issues relating to alcohol and drug use. Other exercises might include more-general problem solving or responding to emergencies. Not only do these programs attempt to improve family communication, the parents are placed in the roles of teacher of drug facts and coordinator of family action, thus strengthening their knowledge and skills.

One group that began in Florida and has become active nationwide is PRIDE (Parent Resources and Information on Drug Education). They sponsor speakers, provide information about the dangers of drugs, and provide an opportunity for communication among groups of concerned parents across the United States.

Community Programs

There are two basic reasons for trying to organize prevention programs at the community level. The first is that a coordinated approach using schools, parent and peer groups, civic organizations, police, newspapers, radio, and television can have a much greater impact than an isolated program that occurs only in the school, for example. Another reason is that drug-abuse prevention and drug education are controversial and emotional topics. Parents might question the need for or the methods used in drug education programs in the schools. Jealousies and mistrust about approaches can separate schools, police, church, and parent groups. A program that starts by involving all these groups in the planning stages is more likely to receive widespread community support. Clearly, the spread of the DARE program in the schools is based partly on the fact that it demonstrates and encourages cooperation between the police and the schools, as well as encouraging some level of parental involvement.

Community-based programs can bring other resources to bear. For example, the city council and local businesses can be involved in sponsoring alcohol-free parties, developing rec-

reational facilities, and arranging field trips so that when the school-based program talks about alternatives, the alternatives are real. The public media can be enlisted not only to publicize public meetings and programs but also to present drug- and alcohol-related information that reinforces what is learned in the other programs. Specific problems such as driving while intoxicated can be addressed publicly and attacked from several directions (e.g., publicity, education, police practices, parent awareness, vendor awareness).

A number of organized community programs have been attempted.[23] Probably none has ever met all its goals, and of necessity each community comes up with a different program. Under the circumstances, it is impossible to evaluate the general approach, but the assumption is that, the broader the bases of support and involvement for prevention programs, the more effective they are likely to be.

Prevention in the Workplace

As a part of its efforts to reduce the demand for drugs, the federal government has encouraged private employers, especially those who do business with the government, to adopt policies to prevent drug use by their employees. Increasingly, these policies include random urine screens. In 1989, rules went into effect requiring all companies and organizations who obtain grants or contracts from the federal government to adopt a "drug-free workplace" plan. The exact nature of the plan is up to the company, but guidelines have been produced by the Department of Labor. Modeled after the Education Department's book, the Labor Department's is called *What Works: Workplaces without Drugs.*[24] At a minimum they expect employers to state clearly that drug use on the job is unacceptable and to notify employees of the consequences of violating company policy regarding drug use. The ultimate goal is not to catch drug users and fire them but to prevent drug use by making it clear that it is not condoned.

WHAT SHOULD WE BE DOING?

By now you have picked up some ideas for things to do, as well as some things to avoid doing. But the answer as to what needs to be done in a particular situation depends on the motivations for doing it. Most states require drug and alcohol abuse prevention education as part of a health curriculum, for example. If that is the primary motive for doing something, and if there doesn't seem to be a particular problem with substance abuse in the schools, then the best thing would probably be to adopt one of the modern curricula that have been developed for this purpose, make sure the teachers and other participants are properly trained in it, and go ahead. In selecting among the curricula, a sensible, balanced approach that combines some factual information with social skills training, perhaps integrated into the more general themes of health, personal values, and decision making, would be appropriate. The three mentioned above under "Programs that work" would fit this general description, and each deserves a careful look. Above all, avoid sensational scare stories, "preachy" approaches from the teacher to the student, and having untrained personnel develop their own curricula. Another good thing to avoid is the inadvertent demonstration of how to do things you don't want them to do—that is, don't show them how they shouldn't put beans in their noses!

If, on the other hand, there is a public outcry about the "epidemic" of drugs and alcohol abuse in the community, speakers have come around inflaming passions, and there is a widespread fervor to "do something about it," this presents both a danger and an opportunity. The danger is that this passionate group might attack and undermine efforts already being made in the schools, substituting scary, preachy, negative approaches that can have negative consequences. The opportunity lies in the possibility that this energy can be organized into a community planning effort, out of which could develop cooperation, increased parent understanding, a focus on family communication, interest in the lives of the community's young people, and increased recreational and creative opportunities.

The key to making this happen is convincing the aroused citizenry of the possibly negative consequences of doing what seems obvious and selling them on the idea of studying what needs to be done. A good place to start might be by writing to the Center for Substance Abuse Prevention, 5600 Fishers Lane, Rockville, MD 20857. This agency produces updated materials for groups interested in developing drug and alcohol abuse prevention programs, provides technical assistance and training to communities interesting in developing programs, and also offers Community Partnership Grants.

SUMMARY

- ▲ We may distinguish between education programs with the goal of imparting knowledge and prevention programs aimed at modifying drug-using behavior.
- ▲ Most of the research over the past thirty years has failed to demonstrate that prevention programs can produce clear, meaningful, long-lasting effects on drug-using behavior.
- ▲ The affective education programs of the 1970s have been criticized for being too value-free.
- ▲ Based on the success of the social influence model in reducing cigarette smoking, a variety of school-based prevention programs have used the same techniques with illicit drugs.

- The DARE program has been adopted rapidly and widely, in spite of limited research evaluating its impact on drug-using behavior.
- Current school-based approaches use refusal skills, countering advertising, public commitments, and teen leaders. Several of these programs have been demonstrated to be effective.
- Other nonschool programs might be peer-based through after-school groups or activities, parent-based through parent and family training, or community-based.

REVIEW QUESTIONS

1. What is the distinction between secondary and tertiary prevention?
2. What is the knowledge-attitudes-behavior model, and what information first called it into question?
3. What were three of the training approaches used in values clarification programs?
4. Distinguish between student assistance programs and peer counseling.
5. What were the five successful components of the social influence model for smoking prevention?
6. In project ALERT, what was the impact of using teen leaders to assist the instructors?
7. What distinguishes DARE from other similar programs based on the social influence model?
8. What do ALERT, STAR, and Life Skills Training have in common, besides their effectiveness?
9. What are some of the "parenting" skills that might be taught and practiced in a prevention program?
10. What is meant by the "Drug-Free Workplace" program?

Related Internet Sites on Breaking the Cycle

Prevention Online: http://www.health.org/

Join Together Online: http://www.join together.org/jto/

D.A.R.E. America: http://www.dare-america.com/

Center on Addiction and Substance Abuse: http://www.casacolumbia.org/

And of course the *Drugs, Society, and Human Behavior* home page: http://www.uwyo.edu/A&S/psyc/dshb.htm

REFERENCES

1. Goodstadt MS: Alcohol and drug education: models and outcomes, *Health Education Monographs* 6:263–278, 1978.
2. Swisher JD and others: Drug education: pushing or preventing? *Peabody J Education* 49:68–75, 1971.
3. Swisher JD and others: A comparison of four approaches to drug abuse prevention at the college level, *J Coll Stud Personnel* 14:231–235, 1973.
4. How U.S. is smashing "hard drug" rings: interview with John R. Bartels, Jr, Administrator of Drug Enforcement, Department of Justice, *US News and World Report,* pp 38–41, April 1, 1974.
5. Drug education is linked to use, *New York Times,* Dec 3, 1972.
6. Blum RH, Blum E, Garfield E: *Drug education: results and recommendations,* Lexington, Mass, 1976, DC Heath.
7. Swisher JD: Prevention issues. In DuPont RI, Goldstein A, O'Donnell J, editors: *Handbook on drug abuse,* Washington, DC, 1979, NIDA, US Government Printing Office.
8. Schaps E and others: *The Napa drug abuse prevention project: research findings,* Washington, DC, 1984, DHHS Pub No (ADM)84-1339, US Government Printing Office.
9. Prevention research. In *Drug abuse and drug abuse research,* Washington, DC, 1984, DHHS Pub No (ADM)85-1372, US Government Printing Office.

10. US Department of Education: *What works: schools without drugs,* Washington, DC, 1987.

11. Evans RI: Smoking in children: developing a social psychological strategy of deterrence, *Prev Med* 5:122–127, 1976.

12. Flay BR: What we know about the social influences approach to smoking prevention: review and recommendations. In Bell CS, Battjes R, editors: *Prevention research: deterring drug abuse among children and adolescents,* Washington, DC, 1985, NIDA Research Monograph 63, DHHS Pub No (ADM)85-1334, US Government Printing Office.

13. McCarthy WJ: The cognitive developmental model and other alternatives to the social skills deficit model of smoking onset. In Bell CS, Battjes R, editors: *Prevention research: deterring drug abuse among children and adolescents,* Washington, DC, 1985, NIDA Research Monograph 63, DHHS Pub No (ADM)85-1334, US Government Printing Office.

14. Glynn K, Leventhal H, Hirschman R: A cognitive developmental approach to smoking prevention. In Bell CS, Battjes R, editors: *Prevention research: deterring drug abuse among children and adolescents,* Washington, DC, 1985, NIDA Research Monograph 63, DHHS Pub No (ADM)85-1334, US Government Printing Office.

15. Aniskiewicz R, Wysong E: Evaluating DARE: drug education and the multiple meanings of success, *Policy Studies Review* 9:727–747, 1990.

16. Ennet ST and others: Long-term evaluation of Drug Abuse Resistance Education, *Addict Behav* 19:113, 1994.

17. Ennett ST and others: How effective is Drug Abuse Resistance Education? A meta-analysis of Project DARE outcome evaluations, *Am J Public Health* 84:1394, 1994.

18. Ellickson PL, Bell RM: Drug prevention in junior high: a multi-site longitudinal test, *Science* 247:1299–1305, 1990.

19. Johnson,CA, MacKinnon DP, Pentz MA: Breadth of Program and Outcome Effectiveness in Drug Abuse Prevention, *American Behavioral Scientist* 39:884, 1996.

20. Botvin GJ, Schinke SP: Effectivness of Culturally Focused and Generic Skills Training Approaches to Alcohol and Drug Abuse Prevention Among Minority Adolescents: Two-Year Follow-Up Results, *Psych Addictive Behaviors* 9:183, 1995.

21. Resnik HS, Gibbs J: Types of peer program approaches. In Gardner SE, editor: *Adolescent peer pressure: theory, correlates, and program implications for drug abuse prevention,* Washington, DC, 1981, DHHS Pub No (ADM) 81-1152, US Government Printing Office.

22. Parent education. In *Prevention plus: involving schools, parents, and the community in alcohol and drug education,* Washington, DC, 1984, DHHS Pub No (ADM)84-1256, US Government Printing Office.

23. Community approaches. In *Prevention plus: involving schools, parents, and the community in alcohol and drug education,* Washington, DC, 1984, DHHS Pub No (ADM) 84-1256, US Government Printing Office.

24. US Department of Labor: *What works: workplaces without drugs,* Washington, DC, 1989.

ASSESS YOURSELF!

Alternatives to Drug Use

How many things do you do that may be seen as ways of achieving some of the same things people achieve by taking drugs? List your hobbies, sports activities, and recreational activities down the side of the page, and then check underneath each "goal" whether that activity meets that goal for you.

Are some of your activities currently closely related to alcohol or other drug use? Are there goals that your current activities are not meeting? A review of this sheet might give you some ideas about your own vulnerability to psychoactive drug use or abuse.

GOALS

ACTIVITIES:	Excitement, "rush" of adrenaline	Relaxation "time out"	Altered state of consciousness
_____	_____	_____	_____
_____	_____	_____	_____
_____	_____	_____	_____
_____	_____	_____	_____
_____	_____	_____	_____

A

Drug Names

acetaminophen: OTC analgesic. Similar to aspirin in its effects.

acetophenazine: Tindal. Antipsychotic.

acetylsalicylic acid: aspirin. OTC analgesic.

Adapin: doxepin. Tricyclic antidepressant.

alprazolam: Xanax. Benzodiazepine sedative.

Alurate: aprobarbital. Barbiturate sedative-hypnotic.

Amanita muscaria: Hallucinogenic mushroom.

amitriptyline: Elavil, Endep. Tricyclic antidepressant.

amobarbital: Amytal. Barbiturate sedative-hypnotic.

amoxapine: Asendin. Tricyclic antidepressant.

amphetamine: Benzedrine. CNS stimulant and sympathomimetic.

Amytal: amobarbital. Barbiturate sedative-hypnotic.

Anavar: oxandrolone. Anabolic steroid.

angel dust: Street name for PCP.

Antabuse: disulfiram. Alters metabolism of alcohol; used to treat alcoholism.

aprobarbital: Alurate. Barbiturate sedative-hypnotic.

Artane: trihexyphenidyl. Anticholinergic used to control extrapyramidal symptoms.

Asendin: amoxapine. Tricyclic antidepressant.

aspirin: acetylsalicylic acid. OTC analgesic.

Ativan: lorazepam. Benzodiazepine sedative.

atropine: Anticholinergic.

Aventyl: nortriptyline. Tricyclic antidepressant.

belladonna: Poisonous anticholinergic plant.

Benzedrine: amphetamine. CNS stimulant and sympathomimetic. Brand name no longer used.

benzodiazepines: Class of sedative-hypnotics that includes diazepam (Valium).

benztropine: Cogentin. Anticholinergic used to control extrapyramidal symptoms.

bromide: Group of salts with sedative properties.

bupropion: Wellbutrin. Atypical antidepressant.

butabarbital: Butisol. Barbiturate sedative-hypnotic.

Butisol: butabarbital. Barbiturate sedative-hypnotic.

caffeine: Mild stimulant found in coffee and in OTC preparations.

Catapres: clonidine. Antihypertensive drug shown to reduce narcotic withdrawal symptoms.

chloral hydrate: Noctec. Nonbarbiturate sedative-hypnotic.

chlordiazepoxide: Librium. Benzodiazepine sedative.

chlorpheniramine maleate: OTC antihistamine.

chlorpromazine: Thorazine. Antipsychotic.

chlorprothixene: Taractan. Antipsychotic.

Cibalith: lithium citrate. Salt used in treating amnia and bipolar affective disorders.

clenbuterol: An alpha-2 adrenergic agonist developed to treat asthma, but used by athletes to build muscle.

clonidine: Catapres. Antihyperintensive drug shown to reduce narcotic withdrawal symptoms.

clorazepate: Tranxene. Benzodiazepine sedative.

clozapine: Clozaril. Atypical antipsychotic.

Clozaril: clozapine. Atypical antipsychotic.

cocaine: CNS stimulant and local anesthetic.

codeine: Narcotic analgesic found in opium.

Cogentin: benztropine. Anticholinergic used to control extrapyramidal symptoms.

Compazine: prochlorperazine. Antipsychotic.

creatine: Natural substance found in meat and fish that might have anabolic properties and is used by athletes.

Cylert: pemoline. Stimulant used to treat ADD with hyperactivity.

Dalmane: flurazepam. Benzodiazepine hypnotic.

Darvon: propoxyphene. Narcotic analgesic.

*Datura***:** Genus of plants, many of which are anticholinergic.

Demerol: meperidine. Narcotic analgesic.

desipramine: Norpramin, Pertofrane. Tricyclic antidepressant.

Desoxyn: methamphetamine. CNS stimulant and sympathomimetic.

Desyrel: trazodone. Atypical antidepressant.

Dexedrine: dextroamphetamine. CNS stimulant and sympathomimetic.

dexfenfluramine: Redux. Appetite suppressant, removed from the market in 1997.

dextroamphetamine: Dexedrine. CNS stimulant and sympathomimetic.

dextromethorphan: OTC cough supressant.

diazepam: Valium. Benzodiazepine sedative.

diethylpropion: Tenuate, Tepanil. Amphetamine-like appetite supressant.

dihydrocodeine: Narcotic analgesic.

Dilaudid: hydromorphone. Narcotic analgesic.

diphenhydramine: Antihistamine.

disulfiram: Antabuse. Alters metabolism of alcohol; used to treat alcoholism.

DMT: dimethyltryptamine. Hallucinogen.

Dolophine: methadone. Narcotic analgesic.

DOM: Hallucinogen.

doxepin: Adapin, Sinequan. Tricyclic antidepressant.

dronabinol: Marinol. Prescription form of delta-9-tetrahydrocannabinol.

Effexor: venlafaxine. Antidepressant (SSRI).

Elavil: amitriptyline. Tricyclic antidepressant.

Endep: amitriptyline. Tricyclic antidepressant.

endorphin: Endogenous substance with effects similar to those of the narcotic analgesics.

enkephalin: Endogenous substance with effects similar to those of the narcotic analgesics.

ephedrine: Sympathomimetic used to treat asthma.

Equanil: meprobamate. Nonbarbiturate sedative-hypnotic.

Eskalith: lithium carbonate. Salt used in treating mania and bipolar affective disorders.

fenfluramine: Pondimin. Appetite suppressant, removed from the market in 1997.

fentanyl: Sublimaze. Potent synthetic analgesic.

flunitrazepam: Rohypnol. Benzodiazepine hypnotic, not sold in the U.S. Known as a "date-rape" drug.

fluoxetine: Prozac. Antidepressant (SSRI).

fluphenazine: Permitil, Prolixin. Antipsychotic.

flurazepam: Dalmane. Benzodiazepine hypnotic.

GHB: gamma hydroxybutyrate. CNS depressant, produced naturally in small amounts in the human brain. Has been used recreationally and, in combination with alcohol, has some reputation as a "date-rape" drug.

Halcion: triazolam. Benzodiazepine hypnotic.

Haldol: haloperidol. Antipsychotic.

haloperidol: Haldol. Antipsychotic.

henbane: Poisonous anticholinergic plant.

heroin: Diacetylmorphine. Narcotic analgesic.

hydrocodone: Narcotic analgesic.

hydromorphone: Dilaudid. Narcotic analgesic.

ibogaine: hallucinogen, also proposed to reduce craving in drug addicts

ibuprofen: analgesic and antiinflammatory.

imipramine: Janimine, Tofranil. Tricyclic antidepressant.

isocarboxazid: Marplan. MAO inhibitor used as antidepressant.

Janimine: imipramine. Tricyclic antidepressant.

Ketalar: ketamine. Dissociative anesthetic.

ketamine: Ketalar. Dissociative anesthetic.

LAAM: L-alpha-acetyl-methadol. Long-lasting synthetic narcotic used in maintenance treatment of narcotic addicts.

laudanum: Tincture (alcohol solution) of opium.

Librium: chlordiazepoxide. Benzodiazepine sedative.

Lithane: lithium carbonate.

lithium carbonate, lithium citrate: Salts used in treating mania and bipolar affective disorders.

Lithobid: lithium carbonate.

lorazepam: Ativan. Benzodiazepine sedative.

loxapine: Loxitane. Antipsychotic.

Loxitane: loxapine. Antipsychotic.

LSD: lysergic acid diethylamide. Hallucinogen.

Ludiomil: maprotiline. Tricyclic antidepressant.

Luminal: phenobarbital. Barbiturate sedative-hypnotic.

mandrake: Anticholinergic plant.

maprotiline: Ludiomil. Tricyclic antidepressant.

Marinol: dronabinol. Prescription form of delta-9-tetrahydrocannabinol.

Marplan: isocarboxazid. MAO inhibitor used as antidepressant.

Mazanor: mazindol. Appetite suppressant.

mazinodol: Mazanor, Sanorex. Appetite suppressant.

MDA: Hallucinogen.

MDMA: Hallucinogen.

Mebaral: mephobarbital. Barbiturate sedative-hypnotic.

Mellaril: thioridazine. Antipsychotic.

meperidine: Demerol. Narcotic analgesic.

mephobarbital: Mebaral. Barbiturate sedative-hypnotic.

meprobamate: Equanil, Miltown. Nonbarbiturate sedative-hypnotic.

mescaline: Hallucinogen found in peyote cactus.

mesoridazine: Serentil. Antipsychotic.

methadone: Dolophine. Narcotic analgesic.

methamphetamine: Desoxyn, Methedrine. CNS stimulant and sympathomimetic.

methaqualone: Quaalude, Sopor. Nonbarbiturate sedative-hypnotic.

methylphenidate: Ritalin. Stimulant used to treat ADD with hyperactivity.

Metrazol: pentylenetetrazol. Convulsant formerly used in convulsive therapy.

Miltown: meprobamate. Nonbarbiturate sedative-hypnotic.

mirtazapine: Remeron. Atypical antidepressant

Moban: molindone. Antipsychotic.

molindone: Moban. Antipsychotic.

morphine: Narcotic analgesic.

naloxone: Narcan. Narcotic antagonist.

naltrexone: Trexan, reVIA. Narcotic antagonist. Used in treating alcoholism.

Narcan: naloxone. Narcotic antagonist.

Nardil: phenelzine. MAO inhibitor used as antidepressant.

Navane: thiothixene. Antipsychotic.

Nembutal: pentobarbital. Barbiturate sedative-hypnotic.

Noctec: chloral hydrate. Nonbarbiturate sedative-hypnotic.

Norpramin: desipramine. Tricyclic antidepressant.

nortriptyline: Aventyl, Pamelor. Tricyclic antidepressant.

Numorphan: oxymorphone. Narcotic analgesic.

olanzepine: Zyprex. Atypical antipsychotic.

opium: Narcotic analgesic.

oxandrolone: Anavar. Anabolic steroid.

oxazepam: Serax. Benzodiazepine sedative.

oxycodone: Percodan. Narcotic analgesic.

oxymorphone: Numorphan. Narcotic analgesic.

Pamelor: nortriptyline. Tricyclic antidepressant.

paraldehyde: Nonbarbiturate sedative-hypnotic.

paregoric: Tincture (alcohol solution) of opium.

Parnate: tranylcypromine. MAO inhibitor used as antidepressant.

paroxetine: Paxil. Antidepressant (SSRI).

Paxil: paroxetine. Antidepressant (SSRI).

PCP: phencyclidine, "angel dust." Hallucinogen.

pemoline: Cylert. Stimulant used to treat ADD with hyperactivity.

pentazocine: Talwin. Narcotic analgesic.

pentobarbital: Nembutal. Barbiturate sedative-hypnotic.

pentylenetetrazol: Metrazol. Convulsant formerly used in convulsive therapy.

Percodan: oxycodone. Narcotic analgesic.

Permitil: fluphenazine. Antipsychotic.

perphenazine: Trilafon. Antipsychotic.

Pertofrane: desipramine. Tricyclic antidepressant.

peyote: Cactus containing mescaline (hallucinogenic).

phencyclidine: PCP, "angel dust." Hallucinogen.

phendimetrazine: Amphetamine-like appetite suppressant.

phenelzine: Nardil. MAO inhibitor used as antidepressant.

phenmetrazine: Preludin. Amphetamine-like appetite suppressant.

phenobarbital: Luminal. Barbiturate sedative-hypnotic.

phentermine: Amphetamine-like appetite suppressant.

phenylpropanolamine (PPA): OTC appetite suppressant.

Pondimin: fenfluramine. Appetite suppressant, removed from the market in 1997.

Preludin: phenmetrazine. Amphetamine-like appetite suppressant.

prochlorperazine: Compazine. Antipsychotic.

Prolixin: fluphenazine. Antipsychotic.

propoxyphene: Darvon. Narcotic analgesic.

protriptyline: Vivactil. Tricyclic antidepressant.

Prozac: fluoxetine. Antidepressant (SSRI).

pseudoephedrine: OTC sympathomimetic.

psilocybin: Hallucinogen from the Mexican psilocybe mushroom.

Quaalude: methaqualone. Nonbarbiturate sedative-hypnotic.

Redux: dexfenfluramine. Appetite suppressant, removed from the market in 1997.

Remeron: mirtazapine. Atypical antidepressant.

Restoril: temazepam. Benzodiazepine hypnotic.

reVIA: naltrexone. Narcotic antagonist used in treating alcoholism.

Risperdal: risperidone. Atypical antipsychotic.

risperidone: Risperdal. Atypical antipsychotic.

Ritalin: methylphenidate. Stimulant used to treat ADD with hyperactivity.

Rohypnol: flunitrazepam. Benzodiazepine hypnotic, not sold in the U.S., known as a "date-rape" drug.

Sanorex: mazindol. Appetite suppressant.

scopolamine: Anticholinergic.

secobarbital: Seconal. Barbiturate sedative-hypnotic.

Seconal: secobarbital. Barbiturate sedative-hypnotic.

Serax: oxazepam. Benzodiazepine sedative.

Serentil: mesoridazine. Antipsychotic.

Sernyl: Former brand name for PCP.

sertraline: Zoloft. Antidepressant (SSRI).

Sinequan: doxepin. Tricyclic antidepressant.

Sopor: methaqualone. Nonbarbiturate sedative-hypnotic.

stanozolol: Winstrol. Anabolic steroid.

Stelazine: trufluoperazine. Antipsychotic.

Sublimaze: fentanyl. Potent synthetic analgesic.

Talwin: pentazocine. Narcotic analgesic.

Taractan: chlorprothixene. Antipsychotic.

temazepam: Restoril. Benzodiazepine hypnotic.

Tenuate: diethylpropion. Amphetamine-like appetite suppressant.

Tepanil: diethylpropion. Amphetamine-like appetite suppressant.

Teslac: testolactone. Anabolic steroid.

testolactone: Teslac. Anabolic steroid.

theophylline: Mild stimulant found in tea; used to treat asthma.

thioridazine: Mellaril. Antipsychotic.

thiothixene: Navane. Antipsychotic.

Thorazine: chlorpromazine. Antipsychotic.

Tindal: acetophenazine. Antipsychotic.

Tofranil: imipramine. Tricyclic antidepressant.

Tranxene: clorazepate. Benzodiazepine sedative.

tranylcypromine: Parnate. MAO inhibitor used as an antidepressant.

trazodone: Desyrel. Atypical antidepressant.

Trexan: naltrexone. Narcotic antagonist.

triazolam: Halcion. Benzodiazepine hypnotic.

trifluoperazine: Stelazine. Antipsychotic.

triflupromazine: Vesprin. Antipsychotic.

trihexyphenidyl: Artane. Anticholinergic used to control extrapyramidal symptoms.

Trilafon: perphenazine. Antipsychotic.

Valium: diazepam. Benzodiazepine sedative.

venlafaxine: Effexor. Antidepressant (SSRI).

Vesprin: triflupromazine. Antipsychotic.

Vivactil: protriptyline. Tricyclic antidepressant.

Wellbutrin: bupropion. Atypical antidepressant.

Winstrol: stanozolol. Anabolic steroid.

Xanax: alprazolam. Benzodiazepine sedative.

Zoloft: Sertraline. Antidepressant (SSRI).

Zyprex: olanzepine. Atypical antipsychotic.

APPENDIX B

Resources for Information and Assistance

FEDERAL GOVERNMENT AGENCIES

National Clearinghouse for Alcohol and Drug
  Information
Office of Substance Abuse Prevention (OSAP)
P.O. Box 2345
Rockville, MD 20852
(301) 468-2600
1-800-729-6686

NIDA Cocaine Hot Line
1-800-662-HELP
Office on Smoking and Health
5600 Fishers Lane
Rockville, MD 20857
(301) 443-1575

Drugs & Crime Data Center
Bureau of Justice Statistics
1600 Research Blvd.
Rockville, MD 20850
1-800-666-3332

ALCOHOL

Alcohol Research Information Service
1106 E. Oakland
Lansing, MI 48906
(517) 485-9900

Alcoholics Anonymous World Services
P. O. Box 459, Grand Central Station
New York, NY 10163
(212) 686-1100

American Council on Alcoholism
5024 Campbell Blvd., Suite H
Whitemarsh Business Center
Baltimore, MD 21236
(301) 529-9200

American Health and Temperance Society
6830 Eastern Ave., N.W.
Washington, D.C. 20012
(202) 722-6736

BACCHUS of the U.S.
(Boost Alcohol Counsciousness Concerning the
  Health of University Students)
P.O. Box 10430
Denver, CO 80210
(303) 871-3068

Licensed Beverage Information Council
1250 I St., Suite 900
Washington, D.C. 20005
(202) 628-3544

MADD (Mothers Against Drunk Driving)
669 Airport Fwy., Suite 310
Hurst, TX 76053
(817) 268-6233

National Alcohol Hot Line
1-800-ALCOHOL

National Council on Alcoholism
12 W. 21st St.
New York, NY 10010
(212) 206-6770

National Woman's Christian Temperance Union
1730 Chicago Ave.
Evanston, IL 60201
(312) 864-1396

RID (Remove Intoxicated Drivers)
P.O. Box 520
Schenectady, NY 12301
(518) 372-0034

SMOKING

ASH (Action on Smoking and Health)
2013 H St., N.W.
Washington, D.C. 20006
(202) 659-4310

Smoking Control Advocacy Resource Center
1730 Rhode Island Ave., N.W.
Washington, D.C. 20036
(202) 659-8475

Tobacco Institute
1875 I St., N.W.
Washington, D.C. 20006
(202) 457-4800

DRUGS

Alcohol and Drug Problems Association of North
  America
444 N. Capitol St., N.W., Suite 706
Washington, D.C. 20001
(202) 737-4340

American Council for Drug Education
204 Monroe St., Suite 110
Rockville, MD 20850
(301) 294-0600

Do It Now Foundation
Box 27568
Tempe, AZ 85285
(602) 257-0797

Drug Policy Foundation
4801 Massachusetts Ave., N.W., Suite 400
Washington, D.C. 20016-2087

Fair Oaks Hospital
19 Prospect St. Box 100
Summit, NJ 07901
(201) 552-7000
1-800-COCAINE

Narcotic Educational Foundation of America
5055 Sunset Blvd.
Los Angeles, CA 90027
(213) 663-5171

National Drug Information Center of Families in
  Action, Inc.
2296 Henderson Mill Rd., Suite 204
Atlanta, GA 30345
(404) 934-6364

National Federation of Parents for a Drug-Free Youth
1423 N. Jefferson
Springfield, MO 65802-1988
(407) 836-3709

NIDA (National Institute on Drug Abuse)
5600 Fishers Lane
Rockville, MD 20857

NORML (National Organization for the Reform of
  Marijuana Laws)
2001 S. St., N.W., Suite 640
Washington, D.C. 20009
(202) 483-5500

PRIDE (Parent Resource Institute for Drug
  Education)
100 Edgewood Ave., Suite 1002
Atlanta, GA 30303
1-800-241-7946

DRUG INFORMATION ON THE INTERNET

There is a great deal of information, opinion, misinformation, and discussion about drugs available on the Internet. It is possible to learn about the latest drug fads, to get involved in arguments about drug policy, and occasionally even to learn some solid facts by browsing on the Internet. But be warned that there is no quality control on many of these computer sites—they represent the ultimate in free expression! You're liable to find such things as a bogus recipe for making LSD from Foster's Beer, warnings about water addiction, and other foolishness mixed in with potentially useful information, so take care! Brief lists of some relevant internet sites are found in the Web Watch in each chapter.

abstinence Refraining completely from the use of a drug or alcohol. Complete abstinence from alcohol means no drinking at all. Abstinence syndrome: see *withdrawal syndrome*.

abstinence violation effect The tendency of a person who has been abstaining (as from alcohol), and "slips," to go on and indulge fully, because the rule of abstinence has been broken anyway.

acetaldehyde The chemical product of the first step in the liver's metabolism of alcohol. It is normally present only in small amounts because it is rapidly converted to acetic acid.

acetylcholine Neurotransmitter found in the parasympathetic branch and in the cerebral cortex.

acute In general, "sharp." In medicine, "rapid." Referring to drugs, the short-term effects or effects of a single administration, as opposed to *chronic*, or long-term, effects of administration.

additive effects When the effects of two different drugs add up to produce a greater effect than either drug alone. As contrasted with *antagonistic* effects in which one drug reduces the effect of another or *synergistic* effects in which one drug greatly amplifies the effect of another.

adenosine A chemical believed to be a neurotransmitter in the CNS, primarily at inhibitory receptors. Caffeine might act by antagonizing the normal action of adenosine on its receptors.

ADHD Attention deficit hyperactivity disorder, a learning disability. Terminology of the *DSM-IV*.

affective disorder A disorder of mood or emotion, in contrast to disorders of thought. Depression, mania, and bipolar (formerly manic-depressive) disorders are examples.

affective education In general, education that focuses on emotional content or emotional reactions, in contrast to *cognitive* content. In drug education, one example would be learning how to achieve certain "feelings" (of excitement or belonging to a group) without using drugs.

aftercare In drug or alcohol treatment programs, the long-term follow-up or maintenance support that follows a more intense period of treatment.

AIDS Acquired immunodeficiency syndrome, a disease in which the body's immune system breaks down, leading eventually to death. Because the disease is spread through the mixing of body fluids, it is more prevalent in intravenous drug users who share needles. The infectious agent is the human immunodeficiency virus (HIV).

alcohol Generally refers to grain alcohol, or ethanol, as opposed to other types of alcohol (for example, wood or isopropyl alcohol), which are too toxic to be drinkable.

alcohol abuse In the *DSM-IV*, defined as a pattern of pathological alcohol use that causes impairment of social or occupational functioning. Compare with *alcohol dependence*.

alcohol dehydrogenase The enzyme that metabolizes almost all of the alcohol consumed by an individual. It is found primarily in the liver.

alcohol dependence In the *DSM-IV*, alcohol dependence is considered a more serious disorder than alcohol abuse, in that dependence includes either tolerance or withdrawal symptoms.

alcoholic personality Personality traits, such as immaturity and dependency, that are frequently found in alcoholics in treatment. Many of these consistent traits might be a result of years of heavy drinking rather than a cause of alcoholism.

Alcoholics Anonymous A worldwide, loosely organized group of alcoholics who try to help each other abstain from the use of alcohol.

alcoholism The word has many different definitions and therefore is not a precise term. Definitions might refer to pathological drinking behavior (e.g.,

469

remaining drunk for two days), to impaired functioning (e.g., frequently missing work), or to physical dependence. See *alcohol abuse* and *alcohol dependence*.

alternatives (to drugs) Assuming that there are motives for drug use, such as the need to be accepted by a group, many prevention and treatment programs teach alternative methods for satisfying these motives.

Alzheimer's disease A progressive neurological disease that occurs primarily in the elderly. It causes loss of memory and then progressively impairs more aspects of intellectual and social functioning. Large acetylcholine-containing neurons of the brain are damaged in this disease.

Amanita muscaria The fly agaric mushroom, widely used in ancient times for its hallucinogenic properties.

amotivational syndrome A hypothesized loss of motivation that has been attributed to chronic marijuana use.

anabolic Promoting constructive metabolism; building tissue.

anabolic steroids Substances that increase anabolic (constructive) metabolism, one of the functions of male sex hormones. The result is increased muscle mass.

analgesic Pain-relieving. An analgesic drug produces a selective reduction of pain, whereas an *anesthetic* reduces all sensation.

anandamide A naturally occurring brain chemical with marijuana-like properties.

androgenic Masculinizing.

anesthetic Sense deadening. An anesthetic drug reduces all sensation, whereas an *analgesic* drug reduces pain.

angel dust A street name for phencyclidine (PCP).

animism The belief that objects and plants contain spirits that move and direct them.

Antabuse Brand name for dusulfiram, a drug that interferes with the normal metabolism of alcohol so that a person who drinks alcohol after taking disulfiram will become quite ill. Antabuse interferes with the enzyme aldehyde dehydrogenase so that there is a buildup of acetaldehyde, the first metabolic product of alcohol.

antecedents In the context of chapter 1, behaviors or individual characteristics that can be measured before drug use and might therefore be somewhat predictive of drug use. These are not necessarily causes of the subsequent drug use.

anticonvulsant A drug that prevents or reduces epileptic seizures.

antidepressant A group of drugs used in treating depressive disorders. The MAO inhibitors, the tricyclics, and the SSRIs are the major examples.

antihistamines A group of drugs that act by antagonizing the actions of histamine at its receptors. Used in cold and sinus remedies and in OTC sedatives and sleep aids.

antiinflammatory Reducing the local heat, swelling, and redness caused by injury or infection. Aspirin has antiinflammatory properties.

antipsychotics A group of drugs used to treat psychotic disorders, such as schizophrenia. Also called neuroleptics or major tranquilizers.

antipyretic Fever-reducing. Aspirin is a commomly used antipyretic.

antitussive Cough-reducing. Narcotics have this effect. OTC antitussives generally contain dextromethorphan.

anxiety disorders Mental disorders characterized by excessive worry, fears, avoidance, or a sense of impending danger. At pathological levels, these disorders can be debilitating.

anxiolytics Drugs, such as Valium, used in treatment of anxiety disorders. Literally, "anxiety-dissolving."

aphrodisiac Any substance that is said to promote sexual desire.

aspirin Originally Bayer's brand name for acetylsalicylic acid, now a generic name for that chemical.

assassin The story is that this term for a hired killer is derived from a hashish-using cult, the hash-shiyya.

ataxia Loss of coordinated movement; for example, the staggering gait of someone who has consumed a large amount of alcohol.

attention deficit hyperactivity disorder A learning disability accompanied by hyperactivity. More common in male children. This *DSM-IV* diagnostic category replaces *hyperkinetic syndrome* and *minimal brain dysfunction*.

autonomic nervous system The branch of the peripheral nervous system that regulates the visceral, or automatic, functions of the body, such as heart rate and intestinal motility. In contrast to the *somatic*, or voluntary, nervous system.

aversion therapy A form of treatment that attempts to suppress an undesirable behavior by punishing each instance of the behavior. For example, the drinking of alcohol might be punished by electric shocks or by a drug that causes nausea.

BAC Blood alcohol concentration, also called blood alcohol level (BAL). The proportion of blood that consists of alcohol. For example, a person with a BAC of 0.10 percent has alcohol constituting one-tenth of 1 percent of the blood and is legally intoxicated in all states.

balanced placebo A research design in which alcohol is compared with a placebo beverage, and subjects either believe they are drinking alcohol or believe they are not.

barbiturate A major class of sedative-hypnotic drugs, including amobarbital and sodium pentothal.

basal ganglia A part of the brain containing large numbers of dopamine synapses. Responsible for maintaining proper muscle tone as a part of the *extrapyramidal motor system*. Damage to the basal ganglia, as in Parkinson's disease, produces muscular rigidity and tremors.

behavioral tolerance Repeated use of a drug can lead to a diminished effect of the drug (tolerance). When the diminished effect occurs because the individual has learned to compensate for the effect of the drug, it is called behavioral tolerance. For example, a novice drinker might be unable to walk with a BAC of 0.20 percent, whereas someone who has practiced walking while intoxicated would be able to walk fairly well at the same BAC.

behavioral toxicity Refers to the fact that a drug can be toxic because it impairs behavior and amplifies the danger level of many activities. The effect of alcohol on driving is an example.

benzodiazepine The group of drugs that includes Valium (diazepam) and Librium (chlordiazepoxide). They are used as *anxiolytics* or *sedatives*, and some types are used as sleeping pills.

benzoylecgonine A metabolite of cocaine that can be detected in urine samples.

bhang A preparation of cannabis (marijuana) that consists of the whole plant, dried and powdered. The weakest of the forms commonly used in India.

binding The interaction between a molecule and a receptor for that molecule. Although the molecules float onto and off the receptor, there are chemical and electrical attractions between a specific molecule and its receptor so that there is a much higher probability that the receptor will be occupied by its proper molecule than by other molecules.

bioavailability The availability of molecules of a drug at the site of the drug's action in the body. An important concept in comparing different brands of the same generic drug, because one preparation might dissolve better or be absorbed more readily than the other, thus producing greater bioavailability.

bipolar disorder One of the major affective, or emotional, disorders. Periods of mania and periods of depression have occurred in the same individual. Also called *manic-depressive illness*.

blackout A period of time during which a person was behaving, but of which the person has no memory. The most common cause of this phenomenon is excessive alcohol consumption, and blackouts are considered to indicate pathological drinking.

black tar A type of illicit heroin usually imported from Mexico.

blood alcohol concentration A measure of the concentration of alcohol in the blood, expressed in grams per 100 ml (percentage).

blood-brain barrier Refers to the fact that many substances, including drugs, that can circulate freely in the blood do not readily enter the brain tissue. The major structural feature of this barrier is the tightly jointed epithelial cells lining blood capillaries in the brain. Drug molecules cannot pass between the cells but must instead go through their membranes. Small molecules and molecules that are lipid- (fat-) soluble cross the barrier easily. Obviously, all psychoactive drugs must be capable of crossing the blood-brain barrier.

brain stem The medulla oblongata, pons, and midbrain. Located between the spinal cord and the forebrain, and generally considered to contain the "oldest" (in an evolutionary sense) and most primitive control centers for such basic functions as breathing, swallowing, and so on.

brand name The name given to a drug by a particular manufacturer and licensed only to that manufacturer. For example, *Valium* is a brand name for diazepam. Other companies may sell diazepam, but Hoffman-LaRoche, Inc. owns the name *Valium*.

bright Light-colored, flue-cured tobacco. Compare with *burley*.

British system Generally refers to the fact that heroin addicts in Great Britain may register as addicts and be prescribed legal narcotics, including heroin.

burley Dark-colored, air-cured tobacco. Compare with *bright*.

caffeinism Habitual use of large amounts of caffeine, usually in coffee.

Camellia sinesis The plant from which tea is made.

Cannabis Genus of plants known as marijuana, or hemp. Includes *C. indica* and *C. sativa*.

carbon monoxide A poisonous gas found in cigarette smoke.

catheter A piece of plastic or rubber tubing that is inserted into a vein or other structure.

central nervous system Brain and spinal cord.

charas A preparation of cannabis, or marijuana, that is similar to hashish. The most potent form of marijuana commonly used in India.

chemical name For a drug, the name that is descriptive of its chemical structure. For example, the chemical name *sodium chloride* is associated with the *generic* name *table salt*, of which there may be several *brand* names, such as *Morton's*.

China white A street name for one of the potent synthetic narcotics.

chipper An individual who uses heroin occasionally.

chronic Occurring over time. Chronic drug use is long-term use; chronic drug effects are persistent effects produced by long-term use.

chronic obstructive lung disease A group of disorders that include emphysema and chronic bronchitis. Cigarette smoking is a major cause of these disorders.

cirrhosis A serious, largely irreversible, and frequently deadly disease of the liver. Usually caused by chronic heavy alcohol use.

coca The plant *Erythroxylon coca*, from which cocaine is derived. Also refers to the leaves of this plant.

cocaethylene A potent stimulant formed when cocaine and alcohol are used together.

cocaine hydrochloride The most common form of pure cocaine; it is stable and water soluble.

coca paste A paste derived from the coca leaf in the process of making cocaine. It is sometimes smoked in South and Central America and Mexico.

codeine A narcotic chemical present in opium.

Coma A state of unconsciousness from which the individual cannot be aroused.

congeners In general, members of the same group. With respect to alcohol, the term refers to other chemicals that are produced in the process of making a particular alcoholic beverage.

controlled drinking The concept that individuals who have been drinking pathologically can be taught to drink in a controlled, nonpathological manner.

controlled substance A term coined for the 1970 federal law that revised previous laws regulating *narcotics and dangerous drugs*. Heroin and cocaine are examples of controlled substances.

correlate A variable that is statistically related to some other variable, such as drug use.

crack A smokable form of cocaine. Also called *rock*.

crank Street name for illicitly manufactured methamphetamine.

crash Originally referred to the rapid emotional descent after a binge of amphetamine use. One symptom is prolonged sleep, and eventually sleeping in general was referred to as crashing.

crystal meth Street term for a form of methamphetamine crystals, also called *ice*.

cumulative effects Drug effects that increase with repeated administrations, usually due to the buildup of the drug in the body.

DARE Drug Abuse Resistance Education, the most popular prevention program in schools.

date-rape drug A substance given to someone without her knowledge to cause unconsciousness in order to have nonconsensual sex. Rohypnol and GHB have become known for such use. A 1996 U.S. law provides serious penalties for using drugs in this manner.

Datura A plant genus that includes many species used for their hallucinogenic properties. These plants contain anticholinergic chemicals.

DAWN Drug Abuse Warning Network, a federal government system for reporting drug-related medical emergencies and deaths.

DEA United States Drug Enforcement Administration.

delirium tremens Alcohol withdrawal symptoms, including tremors and hallucinations.

demand reduction Efforts to control drug use by reducing the demand for drugs, as opposed to efforts aimed at reducing the supply of drugs. Demand reduction efforts include education and prevention programs, as well as increased punishments for drug users.

depressant Any of a large group of drugs that generally depress the CNS and at high doses induce sleep. Includes alcohol, the barbiturates, and other sedative-hypnotic drugs.

depression A major type of mood disorder.

detoxification The process of allowing the body to rid itself of a large amount of alcohol or another drug. Often the first step in a treatment program.

deviance Behavior that is different from established social norms and that social groups take steps to change.

diagnosis The process of identifying the nature of an illness. A subject of great controversy for mental disorders.

distillation The process by which alcohol is separated from a weak alcohol solution to form more concentrated distilled spirits. The weak solution is heated and the alcohol vapors are collected and condensed to a liquid form.

dopamine A neurotransmitter found in the basal ganglia and other regions of the brain.

dose-response curve A graph showing the relationship between the size of a drug dose and the size of the response (or the proportion of subjects showing the response).

drug Any substance, natural or artificial, other than food, that by its chemical nature alters structure or function in the living organism.

drug abuse Use of a drug in such a manner or in such amounts or in situations such that the drug use causes problems or greatly increases the chance of problems occurring.

drug disposition tolerance The reduced effect of a drug that can result from more rapid metabolism or excretion of the drug.

drug misuse Use of prescribed drugs in greater amounts than, or for purposes other than, those prescribed by a physician or dentist.

drug therapy The use of a drug in an effort to treat an illness.

DSM-IV *Diagnostic and Statistical Manual of Mental Disorders*, fourth edition, published by the American Psychiatric Association. It has become a standard for naming and distinguishing among mental disorders.

dysentery A bowel infection that causes severe diarrhea, pain, and fever.

Ecstasy Street name for the hallucinogen MDMA. Also called "XTC."

ECT Electroconvulsive therapy, or electroconvulsive shock treatment. A procedure in which an electrical current is passed through the head, resulting in an epileptic-like seizure. Although this treatment is now used infrequently, it is still considered to be the most effective and rapid treatment for severe depression.

ED$_{50}$ The effective dose for half the subjects in a drug test.

effective dose The dose of a drug that produces a certain effect in some percentage of the subjects. For example, an ED$_{50}$ produces the effect in 50 percent of the subjects. Note that the dose will depend on the effect that is monitored.

EMIT Enzyme multiplied immunoassay test. The most commonly used urine-screening technique for detecting the presence of various drugs.

emphysema A lung disease in which tissue deterioration results in increased air retention and reduced exchange of gases. The result is difficulty breathing and shortness of breath. An example of a *chronic obstructive lung disease*, often caused by smoking.

employee assistance program A program within a company or organization that provides counseling and/or treatment services to employees.

endorphins Opiate-like chemicals that occur naturally in the brains of humans and other animals. There are several proper endorphins, and the term is also used generically to refer to both the endorphins and the enkephalins.

enkephalins Opiate-like chemicals that occur naturally in the brains of humans and other animals. The enkephalins are smaller molecules than the endorphins.

enzyme A large organic molecule that works to speed up a specific chemical reaction. Enzymes are found in brain cells, where they are needed for most steps in the synthesis of neurotransmitter molecules. They are also found in the liver, where they are needed for the metabolism of many drug molecules.

ephedrine A drug derived from the Chinese medicinal herb *ma huang* and used to relieve breathing difficulty in asthma. A sympathomimetic from which amphetamine was derived.

epilepsy A disorder of the nervous system in which recurring periods of abnormal electrical activity in the brain produce temporary malfunction. There might or might not be loss of consciousness or convulsive motor movements.

ergogenic Energy-producing. Refers to drugs or other methods (e.g., blood doping) designed to increase an athlete's energy output.

ergotism A disease caused by eating grain infected with the ergot fungus. There are both psychological and physical manifestations.

ethical In pharmacy, medicines dispensed only by prescription.

expectancies Learned beliefs about the effects of alcohol or another drug.

extrapyramidal system A motor control system in the central nervous system that is responsible for maintaining muscle tone and posture. Parkinson's disease causes damage to this system. Antipsychotic drugs also interfere with the extrapyramidal system, often producing symptoms similar to those of Parkinson's disease.

false transmitter One method by which a drug can affect the nervous system. The drug is taken into a neuron and acted on by enzymes to produce a substance resembling the natural neurotransmitter but differing from it functionally.

FAS Fetal alcohol syndrome.

FDA United States Food and Drug Administration.

fen-phen A combination of two prescription weight-control medications, fenfluramine and phentermine. No longer prescribed, due to concerns with toxicity to heart valves.

fermentation The process by which sugars are converted into grain alcohol through the action of yeasts.

fetal alcohol effect Individual developmental abnormalities associated with the mother's alcohol use during pregnancy.

fetal alcohol syndrome Facial and developmental abnormalities associated with the mother's alcohol use.

fibrocystic breast disease A benign (noncancerous) but painful disorder characterized by lumps (fibrocysts) in the breasts. There is controversy as to whether caffeine consumption is related to this problem.

flashback An experience reported by some users of LSD in which portions of the LSD experience recur at a later time without the use of the drug.

fly agaric mushroom *Amanita muscaria*, a hallucinogenic mushroom that is also considered poisonous.

freebase In general, when a chemical salt is separated into its basic and acidic components, the basic component is referred to as the free base. Most psychoactive drugs are bases that normally exist in a salt form. Specifically, the salt cocaine hydrochloride can be chemically extracted to form the cocaine free base, which is volatile and can therefore be smoked.

functional disorder A mental disorder for which there is no known organic cause. Schizophrenia is a form of psychosis that is considered to be a functional disorder.

GABA An inhibitory neurotransmitter; gamma-aminobutyric acid.

ganja A preparation of *cannabis* (marijuana) in which the most potent parts of the plant are used.

gateway substances Substances such as alcohol, tobacco, and sometimes marijuana that most users of illicit substances will have tried before their first use of cocaine, heroin, or other less widely used illicit drugs.

generic name For drugs, a name that specifies a particular chemical without being chemically descriptive. As an example, the *chemical name*, sodium chloride, is associated with the *generic name*, table salt, of which there may be several *brand names*, such as Morton's.

genetic marker A chemical or physiological characteristic that is known to be caused by a particular gene and that is highly correlated with some disease state.

GRAE "Generally recognized as effective;" a term defined by the FDA with reference to the ingredients found in OTC drugs (see also *GRAS*).

GRAHL "Generally recognized as honestly labeled" (see *GRAE* and *GRAS*).

grain neutral spirits Ethyl alcohol distilled to a purity of 190 proof (95 percent).

grand mal An epileptic seizure that results in convulsive motor movements and loss of consciousness.

GRAS "Generally recognized as safe;" a term defined by the FDA with reference to food additives and the ingredients found in OTC drugs.

hallucinogen A drug such as LSD or mescaline that produces profound alterations in perception.

hashish A potent preparation of *cannabis* (marijuana).

hash oil A slang term for oil of cannabis, a liquid extract from the marijuana plant.

henbane A poisonous plant containing anticholinergic chemicals and sometimes used for its hallucinogenic properties. *Hyoscyamus niger*.

heroin Originally Bayer's name for diacetylmorphine, a potent narcotic analgesic synthesized from morphine.

HIV Human immunodeficiency virus. The infectious agent responsible for AIDS.

homeostasis A state of physiological balance maintained by various regulatory mechanisms.

hormone A chemical substance formed in one part of the body that stimulates action in another part of the body.

human growth hormone A pituitary hormone responsible for some types of giantism.

hyperactive Refers to a disorder characterized by short attention span and a high level of motor activity. The *DSM-IV* term is *attention-deficit hyperactivity disorder*.

hypnotic Sleep-inducing. For drugs, refers to sleeping preparations.

hypodermic syringe A device to which a hollow needle can be attached so that solutions can be injected through the skin.

hypothalamus A group of nuclei found at the base of the brain, just above the pituitary gland.

ibogaine Hallucinogen that has been shown to reduce self-administration of cocaine and morphine in rats and is proposed to reduce craving in drug addicts.

ibuprofen An aspirin-like analgesic and antiinflammatory.

ice The street name for crystals of methamphetamine hydrochloride.

immunoassay A method for measuring an organic chemical by inducing an animal to develop an antibody to it, then purifying the antibody and using it to measure the chemical in another tissue sample.

IND Approval to conduct clinical investigations on a new drug, filed with the FDA after animal tests are complete.

indole A type of chemical structure. The neurotransmitter serotonin and the hallucinogen LSD both contain an indole nucleus.

inhalants Any of a variety of volatile solvents or other products that can be inhaled to produce intoxication.

insomnia Inability to sleep. The most common complaint is difficulty falling asleep. Often treated with a hypnotic drug.

interferon A chemical produced by the body in response to viral infections. Interferon treatments have been shown to reduce the risk of catching a cold.

intramuscular A type of injection in which the drug is administered into a muscle.

intravenous A type of injection in which the drug is administered into a vein.

kretek A clove cigarette.

laissez-faire A theory that government should not interfere with business or other activities.

LD_{50} The lethal dose for half the animals in a test.

lethal dose The dose of a drug that produces a lethal effect in some percentage of the animals on which it is tested. For example, LD_{50} is the dose that would kill 50 percent of the animals to which it was given.

leukoplakia A whitening and thickening of the soft tissues of the mouth. The use of chewing tobacco is associated with an increase in leukoplakia, considered to be a "precancerous" tissue change.

limbic system A system of various brain structures that are involved in emotional responses.

lipid solubility The tendency of a chemical to dissove in oil, as opposed to in water.

lithium A highly reactive metallic element, atomic number 3. Its salts are used in the treatment of mania and *bipolar disorder*.

liver microsomal enzyme An enzyme associated with a particular subcellular component (the microsomal fraction) of liver cells. There are many such enzymes that are important for drug metabolism.

longitudinal A study done over a period of time (months or years).

look-alikes Drugs sold legally, usually through the mail, that are made to look like controlled, prescription-only drugs. The most common types contain caffeine and resemble amphetamine capsules or tablets.

ma huang A Chinese herb containing ephedrine, which is a sympathomimetic drug from which amphetamine was derived.

major depression A serious mental disorder characterized by a depressed mood. A specific diagnostic term in the *DSM-IV*.

malting The process of wetting a grain and allowing it to sprout, to maximize its sugar content before fermentation to produce an alcoholic beverage.

mandrake *Mandragora officinarum*, a plant having a branched root that contains anticholinergic chemicals. Now classed among the other anticholinergic hallucinogens, this plant was widely believed to have aphrodisiac properties.

marijuana Also spelled marihuana; dried leaves of the cannabis plant.

MDMA Methylenedioxy methamphetamine, a catechol hallucinogen related to MDA. Called "Ecstasy" or "XTC" on the street.

medial forebrain bundle A group of neuron fibers that projects from the midbrain to the forebrain, passing near the hypothalamus. Now known to contain several chemically and anatomically distinct pathways, including dopamine and norepinephrine pathways.

medical model With reference to mental disorders, a model that assumes that abnormal behaviors are *symptoms* resulting from a *disease*.

mental illness A term that, to some theorists, implies acceptance of a medical model of mental disorders.

mesolimbic pathway A group of dopamine-containing neurons that have their cell bodies in the midbrain and their terminals in the forebrain, on various structures associated with the limbic system. Believed by some theorists to be important in explaining the therapeutic effects of antipsychotic medications. Also believed by some theorists to be important for many types of behavioral reinforcers.

metabolism (of drugs) The breakdown of drug molecules by enzymes, often in the liver.

metabolite A product of enzyme action on a drug.

methadone maintenance A program for treatment of narcotic addicts in which the synthetic drug methadone is provided to the addicts in an oral dosage form, so that they can maintain their addiction legally.

Mexican brown A form of heroin that first appeared on American streets in the mid 1970s. Because the heroin is made from the hydrochloride salt of morphine, it is brown in its pure form.

moist snuff A type of oral smokeless tobacco that is popular among young American men. A "pinch" of this chopped, moistened, flavored tobacco is held in the mouth, often between the lower lip and the gum.

monoamine oxidase (MAO) inhibitor A drug that acts by inhibiting the enzyme monoamine oxidase (MAO). Used as an antidepressant.

morphinism An older term used to describe dependence on the use of morphine.

motivational interviewing A technique for encouraging alcoholics or addicts to seek treatment by first assessing their degree of dependence and then discussing the assessment results. Direct confrontation is avoided.

narcolepsy A form of sleep disorder characterized by bouts of muscular weakness and falling asleep involuntarily. The most common treatment employs stimulant drugs such as amphetamine to maintain wakefulness during the day.

narcotic See *opiate*.

narcotic antagonists Drugs that can block the actions of narcotics.

Native American Church A religious organization active among American Indians, in which the hallucinogenic peyote cactus is used in conjunction with Christian religious themes.

NDA In FDA procedures, a New Drug Application. This application, demonstrating both safety and effectiveness of a new drug in both animal and human experiments, must be submitted by a drug company to the FDA before a new drug can be marketed.

neuroleptic A general term for the antipsychotic drugs (also called *major tranquilizers*).

neurosis A type of mental disorder, mostly now referred to as *anxiety disorders*.

neurotransmitter A chemical that is released by one neuron and that alters the electrical activity in another neuron.

Nicotiana Any of several types of tobacco plant, including *N. tobacum* and *N. rustica*.

nicotine The chemical contained in tobacco that is responsible for its psychoactive effects and for tobacco dependence.

nigrostriatal pathway A group of dopamine-containing neurons that have their cell bodies in the *substantia nigra* of the midbrain and their terminals in the *corpus striatum* (basal ganglia), which is part of the extrapyramidial motor system. It is this pathway that deteriorates in Parkinson's disease and on which antipsychotic drugs act to produce side effects resembling Parkinson's disease.

nitrosamines A group of organic chemicals, many of which are highly carcinogenic. At least four are found only in tobacco, and these might account for much of the cancer-causing property of tobacco.

nonspecific effects Effects of a drug that are not changed by changing the chemical makeup of the drug. Also referred to as placebo effects.

norepinephrine A neurotransmitter that might be important for regulating waking and appetite.

NORML The National Organization for the Reform of Marijuana Laws.

NSAIDs Nonsteroidal antiinflammatory drugs, such as ibuprofen and naproxen.

nucleus basalis A group of large cell bodies found just below the basal ganglia and containing acetylcholine. These cells send terminations widely to the cerebral cortex. In Alzheimer's disease, there is a loss of these neurons and a reduction in the amount of acetylcholine in the cortex.

opiate One of a group of drugs similar to morphine, also referred to as narcotics, and used medically primarily for their analgesic effects. The Greek root for *narcotics* meant "numbness," and in early pharmacology writings the term was used for many psychoactive drugs that were thought to reduce pain or dull the senses. Also, by extrapolation from the Bureau of Narcotics, the term *narcotic* came into popular use to refer to any illegal drug (now replaced by the term *controlled substance* in legal writings).

opiate antagonist Any of several drugs that are capable of blocking the effects of drugs. Used in emergency medicine to treat overdose, and in some addiction treatment programs to block the effect of any illicit opiate that might be taken. Nalorphine and naltrexone are examples.

opium A sticky substance obtained from the seed pods of the opium poppy and containing the narcotic chemicals morphine and codeine.

organic disorder For mental disorders, those with a known physical cause (e.g., psychosis caused by long-term alcohol use).

OTC Over-the-counter. OTC drugs are those drugs that can be purchased without a prescription.

Papaver somniferum The opium poppy.

paraphernalia In general, the equipment used in some activity. Drug paraphernalia might include such items as syringes, pipes, scales, or mirrors.

parasympathetic The branch of the autonomic nervous system that has acetylcholine as its neurotransmitter and, for example, slows the heart rate and activates the intestine.

Parkinson's disease A disease of the extrapyramidal motor system, specifically involving damage to the nigrostriatal dopamine system. Early symptoms include muscular rigidity, tremors, a shuffling gait, and a masklike face. Occurs primarily in the elderly.

passive smoking Inhalation of tobacco smoke from the air by nonsmokers.

patent medicines Proprietary medicines. Originally referred to medicines that were in fact treated as inventions and patented in Great Britain. In America, the term came to refer to medicines sold directly to the public.

PCP Phenycyclidine; 1-(1-phenylcyclohexl) piperidine. The brand name Sernyl is no longer in use because it is not legally available for human use. This hallucinogen is often referred to as "angel dust."

PDR *Physician's Desk Reference*, a book listing all prescription drugs and giving prescribing information about each. Updated yearly.

pekoe A grade of tea.

peptide A class of chemicals made up of sequences of amino acids. Enkephalins are small peptides containing only five amino acids, whereas large proteins may contain hundreds.

peyote A hallucinogenic cactus containing the chemical mescaline.

phantastica Hallucinogens that produce altered perceptions but do not generally impair communication with the real world.

pharmacodynamic tolerance Reduced effectiveness of a drug resulting from an altered tissue reaction to the drug.

phenothiazines A group of chemicals that includes several antipsychotic medications.

physical dependence Defined by the presence of a consistent set of symptoms when use of a drug is stopped. These withdrawal symptoms imply that homeostatic mechanisms of the body had made adjustments to counteract the drug's effects and without the drug the system is thrown out of balance.

placebo An inactive drug, often used in experiments to control for nonspecific effects of drug administration.

postsynaptic Refers to structures associated with the neural membrane on the receiving side of a synapse.

potency Relates to how little of a drug is required to produce a given effect.

precursor Something that precedes something else. In biochemistry, a precursor molecule may be acted upon by an enzyme and changed into a different molecule. For example, the dietary amino acid tryptophan is the precursor for the neurotransmitter serotonin.

prodrugs Drugs that are administered in an inactive form and become effective after they are chemically modified in the body by enzymes.

Prohibition The period 1920–1933 during which the sale of alcoholic beverages was prohibited in the United States.

proof A measure of a beverage's alcohol content; twice the alcohol percentage.

proprietary A medicine that is marketed directly to the public. Also called *OTC, patent,* or *nonprescription* medicines.

prostaglandins Local hormones, some of which are synthesized in response to cell injury and are important for initiating pain signals. Aspirin and similar drugs inhibit the formation of prostaglandins.

protein binding The combining of drug molecules with blood proteins.

psychedelic Another name for hallucinogenic drugs. Has a somewhat positive connotation of mind viewing or mind clearing.

psychoactive A term used to describe drugs that have their principal effect on the CNS.

psychological dependence A strong tendency to repeat the use of a drug.

psychopharmacology Science that studies the behavioral effects of drugs.

psychosis A type of mental disorder characterized by a loss of contact with reality and by deterioration in social and intellectual functioning.

psychotomimetic Another name for hallucinogenic drugs. Has a negative connotation of mimicking psychosis.

quid A piece of something to be chewed, such as a wad of chewing tobacco.

receptors Locations at which neurotransmitters or drugs bind, perhaps triggering a physiological response.

reinforcement The process of strengthening a behavioral tendency by presenting a stimulus contingent on the behavior. For example, the tendency to obtain and take a drug might be strengthened by the stimulus properties of the drug that occur after it is taken, thus leading to psychological dependence.

reuptake One process by which neurotransmitter chemicals are removed from synapses. The chemical is taken back up into the cell from which it was released.

Reye's syndrome A rare brain infection that occurs almost exclusively in children and adolescents. There is some evidence that it is more likely to occur in children who have been given aspirin during a bout of flu or chickenpox.

risk factors Behaviors, attitudes, or situations that correlate with, and might indicate the development of, a deviance-prone lifestyle that includes drug or alcohol abuse. Examples are early alcohol intoxification, absence from school, and perceived peer approval of drug use.

rock Another name for *crack*, a smokable form of cocaine.

salicylate A class of chemicals that includes aspirin.

schizophrenia A chronic psychotic disorder for which the cause is unknown.

sedative A drug used to calm a person, reducing stress and excitement.

serotonin A neurotransmitter found in the raphe nuclei that might be important for impulsivity and depression.

sidestream smoke Smoke that comes off a cigarette or cigar from the ash.

sinsemilla A process for growing marijuana that is especially potent in its psychological effects because of a high THC content.

smokeless tobacco Various forms of chewing tobacco and snuff.

social influence model A prevention model adapted from successful smoking-prevention programs.

somatic system The part of the nervous system that controls the voluntary, skeletal muscles, such as the large muscles of the arms and legs.

specific effects Those effects of a drug that depend on the amount and type of chemical contained in the drug.

speed A street term used at one time for cocaine, then for injectable amphetamine, and later for all types of amphetamine. Probably shortened from *speedball.*

SSRI Selective serotonin reuptake inhibitor; a class of antidepressants that includes Prozac.

stages of change Theoretical description of the cognitive stages through which an addict would go in moving from active use to treatment and abstinence: precontemplation, contemplation, preparation, action, and maintenance

stimulant Any of a group of drugs that has the effect of reversing mental and physical fatigue.

street value The theoretical value of an amount of drugs if sold in small quantities on the street.

subcutaneous Under the skin. A form of injection in which the needle penetrates through the skin (about $3/_8$ inch) but does not enter a muscle or vein.

sulfanilamide A type of antibiotic.

sympathetic nervous system A branch of the autonomic nervous system that contains norepinephrine as its neurotransmitter and, for example, increases heart rate and blood pressure.

sympathomimetic Any drug that stimulates the sympathetic nervous system, for example, amphetamine.

symptom In medical terms, some abnormality that indicates a disease. When applied to abnormal behavior, seems to imply a medical model in which some unseen disease causes the abnormal behavior.

synesthesia A phenomenon in which the different senses become mixed, for example, a sound is "seen." Might be reported by a person taking hallucinogens.

synthesis Formation of a chemical compound. For example, some neurotransmitter chemicals must be synthesized within the neuron.

tachyphylaxis A rapid form of tolerance in which a second dose of a drug has a smaller effect than a first dose taken only a short time before.

tar With regard to tobacco, a complex mixture of chemicals found in cigarette smoke. After water, gases, and nicotine are removed from the smoke, the remaining residue is considered to be tar.

tardive dyskinesia Movement disorders that appear after several weeks or months of treatment with antipsychotic drugs, and that usually become worse if use of the drug is discontinued.

temperance With reference to alcohol, temperance originally meant moderation. Eventually the temperance movement adopted complete abstinence as its goal and prohibition as the means.

tetrahydrocannabinol The most active of the many chemicals found in cannabis (marijuana).

THC Tetrahydrocannabinol.

theobromine A mild stimulant similar to caffeine and found in chocolate; a xanthine.

theophylline A mild stimulant similar to caffeine and found in tea; a xanthine.

tolerance The reduced effectiveness of a drug after repeated administration.

toxic Harmful, destructive, or deadly.

tricyclics A group of chemicals used in treating depression.

truth serum Any drugs used to "loosen the tongue," in association with either psychotherapy or interrogation. Although people might speak more freely after receiving some drugs, there is no guarantee that anything they say is true.

uptake The process by which a cell expends energy to concentrate certain chemicals within itself. For example, precursor substances to be synthesized into neurotransmitters must be taken up by the neuron.

values clarification A type of affective education that avoids reference to drugs but focuses on helping students define and defend their own values.

Wernicke-Korsakoff syndrome Chronic mental impairments produced by heavy alcohol use over a long period of time.

wine cooler A beverage made from mixing wine with a fruit-based soft drink.

withdrawal syndrome The set of symptoms that occur reliably when someone stops taking a drug; also called *abstinence syndrome*.

xanthine The chemical class that includes caffeine, theobromine, and theophylline.

CREDITS

PHOTO

Section Openers

One and Two: PhotoDisc/Health and Medicine; **Three:** PhotoDisc/Health and Medicine II; **Four and Five:** Photo-Disc/Health and Medicine; **Six:** Photo-Disc/Science, Technology, Medicine; **Seven:** PhotoDisc/Health and Medicine.

Chapter 1

p.3 (both), p.6, p.17: © McGraw-Hill Higher Education; **p.20:** © H. Armstrong Roberts.

Chapter 2

p.26, p.28: © McGraw-Hill Higher Education; **p.30:** © Annie Griffiths Belt/Corbis Images.

Chapter 3

p.44: © Dennis MacDonald/PhotoEdit; **p.49:** © McGraw-Hill Higher Education.

Chapter 4

p.58: North Wind Picture Archives; **p.59:** National Institutes of Health/Corbis; **p.67:** courtesy of Federal Drug Enforcement Administration; **p.72:** © McGraw-Hill Higher Education; **p.75:** © Charles Gupton/Stock Market; **p.77:** © Amy C. Etra/PhotoEdit; **p.79:** © Michael Okoniewski/The Image Works.

Chapter 5

p.98: © McGraw-Hill Higher Education; **Figure 5.10:** © H. Sochurek, Medichrome/Stock Shop, Inc.; **Figure 5.11:** © Tom & Dee Ann McCarthy/PhotoEdit.

Chapter 6

p.121(both): © McGraw-Hill Higher Education; **p.123(left):** Wolff Communications; **p.123(right):** © McGraw-Hill Higher Education; **p.128:** © W Bertsch/H. Armstrong Roberts.

Chapter 7

p.135: © Gregory G. Dimijian/Photo Researchers, Inc.; **p.139:** © Tony Savino/The Image Works; **p.140(left):** © Johnny Crawford/The Image Works; **p.140(right):** © Charles Steiner/The Image Works; **p.144:** © PhotoEdit; **p.145:** © Alon Reininger/Unicorn Stock Photos; **p.150:** © Michael Newman/PhotoEdit.

Chapter 8

p.166, p.167, p.168, p.170: Drug Enforcement Agency (DEA)/U.S. Department of Justice; **p.179:** © Stewart Halperin Photography.

Chapter 9

p.195: © Robert W. Ginn/Unicorn Stock Photos; **p.200:** © McGraw-Hill Higher Education.

Chapter 10

p.209, p.210, p.213: © McGraw-Hill Higher Education; **Figure 10.4:** Fletcher, C.D.M. and McKee, P.H. An Atlas of Gross Pathology. © 1987 Mosby-Wolfe Europe Limited, London, UK; **p.214:** © McGraw-Hill Higher Education; **Figure 10.5:** © David Young-Wolff/PhotoEdit; **p.216:** © Stewart Halperin Photography; **p.218, p.228 (both):** © McGraw-Hill Higher Education.

Chapter 11

p.240: Bettmann Archive; **p.246:** © Jeff Greenberg/Unicorn Stock Photos; **p.250(left)** © Will & Deni McIntyre/Photo Researchers, Inc.; **p.250(right):** © PhotoEdit.

Chapter 12

p.267: © Andrew Lichtenstein/The Image Works; **p.269:** © Lee Snider/The Image Works; **p.272:** © Adam Jones/Photo Researchers, Inc.; **p.275:** © Michael Greenlar/The Image Works; **p.276:** © Jonathan Nourok/PhotoEdit; **p.280(left):** © Conor Caffrey/SPL/Photo Researchers, Inc.; **p.280(right):** © Bob Daemmrich/The Image Works.

Chapter 13

p.291, p.293: © McGraw-Hill Higher Education/Bob Coyle, photographer; © **p.294:** © Jim Shippee/Unicorn Stock Photos; **p.296:** North Wind Picture Archives; **p.297, p.298:** © McGraw-Hill Higher Education/Bob Coyle, photographer.

Chapter 14

p.315: © Will & Deni McIntyre/Photo Researchers, Inc.; **p.316:** © McGraw-Hill Higher Education/Bob Coyle, photographer; **p.317:** © Michael Newman/PhotoEdit; **p.329:** © Bonnie Kamin/PhotoEdit.

Chapter 15

p.336(both): DEA/U.S. Dept. of Justice; **p.346:** © A. Dex/Publiphoto/Photo Researchers, Inc.; **p.354:** © D. Esbin-Anderson/The Image Works.

Chapter 16

p.396: © McGraw-Hill Higher Education/Red Diamond Stock Photos; **p.367, p.373, p.380:** DEA/U.S. Dept. of Justice; **p.382:** © McGraw-Hill Higher Education/Red Diamond Stock Photos; **p.384:** DEA/U.S. Dept. of Justice; **p.385:** Corbis-Bettmann; **p.390:** DEA/U.S. Dept. of Justice; **p.395:** © K.G. Vock/Okapia/Photo Researchers, Inc.

Chapter 17

p.402, p.403, p.404: DEA/U.S. Dept. of Justice; **p.419:** © Richard Hutchings/Photo Researchers, Inc.

Chapter 18
p.433: © SPL/Photo Researchers, Inc.

Chapter 19
p.449: © PhotoEdit; **p.451:** © Tony Freeman/PhotoEdit; **p.456:** © David K. Crow/PhotoEdit.

LINE ART

Chapter 3
p.46: Reprinted with permission from the *Diagnostic and Statistical Manual of Mental Disorders*, Fourth Edition. Washington, DC, American Psychiatric Association, 1994.

p.52: Reprinted with permission of Alcoholics Anonymous World Services, Inc.

Chapter 7
p.157: Reprinted with permission from the *Diagnostic and Statistical Manual of Mental Disorders*, Fourth Edition. Washington, DC, American Psychiatric Association, 1994.

Chapter 9
p.186, 187, 188: Reprinted with permission from the *Diagnostic and Statistical Manual of Mental Disorders*, Fourth Edition. Washington, DC, American Psychiatric Association, 1994.

Chapter 11
p.262: Reprinted with permission of Alcoholics Anonymous World Services, Inc.

Chapter 16
p.377: From Cohen SL: Lysergic acid diethylamide: Side effects and complications, *Journal of Nervous and Mental Disease* 130:30–40, 1960. © 1982 Williams & Wilkins.

Chapter 18
p.430: © Tribune Media Services, Inc. All Rights Reserved. Reprinted with permission.

INDEX

A

Absenteeism, and drug use, *15*
Abstinence
    in alcoholism treatment, 258–59
    defined, 47, 48
Abstinence syndrome, for
        narcotics, 353*t*
Abstinence violation effect, 253
Academic achievement, and
        drug use, *15*
Acetaldehyde, 219, 256
Acetaminophen
    annual mentions in DAWN, 27*t*
    in cold remedies, 326, 327*t*
    over the counter, 323, 329*t*
Acetylcholine, 94, 99
Acetylsalicylic acid, 319, 329*t*
Acquired immunodeficiency syndrome
        (AIDS). *See* HIV/AIDS
Action stage, of change, 47
Active metabolites, 128, 129
Active placebo effects, 435–36
Active treatment, 49
Acute toxicity, 24, *25*, 354–55
Addiction
    causes of, 42–45
    defining, *5*, 30–31, 37–38
    diagnosing, 45–46
    and early drug law enforcement, 66
    Internet sites on, 54
    lifestyle of, 355–58
    maturing out of, 356
    processes involved in, 38–39
    public image of, 39–41, 340–41,
        343–44
    treatments for, 46–53, 254–59,
        358–63
Adenosine, effects of xanthines
        on, 303–4
Administration routes, of drugs, 120–23

Adrenaline, effect of nicotine on, 282
Advertising
    of alcohol, 243
    countering, 453
    requirements for, 63
    of tobacco, 276, 286, 453
Aerosols, 180*t*
Affective education model, 447–49
Aftercare, 49–50
Aggression
    and alcohol, 32, 249–50
    amphetamines and, 160
    and serotonin, 99
    and steroid use, 437
Agonistic actions of drugs, 103
Agranulocytosis, with clozapine use, 192
AIDS. *See* HIV/AIDS
Alcohol
    advertising of, 243
    annual mentions in DAWN, 27*t*
    behavioral effects of, 221–25, 247–50
    consumption patterns by state, 207,
        244–47
    "demonization" of, 239
    dependence potential of, 31*t*
    forms of, 210–18
    history of use in U.S., 238–44
    interaction with cocaine, 127, 142
    interaction with narcotics, 355
    interaction with sedative-hypnotics,
        174, 179
    Internet sites on, 236, 260
    metabolism of, 218–20
    methods of producing, 208–10
    physiological effects of, 220–25,
        227–28
    and pregnancy, 233–35
    rate of use by age, 12*t*
    and sexual behavior, 225–26
    taxes on, 242
    tolerance for, 222
    toxic effects of, 228–33, 256
    use by college students, 11*t*, 246–47
    and violent crime, 32, 249–50
    withdrawal from, 226–27

Alcohol-content labeling, 221
Alcohol dehydrogenase, 219
Alcoholic dementia, 230
Alcoholics Anonymous (AA)
    creation of, 251
    and disease model of addiction,
        44–45
    treatment approach of, 254–56
    twelve steps of, *52*
Alcoholism
    blackouts and, 225
    brain damage from, 230
    disease model of, 251–52, 254–56
    diseases of, 230, 231–32
    effect of Prohibition on, 242
    and fetal alcohol syndrome, 233–35
    and hormone disorders, 228
    identifying, 250–52
    and immunity, 232–33
    physical symptoms, 229–30
    risk factors for, 252–54
    treating, 254–59
    withdrawal from, 226–27
Aldehyde dehydrogenase, 256
Ale, 211
Allergies, OTC remedies for, 327
All-or-none response, 115
Alpert, Richard, 372–73
Alprazolam (Xanax)
    annual mentions in DAWN, 27*t*
    as antianxiety drug, 170, 173
    dependence potential of, 176
    half-life of, 173*t*
Alternatives to drug use, in drug
        education, 447–48, 449*t*, *450*
Alzheimer's disease, *98*, 99
Amanita muscaria, 395–97
American Medical Association (AMA),
        position on marijuana, 409, 423
Amino acids, in nutritional
        supplements, *436*
Amitriptyline (Elavil), dose range of,
        27*t*, 194*t*
Amobarbital (Amytal), 167*t*
Amotivational syndrome, 420, *421*

Page numbers in *italics* indicate
illustrations or boxed material; page
numbers followed by *t* indicate tables.

482

Amoxapine (Asendin), 194*t*
Amphetamines
  beneficial uses of, 153–60
  on controlled substance
      schedule, 69*t*
  dependence potential of, 31*t*, 161–62
  excretion of, 128
  history of use, 147–51
  illicit production of, 162
  molecular structure of, *152*
  performance-enhancing effects of,
      430, 431, 433–34
  pharmacology of, 104, 151–53
  toxic reactions to, 160–61
Amyl nitrite, 180
Anabolic effects, 435
Anabolic steroids. *See* Steroids
Analgesics
  in cold remedies, 326, 327*t*
  narcotic, 350*t*
  over the counter, 302*t*, 318–24
Anandamide, *410*, 411
Androgenic effects, 435
Anesthesia
  abuse of, 180
  alcohol for, 220
  cocaine for, 136, 141
Angel dust, 390
Animal studies, 64, 116–18
Animism, 366, 367
Anslinger, Harry, 67, 358, 406
Antabuse. *See* Disulfiram (Antabuse)
Antagonistic actions, 103
Antecedents, 15
Antianxiety drugs
  benzodiazepines, 170–72
  development of, 168–69
  half-life of, 173*t*
  medical use of, 173–75, 186–87
Antibiotics, 7
Anticholinergic drugs, synthetic, 394–95
Anticoagulant effects of aspirin, 321–22
Anticonvulsant effects of cannabis, 415
Antidepressants
  actions of, 195–97
  for cocaine dependence
      treatment, 146
  interactions with other drugs, 127
  physical effects of, 113
  types of, 193–95
Antidiuretic hormone (ADH), 228
Antihistamines
  in cold remedies, 326–27
  in OTC sleep aids, 316–17
Antipsychotics
  actions of, 105, 112–13
  characteristics of, 190–93

Antipsychotics—cont'd
  development of, 8
  variations of, 191*t*
Anxiety disorders, 185–87
Anxiolytics. *See* Antianxiety drugs
Appetite, effect of smoking on, 283
Appetite suppressants, 148, 151, 315–16
Aprobarbital (Alurate), 167*t*
Aquarian age, 8–9
Artificial Paradises, 405–6
Aspirin
  annual mentions in DAWN, 27*t*
  development of, 318–19
  physical effects of, 321–23
  therapeutic use of, 319–21
Assassins, 405, 408
Association Against Prohibition, 242
Ataxia, 115
Athletes, influence of, 428–29
Athletics
  beta-2 agonist use in, 439–40
  creatine use in, *439*, 440
  drug-related Internet sites for, 441
  drug testing in, 431
  historical use of drugs in, 429–33
  steroid use in, 431–32, 435–38
  stimulant use in, 160, 433–35
Atropine, 392–93
Attention-deficit hyperactivity disorder
      (ADHD), 156–58
Autonomic nervous system, 94
Avicenna, 336
Axons, chemical signaling in, *90*
Ayahuasca, 382

B

Babies, damaged by crack, *26*, 143, 144
Balanced placebo design, 253
Ballot initiatives on marijuana, *416*, 417
Balzac, Honoré de, 304
Barbital (Veronal), 69*t*, 167*t*
Barbiturates, 166
  as anticonvulsants, 176
  on controlled substance schedule, 69*t*
  dependence potential of, 168, 176–78
  history of use, 167–68
  tolerance for, 168
  toxicity reactions, 178–79
  types of, 167*t*
  withdrawal from, 178
Basal ganglia, 95
Baudelaire, Charles-Pierre, 405
Bayer Company, 319
Beer
  consumption trends, *212*
  labeling of, 221

Beer—cont'd
  manufacture of, 210–12
  and prohibition, 243
Behavior, and brain chemistry, 105–6
Behavioral tolerance, 128–29, 352
Behavioral toxicity, 24, *25*
Behavioral treatments for
      alcoholism, 257
Belladonna, 392–93
Benign breast disease, 307
Benzedrine, 148, 149
Benzocaine, 316
Benzodiazepines, 166
  as anticonvulsants, 176
  dependence potential of, 176–78
  history of use, 170–72
  as hypnotics, 175–76
  mechanisms of action, 172–73
  toxicity reactions, 178–79
  withdrawal from, 178
Benzopyrene, 419
Beta-2 agonists, 439–40
Beta-endorphin, 350
Betty Ford Clinic, 51
Bhang, 403
Binge drinking, 257
Biochemical theories of behavior, 105–6
Biology, and addiction, 43
Biopsychosocial perspective of
      addiction, 45
Bipolar disorder, 187, 198
Birth defects, 307. *See also* Pregnancy;
      Reproduction
Biruni, 336
Blackouts, 225
Black tar, 346, 357
Bleeding, aspirin's effect on, 321–22
Blood, drug transport in, 123–25
Blood alcohol concentration, 221–25
Blood-brain barrier, 95, 125
Blood vessels, autonomic effects on, 94*t*
Body weight, and blood alcohol
      concentration, 223*t*
Boggs amendment, 67
Boston Tea Party, 295–96
Bourbon, 217
Brain
  action of cocaine on, 140
  chemical pathways of, 97–100
  damage from alcohol abuse, 230
  damage from marijuana use, 420–21
  imaging technologies for, 106–7
  opiate receptors in, 349–50
  structures of, 94–97
Brain stem, 96
Brand names of drugs, 110
Breathing, autonomic effects on, 94*t*

Breweries, 211
Bright tobacco, 269
British East India Company, 338
Bromides, 166
Bronchi, autonomic effects on, 94t
Buckley, William F., 423
Buffering of aspirin, 320
Bufotenin, *396, 397*
Buprenorphine, 52, 146
Bupropion (Wellbutrin), 194t
Bureau of Land Management, 78
Bureau of Narcotics
    creation of, 67
    uniform law on cannabis, 408
Burley tobacco, 269
Butabarbital (Butisol), 167t
Butyl nitrite, 180

C

Cade, John, 197
Caffeine
    behavioral effects of, 304–6
    common sources of, 302, 303t
    dependence potential of, 31t, 303, *305*
    Internet sites on, 309
    OTC use of, 302, 314, 329t
    pharmacology of, 302–6
    physiological effects of, 304, 429, 434
    potential risks of, 306–8
    removing from coffee, 293
    in soft drinks, 300, 301
    in tea, 297
    withdrawal from, 303
Caffeinism, 308
Camel cigarettes, 268
Cancer
    and alcohol, 232
    and caffeine, 307
    and smoking, 276–77
Cannabinoids, 410
Cannabis
    dependence potential of, 417–18
    history of use, 404–9
    medical uses of, 414–17
    pharmacology of, 410–14
    regulation of, 408–9
    toxicity potential of, 418–21
    types of, 401–4
    See also Marijuana
Cannabis buyers clubs, *416*
Carbohydrate loading, *436*
Carbohydrates, in nutritional
        supplements, *436*
Carbon monoxide
    in cigarettes, 270
    in marijuana, 419

Cardiovascular disease, 276–77
Cardiovascular system
    effect of alcohol on, 232
    effect of caffeine on, 304, 307–8
    effect of cocaine on, 142
    effect of marijuana smoking on, 412
    effect of smoking on, 276–77, 282–83
    effect of steroids on, 438
Carter's Little Liver Pills, 63
Catecholamines, 106, 151, 153
Cell membrane, effects of drugs on, 126
Central Intelligence Agency (CIA), LSD
        research by, 371–72
Central nervous system, 93
Cerebral atrophy, 420–21
Cerebral cortex, 95, *96*
Cerletti, Ugo, 189
Charas, 402
Cheek, J. O., 293
Chemical dependency programs, 51–52
Chemical messengers, 89–93
Chemical names of drugs, 110
Chemotherapy, and marijuana smoking,
        415–16
Chewing tobacco, development of,
        266–67, 273–74
Children, and cigarette advertising, 286
Chloral hydrate, 69t, 166
Chlordiazepoxide (Librium)
    in alcohol detoxification, 227
    dependence potential of, 176, 178
    development of, 170
    half-life of, 173t
    time course of, *171*
Chlorpheniramine maleate, 326,
        327t, 329t
Chlorpromazine (Thorazine)
    as antipsychotic, 190
    dose range of, 191t
    effect on DOM, 387
    as LSD antagonist, 376
Chocolate, 297–98, 299t
Cholecystokinin, 316
Chromosome damage, and LSD, 379–80
Chronic diseases, from alcohol
        abuse, 230
Chronic obstructive lung disease, 277
Chronic toxicity, 24, *25*, 355
Chute, Anthony, 265
Cigarettes
    advertising of, 286
    dependence potential of, 31t
    development of, 267–68
    as gateway substances, 16–17
    low tar and nicotine, 270–71
    production of, 268–70
    rate of use by age, 12t

Cigarettes—cont'd
    sales of, *271*
    smokeless, 287
    use by adolescents, 12t, 452–53
    use by college students, 11t
    See also Smoking; Tobacco
Cigars
    development of, 267–68
    usage trends, 274
Cirrhosis, 231–32
Clark, Walter, 371
Clenbuterol, 439–40
Clinics, for narcotic addicts, 343, 358,
        361, 362–63
Clonidine, 352–53
Clorazepate (Tranxene), 173t
Clozapine (Clozaril), 191t, *192*
Coca, early use of, 135–36
Coca-Cola, 136, 299–301
Cocaethylene, 127, 142
Cocaine
    action on neurotransmitters, 104
    anesthetic properties of, 6
    annual mentions in DAWN, 27t, 145
    chemical structure of, 140
    in Coca-Cola, 299–301
    deaths from, 27t, 28–29, 142
    defined, 59
    dependence potential of, 31t, 142–43
    early history of use and abuse, 58,
        135–39
    forms of, 139
    interactions with alcohol, 127, 142
    Internet sites on, 163
    paraphernalia for, 73
    pharmacology of, 139–41
    physical effects of, 141
    popularity of, 9–10, 138–39, 141,
        145–46
    production and smuggling of, 145
    rate of use by age, 12t
    reproductive effects of, 143, 144
    toxic reactions to, 142, 146
    treatment for dependence, 146–47
    use among college students, 11t, 145
    use in sports, 429, 433, 434
Cocaine hydrochloride, 139
Cocoa, 298
Codeine
    annual mentions in DAWN, 27t
    on controlled substance
        schedule, 69t
    as cough suppressant, 351
    discovery of, 339
    molecular structure of, 348, *349*
    recommended dosage, 350t
Codependency, 43–44

Coffee
  caffeine content of, 299t
  decaffeinated, 293
  history of use, 290–94
  instant, 293
Coffeehouses, 291–92
Cognitive developmental approach, to
      smoking prevention, 454
Cohoba snuff, 381
Colds
  causes and symptoms of, 324–25
  OTC remedies for, 302t, 325–27
Coleridge, Samuel Taylor, 337
College students, use of alcohol by,
      11t, 246–47
Columbus, Christopher, 264
Comatose, 116
Commission on Marijuana and Drug
      Abuse, 423
Commitment, involuntary, 200–201
Communication skills instruction, in
      drug education, 448–49
Community programs, for drug abuse
      prevention, 458
Compassionate use, 76, 415, 416–17
Comprehensive Drug Abuse Prevention
      and Control Act, 68–70, 423
Compulsive behavior, and
      amphetamines, 161
Comtrex, 327t
Concentration, and drug effects, 118–20
Conditioned reflexes, to narcotics, 352
Confessions of an English Opium
      Eater 337
Congeners, 217, 229
Conservatism, social, 9
Contac, 327t
Contemplation stage of change, 47
Contingency contracting, 146–47
Contraceptives, oral, 8
Controlled drinking, 47, 48, 257–59
Controlled substances, 69t, 70
Controlled Substances Act, 68–70
Convulsive therapy, 189
Coping skills, 257, 448
Coronaviruses, 324
Correlate, 13
Correlations, of personal characteristics
      with drug use, 12–14, 15
Corruption of drug enforcement
      officers, 78–79
Cortez, Hernando, 298
Cough suppressants
  narcotics as, 351
  over the counter, 326, 327t, 329, 351
Council for Tobacco Research, 276
Count of Monte Cristo, The, 405

Crack
  combining with heroin, 347–48
  dependence potential of, 31t
  development of, 139
  patterns of use, 145–46
  use among college students, 11t
Crack babies, 26, 143, 144
Cranial nerves, 93
Crank. See Methamphetamine
Creatine, 439, 440
Creativity, and LSD, 379
Crime
  and drug abuse, 31–35, 343–44
  and marijuana, 406, 407–8
Culture, and alcohol use, 244
Cumulative effects, 120, 121
Cyclazocine, 359
Cylert, 159–60

D
Date-rape drug, 172
Datura, 393–94
Deactivation, 119, 126–28
Deaths from drug abuse, 27, 28
Decaffeination, 293
Decongestants, 326, 327t
Dehydration, and hangover, 229
Delirium tremens, 226
Delta-9-tetrahydrocannabinol (THC)
  as active ingredient in
      cannabis, 402–3
  behavioral effects of, 412–14
  classification of, 76
  medical uses of, 415–17
  molecular structure of, 410
  physical effects of, 410–12
  toxicity potential of, 418–21
  See also Cannabis; Marijuana
Demonization of alcohol, 239
Dependence
  physical, 38–39
  psychiatric diagnosis of, 46
  psychological, 40, 161–62, 353, 418
Dependence potential
  of amphetamines, 161–62
  of barbiturates, 168
  of cocaine, 142–43
  and drug actions, 171
  of marijuana, 417–18
  of narcotics, 352–54
  of psychoactive drugs, 31t
  of sedative-hypnotics, 176–78
Depressants
  abuse of, 169, 172, 174, 179
  as anticonvulsants, 176
  beneficial uses of, 173–76

Depressants—cont'd
  dependence potential of, 176–78
  examples of, 112
  history of use, 166–72
  interactions with other drugs, 127
  mechanisms of action, 172–73
  physical effects of, 111–12, 133, 165
  respiratory depression from, 127
  toxicity reactions, 178–79
  withdrawal from, 178
Depression
  described, 187
  electroconvulsive therapy for, 197
  and serotonin, 100
  treatment with amphetamines, 153
De Quincey, Thomas, 337–38
Designer drugs, 357, 387
Desipramine (Norpramin), 194t
Detoxification, 48–49, 226, 256
Deviant drug use, 4–5
Deviant subcultures, and drug use, 14, 19
"Devil drugs," 333
Dexamethasone suppression test, 197
Dexedrine, 151
Dexfenfluramine (Redux), 155, 156
Dextromethorphan
  in cold remedies, 326, 327t, 329
  as cough suppressant, 351
Diagnostic and Statistical Manual
      (DSM-IV)
  alcoholism in, 252
  and addiction, 45–46
  and caffeine dependence, 305
  classifications of mental illness,
      185–88
  recognition of ADHD, 156–57
Diarrhea, treatment with narcotics,
      334, 351
Diazepam (Valium)
  annual mentions in DAWN, 27t
  dependence potential of, 31t,
      176, 178
  half-life of, 173t
  history of use, 170–71
  time course of, 171
  toxicity reactions, 179
Diazepam-binding inhibitor peptide, 173
Diethylene glycol, 62
Digestive tract, effect on drugs, 120–21
Dihydrocodeine, 350t
Dimethyltryptamine (DMT), 381–82
Diphenhydramine, 317, 329t
Director of National Drug Control
      Policy, 70
Disease
  addiction as, 44–45, 251–52, 254–56
  drug treatments for, 7–8

Distilled spirits
  early movements against, 239–40
  invention of, 209–10
  manufacture of, 215–17
Disulfiram (Antabuse), 52, 256
Diuretics, caffeine in, 302t
d-lysergic acid diethylamide (LSD)
  adverse reactions to, 376–78
  on controlled substance schedule, 69t
  dependence potential of, 31t
  discovery of, 369–70
  misconceptions about, 379–80
  molecular structure of, 368
  perceptual effects of, 375–76
  pharmacology of, 374–75
  potency of, 118
  recreational use of, 372–74
  research on, 370–72
DOM, 383, 387
Dopamine
  brain pathways for, 97–99
  effect of antipsychotics on, 191–92
  effect of cocaine on, 140
  effect of tobacco on, 285
  molecular structure of, 152, 383
  synthesis of, 101
Doping, and athletics, 429–30
Dosage, relation to effects, 6, 114–18
Dose-response curve, 114
Double-blind experiments, 114
Doxepin (Sinequan), 194t
D-propoxyphene, 27t
Drinking
  controlled, 47
  See also Alcohol; Alcoholism
Drinking age, 243
Dristan, 327t
Driving
  and marijuana use, 418–19
  under the influence of alcohol,
    247–49
Dronabinol (Marinol), 76, 416
Drug abuse
  and crime, 31–35
  deaths from, 25, 27t
  defined, 5
  influence of peers, parents, and
    community on, 456–58
  interventions for, 47 (see also
    Treatment)
  and lifestyle patterns, 355–58
  prevention stages, 445–46
  psychiatric diagnosis of, 46
  school prevention programs, 446–56
  treatments for, 46–53
  victims of, 24
  See also specific drugs
Drug Abuse Control Amendments, 68

Drug Abuse Reporting Program
    (DARP), 51
Drug Abuse Resistance Education
    (DARE), 454–55
Drug Abuse Warning Network
    (DAWN), 25–27
Drug addiction. See Addiction;
    Dependence potential
Drug czar, 70
Drug dependence, Internet sites on, 182
Drug disposition tolerance, 128, 129
Drug education, 444–47. See also
    Prevention programs
Drug enforcement. See Regulation
    of drugs
Drug Enforcement Agency (DEA)
  creation of, 68
  efforts against cocaine smuggling, 145
  foreign activities of, 78
Drug-free schools program, 449–51
Drug-free zones, 73
Drug-Induced Rape Prevention and
    Punishment Act, 172
Drug interactions, 127
Drug misuse, 5
Drug paraphernalia, 73–74
Drugs
  abusing (see Drug abuse)
  actions on brain, 100–105, 108
  addiction to (see Addiction;
    Dependence potential)
  antipsychotic, 8
  categories of, 110–13
  deactivation of, 119, 126–28
  defining, 4, 59, 87
  effectiveness of, 63
  effects of, 113–20, 125–26 (see also
    specific drugs)
  identifying, 113
  illicit, 4, 33–35
  interactions with other drugs, 127
  marketing, 63–65
  methods of taking, 120–23, 141
  misuse of, 5
  naming, 110
  over the counter (see Over-the-
    counter drugs)
  prescription (see Prescription drugs)
  psychoactive (see Psychoactive drugs)
  regulation of (see Regulation of drugs)
  testing, 63–65, 114
  tolerance for (see Tolerance)
  toxicity of (see Toxicity)
  transport to tissues, 123–25
  wartime uses of, 148–49
  See also Drug abuse; Drug use
Drug selling, penalties for, 70
Drug testing, 74–76

Drug use
  alternatives to, 449t, 450
  analyzing, 2–4
  antecedents of, 14–18
  correlates of, 12–14, 15
  current extent of, 10–12
  deviant, 4–5
  gateway substances for, 16–17
  history of, 7–10
  laissez-faire approach to, 23–24
  motives for, 18–20, 21
  perspectives of, 1
  risk factors for, 14, 15, 16
  social influences on, 7–9, 21
  and socioeconomic status, 13–14
Drug Use Forecasting Program, 33
Duke, James Buchanan, 269
Dumas, Alexander, 405
Dutch East India Company, 295
Dysfunctional families, and
    addiction, 43–44

E

Ebers papyrus, 335
Education, and drug use, 15
Effective dose, 116–17
Effectiveness criteria for drugs, 63, 312
Eighteenth Amendment, 65–66
Electroconvulsive therapy, 189, 197
Electrolyte drinks, 437
Elixir Sulfanilimide, 62
Ellis, Havelock, 386
Emergency room visits, 25, 27t
Emphysema, 285
Employees, urine testing of, 74
Enabling behavior, 43–44
Endorphins
  brain pathways for, 100
  discovery of, 350
  and placebo effects, 114
English East India Company, 294–95
Enkephalins, 349–50
Enzyme multiplied immunoassay test
    (EMIT), 74–75
Enzymes
  metabolic actions of, 103, 104, 126–28
  for metabolizing alcohol, 219–20
  role in neurotransmitter
    synthesis, 102
  synthetic, 102
Ephedrine, 147–48
  in cold remedies, 326, 327t
  in look-alike drugs, 315
  molecular structure of, 152
Epilepsy, 176
Ergogenic drugs, 430
Ergot fungus, 369–70

Ergotism, 369
Expectancies, 246
Experiments, double-blind, 114
"Extreme" beverages, 301–2

F

Families, alcoholism in, 43–44
Family interaction approaches to drug
    education, 457–58
Fats, in nutritional supplements, *436*
Fatty liver, 231
Federal Aviation Administration, 78
Federal Narcotics Control Board, 66
Fenfluramine (Pondimin), 99, 155, 156
Fen-Phen, 155, 156
Fentanyl, 348, 350*t*, 357
Fermentation, 208–9
Fetal alcohol effect, 234
Fibrocystic breast disease, 307
Fight or flight response, 94
Filter cigarettes, 268, 270
Financial Crimes Enforcement
    Network, 78
Flashbacks, 378
Flue-curing, 269
Fluffing, 270
Flunitrazepam (Rohypnol), 172
Fluoxetine (Prozac)
    and depression, 100
    development of, 195
    dose range of, 194*t*
    effect on MDMA, 388
    popularity of, 196
Fluphenazine (Permitil), of, 191*t*
Flurazepam (Dalmane), 173*t*, 175
Food, Drug, and Cosmetic Act
    passage of, 62
    recognition of prescription drugs, 313
Food and Drug Administration (FDA)
    creation of, 62
    drug review procedures of, 63–65,
        311–13
Football, drug use in, 431
Foreign policy, and drug
    enforcement, 78, 79
Freebase, 139
Freedom, effect of drug enforcement
    on, 79–80
"French connection," 345
Freud, Sigmund, 136–37

G

Galen, 335
Gamma alcoholism, 256
γ-aminobutyric acid (GABA)
    actions of, 93
    and brain pathways, 100

γ-aminobutyric acid (GABA)—cont'd
    effect of alcohol on, 129, 220
    effect of depressants on, 173, 220
Gamma-hydroxybutyrate (GHB),
        174, 175
Gangrene, and ergotism, 369
Ganja, 402
Gas chromatography/mass spectrometry
        (GS/MS), 74–75
Gaseous anesthetics, 180
Gastrointestinal system, effect of
        narcotics on, 351
Gateway substances, 16–17
Gautier, Théophile, 405
Gender, and alcohol consumption, 246
Generalized anxiety disorder, *186*
Generally recognized as safe
        (GRAS), 312
General paresis, 189
Generic drugs, FDA approval of, 110
Generic names, of drugs, 110
Generic wines, 213
Genetic marker for alcoholism, 254, 255
Gin, 216
Glaucoma, marijuana smoking for, 415
Glue sniffing, 181
Good Friday study, 381
Grain neutral spirits, 216
Growth, manipulating, 438–39
Gymnastics, hormone use in, 438

H

Hair, drug screening from, 75–76
Hallucinogens
    anticholinergic, 392–95
    catechol, 382–92
    examples of, *112*
    indole, 368–82
    Internet sites on, 398
    LSD, 369–80
    physical effects of, 112
    regulation of, 68
    use among college students, 11*t*
Haloperidol (Haldol)
    dose range of, 191*t*
    movement disorders from, 193
    for psychoses, 105
Halsted, W. S., 136
Hangover, 228–30
Hard-core users, *19*
Harm reduction model of drug
        control, *362*
Harrison Act
    enforcement of, 65–68, 138, 342–44
    passage of, 60–61
Hashish
    annual mentions in DAWN, 27*t*

Hashish—cont'd
    history of use, 404–9
    origin of, 402
    use among college students, 11*t*
    See also Cannabis
Hash oil, 403, 404
Headache, and caffeine, 305–6
Heart, effects of cocaine on, 142
Heart attacks, and aspirin, 321
Heart disease
    and alcohol, 232
    and caffeine, 307–8
Heart rate, autonomic effects on, 94*t*
Heffter, Arthur, 385
Hemp, 402
Henbane, 393
Hepatitis, alcoholic, 231
Heredity, and addiction, 43–44, 253–54
Heroin
    addict's lifestyle, 355–58
    anesthetic properties of, 6
    annual mentions in DAWN, 27*t*
    changing addict population,
        344–45, 346
    on controlled substance schedule, 69*t*
    deaths from, 28–29
    dependence potential of, 31*t*, 340
    development of, 340
    diamorph, 350*t*
    medical use of, *343*, 361–63
    misconceptions about, 356–57
    molecular structure of, 348, *349*
    sources of, 345–46, *347*
    withdrawal from, 353*t*, 357
Heroin chic, 346
Hicks, Thomas, 429
High-density lipoproteins (HDL), 232
High school students
    marijuana use among, 422
    smoking among, *272*
Hiring, urine testing in, 74
HIV/AIDS
    among drug abusers, 29–30
    new drugs for, 65
Hofmann, Albert, 369–70, 380, 381
Hogsheads, 269
Homelessness, and mental illness, *201*
Homeostasis, 89
Homicide, and alcohol, 249
Hormone receptor blocking drugs, 438
Hormones
    actions of, 89, *90*
    effect of alcohol on, 228
    use in sports, 431–32, 435–38
House-to-house surveys, 12
Human growth hormone, 438
Human immunodeficiency virus (HIV).
        See HIV/AIDS

Huxley, Aldous, 386
Hydrocodone, 350*t*
Hydrogen cyanide, in marijuana, 419
Hydromorphone, 350*t*
Hyperactivity
   and caffeine, 306
   treatment with amphetamines,
      156–58
Hypnotics
   defined, 165
   half-life of, 173*t*
   medical use of, 175–76
Hypodermic syringe
   impact on morphine use, 339
   introduction of, 58
Hypothalamus, functions of, 95–96

I

Ibogaine
   as addiction treatment, *391*
   effects of, 52–53
Ibotenic acid, 397
Ibuprofen, annual mentions in DAWN,
      27*t*, 323–24
Ice, 151. *See also* Methamphetamine
Illicit drugs, defined, *4*, 33–35
Imipramine (Tofranil), 194*t*, 198*t*
Immune system
   alcohol's effects on, 232–33
   effects of marijuana on, 420
Indole hallucinogens
   DMT, 381–82
   LSD, 369–80
   molecular structure of, 368–69
   morning glory, 381
   psilocybin, 380–81
Inhalants, 166
   preventing abuse of, *452*
   types of, 179–82
   use among college students, 11*t*
Inhalation, advantages and
      disadvantages of, 122
Inhalers, amphetamines in, 148, 149
Injection
   advent of, 339, 343
   and addiction, 353, 354
   by heroin addicts, described, 355–56
   HIV/AIDS spread by, 29–30
   methods of, 121–22
Insanity, and marijuana use, 420
Insomnia, 175–76, 177
Institute of Medicine, 417
Insulin-shock therapy, 189
Interactions between drugs, 127
International programs for drug
      enforcement, 78

Internet sites
   addiction, 54
   alcohol, 236, 260
   caffeine, 309
   cocaine and methamphetamine, 163
   drug actions, 108
   drug dependence, 182
   drug regulation, *82*
   drugs and crime, *36*
   drugs in sports, 441
   drug toxicity, *36*
   drug use, *22*
   hallucinogens, 398
   marijuana, 425
   opiates, 364
   OTC drugs, 330
   pharmacology, 130
   prevention, 460
   psychopharmacology, 182
   psychotherapeutic drugs, 202
   tobacco, 288
Interventions, 47. *See also* Treatment
Intestines, autonomic effects on, 94*t*
Intoxication, and blood alcohol
      concentration, 221–25
Intramuscular injections, 122
Intravenous injection, 121
Iproniazid, 193–94
Iron, in nutritional supplements, *437*
Isoniazid, 193–94

J

James, William, 386
Jaundice, and cirrhosis, 231–32
Jellinek, E. M., 256
Jimsonweed, 394
Joe Camel, 286
Jones-Miller Act, 66
"Just Say No!" model, 449

K

Kefauver, Estes, 63
Ketamine, 31*t*, 389
Kidneys, excretion of drugs by, 126
Knowledge-attitudes-behavior
      model, 446–47

L

Labeling, of OTC drugs, 313
Laborit, Henri, 190
Lager, 210
LaGuardia, Fiorello, 409
Laissez-faire approach to drug
      use, 23–24

L-alpha-acetyl-methadol
      (LAAM), 360–61
Laudanum, 336–37
L-dopa, 105
League of Spiritual Discovery, 373
Leary, Timothy, and LSD, 372–74, 408
Le Club de Hachischins, 405
Legare, D., 265
Lethal dose, 117–18
Leu-enkephalin, 349–50
Leukoplakia, 274
l-hyoscyamine, in anticholinergic
      hallucinogens, 392, 393
Librium. *See* Chlordiazepoxide (Librium)
Life Skills Training Program, 456
Limbic system, functions of, 96
Lipid solubility, 120, 167
Lipton, Thomas, 297
Liqueurs, 217
Liquor. *See* Alcohol; Distilled spirits
Lithium, 197–98
Liver
   action on drugs, 121, 126–28
   alcohol-induced disorders of, 231–32
   alcohol metabolism in, 219–20
   damage from acetaminophen, 323
   metabolism of nicotine, 282
Liver microsomal enzymes, 127
Local government, drug regulation
      by, 70–73
Locus ceruleus, 99
Longitudinal studies, 16, 17
Look-alike drugs, 150–51, 314–15
Loose-leaf tobacco, 273
Lorazepam (Ativan), 173*t*
Loxapine (Loxitane), 191*t*
LSD. *See* d-lysergic acid
      diethylamide (LSD)
Lung cancer
   and cigarettes, 276–77
   and marijuana, 419
Lungs, effect of marijuana smoking
      on, 412, 419

M

Magnetic resonance imaging
      (MRI), 106–7
Mainlining. *See* Injection
Maintenance stage of change, 47
Malaria therapy, for general
      paresis, 189
Malting, 209
Malt liquor, 211
Mandrake, 393
Mandrax, 169
Mania, treatment with lithium, 197–98

Manic-depressive episode, *DSM-IV* criteria for, *188*
Manic episode, *DSM-IV* criteria for, *188*
Mariani, Angelo, 136
Mariani's Coca Wine, 429
Marijuana
 annual mentions in DAWN, 27*t*
 on controlled substance schedule, 69*t*, 416
 defined, 7
 dependence potential of, 31*t*, 417–18
 history of use, 404–9, 422–24
 Internet sites on, 425
 medical uses of, 414–17
 origin of, 401–4
 pharmacology of, 410–14
 potency of, 404
 rate of use by age, 12*t*
 regulation of, 67, 408–9, 423–24
 screening tests for, 75
 society's attitudes about, 422–24
 special status of, *76*, 113
 studies of, 409, 411–14
 tolerance for, 414*t*, 417
 toxicity potential of, 418–21
 usage trends of, 11–12, 409, 422
 See also Cannabis
Marijuana Tax Act, 67, 408–9, 422–23
Marinol, 416
Masculinization, and steroid use, 432, 435, 438
Maturing out, of addicts, 356
Maxwell House coffee, 293
McCarthy, Joseph, 67–68
MDA, *383*, 387
MDMA
 dependence potential of, 31*t*
 effects of, 387–88
 molecular structure of, *383*
Medication-assisted treatment, 52–53
Medicine
 drugs as, 7–8
 patent (*see* Patent medicines)
 tobacco as, 265
Medulla, 96
Memory, effects of marijuana on, 413–14
Mental disorders, chemical causes of, *105*
Mental hospitals, effect of drug treatments on, 199–201
Mental illness
 classification of, 185–88
 evolution of treatment for, 188–98, 199–201
 and homelessness, *201*
 medical model of, 184–85

Mental performance, effects of amphetamines on, 159–60
Meperidine, 350*t*
Mephobarbital (Merbaral), 167*t*
Meprobamate, 168–69
Meridia. *See* Sibutramine (Meridia)
Mescal beans, 384
Mescal buttons, 383
Mescaline
 dependence potential of, 31*t*
 molecular structure of, *383*
 nonreligious use of, 385–86
 pharmacology of, 386–87
 religious use of, 382–85
Mesolimbic dopamine pathway, 99
Mesoridazine (Serentil), 191*t*
Metabolism
 of alcohol, 218–20
 of drugs, 126–28
 of neurotransmitters, 103, *104*
 and smoking, 283
Met-enkephalin, 349–50
Methadone
 for addiction treatment, 359–60
 annual mentions in DAWN, 27*t*
 effectiveness of, 53
 recommended dosage, 350*t*
 withdrawal from, 352, 353*t*
Methamphetamine
 annual mentions in DAWN, 27*t*
 on controlled substance schedule, 69*t*
 illicit production of, 162
 injection of, 150
 Internet sites on, 163
 molecular structure of, *152*
 resurgence of popularity, 151
 wartime use in Japan, 148–49
Methapyrilene, 316–17
Methaqualone, 169–70
Methylene chloride, 293
Methylphenidate (Ritalin), 158
Mexican brown, 346
Midbrain, 96
Migraine, effect of caffeine on, 304, 305–6
Military
 heroin addiction in Vietnam, 344–45
 LSD research by, 371–72
 urine testing in, 74
 in war on drugs, 77
Milk chocolate, 298
Miltown, 168
Minerals, in nutritional supplements, *437*
Minimal brain dysfunction, 156
Mirtazapine (Remeron), 194*t*

Miscarriage, 280, 307
Mitchell, Weir, 386
Model glue, sniffing, 181
Moist snuff, 273
Molindone (Moban), 191*t*
Monitoring the Future Project, 11
Monkeys
 drug research with, 40–41
 effects of marijuana on, *421*
Monoamine oxidase (MAO), 285
Monoamine oxidase (MAO) inhibitors, 193–94
Mood
 catecholamine theory of, 106
 disorders of, 187, *188*
 effect of steroids on, 436–37
 ranges of, *154*
Morning glory, 381
Morphine
 annual mentions in DAWN, 27*t*
 on controlled substance schedule, 69*t*
 dependence potential of, 31*t*, 137
 discovery of, 339–40
 early history of abuse, 58
 molecular structure of, 348, *349*
 as pain reliever, 351
 recommended dosage, 350*t*
 withdrawal from, 353*t*, 357
Motivation
 for drug use, 18–20
 effect of marijuana use on, 420
Motivational interviewing, 47
Movement disorders, from antipsychotics, 192–93
MPPP, 357
MPTP, 357
Mucous membranes, absorption of drugs through, 123
Murder, and alcohol, 249
Muscarine, 397
Muscimol, 397

N

Naloxone, 349, 359
Naltrexone
 for alcoholism, 256–57
 effects of, 52
 for heroin addiction, 349, 359, 363
Napoleon, 405
Narcolepsy, 148, 155–56
Narcosis therapy, 189
Narcotic antagonists
 discovery of, 348–49
 treatment with, 358–59
Narcotic Drug Control Act, 68

Narcotics
beneficial uses of, 351
dependence potential of, 352–54
interaction with alcohol, 355
Internet sites on, 364
misconceptions about, 356–57
regulation of, 65–70
respiratory depression from, 127
tolerance for, 352
toxic effects of, 354–55
treatment for addicts, 358–63
withdrawal from, 352–53, 357
See also Opiates
Narcotics Division, 65–67
Narcotic triad, 355
Nasal decongestants, 326, 327t
National Collegiate Athletic Association
(NCAA) drug ban, 433
National Drug Control Strategy
review, 77–78
National Football League (NFL) drug
ban, 431
National Institute of Mental
Health (NIMH)
marijuana research, 411
review of LSD research, 371
National Organization for the Reform of
Marijuana Laws, 416, 423
National Park Service, 78
Native American Church, 384–85
Natural highs, 447–48, *450*
Nausea
and hangover, 229
marijuana smoking for, 415–16
from narcotics, 355, 356, 357
Needle exchange programs, 29–30, *362*
Needle freaks, 354
Needles, sharing, 29, 122. *See also*
Hypodermic syringe; Injection
Negative reinforcement, 353
Nervous system
chemical signaling in, *90,* 91–93
natural opiates in, 349–51
parts of, 93–94
Netazodone (Serzone), 194t
Neuroleptic drugs, 190
Neurons
chemical signaling in, *90*
effects of drugs on, 126
Neurotransmitters
actions of, 91–93
effects of drugs on, 103–5, 126,
195–96, 285
life cycle of, 100–103
production of, 96
New drug application, 62

New York Academy of Medicine, 409
Nicot, Jean, 265
Nicotiana rustica, 266, 267
Nicotiana tobacum, 266, 267
Nicotine
action on neurotransmitters, 104
in Alzheimer's research, *98*
dependency potential of, 284–85
derivation of term, 265
non-tobacco products containing, 287
pharmacology of, 281–85
Nicotinic receptors, *98*
Nigerian connection, *348*
Nigrostriatal dopamine pathway, 97–99
Nitrites, abuse of, 180–81
Nitrosamines
in marijuana, 419
in smokeless tobacco, 274
Nitrous oxide, 180
Nonprescription Drug Advisory
Committee, 313
Nonspecific effects of drugs, 113–14
Nonsteroidal antiinflammatory drugs
(NSAIDs), 324
Norepinephrine
brain pathways for, 99
function of, 94
molecular structure of, *152*
synthesis of, *101*
Normative education, 453
Nortriptyline (Pamelor)
annual mentions in DAWN, 27t
dose range of, 194t
Novocaine, 141
Nucleus basalis, 99
Nutritional supplements, and
athletics, *436*

O

Obesity, treatment with amphetamines,
150, 154–55
Obsessive-compulsive disorder, *186*
Odyssey, reference to opium in, 335
Olanzepine (Zyprex), 191
Olson, Frank, 372
Olympics, early drug use in, 430
Omnibus Crime Control Act of
1990, 438
Omnibus Drug Act, 70
Operation Golden Flow, 345
Opiate receptors, 349–50
Opiates
addiction to, 340–42
beneficial uses of, 351
examples of, *112*

Opiates—cont'd
hazards of, 352–58
history of use, 334–48
Internet sites on, 364
natural, 349–51
pharmacology of, 348–51
physical effects of, 112
sources of, 345–46, *347*
synthetic, 348, 350t
treatment for addicts, 358–63
Opium
dependence potential of, 31t
early regulation of, 57–58, 65
history of use, 334–48
origins of, 335
Opium Wars, 338–39
Oral administration, methods of, 120–21
Oral contraceptives, 8
Orphan Drug Act, 64
Outpatient treatment programs, 53
Overdose, 355
Over-the-counter drugs
analgesics, 318–24
caffeine in, 302, 314, 329t
choosing, 327–29
cold and allergy products, 324–27
federal regulation of, 311–13
Internet sites on, 330
most common ingredients of, 329t
versus prescription drugs, 313–14
psychoactive, 314–17
sleep aids, 316–17
stimulants, 314–15
for weight control, 315–16
Oxazepam (Serax), 173t
Oxycodone, 350t
Oxymorphone, 350t

P

Pain relievers
heroin as, 343
natural, 349–51
opiates as, 351
over the counter, 318–24
synthetic opiates, 348, 350t
Pall Mall cigarettes, 268
Panic disorder, *DSM-IV* criteria for, *186*
Panic reactions
and LSD, 377
and marijuana, 419
Paracelsus, 336
Paraldehyde
on controlled substance schedule, 69t
history of use, 166, 189
Paranoid psychotic reactions, 148, 161

Paraphernalia, regulation of, 73–74
Parasympathetic branch of autonomic
        nervous system, 94
Paregoric, 351
Parent Resources and Information on
        Drug Education (PRIDE), 458
Parents
    in drug education, 457–58
    influence on drug use, 15, 17–18
Parkinson's disease
    drug treatments for, 105, 192–93
    effects of, 95, 192–93
Paroxetine (Paxil), 194t, 195
Passive smoking, 278–79
Patent medicines
    cocaine in, 138, 341
    and early drug abuse, 58–59, 341
    and opiate addiction, 341
Patents, on drugs, 64–65, 110
PCP
    on controlled substance schedule, 69t
    dependence potential of, 31t, 390
    development and history of use,
        388–91
    pharmacology of, 391–92
Peer counseling, 452
Peer programs, for drug education, 457
Peers, influence on drug use, 15, 17–18
Pekoe tea, 296
Penny universities, 292
Pentazocine, 350t
Pentobarbital (Nembutal), 167t
Peripheral nerves, 93
Perphenazine (Trilafon), 191t
Personality
    and addiction, 43
    and alcoholism, 252
    and drug use, 14, 15
Personal skills instruction, 448–49
Peyote, 382–86
Phantastica, 367–68
Pharmaceuticals, early regulation
    of, 61–65
Pharmacist-recommended drugs, 314
Pharmacodynamic tolerance, 129
Pharmacology, Internet sites on, 130
Phenacetin, 323
Phenelzine (Nardil), 194t
Phenobarbital (Luminal), 167t, 171
Phenothiazines, 190–93
Phentermine, 155, 156
Phenylpropanolamine (PPA)
    molecular structure of, 152
    OTC use of, 315–16, 329t
Phobias, 186
Phosphate loading, 437

Physical dependence, 38–39
Physicians, and opiate addiction,
        341–42, 343
Physician's Desk Reference (PDR), 113
Physiological toxicity, 24, 25
Physiology, and addiction, 43
Pituitary gland, actions of, 89, 95–96
Placebo effect, 113–14
    and balanced placebo design, 253
    and marijuana use, 412–14
    for pain, 318
    of steroids, 435–36
Plants, as source of drugs, 109–10
Police, search authority of, 72
Pondimin. See Fenfluramine
        (Pondimin)
Pons, 96
Poppers, 180–81
Positive reinforcement, 353
Positron emission tomography
        (PET), 106
Possession of drugs, penalties for, 66,
        68, 69–70
Posttraumatic stress disorder, 186
Postwar era, social influences on
        drug use, 7–9
Potency, 118, 119
Precontemplation stage, of change, 47
Precursors of neurotransmitters, 101–2
Pregnancy
    and alcohol, 233–35
    and aspirin, 321
    and caffeine, 307
    and cocaine, 143, 144
    and marijuana, 419–20
    and smoking, 274–75, 279–81
Preparation stage, of change, 47
Prescription Drug Marketing Act, 64
Prescription drugs
    effectiveness of, 63
    recognition of, 62, 313
    state regulation of, 70–73
    testing, 63–65
Pressure resistance strategies, 449
Prevention programs
    Internet sites on, 460
    parent and community involvement,
        456–58
    in schools, 446–56
    stages of, 445–46
Primary prevention programs, 445
Prison populations, impact of drug laws
    on, 71, 78
Private employers, urine testing by, 74
Problem solving, as values clarification
    strategy, 448

Procaine, 141
Prochlorperazine (Compazine), 191t
Prodrugs, 128, 129
Prohibition, 65–66, 240–43
Project ALERT, 455
Project STAR, 456
Proof, of alcohol, 210
Propoxyphene, 350t
Prostaglandins, aspirin's effects
        on, 322
Protein binding, 123–25
Protriptyline (Vivactil), 194t
Prozac. See Fluoxetine (Prozac)
Pseudoephedrine, 326, 327t, 328, 329t
Psilocybin
    dependence potential of, 31t
    effects of, 380–81
    Leary's use of, 372–73
    molecular structure of, 368
Psychedelic, origin of term, 367
Psychoactive, defined, 7
Psychoactive drugs
    actions in brain, 100–105
    classes of, 111–13
    defined, 6
    dependence potential of, 31t
    effects of, 125–26
    interactions between, 127
    methods of taking, 120–23
    over the counter, 314–17
    principles of, 4–7
    tolerance for (see Tolerance)
Psychological dependence
    and addiction, 40
    on amphetamines, 161–62
    on marijuana, 418
    on narcotics, 353
Psychological inoculation, 449, 453
Psychology, cannabis used in
        research, 406
Psychopharmacology, 8, 9, 182
Psychoses
    described, 187
    drug treatments for, 190–93
    and LSD, 377–78
    and marijuana use, 420
Psychotherapeutics
    examples of, 112
    Internet sites on, 202
    physical effects of, 112
    See also Antianxiety drugs;
        Antidepressants; Antipsychotics
Psychotomimetic drugs, 367
P300 wave, 254
Pupils, autonomic effects on, 94t
Pure Food and Drugs Act, 59–60, 61–62

Q

Quaaludes, 169–70
Quid, 273

R

Rape, and drug abuse, 172
Raphe nuclei, and serotonin
       pathways, 99
Rapid opiate detoxification, 363
Reaction time, effects of marijuana
       on, 414, 418
Rebelliousness, and drug use, 19
Receptors
   of neurons, 102–3, 126
   on target cells, 91–93
Reconstituted tobacco, 270
Redux. *See* Dexfenfluramine (Redux)
Reese, Jeff, *439*
Reformism, 57
Refusal skills, 449, 453
Regulation of drugs, 35
   early history of, 56–61, 138–39
   federal expenditures on, 78
   impact of, 76–80
   Internet sites about, *82*
   narcotics and controlled substances,
      65–70
   over-the-counter, 311–13
   pharmaceutical safety, 61–65
   screening programs, 74–76
   state and local, 70–74
Reinforcement
   and addiction, 39, 41
   brain centers for, 99
   for drug use, 19–20
Relapses, preventing, 49–50
Religious commitment, and drug
      use, *15*
Reproduction
   effect of caffeine on, 307
   effect of cocaine on, 143, 144
   effect of marijuana on, 419–20
   See also Pregnancy
Research
   double blind, 114
   for FDA approval, 63–65
   See also Testing
Residential treatment approaches, 50–52
Respiratory center, 96
Respiratory depression
   from barbiturates, 168
   from drug interactions, 127
   from narcotics, 354–55
Reuptake, 103, 104
Reye's syndrome, 322
Rhinoviruses, 324

Risk factors
   for alcoholism, 252–54
   for drug use, 14, *15, 16*
Risperidone (Risperdal), 191
Ritalin. *See* Methylphenidate (Ritalin)
Robberies, for drug money, 32–33
Rock. *See* Crack
Rohypnol, 172
Roid rage, 437
Rolfe, John, 266
Runner's high, 351
Rush, Benjamin, 239
Rye whiskey, 217

S

Safety, regulating, 62, 312
Safety margin, 118, 119
Saint Anthony's fire, 369
Sakel, Manfred, 189
Salem witch trials, 369
Salicylates. *See* Aspirin
Salicylic acid, 319
Sandoz Laboratories, and early LSD
      research, 369, 370, 371
Schedules of controlled substances, 69*t*
Schizophrenia, 187. *See also* Psychoses
School-based prevention programs
   affective education, 447–49
   DARE, 454–55
   drug-free schools, 449–51
   effectiveness of, 449, 455–56
   "Just Say No!" 449
   knowledge-attitudes-behavior model,
     446–47
   peer counseling, 452
   social influence model, 452–54
   student assistance programs, 451–52
Schools, drug-free zones around, 73
Scopolamine
   in anticholinergic hallucinogens,
     392, 393
   in OTC sleep aids, 316–17
Screening programs, urine testing, 74–76
Searches, laws governing, *72*
Secobarbital (Seconal), 167*t, 171*
Secondary prevention programs, 445–46
Sedative-hypnotics
   abuse of, 169, 172, 174, 179
   as anticonvulsants, 176
   beneficial uses of, 173–76
   dependence potential of, 176–78
   history of use, 166–72
   mechanisms of action, 172–73
   toxicity reactions, 178–79
   use in narcosis therapy, 189
   withdrawal from, 178

Sedatives
   defined, 165
   over the counter, 316–17 (*see also*
     Hypnotics)
   uses of, 173–75
Selective serotonin reuptake
      inhibitors, 195
Self-concept exercises, *448*
Sernyl. *See* PCP
Serotonin
   action of cocaine on, 140
   brain pathways for, 99
   effect of hallucinogens on, 374–75
   effect of SSRIs on, 195
   and indole hallucinogens, 368–69
Sertraline (Zoloft), 194*t,* 195
Sertürner, Frederich, 339
Sex hormones, use in sports, 438
Sexual activity, effects of alcohol
      on, 225–26
Shamans, 367
Shen Nung, 404–5, 414
Sherley amendment, 61
Sherry, 214
Short-term memory, effects of marijuana
      on, 413–14
Sibutramine (Meridia), 156
Side effects, testing for, 118, 119
Sidestream smoke, 278–79
Simpson, Tommy, 431
Sinsemilla, 402–3
Skin patches
   for drug administration, 122–23
   nicotine, 287
Skin popping, 122, 356
Sleep aids, over the counter, 316–17. *See
     also* Hypnotics
Sleep disorders, treatment with
      amphetamines, 155–56
Sleeping pills. *See* Hypnotics
Smart pills, amphetamines as, 158–60
Smokeless tobacco, 266–67, 273–74
Smoking
   by adolescents, 452–53
   cessation techniques, 278, 285–87
   and health, 276–81
   introduction to China, 338
   in other countries, 279
   passive, 278–79
   and pregnancy, 279–81
   prevention education, 453–54
   trends in, 271–73
   See also Tobacco
Snorting, of cocaine, 141
Snuff, 266
Social influence model of drug
      education, 452–54

Social skills instruction, 448–49
Socioeconomic status, and drug use, 13–14
Sodium bicarbonate, and athletic performance, *437*
Soft drinks
  development of, 299–302
  per capita consumption, 292
Solpidem (Ambien), 176
Solvents, abuse of, 180*t*, 181–82
Soma, 395
Somatic nervous system, 93
Somatic pain, 318
Sopor. *See* Methaqualone
Specific effects, 114
Speed. *See* Amphetamines
Speedball, 149
Spinal nerves, 93
Spontaneous abortion
  and caffeine, 307
  and smoking, 280
Sports, drug-related Internet sites for, 441. *See also* Athletics
Stacking, of steroids, 435
Stages of change, 47
Stages of prevention, 445*t*
Stamp Act of 1765, 295
Starch blockers, 316
States, drug regulation by, 70–73
Steroids
  physical effects of, 437–38
  psychological effects of, 436–37
  regulation of, 438
  use in sports, 431–33, 435–38
Stimulants
  examples of, *112*
  interactions with other drugs, 127
  over the counter, 302*t*, 314
  performance-enhancing effects of, 429–30, 433–35
  physical effects of, 111, 133, *159*
  types of, 134
  use among college students, 11*t*
  See also Amphetamines
Stomach, autonomic effects on, 94*t*
Stone, Edward, 318–19
STP, 387
Stress, and pain relief, 318
Strychnine, early use in sports, 429
Student assistance programs, 451–52
Subcutaneous injections, 122
Substance abuse, psychiatric diagnosis of, *46*
Substance disorders, psychiatric diagnosis of, *46*
Sudden infant death syndrome (SIDS), 280

Suicide
  and alcohol, 250
  attempting, 27, 168
  and LSD, 377*t*
  and serotonin, 99–100
Sulfa drugs, 62
Sulfanilamide, 62
Sullivan, John L., 268
Sunday, Billy, 242
Support groups, for parents in drug education, 457
Surgeon General's Report on Smoking and Health, 272
Surveys, of drug use, 10–12
Sweat glands, autonomic effects on, 94*t*
Sydenham, Thomas, 336–37
Sympathetic branch, of autonomic nervous system, 94
Sympathomimetic drugs, 94, 148
Synanon, 50–51
Synapses
  action of drugs on, 102–3, 126
  neurotransmitters and, 91, *92*
Synesthesia, and LSD, 376
Synthesis, of neurotransmitters, *101*, 102
Synthetic enzymes, and neurotransmitter synthesis, *102*
Systematic desensitization, 146

T

Tar
  in cigarettes, 270
  in marijuana, 419
Tardive dyskinesia, 193
Target cells, 89, *90*
Task Force on Drug Abuse, 345
Taxes
  on alcohol, 242, 243–44
  on tea, 292
  on tobacco, 276
Tea
  caffeine content of, 299*t*
  cultivation and marketing of, 296–97
  history of use, 294–96
  taxes on, 292
Tea bags, 296–97
Teen leaders, in drug abuse prevention, 453
Temazepam (Restoril), 173*t*
Temperance, 239–40
Tentative Final Monographs, 312
Tertiary prevention programs, 445*t*, 446
Testing
  of dosage effects, 114–18
  double blind, 114

Testing—cont'd
  for FDA approval, 63–65
  methods of, 74–76
Testosterone, 431–32, 435
Tetracycline, 120–21
Thalidomide, 63
THC. *See* Delta-9-tetrahydrocannabinol (THC)
Theobromine, 299
Theophylline, 297
Therapeutic communities, 50–51, 53
Therapeutic index, 118, 119
Thiopental sodium, 189
Thioridazine (Mellaril), 191*t*
Thiothixere (Navane), 191*t*
Thirst, and hangover, 229
Threshold concentration, 119
Time course, 118–20, *171*
Time-release preparations, 120
Toadlicking, *396*
Tobacco
  advertising, 276, 286
  current products, 268–74
  dependency potential of, 283–85
  and health, 276–81
  history of use, 264–68, 338
  Internet sites on, 288
  revenues from, 275–76
  smokeless, 266–67, 273–74
  social mores about, 274–75
  use by adolescents, 452–53
Tolerance
  and addiction, 38, 39
  for alcohol, 222
  for barbiturates, 168
  for caffeine, 302–3
  for narcotics, 352
  mechanisms of, 128–29
Topical application, 122–23
Toxicity, 24–30
  acute, 354–55
  chronic, 355
  and dosage, 116, 117–18
  See also specific drugs
Tracking behavior, effects of marijuana on, 414
Trade and Revenue Act of 1767, 295
Traffic fatalities, alcohol related, 247–49
Transient ischemic attack, 321
Transportation workers, urine testing for, 74
Tranylcypromine (Parnate), 194*t*
Trazodone (Desyrel), 194*t*
Treatment
  for alcoholism, 254–59
  approaches to, 50–53
  effectiveness of, 53, 259

Treatment—cont'd
goals of, 48–50
for narcotic addictions, 358–63
Triazolam (Halcion), as hypnotic, 173*t*, 175, 176
Tricyclic antidepressants, 194–95
Trifluoperazine (Stelazine), 191*t*, 193
Truth serum, 189
Tuberculosis, and antidepressant development, 193–94
Twelve Steps of Alcoholics Anonymous, *255*
Twin studies, of alcoholism, 253–54
Tylenol Cold, 327*t*
Tyramine, effect of MAO inhibitors on, 194
Tyrosine, in norepinephrine synthesis, *101*

U

Uniform Controlled Substances Act, 73
Unimed, Inc., 416
Unipolar disorders, 198*t*
United States Pharmacopeia (USP), 110
Uptake, 101
Urine testing, 74–76
U.S. Department of Agriculture, drug regulation by, 61, 78
U.S. State Department, involvement in war on drugs, 78
U.S. Treasury Department, drug regulation by, 61

V

Vaccines, development of, 7
Valium. *See* Diazepam (Valium)
Values clarification, 447, *448*
Varietals, 213
Vaughn, William, 265

Venlafaxine (Effexor), 194*t*, 195
Ventricular fibrillation, from cocaine use, 142
Vesicles, in neurons, 102
Vietnam War, effect on heroin use, 344–45
Violence
and alcohol, 249–50
and amphetamines, 160
and drug abuse, 31–35
and marijuana, 407–8
and PCP use, 390–91
and steroid use, 437
Viruses, and colds, 324–25
Visceral pain, 318
Vitamins, in nutritional supplements, *436–37*
Vodka, 216
Volatile solvents, 180*t*, 181–82
Volstead, Andrew, 241
Vomiting center, 96
von Meduna, Ladislas, 189

W

Warning labels, 274, *278*
War on drugs, 76–80, 145
Washington, George, 266
Water, and athletic performance, *437*
Websites. *See* Internet sites
Weight, and blood alcohol concentration, 223*t*
Weight control
amphetamines for, 150, 154–55
OTC products for, 315–16
in sports, *439*
Wernicke-Korsakoff syndrome, 230
What Works: Schools Without Drugs, 450
What Works: Workplaces Without Drugs, 458

Whiskey Rebellion, 56
Whisky, 215
Wiley, Harvey, 61
Wine consumption trends, *215*
Wine coolers, 214–15
Wine making, 212–15
Winston cigarettes, 268
Witchcraft, and belladonna, 392–93
Withdrawal
from alcohol dependence, 129
from amphetamines, 161
from caffeine, 303
from cocaine, 142–43, 146
from methadone, 352
from narcotics, 352–53, 357
and physical dependence, 38–39, 41, 48
from sedative-hypnotics, 178
Withdrawal syndrome, 38–39
Women
effect of steroids on, 432, 438
smoking by, 272–73, 274–75
Wood, Alexander, 339
Workplace, drug abuse prevention in, 458
Wrestling, and dangerous weight loss, *439*
Wright, Hamilton, 60

X

Xanax. *See* Alprazolam (Xanax)
Xanthines, 290, 291, 302

Y

Yuppies, 9–10